Energy Metabolism

Tissue Determinants and Cellular Corollaries

Energy Metabolism

Tissue Determinants and Cellular Corollaries

Editors

John M. Kinney, M.D.
Visiting Professor and
* Physician*
The Rockefeller University
* and Professor of Surgery*
St. Luke's/Roosevelt
* Hospital Center*
New York, New York

Hugh N. Tucker, PH.D.
Research and Development
Clintec Technologies Inc.
Deerfield, Illinois

RAVEN PRESS   NEW YORK

Raven Press, Ltd., 1185 Avenue of the Americas, New York, New York 10036

Made in the United States of America

Library of Congress Cataloging in Publication Data

Clintec International Horizons Conference (1st : 1991 : Amsterdam, Netherlands)
    Energy metabolism : tissue determinants and cellular corollaries / the First Clintec International Horizons Conference : editors, John M. Kinney and Hugh N. Tucker.
        p.   cm.
    Proceedings of a conferences held in Amsterdam, May 5–9, 1991.
    Includes bibliographical references and index.
    ISBN 0-88167-871-6
    1. Energy metabolism—Congresses. 2. Indirect calorimetry—Congresses. 3. Diet therapy—Congresses. 4. Nutrition—Congresses. I. Kinney, John M., 1921–   . II. Clintec International Inc. III. Title.
        [DNLM: 1. Energy Metabolism—congresses.   QU 125 C6407e 1991]
    QP176.C54   1991
    612.3′9—dc20
    DNLM/DLC
    for Library of Congress   91-37137
                                                                          CIP

9   8   7   6   5   4   3   2   1

Contents

v

Contributing Authors

Arne Astrup, M.D., Dr. Sci.
*Research Department of Human
  Nutrition
The Royal Veterinary and Agricultural
  University
25 Rolighedsvej
1958 Frederiksberg, Denmark*

Alison E. Black
*MRC Dunn Clinical Nutrition Centre
100 Tennis Court Road
Cambridge CB2 1QL, United Kingdom*

Niels Juel Christensen, M.D.
*Department of Internal Medicine and
  Endocrinology
Herlev Hospital
University of Copenhagen
Copenhagen, Denmark*

B. Crabtree, Ph.D.
*Rowett Research Institute
Bucksburn
Aberdeen AB2 9SB, United Kingdom*

Erik Diaz
*MRC Dunn Clinical Nutrition Centre
100 Tennis Court Road
Cambridge CB2 1QL, United Kingdom*

J. V. G. A. Durnin, Ph.D.
*Institute of Physiology
University of Glasgow
Glasgow G12 8QQ, United Kingdom*

Neile K. Edens, Ph.D.
*The Rockefeller University
1230 York Avenue
New York, New York 10021*

Richard Edwards, M.D.
*Department of Medicine
University of Liverpool
P.O. Box 147
Liverpool L69 3BX, United Kingdom*

M. Elia, M.D.
*MRC Dunn Clinical Nutrition Centre
100 Tennis Court Road
Cambridge CB2 1QL, United Kingdom*

Eleuterio Ferrannini, M.D.
*CNR Institute of Clinical Physiology
University of Pisa
Pisa, Italy*

J. P. Flatt, Ph.D.
*Department of Biochemistry
University of Massachusetts Medical
  School
Worcester, Massachusetts 01655*

Keith N. Frayn, Ph.D.
*Sheikh Rashid Diabetes Unit 6
Radcliffe Infirmary
Oxford OX2 6HE, United Kingdom*

Naomi K. Fukagawa
*Department of Pediatrics and Medicine
Beth Israel Hospital and Harvard
  Medical School
Boston, Massachusetts 02215*

David G. Gadian, Ph.D.
*Department of Biophysics
Hunterian Institute
The Royal College of Surgeons of
  England
35–43 Lincoln's Inn Fields
London WC2A 3PN, United Kingdom*

Gail R. Goldberg
*MRC Dunn Clinical Nutrition Centre
100 Tennis Court Road
Cambridge CB2 1QL, United Kingdom*

Roger C. Harris, Ph.D.
*Department of Comparative Physiology
Animal Health Trust
Newmarket
Suffolk CB8 7DW, United Kingdom*

Jan Henriksson, M.D., Ph.D.
Department of Physiology III
Karolinska Institute
Box 5626
S-114 33 Stockholm, Sweden

Jules Hirsch, M.D.
The Rockefeller University
1230 York Avenue
H-26
New York, New York 10021

Eric Hultman, Ph.D.
Institute of Clinical Chemistry II
Huddinge University Hospital
C262
S-14186 Huddinge, Sweden

W. P. T. James, Ph.D.
Rowett Research Institute
Greenburn Road
Bucksburn, Aberdeen, United Kingdom
AB2 9SB

Eric Jéquier, M.D.
Institute of Physiology
The University of Lausanne
Rue du Bugnon 7
1005 Lausanne, Switzerland

J. M. Kelly
Department of Animal and Poultry
Science
University of Guelph
Guelph, Ontario, Canada N1G 2W1

John M. Kinney, M.D.
The Rockefeller University
1230 York Avenue
New York, New York 10021 and
St. Luke's/Roosevelt Hospital Center
New York, New York 10025

Rudolph L. Leibel, M.D.
The Rockefeller University
1230 York Avenue
New York, New York 10021

Ian A. Macdonald, Ph.D.
Department of Physiology and
Pharmacology
Queen's Medical Centre
Nottingham NG7 2UH, United
Kingdom

L. P. Milligan, Ph.D.
Department of Animal and Poultry
Science
University of Guelph
Guelph, Ontario, Canada N1G 2W1

Peter R. Murgatroyd
MRC Dunn Clinical Nutrition Centre
100 Tennis Court Road
Cambridge CB2 1QL, United Kingdom

E. A. Newsholme, Ph.D.
Department of Biochemistry
Cellular Nutrition Research Group
University of Oxford
South Parks Road
Oxford OX1 3QU, United Kingdom

H. S. Park
Department of Animal and Poultry
Science
University of Guelph
Guelph, Ontario, Canada N1G 2W1

M. Parry-Billings, Ph.D.
Department of Biochemistry
Cellular Nutrition Research Group
University of Oxford
South Parks Road
Oxford OX1 3QU, United Kingdom

F. Xavier Pi-Sunyer, M.D.
Division of Endocrinology, Diabetes,
and Nutrition
Obesity Research Center
Columbia University at St. Luke's/
Roosevelt Hospital Center
Amsterdam Avenue at 114th Street
New York, New York 10025

Andrew M. Prentice, M.D., Ph.D.
MRC Dunn Clinical Nutrition Centre
100 Tennis Court Road
Cambridge CB2 1QL, United Kingdom

Eric Ravussin, Ph.D.
Clinical Diabetes and Nutrition Section
National Institute of Diabetes and
  Digestive and Kidney Diseases
National Institutes of Health
4212 North Sixteenth Street
Room 541
Phoenix, Arizona 85016

Russell Rising, Ph.D.
Clinical Diabetes and Nutrition Section
National Institute of Diabetes and
  Digestive and Kidney Diseases
National Institutes of Health
4212 North Sixteenth Street
Room 541
Phoenix, Arizona 85016

Nancy J. Rothwell, Ph.D.
Department of Physiological Sciences
University of Manchester
Manchester M13 9PT, United Kingdom

Karen R. Segal, Ed.D.
Division of Pediatric Cardiology
Mount Sinai School of Medicine
New York, New York 10029

Bakary J. Sonko
MRC Dunn Clinical Nutrition Centre
100 Tennis Court Road
Cambridge CB2 1QL, United Kingdom

R. James Stubbs
MRC Dunn Clinical Nutrition Centre
100 Tennis Court Road
Cambridge CB2 1QL, United Kingdom

Hugh N. Tucker, Ph.D.
Research and Development
Clintec Technologies Inc.
Deerfield, Illinois 60015

Robert R. Wolfe, Ph.D.
Metabolism Unit
Shriners Burns Institute
Departments of Anesthesiology and
  Surgery
The University of Texas Medical Branch
Galveston, Texas 77550

Vernon R. Young, Ph.D., D.Sc.
School of Science and Clinical Research
  Center
Massachusetts Institute of Technology
Cambridge, Massachusetts 02139 and
Shriners Burns Institute
Boston, Massachusetts 02114

Yong-Ming Yu
Shriners Burns Institute
51 Blossom Street
Boston, Massachusetts 02114

Preface

The First Clintec International Horizons Conference was organized to create bridges between several areas of research that do not ordinarily have the occasion to meet. The intent was to catalyze new thought on the relationship of energy metabolism to clinical nutrition. An appreciation of energy stores, energy balance, and regulation of energy metabolism during the altered metabolic condition of patients in the intensive care environment is critical to the advancement of current medical practice. Linkage of the common concepts of nutrition support, nitrogen balance, and weight loss with the less frequently discussed concepts of cellular energetics and energy balance will begin to bring more understanding to the field. Advances in the therapeutic use of clinical nutrition will be predicated upon the application of appropriate fuel mixes and substrates to sustain metabolism and cellular function.

The five sessions of the conference were spread over four days to allow time for review of indirect calorimetry, energy requirements and storage, neurohormonal and muscle tissue influences on thermogenesis, and cellular energy expenditure. The schedule was constructed with periods for discussion and session overviews. Each participant was asked to summarize their current work and to discuss aspects of energy metabolism related to their specific fields of research.

The conference environment was kept intimate with no audience other than the invited speakers in order to encourage free comment and communication among participants. Each participant's manuscript was submitted prior to the conference to allow for review and comment by an assigned discussant during the conference. Additionally, audio recordings of the proceedings allow this volume to include not only the formal papers and discussants' reviews, but also portions of the open discussion by participants.

The Tuinzaal conference room at the Pulitzer Hotel in Amsterdam became a reaction chamber for new thought and a place for the meeting of minds from diverse areas of research. The extensive review of divergent fields and presentation of the newest work by each participant led to the synergy of thought and insightful deliberation that is evident in the content of this volume. The participant consensus was that the conference was successful in stimulating the presenters to reflect on new aspects or interpretations of their research findings. These interactions served to demonstrate that the future can hold great promise for improvements in patient care.

Clintec International Inc. and the Clintec Nutrition Companies worldwide are grateful to be associated with such an exciting opportunity and to have been the catalyst for the symposium resulting in this text. We are extremely appreciative of Dr. John Kinney's insistence in meeting format and perseverance throughout the planning process without which this opportunity would have never occurred. It is hoped that the availability of these proceedings in published form will spark new creative thinking by others concerning the special relevance of energy metabolism to clinical practice and will inspire research programs that will extend the clinical nutrition field to areas at and beyond the horizon.

Hugh N. Tucker, PH.D.
Clintec Technologies Inc.
Affiliated with Baxter
Healthcare Corporation
and Nestlé S.A.

Introduction

The First Clintec International Horizons Conference on "Energy Metabolism: Tissue Determinants and Cellular Corollaries" was held in Amsterdam on May 5–9, 1991. This volume represents the subjects which were presented and discussed at that conference. Each chairman of the five sessions was invited to write an overview of his session and to provide a personal perspective on the present status of our understanding in the particular subject area.

We all agree that energy metabolism is central to life, yet our quantitative knowledge of how the successive steps in energy exchange are related remains very incomplete. The measurement of human energy expenditure is usually a calculation based upon gas exchange and nitrogen excretion. These calculations were presented a century ago, yet, the details of interpretation are still being worked out today.

The history of this indirect approach to energy expenditure has seen remarkable fluctuations of interest over the past century. The period of 1890 to 1925 represented a flowering of interest in human calorimetry, which was extremely productive. By the early 1900s, the concept of indirect calorimetry had spread from the German laboratories of Voit and Rubner to many parts of Europe, as well to the United States. The 1920s represented a turning point in this interest. The textbook of Lusk, *The Science of Nutrition* was popular at that time and contained extensive material on calorimetry. A few years later, the first edition of MacCollum's *Textbook of Nutrition* was published, and remained dominant in the field for 20 years. This book did not mention calorimetry, since the major emphasis had shifted to vitamins and enzymes.

The famous 1924 studies of DuBois on basal metabolic rate helped to establish the BMR as important for evaluating thyroid dysfunction. However, the BMR had little influence on the care of other conditions. The utilization of the BMR disappeared around 1950 when chemical measurements related to iodine metabolism were introduced to evaluate thyroid disease. Hospital BMR laboratories were dismantled, and between 1950 and 1975 it was not possible to obtain any form of indirect calorimetry in most hospitals. During the 1970s there was a resurgence of clinical interest in indirect calorimetry, but convenient equipment for the measurement of gas exchange was not available. This was a tremendous impetus to the development of new measurement equipment which could be rolled to the bedside, and helped to move attention from the basal metabolic rate to resting energy expenditure.

The new interest in calorimetry was the result of stimuli from four sources: stress testing and sports medicine, new interest in obesity, rapid growth in critical care medicine, and nutritional support for hospital patients. The 1980s saw a rapid growth in measurement devices for indirect calorimetry, new types of exercise equipment and specialized facilities for intensive care, together with advanced products for nutritional support. Today, the long and colorful history of gas exchange and calorimetry is entering a new era. Long established as a research measurement, indirect calorimetry is struggling to find its proper role in clinical care.

Modern medical education has added to the difficulty of gaining a quantitative appreciation of energy flow through the body. Separate disciplines teach the medical student about food intake, body composition, intermediary metabolism, cardiopulmonary function, cell physiology, organ and tissue function, and thermal metabolism. The energy requirements in each of these areas are seldom presented in terms which relate to the total energy expenditure. As modern science reveals more and more of the intimate detail of cells and tissues, the physician must always strive to consider new findings as part of the overall movement of energy without which each patient can not survive and recover.

The clinical physiologist considers energy expenditure as

$$TEE = BMR + TEF + ACT$$

where the thermic effect of food (TEF) and physical activity (ACT) each contribute to energy expenditure beyond the basal metabolic rate.

The cell physiologist views the energy expenditure quite differently; namely, the sum of at least three processes:

$$TEE = \begin{array}{ccc} MEMBRANE & PROTEIN & METABOLIC \\ TRANSPORT & TURNOVER & CYCLES \end{array}$$

It is important to find the common ground between these two approaches to energy expenditure. Part of the Clintec Horizons conference was devoted to the search for this common ground. However, the future suggests that physicians, as well as medical scientists, will need to understand energy expenditure in terms of organ and tissue work if the maximum therapeutic opportunities for nutrition (with or without pharmacologic intervention) are to be realized.

John M. Kinney, M.D.

Energy Metabolism: Tissue Determinants and
Cellular Corollaries, edited by J. M. Kinney
and H. N. Tucker. Raven Press, Ltd.,
New York © 1992.

Equations and Assumptions of Indirect Calorimetry: Some Special Problems

Eleuterio Ferrannini

CNR Institute of Clinical Physiology at the University of Pisa, Pisa, Italy

Indirect calorimetry is the method by which measurements of respiratory gas exchange (oxygen consumption, VO_2, and carbon dioxide production, VCO_2) are used to estimate the type and amount of substrate (carbohydrate and lipid) oxidized and the amount of energy produced by biologic oxidations. Several recent reviews have dealt with the principles and applications of indirect calorimetry in more or less detail (1–4), and the reader is referred to those articles for basic information. In the present chapter, I shall deal with certain issues inherent in both the theory and application of indirect calorimetry, in an attempt to integrate my previous contribution to this subject (3).

INDIRECT CALORIMETRY AND THE FICK PRINCIPLE

If the whole organism is assimilated to one big compartment containing all living cells, bathed by a homogeneous extracellular fluid and renewed by a constant blood flow (Fig. 1), then input-output analysis can be applied to this idealized system to measure VO_2 and VCO_2. The O_2 and CO_2 concentrations having been measured in both the inlet and outlet, and the flow-through being known, the product of O_2 and CO_2 concentration differences by the flow rate gives VO_2 and VCO_2, respectively. The constraints for such a calculation are (A) that cells remove O_2 from the inflow and add CO_2 to the outflow at a constant rate (i.e., cellular metabolism is stable); (B) that O_2 and CO_2 levels in the inflow are constant; and (C) that the flow rate through the system is constant. The anatomical equivalent of the open system in Fig. 1 is shown in Fig. 2: cardiac activity provides the flow (cardiac output), the inlet to the cell compartment is the left ventricle (arterial blood perfusing organs and tissues), and the outlet from the cell compartment is the right heart (mixed venous blood refluent from organs and tissues). The pulmonary circulation interposed between the two sections of the heart provides a constant supply of O_2 and a large diffusion surface for excess CO_2. By measuring O_2 and CO_2 levels in the aorta (or

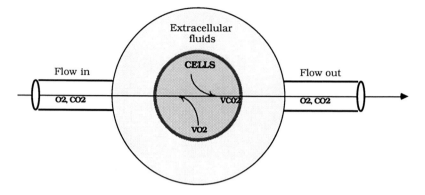

FIG. 1. Diagram of a cellular system with its blood supply. O_2 and CO_2 are oxygen and carbon dioxide concentrations; VO_2 and VCO_2 are rates of oxygen consumption and carbon dioxide production, respectively.

any other accessible artery) as well as in the right cardiac chambers and calculating cardiac output (CO), one can calculate VO_2 and VCO_2 as follows:

$$VO_2 = CO \text{ (arterial } O_2 - \text{ mixed venous } O_2) \qquad [1]$$

$$VCO_2 = CO \text{ (arterial } CO_2 - \text{ mixed venous } CO_2) \qquad [2]$$

Indeed, in 1870 Fick proposed to measure VO_2 from gas exchange and the transpulmonary O_2 gradient by heart catheterization and to calculate CO from Eq. 1 (5). Indirect calorimetry avoids cardiac catheterization by assuming that ambient air is the only source of O_2 as well as the only sink for metabolic CO_2. Thus, by measuring the fractional O_2 and CO_2 concentrations in inspired (FI) as well as expired (FE) air flow, one can calculate VO_2 and VCO_2 as follows:

$$VO_2 = (FIO_2 - FEO_2) \text{ Ve} \qquad [3]$$

$$VCO_2 = (FICO_2 - FECO_2) \text{ Ve} \qquad [4]$$

Once gas concentrations are reduced to STPD conditions and corrected for fractional gas mixing (Haldane's correction), simple spirometric measurements of ventilatory rate (Ve) make it possible to obtain VO_2 and VCO_2 noninvasively.

It should be noted that Eqs. 1 and 3 must both estimate the "true" VO_2 within the limits of precision of the respective technical procedures (CO and whole-blood O_2 concentrations versus Ve and respiratory O_2 tension) because ambient air is in fact the only source of oxygen for the organism. This is not the case for VCO_2, because small amounts of metabolic CO_2 can be lost via other routes (e.g., skin, mucosae, secretions, bone). Thus, both Eqs. 2 and 4 underestimate VCO_2 to the extent that CO_2 is lost to the environment directly from the interstitia (without entering the venous circulation).

When both methods (Fick principle and indirect calorimetry) are applied simul-

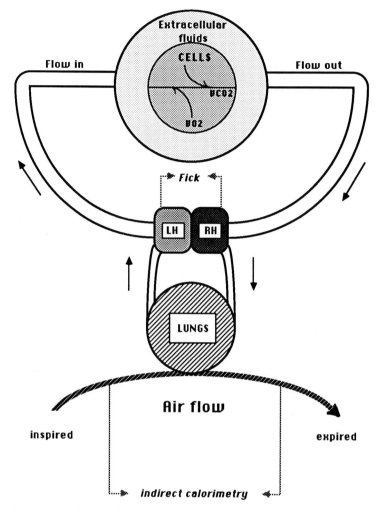

FIG. 2. The diagram of Fig. 1 is here extended to include the heart (RH, right heart; LH, left heart) and lungs.

taneously in the same subjects, the measures of VO_2 are highly correlated (Fig. 3), although the Fick method slightly underestimates calorimetry (by 3% P < 0.01). In contrast, the measures of VCO_2 are definitely lower with Fick than with calorimetry (Fig. 3) (by 12%, P < 0.001, (Table 1). At least in part, this systematic difference may reflect the fact that 60% to 70% of bronchial venous return flows into the pulmonary veins (the remainder being a tributary of the vena cava), thereby diluting the O_2, and enriching the CO_2, contents of arterial blood (6). More importantly, the calorimetric estimates of VCO_2 are three times more precise than whole-blood arteriovenous CO_2 differences (Table 1 and Fig. 3) despite the use of a comprehensive

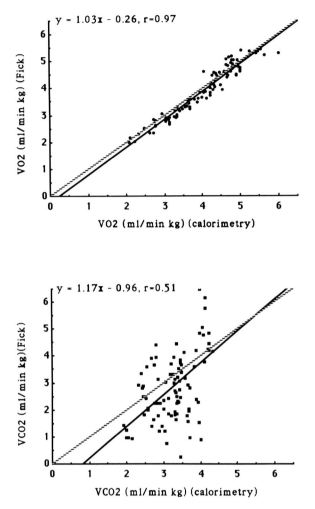

FIG. 3. Relationship between oxygen consumption (VO₂) and carbon dioxide production (VCO₂) as measured by Fick method and indirect calorimetry. The dotted line is the identity line.

correction (for pH, hemoglobin concentration, and O_2 saturation) to convert plasma CO_2 tension into whole-blood CO_2 concentration (7). This result confirms the known difficulty to obtain consistent, reproducible blood CO_2 measurements. As a consequence, the respiratory quotient (VCO_2/VO_2) is poorly estimated by the Fick method (Fig. 4). The calorimetric RQ estimates range between 0.69 and 1.00, i.e., over a fully physiologic range, whereas the corresponding Fick estimates spread to obviously impossible values (0.16 to 1.8). Energy expenditure, on the other hand, being predominantly dependent on VO_2, is estimated with similar precision by both methods (Table 1 and Fig. 4).

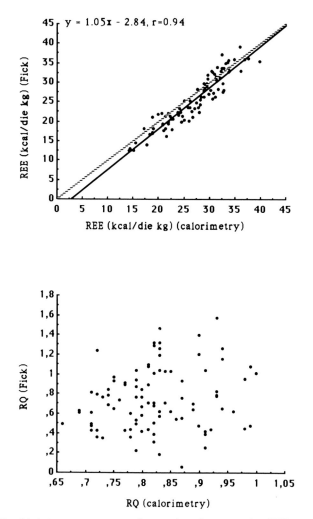

FIG. 4. Relationship between energy expenditure and respiratory quotient (RQ) as calculated from the data in Fig. 3 (Fick method versus indirect calorimetry).

Burning ethyl alcohol in a 40-liter canopy in our hands yielded measurements of VO_2 having a precision of 3.1% and an accuracy of 4.3%, whereas VCO_2 measures had a precision of 3.9% and an accuracy of 4.7% (8). Thus, one can calculate that roughly one-fifth of the overall variability of calorimetric VO_2 and VCO_2 readings (Table 1) is due to the technique, the remainder reflecting interindividual variation and time-related fluctuations. Furthermore, using the same canopy system in a group of healthy volunteers, we found day-to-day reproducibility to average 2.6% for VO_2 and 3.3% for VCO_2 (9). On the other hand, the Fick method, which can be employed to study regional gas exchange by catheterizing the arterial and venous ends of a

TABLE 1. *Oxygen consumption (VO_2), carbon dioxide production (VCO_2), respiratory quotient (RQ), and energy expenditure (EE) estimated in 31 subjects simultaneously by the Fick method and by indirect calorimetry*[a]

	Fick	Calorimetry
VO_2 (ml/min kg)	3.89 ± 0.10	4.02 ± 0.09[b]
C.V.	(24%)	(22%)
VCO_2 (ml/min kg)	2.87 ± 0.14	3.27 ± 0.06[b]
C.V.	(47%)	(18%)
EE (kcal/die kg)	25.7 ± 0.7	27.1 ± 0.6[b]
C.V.	(25%)	(21%)
RQ (VCO_2/VO_2)	0.746 ± 0.03	0.825 ± 0.008[b]
C.V.	(42%)	(10%)

[a] C.V., coefficient of variation. Data obtained by the simultaneous use of indirect calorimetry (with a canopy system) and the Fick method (catheterization of the right atrium and aorta, with thermodilution measurements of cardiac output) in 31 postsurgical patients (Brandi et al., unpublished observations).
[b] Significantly different from the mean Fick value ($P < 0.05$ or less) by paired t test.

circulatory region (e.g., forearm or leg), has a typical intraindividual variability (technique plus time-related changes) of 13% to 18% (10).

INDIRECT CALORIMETRY AND THE NONSTEADY STATE

As mentioned previously, the Fick principle, upon which both the Fick method for measuring cardiac output and indirect calorimetry are based, is valid only under steady state conditions. When the system is driven out of a steady state, major problems arise in the interpretation of the data. The O_2 and CO_2 concentrations in inspired air are reasonably constant (or change very slowly in time), but both the ventilatory and the metabolic rate can change quite rapidly. When this happens, the estimates of VO_2 by either the Fick method or calorimetry are not affected in any detectable degree, because the whole-body O_2 stores are very small (estimated at less than one liter) in comparison with O_2 fluxes (about 0.3 l/min in the resting state). Thus, even abrupt changes in cellular O_2 metabolism are promptly translated into equivalent changes in blood O_2 levels or FEO_2. In contrast, the CO_2 (bicarbonate) space is large, and some time is expected to elapse before a change in cellular VCO_2 output becomes a detectable variation of blood CO_2 concentrations or $FECO_2$. Such delay may be variable but, in general, will distort the time course of VCO_2 as measured either across the pulmonary circulation or in expired air.

The most general approach to the nonsteady state is based on the joint use of input-output analysis and information on the inherent kinetics of the system. If the system in question is first probed with a null-mass input (e.g., a tracer), which scans the kinetic characteristics of the whole system without perturbing it, this knowledge can then be exploited to reconstruct the input (i.e., the actual changes) from the output (i.e., the observed response). One has to assume that the system is time invariant and linear, which means that its response to a given input does not depend on the time at which the input is given and that its response to a linear combination of inputs also is linear. Figure 5 exemplifies the relationship between input and output in a linear, time-invariant system under nonsteady state conditions. Each bit of substance appearing in the system from secretion (e.g., cellular VCO_2) will result in a concentration profile in the "sampling" compartment that decays over time as that bit is cleared from the system via all paths of irreversible loss. This disappearance curve (which most commonly has the analytical form of a multiexponential function of time) is the integrated result of all reversible interchanges and irreversible losses in all the compartments of which the system consists. As such, the tracer disappearance curve contains all the dynamic information on the structure of the system, difficult as it may be to read this information in terms of a given number of body compartments connected in a specified array. Input-output analysis simply assumes that any finite input consists of a sum of unitary (delta function) inputs and that the response to each of these deltas is the same (i.e., a complete disappearance curve). Therefore, the overall output response is, at any given time, the sum of the concentration produced by the last delta input plus the residual concentration of the delta input immediately preceding the last one, plus the still smaller residual concentration due to a still older input, and so on. In mathematical terms, one uses the convolution integral:

$$o(t) = i(t) * h(t) \qquad [5]$$

Here o(t) is the output response (i.e., the observed concentration time course), h(t) is the transfer function (i.e., the disappearance curve of a tracer dose of the substance), and i(t) is the actual time course of production of the substance that gave rise to the measured concentrations (the asterisk indicates the convolution integral). The operation by which one reconstructs the input from the output and the transfer function is called deconvolution.

Figure 6 shows the breath disappearance curve of an intravenous bolus of ^{14}C-labeled sodium bicarbonate in a healthy, overnight-fasted subject under resting conditions. It can be seen that a rapid decay phase is followed by a much slower rate of disappearance over a period of 6 hours. This decay curve can be resolved into three exponential components and used to calculate the turnover rate as well as the mean transit time and whole-body pool of CO_2 (the latter two parameters under a noncompartmental assumption; 11). In this subject, CO_2 was being produced at a rate of 9.4 mmol/min (0.21 l/min) and was taking about 87 minutes to transverse a total body pool of 0.8 mol (i.e., a blood-equivalent distribution space of 34.8 l, or 40% of body weight, in which the CO_2 concentration is 23.5 mmol/l). These values are typical for resting healthy subjects (12). It should be mentioned that CO_2 kinetics can also be reconstructed from data obtained following oral administration of a bicarbonate tracer (13) and that a stable rather than radioactive bicarbonate tracer can be safely administered to children. With this approach, for example, it has been possible to estimate the absorption time of oral bicarbonate at about 7 minutes and

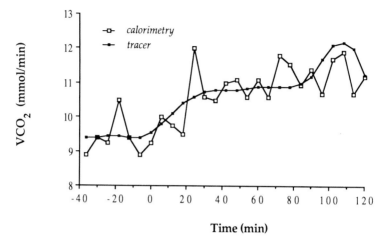

Time (min)

FIG. 8. VCO_2 by indirect calorimetry (open symbols) and by deconvolution of the data in Fig. 7 by the bicarbonate disappearance curve in Fig. 6 (solid symbols).

14). The results (not shown) demonstrated that the breath disappearance curve of this other bolus of tracer bicarbonate was essentially superimposable on that (Fig. 6) recorded under fasting conditions. This is proof that bicarbonate kinetics is not affected by the metabolic perturbation (insulin clamp) applied. During the second study, continuous indirect calorimetry was carried out with the use of a computerized, open-circuit canopy system. The time course of fractional concentration of CO_2 in the expired air ($FECO_2$) was reconstructed from the calorimetric VCO_2 data and smoothed (Fig. 7). This output response of CO_2 concentrations in expired air was then deconvolved by the subject's own transfer function (curve in Fig. 6). The results, graphed in Fig. 8, show that the time course of VCO_2 as reconstructed from tracer data is essentially coincident, if smoother, with the calorimetric VCO_2. It can be seen that either measure of VCO_2 began to rise relatively promptly after the start of insulin infusion, to reach a new apparent plateau some 30 minutes after time zero. This result prompts two considerations. The first is that, although the overall mean transit time of bicarbonate in this subject was 87 minutes, the actual delay between the rise of VCO_2 at the cellular level and its detection in the breath was only one-third of the average transit time. This means that the majority of cellular CO_2 is channeled through relatively fast pathways, whereas only a small fraction of CO_2 molecules takes the longer way through the bicarbonate system. Indeed, from Fig. 6 it can be appreciated that at 30 minutes post-injection the breath bicarbonate counts are about 15% of the peak value. Thus, the combination of relatively fast kinetics for the bulk of cellular CO_2 and the relatively slow rate of change in cellular metabolism (as compared, for instance, with physical exercise) minimizes the delay with which cellular VCO_2 changes are seen at the "breath window."

The other consideration is that the delay measured by collecting expired air is a maximal estimate of the true delay. The latter would be correctly estimated by recording the disappearance curve of tracer bicarbonate in mixed venous blood and by deconvolving this curve by the output CO_2 response also measured in mixed venous blood. This follows from the fact that the transfer function and the actual output response should both be measured upstream to the site of exit of the substance from the system: Such site is the pulmonary arterial circulation before the pulmonary capillary network (Fig. 2). In contrast, when both the transfer function and the output response are measured in expired air, which is a sink for CO_2, a systematic error is introduced. In fact, CO_2 is extracted with relatively low efficiency (~15%) from pulmonary arterial blood, and $FECO_2$ is in equilibrium with the blood CO_2 level on the pulmonary venous side rather than the opposite (pulmonary artery) end of the lung capillaries. Therefore, $FECO_2$ will lag behind cellular VCO_2 by an additional time corresponding to transit and diffusion of the gas through the lung capillary network.

In summary, indirect calorimetry can follow rapid changes in VO_2 faithfully but delays VCO_2 dynamics by a time that depends on individual bicarbonate kinetics and the rate of change in VCO_2. Quick bursts of VCO_2 that rapidly die away may be missed by recording respiratory gas exchange.

INDIRECT CALORIMETRY AND THE METABOLIC MODEL

Indirect calorimetry estimates substrate oxidation rates and energy expenditure starting from measures of respiratory gas exchange. The passage from the latter to the former is made possible by adopting a metabolic model. In such a model, all O_2 disappearing from inspired air is used exclusively for biologic oxidations, with no metabolic source of free O_2, and all CO_2 added to expired air derives solely from the complete combustion of substrates, with no other metabolic sinks for CO_2. Additionally, it is assumed that all the nonprotein urinary nitrogen excreted into the urine results only from the oxidation of free amino acids, the average nitrogen content of which is 16% (3). Any metabolic interconversion that does not involve gas exchange or liberation of urinary nitrogen is not "seen" by the calorimetric technique. Moreover, even for those reactions that do involve respiratory gases, i.e., oxidations, indirect calorimetry estimates only the total net loss of a substrate by oxidation, regardless of any exchange or cycling that the substrate itself or its intermediates undergo along the pathway to complete oxidation. Thus, if there is simultaneous oxidation and de novo synthesis of lipids, calorimetry yields an estimate of fat oxidation which is the algebraic sum of true lipid oxidation and lipid synthesis (2,3). Analogously, if there is concurrent carbohydrate oxidation and glucose new synthesis from alanine, the calorimetry-derived rate of carbohydrate oxidation is the algebraic sum of glucose degradation and synthesis (2,3).

Formal consideration of the impact of de novo lipogenesis, gluconeogenesis from alanine, and ketogenesis on the metabolic model of indirect calorimetry can be found in previous reviews, where equations have been derived for the occurrence of these gas-exchanging metabolic processes in isolation (2) or in various combinations with one another (3).

One problem is the impact of these metabolic processes on the estimates of energy expenditure provided by indirect calorimetry. It has been demonstrated that the presence of net lipid synthesis, although leading to an overestimation of carbohydrate oxidation by the standard calorimetric equation, does not alter energy expenditure as estimated by the standard formula:

$$EE = 3.91\ VO_2 + 1.10\ VCO_2 - 3.34\ N \qquad [6]$$

(in which N is the rate of nonprotein nitrogen excretion in g/min, VO_2 and VCO_2 are in l/min, and EE is in kcal/min). In contrast, the impact of gluconeogenesis on energy estimates has not been formally evaluated. When alanine is taken up by the liver to be converted into glucose, its amino group is split off (deamination), and there is apparent CO_2 fixation at the carbamoyl-phosphate step in the urea synthesis pathway. This leads to an underestimation of CO_2 output and to an excess of nitrogen appearing in the urine. By its assumptions, calorimetry attributes this excess nitrogen to protein oxidation, with its caloric equivalent, and does not take into account the energy (+1.02 kcal/g) required to carry out de novo glucose synthesis, an endergonic process. When both these factors are accounted for, one obtains the following equation:

$$EE = 3.86\ VO_2 + 1.15\ VCO_2 - 3.34\ N - 0.35\ G_a \qquad [7]$$

(in which G_a is the rate of gluconeogenesis from alanine, in g/min). By comparison with the classic Eq. 6, it can be seen that, overall, the latter overestimates energy expenditure by a factor equal to about one-third of the rate of gluconeogenesis from alanine.

Let us consider a healthy male individual of 70 kg who has fasted overnight and undergoes calorimetry in the supine position at 8:00 A.M. His VO_2 and VCO_2 are 0.25 and 0.2 l/min, respectively, and his rate of nonprotein nitrogen excretion into the urine is 20 mg/min. His rate of hepatic glucose production is 150 mg/min, of which 70% is derived from glycogen breakdown and the remaining 30% from gluconeogenesis (15). The gluconeogenic rate is therefore 0.045 g/min. If one uses the standard equations for glycogen, lipid, and protein oxidation (3) and ignores gluconeogenesis, one would calculate a total energy expenditure of 1.132 kcal/min resulting from the oxidation of 46.2 mg/min of glycogen, 45.1 mg/min of fat, and 125 mg/min of protein. In reality, this subject is oxidizing 89.7 mg/min of glycogen and 48.9 mg/min of fat but only 81.3 mg/min of protein, with a total energy expenditure of 1.124 kcal/min, according to the following equations for glycogen oxidation and energy expenditure in the presence of gluconeogenesis from alanine:

$$\text{Glycogen ox.} = 4.09\ VCO_2 - 2.88\ VO_2 - 2.51\ N + 0.93\ G_a \qquad [8]$$
$$EE = 3.92\ VO_2 + 1.10\ VCO_2 - 3.03\ N - 0.34\ G_a \qquad [9]$$

Note that Eq. 8 is the counterpart of Eq. 6 in ref. 3 just as Eq. 9 is the counterpart of Eq. 7 when there is ongoing gluconeogenesis from alanine and the carbohydrate being oxidized is glycogen rather than glucose. Clearly, the overestimation of true energy expenditure owing to the use of the standard rather the the correct equation is very small ($<1\%$) in the previous case. It cannot, however, be excluded that different mixtures of oxidizable substrates may give rise to more significant misjudgments of energy expenditure.

INDIRECT CALORIMETRY AND SUBSTRATE OXIDATION STUDIES

Indirect calorimetry is increasingly used in combination with tracer techniques to study details of substrate oxidation in vivo. Because, in general, tracers are administered into, and sampled from, the blood compartment, they can trace the kinetics of blood-borne substrates, whereas calorimetry estimates whole-body (blood plus tissues) oxidation. Tissue substrates that do not pass through the bloodstream on their way to oxidation are seen by calorimetry (precisely to the extent that their combustion consumes O_2 and releases CO_2) but do not dilute the tracer. Thus, in principle the difference between calorimetric and tracer estimates should reflect phenomena that occur at the tissue level. Obviously, such information is virtually impossible to obtain by any other means. Even tissue biopsy, although as direct a technique as possible, at best can provide a picture of cell metabolism at a given time but does not recover any dynamic element. Serial biopsies are rarely feasible in humans.

Several problems arise when using tracers in combination with indirect calorimetry. First, the directly comparable measure between tracer methods and calorimetry is substrate oxidation. The latter requires the use of a carbon-labeled tracer and the collection of expired tracer CO_2. However, even accurate quantitation of labeled CO_2 excretion misses that fraction of label which is exchanged in the citric acid cycle. For example, when CO_2 is fixed as oxaloacetate in the pyruvate carboxylase reaction, subsequent decarboxylation of oxaloacetate to phosphoenolpyruvate or in the citric acid cycle regenerates the fixed cold CO_2, whereas labeled CO_2 may be randomized at the fumarate step (on account of the reversibility of the malate dehydrogenase reaction). The result is that tracer CO_2 can be fixed without net CO_2 fixation. In general, the higher the ratio of additional inputs (to the Krebs cycle) to acetyl-CoA input, the larger the overestimation of CO_2 production by tracer bicarbonate. A correction factor c has therefore been defined (16) as the ratio of the rate of breath CO_2 excretion (VCO_2) to the rate of appearance of CO_2 ($RaCO_2$) as calculated from tracer CO_2:

$$c = VCO_2/RaCO_2 \qquad [10]$$

Such a correction factor is usually less than unity and accounts for the overestimation of true CO_2 production (VCO_2) brought about by selective labeled CO_2 fixation. It is pertinent to recall here that any CO_2 produced by metabolism but lost, for example, to bone bicarbonate (or to other compartments with very slow turnover) will be missed by both calorimetry and tracer bicarbonate.

By infusing labeled bicarbonate at a constant rate, $RaCO_2$ can be calculated as the ratio of tracer bicarbonate infusion rate (IR) to the specific activity of breath CO_2 ($[*C]O_2sa$) at equilibrium:

$$RaCO_2 = IR/[*C] O_2sa \qquad [11]$$

$RaCO_2$ as derived from Eq. 11 is the rate of appearance computed from isotope dilution measurements at steady state; it is mathematically equivalent to the result obtained when the tracer dose is given as a single intravenous bolus (Fig. 6) and the area under the tracer disappearance curve is computed:

$$RaCo_2 = Dose/\int_0^\infty [*C]O_2 (t) \, dt \qquad [12]$$

When the oxidation of a substrate (e.g., glucose, GL_{ox}) is determined in vivo, a suitable carbon tracer of the substrate ($[*C]GL$) is infused at a constant rate, and the oxidative rate is calculated according to the following precursor-product relationship:

$$GL_{ox} = [*C]O_2sa \cdot VCO_2/[*C]GLsa \cdot c \qquad [13]$$

where $[*C]O_2sa$ is the specific activity of breath $[*C]O_2$, $[*C]GLsa$ is the specific activity of tracer glucose, VCO_2 is carbon dioxide production as measured by indirect calorimetry (an estimate of the true $RaCO_2$), and c is the correction factor. The latter accounts for incomplete recovery in expired air of $[*C]O_2$ derived from $[*C]GL$ oxidation. If, however, $RaCO_2$ is independently measured with a bolus injection or constant infusion of labeled bicarbonate, then Eq. 13 changes:

$$GL_{ox} = [*C]O_2sa \cdot RaCO_2/[*C]GLsa \qquad [14]$$

Here the correction factor is no longer present. If one has accounted for any differential loss of $[*C]O_2$ in a separate experiment, there is no longer a need to use indirect calorimetry to estimate VCO_2 (17). However, one must assume that bicarbonate kinetics are the same when $RaCO_2$ and GL_{ox} are measured by separate experiments. If it is possible to use different carbon tracers for bicarbonate and glucose (e.g., $NaH[^{13}C]O_3{}^-$ and $[1-^{14}C]$-glucose), or if an adequate model for bicarbonate kinetics is available (Cobelli et al., personal communication), one can obtain a reliable measurement of $RaCO_2$ and substrate oxidation in the same experiment.

Finally, I shall illustrate the issue of tissue versus whole-body substrate oxidation by recalculating the data of a study in which the effects of insulin on fat oxidation were investigated with the combined use of indirect calorimetry and $[1-^{14}C]$-palmitate infusion (18). Palmitate is the second most abundant FFA in plasma (25–30% of total FFA), and its kinetics are representative of the total FFA pool (19,20). In a group of healthy volunteers, plasma FFA oxidation was measured with the use of labeled palmitate, both in the fasting state and during graded euglycemic hyperinsulinemia created with the glucose clamp technique (14). Whole-body net lipid oxidation was measured continuously by an open-circuit, computerized canopy system. The dose-response curves of FFA and net whole-body lipid oxidation as a function of pe-

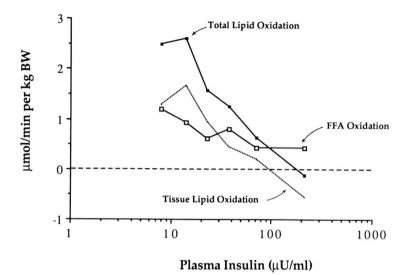

FIG. 9. Dose-response curves for the effect of euglycemic hyperinsulinemia on total lipid, tissue lipid, and plasma FFA oxidation in healthy subjects. The interrupted line represents a null rate of net lipid oxidation (i.e., lipid oxidation = de novo lipid synthesis). Points below the interrupted line indicate net lipogenesis. Data recalculated and drawn from ref. 18.

ripheral plasma insulin concentrations are shown in Fig. 9 together with the dose-response curve (marked as tissue lipid oxidation) calculated as the difference between whole-body lipid and plasma FFA oxidation. Several points are noteworthy. First, in the overnight fasted state, the plasma FFA pool contributes approximately one-half of the total amount of fat that is used as oxidative fuel, the remainder evidently being offered by circulating triglycerides as well as intracellular lipids. Second, FFA oxidation is very sensitive to insulin in vivo (with an apparent ED_{50} of 20 μU/ml) but plateaus relatively soon and is never completely shut off. In contrast, whole-body net lipid oxidation continues to decrease as plasma insulin concentrations are raised into the high physiologic range (up to 220 μU/ml). At plasma insulin of >200 μU/ml, net lipid synthesis occurs (Fig. 9). When tissue lipid oxidation is calculated, it can be seen that, for very small increments in plasma insulin concentrations (+6 μU/ml), tissue lipid oxidation is actually stimulated rather than inhibited, thereby maintaining total net lipid oxidation unchanged in the face of a 25% decrease in plasma FFA oxidation. This apparent paradox probably reflects the fact that the intracellular precursor pool for FFA oxidation (fed by both intracellular and circulating lipids) normally is in excess of the rate of FFA oxidation; as the extracellular FFA input to such pool is cut down by insulin, a larger fraction of the FFA oxidative flux is drawn from the intracellular store. It is only when insulin's inhibitory action begins to involve intracellular (or intercellular) lipolysis that a decrease in tissue lipid oxidation is observed. The other point is that tissue lipid oxidation, after the initial small increase, declines as a linear function of log-transformed plasma insulin concentrations and crosses the zero line (i.e., net tissue lipid synthesis) at plasma insulins of 70 to 80 μU/ml. This finding demonstrates that *physiologic* hyperinsulinemia is capable of inducing net lipid synthesis (i.e., de novo FFA synthesis in excess of concurrent FFA oxidation) in a normal man. This conclusion contrasts with that derived from the total lipid oxidation dose-response curve, which would suggest that net lipid synthesis is seen only at supraphysiologic plasma insulin concentrations (Fig. 9).

CONCLUSIONS

In summary, I have analyzed the relationship between the Fick method and indirect calorimetry as ways to measure respiratory gas exchange both from a theoretical and an experimental viewpoint. In the comparison (and with the necessary specifications), indirect calorimetry fares rather favorably.

Next, I have dealt with the impact of bicarbonate as a time delay in the transfer of changes in cellular CO_2 production to equivalent changes in respiratory CO_2 excretion. In the resting state, calorimetric VCO_2 seems to have a time resolution in the order of 15 to 20 minutes, i.e., adequate to follow most physiologic changes in the pattern of substrate utilization at the whole-body level.

Furthermore, an equation formalizing the impact of gluconeogenesis from alanine on the calorimetric estimation of energy expenditure has been derived. It shows that the presence of significant gluconeogenesis leads to an overestimation of energy expenditure as calculated by standard formulas, but such overestimation is quite small and holds dubious physiologic significance.

Finally, I have described some of the problems that arise when indirect calorimetry is coupled with tracer substrate studies aimed at quantitating the oxidation rate of circulating fuels. A study of combined use of calorimetry and palmitate oxidation kinetics has been taken from the recent literature to exemplify how a correct interpretation of such data can yield a wealth of physiologically meaningful information.

ACKNOWLEDGMENTS

I wish to thank Dr. Riccardo Bonadonna for helping me to understand some points and for letting me reanalyze data from his published work (ref. 18). I also thank Dr. Luigi Brandi for making some of his unpublished data available to me for discussion.

REFERENCES

1. Frayn KN. Calculation of substrate oxidation rates in vivo from gaseous exchange. *J Appl Physiol* 1983;55:628–34.
2. Ben-Porat M, Sideman S, Burzstein S. Energy metabolism rate equation for fasting and postabsorptive subjects. *Am J Physiol* 1983;244:R764–9.
3. Ferrannini E. The theoretical bases of indirect calorimetry: a review. *Metabolism* 1988;37:287–301.

4. Simonson DC, DeFronzo RA. Indirect calorimetry: methodological and interpretative problems. *Am J Physiol* 1990;258:E399–E412.
5. Fick A. Uber die Messung des Blutquantums in den Herzventriken. *Sitz der Physik Med Ges Wurtzburg* 1870:16.
6. Blasi A. Bronchial circulation: anatomical viewpoint. In: Cumming G, Bonsignore G, eds. *Pulmonary circulation in health and disease.* New York: Plenum Press, 1980;19–26.
7. Douglas AR, Jones NL, Reed JW. Calculation of whole blood CO2 content. *J Appl Physiol* 1988;65:473–7.
8. Brandi LS, Frediani M, Oleggini M, Mosca F, Ferrannini E. Evaluation of a computerized, open circuit canopy system for indirect calorimetry. *RINPE* 1986;4:145–52.
9. Oleggini M, Brandi LS, Di Trani M, et al. La produzione di energia a riposo e la misura degli scambi gassosi nel soggetto normale: valutazione mediante calorimetria continua indiretta con sistema a calottina. *RINPE* 1987;5:167–73.
10. Natali A, Buzzigoli G, Taddei S, et al. Effects of insulin on hemodynamics and metabolism in human forearm. *Diabetes* 1990;39:490–500.
11. Distefano JJ, Landaw EM. Multiexponential, multicompartmental, and noncompartmental modeling. I. Methodological limitations and physiological interpretations. *Am J Physiol* 1984;246:R651–64.
12. Barstow TJ, Cooper DM, Sobel E, Landaw EM, and Epstein S. Influence of increased metabolic rate on ^{13}C washout kinetics. *Am J Physiol* 1990;259:R163–71.
13. Armon Y, Cooper DM, Springer C, et al. Oral ^{13}C bicarbonate measurement of CO_2 stores and dynamics in children and adults. *J Appl Physiol* 1990;69:1754–60.
14. DeFronzo RA, Tobin JD, Andres R. Glucose clamp technique: a method for quantifying insulin resistance and secretion. *Am J Physiol* 1979;237:E214–23.
15. Consoli A, Kennedy FP, Miles J, Gerich JE. Determination of Krebs cycle metabolic carbon exchange in vivo and its use to estimate individual contributions of gluconeogenesis and glycogenolysis to overall glucose output in man. *J Clin Invest* 1987;80:1303–10.
16. Issekutz B, Paul P, Miller HI, Bortz WM. Oxidation of plasma FFA in lean and obese humans. *Metabolism* 1968;17:62–73.
17. Kien CL. Isotopic dilution of CO2 as an estimate of CO2 production during substrate oxidation studies. *Am J Physiol* 1989;257:E296–8.
18. Bonadonna RC, Groop LC, Zych K, Shank M, DeFronzo RA. Dose-dependent effect of insulin on plasma free fatty acid turnover and oxidation in humans. *Am J Physiol* 1990;259:E736–50.
19. Hagenfeldt L. Turnover of individual free fatty acids in man. *Fed Proc* 1975;34:2246–9.
20. Hagenfeldt L, Wahren J, Pernow B, and Raf L. Uptake of individual free fatty acids by skeletal muscle and liver in man. *J Clin Invest* 1972;51:2324–30.

Energy Metabolism: Tissue Determinants and Cellular Corollaries, edited by J. M. Kinney and H. N. Tucker. Raven Press, Ltd., New York © 1992.

Energy Expenditure in the Whole Body

M. Elia

Dunn Clinical Nutrition Centre, Cambridge, CB2 1QL, United Kingdom

Over the last century calorimetry has provided important insights regarding the extent to which energy metabolism in humans and other animals responds to food intake, exercise, disease, and the environment. From such information emerged physiologic concepts of energy adaptation and recommendations of energy intake in various circumstances. Naturally, attempts have been made to establish normal values for the various components of energy expenditure, although some of these have not been easy to establish. For example, the energy expended in physical activity by normal free living subjects (or even by hospitalized patients with disease) is not only variable but also difficult to measure. It is only in the last decade that tracer techniques have begun to throw further light on the contribution of physical activity to energy expenditure (1,2). If it can be shown that in certain groups of subjects an increase in energy intake produces an increase in work output, an increase in exploratory behavior, or an improvement in well being, the relationships are of immense physiologic, social, and economic importance.

Emphasis has been given to establishing standards of basal metabolic rate over the last 75 years, partly because this is easier to measure and partly because it is usually the largest component of total energy expenditure (Fig. 1). Of the hundreds of thousands of measurements of basal metabolic rate, some have been used to establish reference standards. It may seem that with such standards available it is a simple matter to assess whether a subject's basal metabolism is normal or abnormal. Figure 2 illustrates the 95% confidence interval (± 2 S.D.) for the basal metabolic rate expressed as a percent of the mean reference values provided by Robertson and Reid (3) and by the Mayo Clinic (4). The percent variation is also similar to that given by Harris and Benedict (5) and by the Schofield reference standards (6). It can be suggested that individuals within this range have a normal overall basal energy expenditure, whereas those outside the range are likely to have an abnormal basal energy metabolism. However, this approach is unsatisfactory for two reasons. First, it is possible for there to be important sequential changes of energy expenditure within the range of normality (up to ~25%), which will be missed from a single measurement. Second, the mean values of energy expenditure predicted by the various reference methods do not always agree. In some cases the discrepancies may be greater than 15% to 20% (equivalent to more than 2 standard deviations above or below the mean value predicted by different reference standards). Systematic

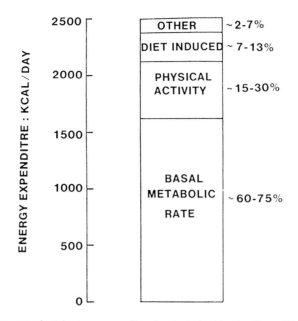

FIG. 1. Components of total energy expenditure in a typical subject leading a "Western" lifestyle. "Physical activity" includes minor movement and the residual effects of exercise. The thermogenic component labeled "other" includes drug-induced thermogenesis (e.g., smoking) and a thermoregulatory component (e.g., energy produced in response to cold). The contribution of various components such as physical activity can vary substantially outside this range in some individuals, such as those who have physically demanding occupations or those who are inactive as a result of disease or hospitalization.

differences ($\pm$10–15%) also exist between the reference standards and the basal energy expenditure of specific populations (see section on race), making it difficult to decide which (if any) of the available standards should be used as the "gold standard." These difficulties are confounded further by the use of surface area to predict the metabolic rate in some standards, weight and height in others, while fat-free mass or an exponent of fat-free mass (or exponents of body weight) is used in others.

In order to identify more clearly the origin of these discrepancies and the basis for using different parameters to predict metabolic rate, a brief historical outline is given in this chapter. It will be seen that over the last century there has been a progressive change in perspective, from an emphasis on heat loss (surface area), to heat production, sites of heat production, and finally mechanisms of heat production in health and disease.

ENERGY METABOLISM AND SURFACE AREA

A unifying theory for explaining differences in heat production by different animals was proposed by Rubner in 1883 (7). The theory, which was dubiously elevated to

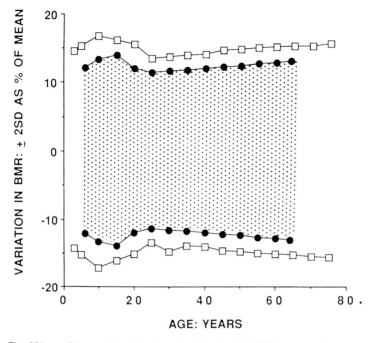

FIG. 2. The 95% confidence interval for basal metabolic rate (BMR) expressed as a percent of mean reference value. Calculated using values provided by Boothby et al. (4) (●——●, inner shaded area) and Robertson and Reid (3) (□——□, outer graph).

the status of a law, had a major impact on reference values for human energy metabolism.

Rubner studied dogs (weighing 3 kg to 31 kg) and related their 24h metabolic rate (measured at 16°C) to their surface area. The dogs he chose came from the short-haired races so that the confounding effects of different hair coverings could be largely eliminated. The results, which indicated a striking similarity in the metabolic rate of different dogs when expressed in relation to surface area (~1,000 kcal/m²/day), formed the basis of the "surface law."

It is surprising that Rubner carried out his dog experiments at 16°C, which is about 10°C below thermoneutrality (Rubner later realized the importance of this and suggested that the metabolic rate of dogs and mammals in general is closer to 615 kcal/m²/day). Indeed, it is probable that dogs shiver when kept at 16°C for prolonged periods of time. Furthermore, dogs are unlikely to remain inactive for 24 hours, especially because they are readily distracted by sound. Finally, it appears that Rubner's surface law emerged without consideration of sex and age, both of which have an influence on the relationship between metabolic rate and body surface area.

Nevertheless, the original work in dogs had a profound effect on concepts of energy metabolism because similar studies were undertaken in other species in order to provide further evidence for the unifying theory of heat loss. Despite substantial variability and some extreme results [a range in metabolic rate of 130–2060 kcal/m²/day; (8)] interest in this area continued. Rubner went on to study the metabolic rate of a fat boy and his brother with the surface law in mind. Clinicians became interested, and it was not long before the massive study from the Mayo Clinic published its reference values for metabolic rate in relation to surface area (4,9). Aub and Dubois (10) published their reference values of metabolic rate in relation to surface area even earlier than this in 1917, and Fleish (11) and Robertson and Reid (3) did so later in 1951 and 1952, respectively.

Controversy over the surface law developed. The theoretical premise on which the theory was based was questioned. The relationship between metabolic rate and surface area was considered to be so variable, both within and between species (8), that several workers regarded the relationship between metabolic rate and body surface area as an empirical one rather than a causal one representing a unified biological principle. (References 8 and 12 provide detailed arguments against the surface law.)

It was argued that instead of exploring the relationship between metabolic rate and heat loss, which was considered to be largely physical, it would be more fruitful to explore the relationship between metabolic rate and the size of tissues that produce heat. Because heat production has both biological and chemical relevance, its source might provide a rational explanation for the irregularities in the surface law.

In humans major factors other than surface area must determine heat production in order to explain the following observations.

1. The basal metabolic rate/m² rises by about 75% between birth and 6–18 months (refs. 13, 14 and Table A1 in Appendix) and then falls by more than 30% in adult life (3,11 and Table A1 in Appendix). With advancing years it decreases even further.
2. Women consistently have a lower basal metabolic rate/m² than men (~10%—see Appendix).
3. At thermoneutrality, which is required for measurements of BMR, major changes in surface area produced by altering the position of the body (e.g., from a fetal to an outstretched position) has little if any effect on metabolic rate.

As will become clear, the major differences in metabolic rate/m² in humans of different sex and age can be explained largely by considering the size and metabolic activity of internal organs, the major sites of heat production.

Perhaps one of the strongest arguments against expressing metabolic rate in relation to surface area concerns the inadequacy of methods for estimating surface area. Of the various anthropomorphic human characteristics, surface area is one of the most difficult to measure. It is therefore normally predicted from weight and height. This estimation implies that the term metabolic rate/m² is also a prediction, irrespective of whether metabolic rate is measured. Clearly errors in estimating the surface area of an individual will result in errors in the value of metabolic rate/m².

THE ESTIMATION OF SURFACE AREA AND ITS IMPLICATIONS FOR HUMAN ENERGY METABOLISM

The first measurement of surface area in humans was made in 1793 by John Abernethy (1764–1831), an anatomist and surgeon and Fellow of the Royal Society, at St. Bartholomew's Hospital, London (15). However, it was not until after the emergence of Rubner's surface law that immense interest in the area developed. Dubois and Dubois (16) were among the early enthusiasts, and they published a formula in 1916. Their work led to a formula for predicting body surface area from weight and height (16). This was to become the most widely used method for estimating surface area, although there are now major doubts about its accuracy in certain individuals.

Dubois and Dubois (16) developed their formula on the basis of both theory and empirical use of mathematical formulas. It is remarkable that the formula that was to find such widespread use was based on measurements of surface area in a group of only nine subjects and one cadaver, which included the following: a malnourished young child with rickets (small for age and height) who died of pneumonia and pertussis; another child aged 12; an emaciated young man with a body mass index of 15.3 kg/m^2; and an obese woman with a body mass index of 41.5 kg/m^2 (16,17). The weight of the group ranged from 6.27 kg to 93.0 kg, the height from 73.2 cm to 184.2 cm, and the measured surface area from 0.3699 m^2 to 1.9 m^2. The Dubois formula predicted the surface area of all the subjects to within ±5%.

However, several other formulas emerged (Table 1), many of which were claimed to be as good as or superior to the Dubois formula. This is not too surprising, since the newer formulas were based on a large number of measurements of surface area (up to several hundred) in adults, children, and infants. Nevertheless, the Dubois formula remains the most widely used, presumably for historic reasons.

The various prediction formulas frequently sought to be universal so that they could apply from infancy (and sometimes fetuses—see ref. 19) to old age, although

TABLE 1. *Some formulas for calculating surface area in humans[a]*

Formula	Year of publication	Reference
SA^b = 71.84W$^{0.425}$H$^{0.725}$	1916	(16)
SA = 74.49W$^{0.427}$H$^{0.718}$	1925	(18)
SA = 3.027 (1,000W)$^{0.7285 - 0.0188Log(1000W)}H^{0.3}$	1935	(19)
SA = 240W$^{0.53}$H$^{0.4}$	1945	(20)
SA = 235W$^{0.51456}$H$^{0.42246}$	1970	(21)
SA = 242.65W$^{0.5378}$H$^{0.3964}$	1978	(22)
SA = 87(H + W) − 2,600	1932	(23)
SA = 168.043(WH)$^{0.5}$	1954	(24)
SA = 10,000 + 100[W + (H − 160)]	1958	(25)

[a] SA, surface area in cm^2 (to convert to m^2, divide by 10,000); W, weight in kg; H, height in cm
[b] The Dubois and Dubois formula

sex and race were not considered. Furthermore, little attention was paid to the potential errors that might arise from the application of these formulas to obese or malnourished patients. Here I have attempted to illustrate possible discrepancies between formulas by applying them to individuals with a different body build. When they are used to estimate the surface area of an adult male weighing 81 kg and having a height of 1.85 m (body mass index 25 kg/m^2), the formulas generally agree with each other to within 1.7% (Table 2). However, when they are used to calculate surface area in obese or lean adults (Table 2), substantial deviation begins to occur, with some differences being as large as 15%.

For a normal child (1.30 m, 271.7 kg), on the 50th percentile of the NCHS percentiles of height and weight, the formulas also agree well with each other, but for smaller children the range in predicted values is large and unacceptable (up to 20–30% difference). It is interesting that for obese adults and for young children the Dubois formula systematically underestimates surface area relative to almost all the other formulas. These discrepancies do not indicate the superiority of one formula over another but merely note that there are differences between them.

In order to assess accuracy, the Dubois formula was used to predict the surface area of various groups of subjects who had their surface area measured directly by triangulation or coating methods (19). The individuals chosen for this analysis (19) had weights and heights similar to those indicated in Table 3 for normal adults and various groups of children. For adults with a height of 175 cm to 185 cm and children with a height of 120 cm to 140 cm, there appears to be little systematic difference between predicted and measured surface area. However, for young children with a height of 70 cm to 80 cm and 55 cm to 65 cm, the Dubois formula underestimates surface area by a mean of about 8%. Other workers have found similar underestimation in individuals with a surface area less than 0.8 m^2. This implies that the mean results obtained by several of the other formulas (Tables 1 and 2) are more correct than those obtained by the Dubois formula.

Table 3 illustrates another interesting point concerned with the prediction of surface area. For children the 95% confidence interval (± 2 S.D.) is about $\pm 15\%$, which is similar to that obtained with the other formulas (data not shown) and similar to the observations of other workers (19–26). This means that the use of the Dubois formula to predict the surface area of individual children may be associated with an error in excess of 20%, because a systematic underestimation of 7% to 9% already exists (see the previous section). In adults the 95% confidence interval was found to be smaller than in children (see Table 2), although in other larger studies it has been shown to be ± 5–10% (26).

The inaccuracies of the surface area prediction formulas (frequently $\pm$ 5%) are sufficiently high to invalidate their use in individual subjects. The inaccuracies are due partly to the application of the same mathematical formulas to subjects of different shapes and partly to the physiologic variation in the gaseous content of lungs and gastrointestinal tract, which alter surface area but not weight and height.

The implications of these conclusions on energy metabolism are twofold. First, because estimates of surface area are only approximate, the results of metabolic

TABLE 2. Percentage difference between surface area predicted by the Dubois and Dubois formula and various other formulas for adults, children and infants[a]

Reference to predication formula (See Table 1)	BMI kg/m²	Adults					Child (male)		Infant (male)		
	ht(m)/wt(kg)	15	25	35	35	45	50th percentile[b]	50th percentile[b]	5th percentile[b]	50th percentile[b]	95th percentile[b]
		1.80/48.6	1.80/81.0	1.80/113.4	1.521/81.0	1.8/145.8	1.30/27.7	0.76/10.1	0.56/3.2	0.56/4.7	0.56/6.7
16		0(a)[c]	0(b)	0(c)	0(d)	0(e)	0(f)	0(g)	0(h)	0(i)	0(j)
18		0.8	0.9	0.9	1.0	1.0	0.9	1.1	1.0	1.1	1.2
19		-5.4	0.7	4.7	8.2	7.7	0.8	9.4	3.4	10.4	16.9
20		-7.1	-2.0	1.5	3.5	4.3	-2.7	4.2	2.0	6.2	10.2
21		-3.7	0.8	3.9	6.0	6.2	1.0	8.5	7.4	11.2	14.7
22		-5.0	0.6	4.5	6.4	7.5	-0.8	5.6	2.6	7.2	11.5
23		7.0	0.2	-1.0	-0.5	-0.1	10.7	10.3	17.0	4.4	-4.4
24		-2.7	1.1	3.7	5.0	5.7	0.4	5.0	3.2	6.2	9.0
25		4.0	0.1	0.8	-2.5	3.2	-2.8	-41.1	—[d]	—[d]	—[d]
Range: lowest		-7.1	-2.0	-1.0	-0.5	-0.1	-2.8	-41.1	-2.6	0	-4.4
highest		7.0	1.1	4.9	8.2	7.5	10.7	26.5	17.0	11.2	16.9

[a] Positive values indicate that the calculated surface area is greater than that predicted by the Dubois and Dubois formula. Negative values indicate that the calculated surface area is smaller than that predicted by the Dubois and Dubois formula (see Table 1 for formula).
[b] Percentiles of weight for height of the National Center of Health Statistics (NCHS).
[c] Surface areas calculated by the Dubois and Dubois formula: (a) 1.6153 m²; (b) 2.0070 m²; (c) 2.3155 m²; (d) 1.7765 m²; (e) 2.5765 m²; (f) 1.0047 m²; (g) 0.4434 m²; (h) 0.2180 m²; (i) 0.2567 m²; (j) 0.2985 m².
[d] These values are clearly incorrect since the value for the lightest child is negative (−80 cm²) and the other two are low to an inconceivable extent (70 cm² and 270 cm²).

TABLE 3. *Errors in the estimation of surface area with the use of the Dubois and Dubois (16) surface area formula[a]*

	Adults[b]	Children		Infants
	1.75 – 1.85 m ($n = 5$)	1.2–1.4 m ($n = 6$)	0.70–0.8 m ($n = 9$)	0.55–0.60 m ($n = 14$)
Height (m)	1.792 ± 0.034	1.33 ± 0.044	0.721 ± 0.168	0.568 ± 0.119
Weight (kg)	67.7 ± 6.22	23.46 ± 3.52	7.95 ± 1.54	4.05 ± 0.94
Surface area (m^2)				
measured[c]	1.8536 ± 0.0513	0.921 ± 0.1451	.4239 ± 0.0659	0.26 ± 0.0414
calculated with Dubois formula	1.8640 ± 0.0534	0.9553 ± 0.0753	0.3837 ± 0.0363	0.2418 ± 0.0261
calculated/ measured × 100	100.4 ± 1.7	102.8 ± 7.3	91.5 ± 7.3	92.4 ± 7.5
% deviation from measured	0.4 ± 1.7	2.8 ± 7.3	−8.5 ± 6.9	−7.6 ± 7.5

Results are expressed as mean ± 1 S.D.
[a] See Table 1 for Dubois and Dubois formula (16).
[b] The body mass index of the adults is 21.14 ± 2.62 kg/m^2.
[c] Individual measurements of weight, height, and surface area (triangulation or coating methods) were taken from the tabulated values given by Boyd (19). Adults 1.75–1.85 m, nos. 100, 101, 102, 110, 215; children 1.2–1.4 m, nos. 84–87, 89, 164; children 0.7–0.8 m, nos. 54–59, 150–153; infants 0.5–0.6 m, nos. 30–33, 36, 39, 40, 48, 137, 140, 142, 145.

rate, expressed in relation to surface area, are also approximate. Therefore, individual comparisons of metabolic rate/unit of true surface area cannot be made with a high degree of certainty. Second, there is a risk involved in comparing measurements of metabolic rate that are expressed in relation to estimates of surface area obtained by different formulas. In this respect it should be remembered that several standard reference tables (3,4,10,11,27) report the metabolic rate of adults and children of all ages, in relation to surface area calculated using the Dubois formula.

To predict metabolic rate it is reasonable on theoretic and empirical grounds to use physical characteristics such as weight or height that are more readily and more accurately measured than surface area. It would appear that surface area has no advantage over weight and height for predicting metabolic rate (ref. 5; E. Pullicino and M. Elia, unpublished material). It is also interesting that as the wave of enthusiasm over Rubner's surface law subsided, new reference standards emerged that used weight, height (± age) as the basis for predicting metabolic rate (6,28–31). Nevertheless, the impact of some of the earlier standards, which were based on surface area (4,10,11), is still felt today. They provide empirical relationships between predicted surface area (indirectly estimated from weight and height) and metabolic rate.

Harris and Benedict (5) withstood pressure from the surface law supporters and in 1919 published their prediction equations in relation to weight and height (Table A6 in Appendix). These standards, which were among the first to be produced, have been extensively used to the present day. Therefore, it is pertinent to consider the origin and shortcomings of these standards.

THE HARRIS BENEDICT STANDARDS (5)

Measurements of metabolic rate were made in 239 individuals (136 M, 103 F, aged 15–73 years). These were made during several 15-minute periods with interims of 15 minutes to 20 minutes. The measurements were frequently repeated on several days in the same subject, and the mean results were calculated. Absence of muscular activity was confirmed by a pneumograph connected to the bed. The smallest motion, imperceptible even to a trained observer, could be detected on the pneumograph. The results of the Harris-Benedict data were actually a combination of results from a series of previous studies. Aware that there may be differences between groups (e.g., athletes and overweight individuals), Harris and Benedict (5) analyzed their data in separate subgroups and provided separate equations for each of them. The standard equations that were to receive widespread use, however, were derived from a combination of all the results.

Evidence then began to accumulate in a number of units that the Harris-Benedict standards for metabolic rate were generally too high, as indicated in Table 4. This was known even to Benedict, who expressed reservations about his own standards—especially those for young women—in 1925 (52) and again in 1928 (32). He suggested that the standards were about 5% too high. He endorsed this later (8) by stating that the metabolism of the women in the Harris-Benedict series (5) "is undoubtedly higher than is true of Caucasian women in general." Remarkably, these warnings were ignored, with the result that the Harris-Benedict standards continue to be used to predict metabolic rate, especially in clinical practice. However, the general over-estimation of the Harris-Benedict standards for women has been repeatedly redis-covered, and evidence has accumulated to indicate that the same is true for men (Table 4).

OTHER REFERENCE STANDARDS (TABLE 5 AND APPENDIX)

The next major standards to emerge were from the Mayo Clinic (4) (Table 5). From a series of more than 80,000 individuals, a selection was made of 639 male and 828 female subjects (total 1,467) aged 6 to 68 years who were considered to have had technically satisfactory basal metabolic rate measurements and no clinically signif-icant abnormality. The study involved children, mainly from Rochester, Minnesota, and adults in various social strata from all parts of the United States. Many of the subjects were normal individuals who asked for routine check-ups. However, some had minor abnormalities such as hernias, ocular defects, and minor injuries that were not considered to affect metabolic rate. Measurements of metabolic rate were ex-pressed in relation to surface area. Unfortunately, details of weight and height of the subjects are not given in the Mayo Clinic report (Boothby et al., 4) in contrast to the Harris-Benedict report (5), so it is impossible to assess the proportion of underweight/overweight individuals involved in the study.

TABLE 4. *Comparison of measurements of metabolic rate obtained by various authors with the Harris Benedict standards (5)*

Place of study	Males n	Males Age range (y)	Females n	Females Age range (y)	% deviation from Harris Benedict prediction Males	Females	Reference
USA	136	16–63	103	15–66	0	0	5
USA	27	21–89	33	15–58	−0.4	−7.3	32
USA	—	—	101	17–39	—	−10.1	33
USA	—	—	100	17–26	—	−2.5	34
USA	—	—	52	17–25	—	−9.9	35
USA	—	—	38	17–26	—	−13	36
USA[a]	59	18–67	68	18–67	−10	−13	37
USA[b]	60	18–32	—	—	−6.4	—	30
USA[c]	—	—	44	18–65	—	−12.8	29
USA[d]	251	19–76	247	20–76	−4.6	−5.1	28
Sweden	64	21–24	19	21–24	−6.7	−6.3	38
Sweden	40	21–27	37	18–30	−8.8	−6.7	39
UK	61	18–49	25	19–63	4.9	−2.1	—[e]
India (Europeans)	—	—	34	20–54	—	−6.3	40
India (Indians)	—	—	26	22–52	−3.4	—	41
(Europeans)	—	—	20	21–39	−8.9	—	41
India	61	18–25	15	19–24	−10.8	−18.2	42
India	60	20–49	—	—	−5.3	—	43
India	—	—	54	17–54	—	−16.9	44
India	24	19–35	52	18–29	−11.7	−15.9	45
India	32	19–32	—	—	−6.8	−6.8	46
China (Chinese)	54	17–59	14	20–58	+1.9	−3.7	47
(Europeans)	5	23–39	21	15–60	−0.3	+1.8	47
China	20	16–36	—	—	−3.5	—	48
China	24	18–51	—	—	+15.8	—	49
Chile	31	19–44	14	18–45	+9.8	14	50
Java (Europeans)	24	19–32	—	—	−6.3	—	51

[a] The age range is for the combined group of males and females.

[b] Includes many obese men. For those with a body mass index (BMI) $<25 (20.4 - 25.0)$ kg/m^2 ($n = 24$), % deviation from Harris and Benedict prediction is −5.7%.

[c] Includes many obese women. For those with a body mass index (BMI) $<25 (18.2 - 25.0)$ kg/m^2 ($n = 24$), % deviation from Harris & Benedict prediction is −13.1%.

[d] These are the calculated mean results for lean and obese individuals. For women 80–100% ideal body wt. (IBW), the % deviation from the Harris Benedict prediction is −4.6%, for 100–119% IBW −6.4%, 120–139% IBW −6%, >140% IBW −3.1%. The corresponding values for men are −1.4%, −3.9%, −3.9%, and −8.7%.

[e] E. Pullicino and M. Elia, unpublished observations.

The same criticism can be made of the Robertson and Reid standards (3) (Table 5; Table A1 in the Appendix), which reported average values of metabolic rate in relation to surface area. The subjects studied were nurses, medical students, staff members of the Middlesex Hospital in London, children attending welfare clinics and on tonsillectomy waiting lists, and members of the public who volunteered to participate in the study after reading newspaper appeals. The subjects were described as normal but it is not clear whether this indicates good health or normal body build (i.e. absence of obesity/undernutrition).

The Fleish standards (Table 5; Table A1 in the Appendix) tabulated results of metabolic rate in relation to surface area and were published in 1951, one year earlier than the Robertson-Reid standards. They were established from measurements made on more individuals (>10,000) than in any other study, but these were obtained by a variety of different workers who had already published their results (often as mean results) in a series of 24 papers. The Fleish standards included measurements made by Aub and Dubois (10), Harris and Benedict (5) and Boothby et al. (4), which formed the basis of earlier standards. The Fleish standards (11) also include the results of Boothby and Sandiford (5,066 females, 1,822 males) (9), which were also partly incorporated into the later standards of Boothby et al. (4). These last standards did not include results that were considered unsatisfactory on technical or clinical grounds. Individual details of some of the subjects incorporated into the Fleish standards can be traced (e.g., ref. 5), but others cannot (e.g., 4).

Following a request from the UN/FAO in 1947, Quenouille et al. published their standards in 1951 (27) from a compilation of results obtained by a variety of workers ($n \geq 8,600$ subjects) in a variety of racial groups (Table 5; Appendix). Their prediction equations did not find widespread use, possibly because they involve cumbersome calculations involving weight, height, surface area, age, humidity, and environmental temperature.

Dissatisfied with the number of available standards, the WHO/FAO/UNU proposed another massive literature search with the aim of selecting individual results of basal metabolic rate that were considered to be satisfactory. A data base of some 7,000 such measurements was established (Table 5), which formed the basis of the 1985 FAO/WHO/UNU or Schofield standards (6). Unlike most previous standards, those of Schofield were established from measurements made on individuals from a variety of different races and countries (USA, Britain, Denmark, Sweden, Japan, China, India, Australia, etc.). The data of Aub and Dubois (10) and Harris and Benedict (5) were also included in the Schofield data base. Attempts were made to exclude subjects with disease, but the exclusion was probably not complete.

Finally, in the last few years, a number of individual units have produced their own prediction equations (28–30) as a result of measurements made in lean and obese individuals. In one of these (28), obese individuals accounted for almost one-half the subjects (Table 5).

TABLE 5. *Subjects and parameters used to establish various standards of basal metabolic rate*

Standard (year) (ref.)	Number			Age (years)		Details of subjects	Parameters needed to predict BMR
	Total	Male	Female	Male	Female		
Aub and Dubois (1917) (10)	?	?	?	14–80	14–80	U.S. subjects. Details not given except for a small subgroup of elderly subjects $n = 6$ aged 77–83 y with a BMI 19.9–25.7 kg/m^2	Age, sex, surface area (reference table)
Harris and Benedict (1919) (5)	239	136	103	16–63	15–73	U.S. subjects. Individual details. Very few overweight individuals.	Age, sex, weight, height (prediction equations)
Boothby et al. (1936) (4)	1,467	639	828	6–64	6–68	U.S. subjects attending Mayo Clinic. No disease or minor abnormalities. No details of weight/height.	Age, sex, surface area (reference table)
Quenouille et al. (1951) (27)[a]	>8,600	?	?	3–>80	3–>80	Various populations (U.S. N. European, Italian, Indian, Chinese, Japanese, and others. No details of weight/height distribution.	Sex, weight, height, surface area (plus correction for age, temperature, and humidity[a]
Fleish (1951) (11)	>10,000	>2,500	>7,000	1–75	1–75	Mainly U.S. subjects compiled from the results of 24 separate studies, including the first 3 on this table. No details of weight/height.	Age, sex, surface area (reference table)

Reference						Variables required
Robertson and Reid (1952) (3)	2,310	987	3–75	3–74	British subjects described as "normal." No details of weight/height.	Age, sex, surface area (reference table)
Schofield (1985) (6)	7,173	4,809	0–>60	0–>60	Various populations (U.S., European, Indian, Japanese, Chinese, Australian, etc.). Underweight individuals included. See text.	Age, sex, weight, height (prediction equations)
Owen et al.[b] (1986, 1987) (29, 30)	104	60	18–82	18–65	U.S. subjects lean and obese. 27% of men and 36% of women have a BMI > 30 kg/m².	Weight (prediction equations)[b]
Mifflin et al.[b] (1990) (28)	498	251	19–78	20–76	U.S. subjects biased toward working class. 49% men and 45% women are obese (>120% ideal body weight). 16% men and 21% women are grossly obese (>140% ideal body weight)	Age, weight, height, (prediction equation)[b]

[a] Separate equations are provided for different racial groups.
[b] These authors also provide equations to predict metabolic rate from fat-free mass (see Table 8).

TABLE 6. *Prediction of BMR in 25-year-old women using*

BMI kg/m²	Height m	Weight kg	Surface area[a] m²	1 Boothby et al. (4)	2 Harris, Benedict (5)	3 Fleish (11)	4 Schofield (6)[b]
15.0	1.75	45.938	1.5452	1,335[e,f]	1,301	1,305	1,219
22.5	1.75	68.906	1.8358	1,586[e,f]	1,521	1,551	1,532
30.0	1.75	91.875	2.0746	1,792	1,741	1,753	1,845[f]
37.5	1.75	114.844	2.2809	1,971	1,960	1,927	2,158[f]
45.0	1.75	137.813	2.4647	2,130	2,180	2,082	2,471[f]
15.0	1.55	36.038	1.2764	1,103	1,170[f]	1,078	1,028[f]
22.5	1.55	54.056	1.5164	1,310	1,341[f]	1,281	1,273
30.0	1.55	72.075	1.7136	1,481	1,513	1,448	1,519[f]
37.5	1.55	90.094	1.8841	1,628	1,687	1,592	1,764[f]
45.0	1.55	108.113	2.0359	1,759	1,859	1,720	2,010[f]

[a] Surface area calculated by the Dubois formula (see Table 1).
[b] Calculated using the equations based on weight and height (see Table A6 in Appendix).
[c] Calculated assuming 75% relative humidity and 70°F, and equation for U.S. and Northern European subjects (see Table A7 in Appendix).

AGREEMENT OR DISAGREEMENT BETWEEN REFERENCE STANDARDS?

As more standards became available, an increasing number of discrepancies were noted. The Fleish standards (11) generally give lower values for the predicted metabolic rate of teenagers and adults than those of Boothby et al. (4) (for 10–30 year old males, 8–9% lower; and for females in the same age range, 2–8% lower). They are also lower than the Aub-Dubois standards (7–14% for subjects aged 15–80 years) but very slightly higher than the Robertson-Reid standards for adults. However, the pattern is not uniform, because the Fleish standards are 5% to 12% lower than the Robertson-Reid standards for children younger than 10.

A comparative assessment of all these methods was undertaken (M. Elia, unpublished data) including the use of recently published predictive equations (28–30) and older ones that are infrequently used today [e.g., 3,10, and 27 and those based on weight$^{0.73}$ such as BMR (kcal/day) = 70.5 weight (kg)$^{0.73}$—ref. 53]. Here only one or two examples from this analysis will be used to highlight some discrepancies.

Table 6 illustrates the extent to which estimates of metabolic rate obtained by ten different methods vary from one another when applied to 25-year-old females with a variety of body mass indices. Although there is considerable agreement between some of the predictions, substantial differences also exist (13–47%). These differences occur even in individuals with a body mass index between 22.5 kg/m² and 30.0 kg/m² (those with an ideal to mildly obese weight). If comparisons are restricted to the more widely used prediction methods (columns 1–4 in Table 6) and to those resulting from the two recent studies (columns 5 and 6), the discrepancy is only

different formulas and reference tables (see Appendix)

5 Mifflin et al. (28)[b]	6 Owen et al. (29)	7 Robertson, Reid (3)	8 Aub, Dubois (10)	9 Quenouille et al. (27)[c]	10 Brody et al. (53)	% variation[d] Columns 1–10[e]	% variation[d] Columns 1–6[f]
1,267	1,125[e,f]	1,261	1,372	1,270	1,152	19	19
1,497	1,290[e,f]	1,498	1,630	1,480	1,549	23	23
1,727	1,455[e,f]	1,693	1,842	1,685	1,911[e]	31	27
1,956	1,620[e,f]	1,861	2,025	1,887	2,249[e]	39	33
2,186	1,784[e,f]	2,011	2,189	2,087	2,570[e]	44	39
1,043	1,054	1,042	1,133[e]	1,112	965[e]	21	14
1,223	1,183[e,f]	1,237	1,347[e]	1,278	1,298	14	13
1,404	1,312[e,f]	1,398	1,522	1,440	1,601[e]	22	16
1,584	1,442[e,f]	1,537	1,673	1,600	1,884[e]	31	22
1,764	1,571[e,f]	1,661	1,808	1,757	2,152[e]	37	28

[d] The % variation is calculated with the highest value as the numerator and the lowest value as the denominator.

[e,f] These indicate the highest and lowest values along a horizontal row ([e] columns 1–10; [f] columns 1–6).

slightly reduced (13–39%). Even if only the results of columns 1 through 4 are compared, substantial discrepancies remain. For an obese individual (height 1.75 m, body mass index 45 kg/m^2), the Schofield standards (column 4) predict a BMR that is 16% higher than that of Boothby et al. (column 1). In contrast, for an abnormally thin individual (1.75 m, body mass index 15 kg/m^2), the standards of Boothby et al. predict a BMR that is 10% higher than the Schofield standards. The trends are better appreciated graphically (Fig. 3).

The differences among the first four prediction methods shown in Table 6—Schofield (6), Boothby et al. (4), Harris-Benedict (5), and Fleish (11)—tend to be smaller when they are applied to a spectrum of individuals with a more normal body mass index (e.g., 20–30 kg/m^2). However, substantial differences may still be found. For example, for a 25-year-old man with a height of 1.65 m and BMI 30 kg/m^2, the Schofield standards predict a metabolic rate that is 13% higher than that calculated by the Fleish standards (1,919 versus 1,702 kcal/day). For a 45-year-old woman with a height of 1.75 and BMI 22.5 kg/m^2, the Boothby standards predict a metabolic rate that is 11% higher than that predicted by the Schofield standards (1,555 versus 1,406 kcal/day).

Similar if not larger differences occur with children, even if the potential problems associated with the use of different formulas to calculate surface area are ignored (see Table 7 and Fig. 4). Although some of the authors of the childhood standards were clearly aware of the effects of undernutrition and overnutrition on metabolic rates (e.g., ref. 54), substantial discrepancies between their reference values and those of others are still found for children with a normal weight and height (Table 7, Fig. 4).

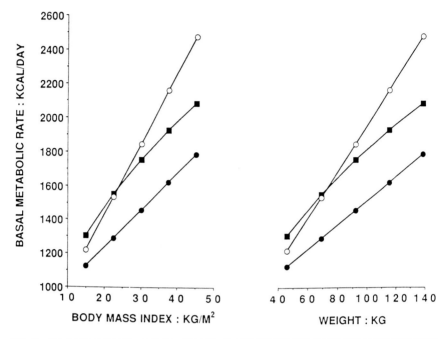

FIG. 3. Prediction of basal metabolic rate in 25-year-old females 1.75 m with different body weights and body mass indices, using three different methods: (O——O, Schofield (6); ■——■, Fleish (11); ●——●, Owen et al. (29). For details see text and Table 6.

The various standards also imply different effects of age on metabolic rate (Table 8). Between the ages of 25 and 65, the Harris-Benedict equations predict a 15% to 21% decrease in BMR for men with the same weight and height (11–16% for females), whereas the equations of Owen et al. (29,30) predict no effect of age (the correlation between age and metabolic rate in this series was very low, so age was excluded from the prediction equations). It should be noted that the authors of several of the reference standards expressed uncertainties about the effects of age on metabolic rate because of the small number of elderly subjects studied. For example, Harris and Benedict (5) cautioned that the effects of age suggested by their equations should be regarded only as tentative. Similar cautions were made about the Schofield standards (6).

As a drawback of using the available standards of metabolic rate to predict the effect of age, all the results were obtained cross-sectionally. In contrast, Keys et al. (57) performed a longitudinal study involving a large number of individuals whose body composition was assessed by densitometry and concluded that aging has only a small effect on metabolic rate (1–2%/decade) (see the section on metabolic rate/kg fat-free mass).

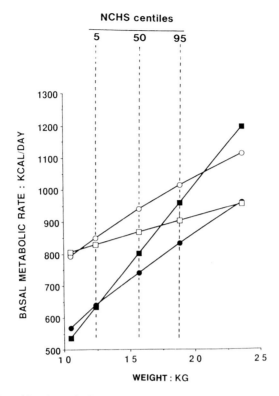

FIG. 4. Prediction of basal metabolic rate in a 3.5-year-old male child 1.0 m with different body weights (corresponding to <5, 5th, 50th, 95th, and >95th percentiles, weight for height, of the NCHS standards) using four different methods: ○———○, Robertson and Reid (3); □———□, Quenouille et al. (27); ■———■, Sherman (55); ●———●, Talbot (54).

POSSIBLE REASONS FOR DISCREPANCIES BETWEEN METABOLIC RATE STANDARDS

The discrepancies between the methods used to predict metabolic rate are almost certainly due to a combination of both biologic and methodologic differences.

Methodologic Differences

It is difficult or impossible to assess retrospectively whether metabolic rate machines used by different workers were adequate with respect to calibration procedures and performance, particularly because no such details are given in some of the papers. Nevertheless, some differences in methodology can be appreciated by considering the selection of data used to establish the Mayo Clinic standards (4) and those used to establish the Robertson-Reid standards (3).

none of the women), measurements were obtained during ten or more test periods. Unfortunately, no information is given about changes in metabolic rate during different periods on the same day or changes on different days.

The reference equations of BMR formulated by Owen et al. (29,30) were derived from individuals that were apparently "familiar with indirect calorimetry." In other studies, particularly those involving analysis of data obtained by a variety of different sources (6,11), the subjects were almost certainly variably accustomed to indirect calorimetry techniques and the surroundings. Sometimes first measurements were used, and at other times, a combination of several measurements. Schofield (6) reported that the metabolic rate of a single-measurement group was not lower than the mean of a series-of-measurements groups, although these comparisons were made cross-sectionally. Others have found only small sequential changes (14).

There are also other differences between the methods used to establish the various standards.

1. The equipment used by various workers differed. In some cases a mouthpiece, noseclip, or an air-sealed face mask was used (29,30). It is uncertain whether the use of this type of equipment in certain sensitive subjects causes some psychological or physical discomfort and produces significantly different results from systems involving free ventilation (ventilated hood in ref. 28; whole body calorimeters in ref. 5). Douglas bags have been used in some studies (e.g., some are incorporated in the Schofield standards, ref. 6), but the interval between sample collection and analysis, which is associated with diffusion of O_2 and CO_2 through the bag, is not always specified.

2. Different environmental temperatures have been used. In the study of Robertson and Reid (3), the ambient temperature was reported to be 20°C; in the study of Owen et al. (29,30), it was 22°C to 24°C. In individual studies incorporated into the Schofield standards (6), it ranged from 16°C to 20°C ($n = 46$—ref. 59), 15°C (winter) to 29°C (summer) ($n = 7$—ref. 60), and 18°C to 28°C depending on the season in India ($n = 891$—ref. 61). Frequently ambient temperature is not reported (nor the type of clothing worn during the test). It is possible that such variations could contribute to small differences in results.

3. The body weight used in the calculations included street clothes in some studies (e.g., 28), whereas in others it did not. In the Robertson-Reid study, nude weight was estimated by allowing 1.4 kg for the clothes worn by men and 1.14 kg for the clothes worn by women. In small individuals these weights are equivalent to about 3% body weight, that is, 3% difference in metabolic rate/kg body weight.

4. Differences in statistical analysis existed (see ref. 6).

5. The equations used to calculate energy expenditure from gaseous exchange is often not stated. Differences in the results obtained by different equations are often small (<2%), but an extensive and critical review by Elia and Livesey (62) suggests that errors in excess of 5% may occur through the use of incorrect equations that are based as erroneous assumptions.

Biologic Differences

Although several studies do not report the physical characteristics of their subjects, there is sufficient information from others to suggest major differences in the populations used to establish the standards.

Body Build

An analysis (M. Elia and A. Kurpad, unpublished data) of the individual data tabulated by Harris and Benedict (5) suggests that only 9% of men and 17% women had a body mass index (BMI) greater than 25 kg/m^2 and that <1% men and <5% women had BMI greater than 30 kg/m^2. In contrast, in the studies of Owen et al. (29,30), 60% of men (56% of the nonathletic women) had a BMI greater than 25 kg/m^2, and 27% (44% nonathletic women) had a BMI greater than 30 kg/m^2. Several of the subjects were grossly obese. Similarly, almost one-half of the individuals studied by Mifflin et al. (28) were considered to be obese (>120% of ideal body weight—Metropolitan Life Insurance tables); 15.9% of males and 20.6% of females were >140% of ideal body weight).

In the Schofield standards (6) no formal information about the distribution of the BMI is given. However, a graph in the report suggests that about one-third of the subjects aged 18 to 30 had a BMI <20 kg/m^2. A substantial number had a BMI below 17 kg/m^2, which suggests the probable presence of chronic protein-energy malnutrition. The number of subjects with grade II or III obesity (BMI > 30 kg/m^2) would appear to be extremely small in this group of subjects.

It is clear that the proportion of underweight and overweight individuals used in various studies differed substantially, and this could contribute significantly to the different predictions obtained by various equations (see also ref. 58).

Race

Most standards of BMR have been derived from studies undertaken in Caucasians. However, the Schofield standards included measurements made on individuals belonging to a variety of races. Of the 114 studies used in deriving these standards, 29 (25%) were from India alone. Others were from Japan, Philippines, China, Singapore, Bangladesh, Burma, Brazil, Chile, etc., but the majority (38%) were from the United States.

Several workers have pointed out that race has an important effect on metabolic rate and that many non-Caucasians have a lower metabolic rate than Caucasians of the same weight and height. Henri and Rees (63) provided data to support this general conclusion (see Table 9 for comparison with Schofield predictions). Quenouille et al. (27) also recognized the importance of race in their analysis of individual and group data and therefore produced separate sets of equations for Asians, Italians, and those from the United States or Northern Europe. In contrast, the general equa-

TABLE 9. *The percentage by which Schofield equations overestimate (+) or underestimate (−) basal metabolic rate in different ethnic groups by sex (18–60)*

Ethnicity	Male		Female	
	Mean %	Sample size	Mean %	Sample size
Philippino	+9.6	82	+0.3	16
Indian	+12.7	48	+12.9	7
Japanese	+8.3	123	+7.9	71
Brazilian	+8.1	122	—	—
Chinese	+8.2	232	+3.4	156
Malay	+9.3	62	—	—
Javanese	+5.1	82	—	—
Mayan	+0.0	68	—	—
Chippewa Indian	−18.5	5	−18.5	5

Reproduced from ref. 63.

tions provided by Schofield (6) do not distinguish between races. It is noteworthy, however, that the Schofield analysis also found that the metabolic rate of Indians is about 10% to 11% lower than that of other groups. Indeed, Indian subjects aged 18 to 30 were reported to have a metabolic rate 14% lower than subjects from the United States and Northern Europe. The reason for the effect of race on metabolic rate is unknown, although it could theoretically be due to differences in body composition, diet, environmental temperature, hormonal differences, and so on.

IMPLICATIONS OF THE DIFFERENT REFERENCE STANDARDS FOR METABOLIC RATE

From the preceding discussion it appears that single age-specific prediction equations for metabolic rate based on weight, height, or surface area cannot be applied universally with a high degree of accuracy. Important discrepancies occur between races and between predictions made by various methods for specific individuals. Indeed, it is possible for a subject's metabolic rate to be classified as normal in relation to one set of standards and abnormal (hypermetabolic or hypometabolic) in relation to another set of standards. Subsequent physiologic concepts and explanations for the abnormal metabolism may depend on the reference method used for the initial comparison. It is, of course, better to make sequential measurements in the same individual than to compare a single measurement with a reference standard. However, in clinical practice this may not be practical, because normal measurements before injury, surgery, sepsis, or other diseases are often not possible.

There is also concern that some standards are inadequate for certain racial groups. It would appear that the various prediction equations have been used uncritically by many workers in a wide variety of circumstances (in cases of undernutrition, overnutrition, and disease and in different racial groups).

At least some of the differences in the prediction equations may be due to differences in body composition between the populations studied. In recent years attempts have been made to establish methods for predicting metabolic rate on the basis of the mass of lean tissues, which are much more metabolically active than adipose tissue. Because it was hoped that this approach would ultimately lead to equations that are more universally applicable (i.e., overcome the difficulties associated with age, sex, and race) the topic is considered in the following section.

FAT-FREE MASS AND METABOLIC RATE

The lower metabolic rate/kg body weight in women compared to men can be explained by the presence of a greater amount of adipose tissue in women, which has a low O_2 consumption relative to other tissues. Indeed, several workers have reported little or no difference in metabolic rate/kg fat-free mass between the sexes (29,64–67). It has therefore been suggested that it might be more useful to express metabolic rate in relation to fat-free mass than in relation to other parameters such as weight and height or surface area. Although not all workers agree on this point (e.g., 30), a variety of formulas describing the relationship between fat-free mass and the metabolic rate of the whole body have emerged (Table 10).

These generally take one of the following two forms:

$$\text{Metabolic rate} = K_1 + K_2\text{FFM}$$

$$\text{Metabolic rate} = K_1 + K_2\text{FFM} + K_3\text{FM}$$

FFM is fat-free mass, FM is fat mass, and K_1, K_2, and K_3 are constants. Because in most formulas K_1 is positive, the calculated metabolic rate per kg fat-free mass decreases as the subject gets bigger (see Table 10 for various formulas and their predictions). In contrast, a variant of the second type of formula, in which K_1 is zero (74,76,77), implies that for a given degree of adiposity (% body fat), whole-body metabolic rate per kg FFM is independent of the size of FFM (see results in Table 10). However, the majority of equations tabulated in Table 10 suggest that metabolic rate/kg FFM (and metabolic rate per kg body weight) depends on the size of fat-free mass, irrespective of whether they were derived from measurements made on individuals with a large or small range of body mass index.

A general difference between the first and second type of formula concerns the degree of obesity. Fat mass (FM) is not a variable in the first type of formula, so the predicted metabolic rate for lean and obese individuals with the same FFM is identical. This is not the case with the second type of formula, which includes FM as a variable. The conflicting implications of these formulas can be resolved only by experimental observation.

When the formulas indicated in Table 10 are used to predict metabolic rate of individuals with the same fat-free mass, the results are found to vary by more than 25% to 50%. This variation (Table 10) is probably due to the way the results have been collected (i.e., the types of methods used for assessing body composition and energy expenditure) and the type of subject studied (Table 11).

TABLE 10. *Prediction of basal metabolic rate (kcal/day) of the whole body from fat-free mass (FFM) (± fat mass, FM) using different formulas*

Author (ref.)	Formula	Fat-free mass (kg)					
		30	40	50	60	70	80
Mifflin et al. (28)	BMR = 19.7 FFM + 413	1,004	1,201	1,398	1,595	1,792	1,989
Owen et al. (30)	BMR = 22.3 FFM + 290	959	1,182	1,405	1,628	1,851	2,074
Owen et al. (29)	BMR = 19.7 FFM + 334	925	1,122	1,319	1,516	1,713	1,910
Cunningham (68)	[a]BMR = 21.6 FFM + 501.6	1,150	1,366	1,582	1,798	2,014	2,230
McNeil et al. (69)	BMR = 21.5 FFM + 329	974	1,189	1,404	1,619	1,834	2,049
Heymsfield et al. (70)	BMR = 21.6 FFM + 302	950	1,166	1,382	1,598	1,814	2,030
Ravussin, Bogardus (71)	[b]BMR = 21.8 FFM + 392	1,046	1,264	1,482	1,700	1,918	2,136
Ravussin et al. (72)	BMR = 20.82 FFM + 471	1,096	1,304	1,512	1,720	1,928	2,137
Pullicino, Elia (unpublished)	BMR = 21.11 FFM + 450	1,083	1,294	1,506	1,717	1,928	2,139
Jensen et al. (73)	BMR = 20.0 FFM + 622	1,222	1,422	1,622	1,822	2,022	2,222
Garby et al. (74)	BMR = 27.88 FFM + 6.4 FM	919[c]	1,225[c]	1,531[c]	1,837[c]	2,144[c]	2,450[c]
Bernstein et al. (75) (K^+)	[d]BMR = 22.05 FFM + 6.36 FM + 188.6	932[c]	1,180[c]	1,427[c]	1,675[c]	1,923[c]	2,170[c]
Bernstein et al. (75) (H_2O)	[d]BMR = 19.02 FFM + 3.72 FM + 190.2	809[c]	1,015[c]	1,221[c]	1,427[c]	1,633[c]	1,839[c]
Range		809–1,222	1,015–1,422	1,221–1,622	1,427–1,837	1,633–2,144	1,839–2,450
% difference (as % lower value)		51%	40%	33%	29%	31%	33%

[a] The corresponding age-related formula is BMR = 21.0 FFM + 601. 2 − 2.6 age.
[b] The corresponding age-related formula is BMR = 21.9 FFM + 441 − 2.4 age (age effect $p = 0.11$).
[c] These values were calculated assuming 30% of body weight is fat.
[d] These two equations are specifically formulated for individuals aged 30. The original equations are BMR = 22.05 FFM + 6.36 FM − 2.08 age (FFM estimated by total body K), and BMR = 19.02 FFM + 3.72 FM + 236.7 age − 1.55 age (FFM estimated from water dilution) (mainly obese).

42

TABLE 11. *Details of subjects and body composition methods used to establish relationships between fat-free mass and basal metabolic rate (see Table 10 for formulas)*

Author (ref.)	Sex	n	Age (y)	BMI kg/m	Fat-free mass (kg)	Method of body composition analysis	Place of study
Mifflin et al. (28)	M, F	498	44.5 ± 14.1 (19–78)	26.9 ± 4.6 (17–42)	58.5 (35–95)	skinfolds	Nevada
Owen et al. (30)	M	60	38 ± 15.6 (21–82)	28.2 ± 7.5 (20.4–58.7)	66 ± 11 (45.2–97.9)	densitometry	Philadelphia
Owen et al. (29)	F	44	35 ± 12.2 (18–65)	37.8 ± 8.6 (18.2–49.6)	49 ± 8.5 (34.3–74.7)	densitometry	Philadelphia
Cunningham (68)	M, F	223	29 ± 11.6 (15–75)	21.3 ± 3.4 (12.3–34.6)	—	formula based on weight and age alone	Boston
McNeil et al. (69)	M	58	30.6 ± 7.9	19.3 ± 2.1	45.2 ± 5.8	skinfolds	—
Heymsfield et al. (70)	M, F	78			—		USA
Ravussin, Bogardus (71)	M, F	249			33–102	densitometry	Arizona
Ravussin et al. (72)	M, F	30	26 ± 7 (22–44)	28.1 ± 6.7 (18–42.7)	56.8 ± 12.7 (36.3–81.3)	densitometry, skinfolds	Lausanne, Switzerland
Pullicino, Elia (unpublished)	M, F	86	27 ± 8 (18–63)	21.2 ± 2.1 (17–25)	51.4 ± 8.2 (33.9 ± 75.4)	skinfolds	Cambridge, England
Jensen et al. (73)	M, F	42	(19–46)	29.1 (<22->35)	55.5 (<45->61)	total body K, water dilution	Rochester, NY
Garby et al. (74)	F	104	32 ± 10.6 (14–60)	34.7 ± 7.4 (16.7–50)	54	densitometry, water dilution, total body K	Middlesex, England
Bernstein et al. (75)	M, F	185	40 ± 12	37	42.1	total body K	New York
Bernstein et al. (75)	M, F	190	40 ± 12	37	61.4	water dilution	New York

METHODS USED TO ASSESS FAT-FREE MASS

In Cunningham's (68) reanalysis of the Harris-Benedict data (5), fat-free mass was estimated using the equations of Moore et al. (78), which are based on weight and age alone. These estimates can at best be regarded as approximate.

Skinfold thicknesses have been used to estimate fat-free mass in some studies, but difficulties must have occurred with some of the measurements, especially those involving grossly obese individuals (Table 11). There may be systematic differences of up to about 10% between estimates of fat-free mass by various bedside methods. The limits of agreement between these bedside methods and either densitometry or isotope dilution techniques frequently vary by about 15% ($\pm 7\%$) (79–81). Bernstein et al. (75) found over 30% mean difference in the estimate of FFM by total body potassium and water dilution techniques in apparently the same group of obese women. The equations relating metabolic rate to body composition therefore vary depending on the body composition technique used (e.g., see the last two equations in Table 10). Webster and Garrow (82) found about 20% difference between the estimate of FFM obtained by densitometry and total body K but used the mean of these two methods plus a water dilution technique to establish a relationship between FFM and BMR (Garby et al., ref. 74, Table 10). Further differences may arise from observer variability. Although the variation in the estimate of fat-free mass by different observers is often less than $\pm 5\%$, this depends on the method used (83) and probably on the type of subject studied.

In some studies energy expenditure has been related to estimates of fat-free mass obtained by densitometry (Table 11). This procedure assumes that fat-free mass has a constant density, which is not entirely true. The fat-free body consists of a variety of different components (water, protein, minerals, and glycogen—all with different densities), which vary in proportion in different individuals and at different times in the same individuals. Osteoporosis, which occurs in advancing years, particularly in women, and which varies in incidence in various races, also has an effect on the density of the fat-free mass. It is a striking example of the effect of race on the density of fat-free mass that some Negroes have been estimated to have no fat (or even a negative amount of fat) by standard densitometric procedures that assume that the density of fat-free mass is 1.1 g/cc. The error is probably due largely to the high bone mineral content in these Negroes, which produces an unusually high density for the fat-free body (84). There is also some uncertainty about the density of fat-free mass in obese individuals because of the increased water content (present in adipose tissue), which tends to reduce the density of the fat-free body, and because of the increased amount of bone mineral, which tends to increase the density of the fat-free body (85).

The estimate of fat-free mass from measurements of total body water depends on there being a constant relationship between total body water and fat-free mass. This is also not true, because the hydration fraction of the fat-free mass may be affected by age and disorders of hydration. Furthermore, the proportion of intracellular to extracellular water changes with age (86,87).

These theoretical difficulties can be reduced by increasing the number of methods used to assess body composition in the same individual. For example, the difficulties associated with bone mineral content can be largely overcome by making measurements of the amount of bone mineral by techniques such as dual photon absorptiometry, and by using them in conjunction with estimates of body composition obtained by densitometry. Further uncertainties about the variable water content of the body can be reduced by including measurements of total body water.

EFFECT OF AGE ON METABOLIC RATE PER KG FAT-FREE MASS

Uncertainties about the effect of age on metabolic rate are due largely to difficulties associated with estimating body composition. Indeed many of the "standard" body composition techniques have never been validated in the elderly.

Although aging might produce a substantial reduction in energy expenditure and fat-free mass, the longitudinal study of Keys et al. (57) suggested that the change in metabolic rate/kg fat-free mass (measured by densitometry) was only 1–2%/decade. However, if the density of the fat-free mass decreased with age as a result of osteoporosis, the percent decrease in metabolic rate/kg fat-free mass would have been greater. In another study in which cross-sectional measurements of densitometry were made in 249 Pima Indians aged 18 to 41, there was a trend toward a lower metabolic rate/kg FFM (1–2% per decade), but the effect was not significant (see footnote to Table 10). A similar overall effect of age was suggested by Cunningham (68) in the reanalysis of the data provided by Harris and Benedict (5). Fukagawa et al. (88) reported that the metabolic rate in a group of elderly men and women (67–75 years old; $n = 20$) was 10% to 13% lower than the rate in a group of young men (18–33 years old; $n = 24$) even after adjusting for fat-free mass, which was estimated by a water dilution technique. These authors also concluded that the differences in metabolic rate between the young and elderly subjects could probably not be accounted for by differences in the hydration fraction of the fat-free mass or the distribution of water between intracellular and extracellular compartments. Other cross-sectional studies have reported either no difference or a lower BMR/kg FFM in the older subjects (89–94). Some of the variability may be related to the lower BMR/kg FFM in inactive individuals compared to active individuals (93) and the differences of the size of the fat-free mass, which was in some cases smaller in the elderly. (This would be expected to increase BMR/kg FFM; see earlier discussion.) However, in at least one study (93) in which FFM was similar in the young and elderly subjects, BMR/kg FFM was significantly lower in the elderly.

PRACTICAL CONSIDERATIONS FOR USING FAT-FREE MASS TO PREDICT METABOLIC RATE

The errors associated with estimating fat-free mass by different observers using different techniques in a wide variety of circumstances limit the use of fat-free mass as the basis of predicting metabolic rate.

Although the use of a combination of body composition techniques (especially the more sophisticated techniques) in the same individual is important in the development of concepts of energy metabolism (e.g., in assessing the effects of aging, obesity, racial differences, etc.), the techniques are likely to have restricted application. The measurements that are likely to find the most widespread use are the simple ones that can be easily obtained and reproduced in a variety of circumstances. The most important measurements are weight and height and derivatives of weight and height such as the body mass index, which provides a general indication of the degree of obesity. It remains to be proved whether predictions of basal metabolic rate based on estimates of fat-free mass have any significant advantages over those based on weight and height, especially if the latter are used to predict metabolic rate within restricted ranges of body mass index.

Finally, if metabolic rate/kg FFM decreases as FFM gets larger, as suggested by several authors (see preceding discussion and results in Table 10), caution should be used in directly comparing results obtained in large and small individuals. A "correction" may be used that takes into account the magnitude of the constant K_1 (see preceding equation and Table 10). The reason for the probable decline in BMR/kg fat-free mass with increasing size is uncertain, but it may be related to the relative size of different organs and tissues. Variations in organ sizes probably also largely explain the differences in metabolic rates of infants, children, and adults (see chapter by Elia, *Organ and Tissue Contribution to Metabolic Rate*).

CONCLUSIONS

The search for universal reference standards or equations for predicting basal metabolic rate has proved to be difficult. Discrepancies between various standards can be explained by differences in methodologic procedures and conditions of testing and by biologic differences (e.g., race, malnutrition/overnutrition, and disease). There may have also been secular changes. Most of the standards used today are based on measurements made in the early part of this century. Since then puberty has occurred earlier, and the height and weight of many populations has tended to increase. This raises questions about the composition of this weight gain and whether this influences the prediction of basal metabolic rate.

If elective procedures or interventions (e.g., nutritional, drug, or hormonal interventions) are carried out it would be sensible to undertake sequential measurements of resting energy expenditure in the same individuals so that preintervention measurements can be directly compared with postintervention measurements. This overcomes the difficulty of individual variation. If this is not possible, as is often the case in clinical practice, the use of reference standards based on the local population (established using the same equipment and techniques as in the study), are preferable to the use of traditional standards. This is particularly important for certain racial groups.

If local standards are not available, then one or more of the traditional standards may be used (see Appendix), although it should be remembered that several of these may be inadequate for patients with disease or malnutrition and in the elderly who accounted for only a small proportion of the original population samples.

Prediction of BMR from estimates of body composition is theoretically attractive, but this is limited by interobserver error and by errors arising from the use of body composition techniques that depend on different assumptions.

If basal metabolic rate is to be predicted from body composition, the measurements should ideally involve the same observers and the same techniques as those used to establish the prediction equations. If different observers or multiple observers are used to assess body composition, the choice of method should take into account not only the accuracy of the technique but also the interobserver variability.

The combined use of different body composition methods in the same individuals (water dilution, densitometry, dual photon absorptiometry, neutron activation) and scanning procedures for assessing individual organs/tissues offers new and exciting possibilities for future research. For example, such an undertaking can help assess whether "adaptations," or changes in energy expenditures with age, malnutrition, and disease, are due to variations in the size of specific organs/tissues or to changes in the metabolic activity of these tissues (see chapter by Elia, *Organ and Tissue Contribution to Metabolic Rate*). There have also been recent and exciting developments for assessing the activity of specific metabolic processes and their contribution to energy expenditure (see chapter by Elia, *Organ and Tissue Contribution to Metabolic Rate*). As a consequence energy expenditure, which in the past has largely been considered in humans as a whole, is now also increasingly being considered in relation to the size and activity of individual tissues and the metabolic processes within tissues that are responsible for heat production.

This appendix provides reference tables and equations used to calculate basal metabolic rate. Results are presented in kcal/day and/or MJ/day.

To convert kcal/day to MJ/day, multiply by 0.004184.
To convert kcal/day to kcal/min, divide by 1,440.
To convert MJ/day to kJ/min, divide by 1.44.

TABLE A1. Standards of basal metabolic rate in infants, children, and adults in relation to surface area^a (kcal/m^2/day)

Age (y)	Males						Females					
	Sherman (13)	Fleish (11)	Robertson, Reid^b (3)	Boothby et al.^{b} (4)	Dubois (56)^c	Aub, Dubois (10)	Sherman (13)	Fleish (11)	Robertson, Reid^b (3)	Boothby et al.^{b} (4)	Dubois (56)^c	Aub, Dubois (10)
Premature infants	600	—	—	—	—	—	600	—	—	—	—	—
0–0.038 (birth–2 weeks)	612–701	—	—	—	—	—	612–701	—	—	—	—	—
0.25	929	—	—	—	—	—	869	—	—	—	—	—
0.5	1,039	—	—	—	—	—	989	—	—	—	—	—
0.75	1,118	—	—	—	—	—	1,099	—	—	—	—	—
1.0	1,140	1,272	—	—	—	—	1,109	1,272	—	—	—	—
1.25	1,154	—	—	—	—	—	1,114	—	—	—	—	—
1.5	1,159	—	—	—	—	—	1,099	—	—	—	—	—
1.75	1,152	—	—	—	—	—	1,097	—	—	—	—	—
2	1,150	1,258	1,442	—	1,442	—	1,090	1,258	1,308	—	1,308	—
3	1,130	1,231	1,390	—	1,390	—	1,039	1,229	1,294	—	1,294	—
4	1,099	1,207	1,351	—	1,351	—	1,020	1,195	1,272	—	1,272	—
5	1,068	1,183	1,301	—	1,296	—	998	1,162	1,243	—	1,228	—
6	1,049	1,159	1,250	1,272	1,255	—	989	1,128	1,205	1,212	1,193	—
7	1,030	1,135	1,202	1,258	1,219	—	970	1,090	1,162	1,164	1,152	—
8	1,010	1,111	1,162	1,236	1,188	—	960	1,046	1,114	1,121	1,109	—
9	998	1,085	1,118	1,198	1,145	—	948	1,027	1,063	1,106	1,078	—
10	979	1,056	1,082	1,152	1,116	—	890	1,020	1,018	1,097	1,058	—
11	934	1,032	1,051	1,132	1,087	—	900–993	1,008	974	1,032	1,008	—
12	924–1,236	1,020	1,024	1,123	1,068	—	917–1,018	991	938	1,054	972	—
13	924–1,063	1,015	1,003	1,116	1,051	—	898–984	967	907	1,020	941	—
14	895–1,063	1,010	984	1,114	1,049	←1,104^d→	878–979	941	883	986	919	—
15	1,087	1,003	967	1,106	1,030		744–830	910	864	953	905	←1032→
16	1,072	994	953	1,092	1,006	◄1032►	744–775	886	847	926	869	
17	1,049	979	941	1,066	972		775	871	838	902	857	◄960►
18	1,030	960	931	1,030	962	◄984	772	862	828	888	850	
19	—	941		1,013			—	852		878		912→

48

Row	(1)	(2)	(3)	(4)	(5)	(6)	(7)	(8)	(9)	(10)	(11)	(12)
20	←888→	847	871	823	847	—	←948→	955	998	922	926	—
21		845	869	818		—		946	989	914		—
22		845	866	816		—		941	982	907		—
23		845	866	816		—		936	977	902		—
24		842	864	814		—		929	972	895		—
25	888	842	864	816	845	—	948	922	967	890	900	—
26		840	862	816		—		916	962	888		—
27		840	862	816		—		912	960	883		—
28		840	862	816		—		907	958	878		—
29		840	859	819		—		905	953	876		—
30		840	859	818	842	—		902	950	874	883	—
31		840	859	816		—		898	948	871		—
32		838	857	814		—		893	943	869		—
33		838	857	811		—		890	941	866		—
34		838	857	809		—		888	938	864		—
35	876	853	854	804	840	—	948	886	934	861	876	—
36		833	854	799		—		883	931	859		—
37		830	854	794		—		881	929	857		—
38		828	854	790		—		881	924	857		—
39		826	852	787		—		878	922	854		—
40		823	852	782	838	—		876	919	852	871	—
41			852	←780		—			917	←828		—
42			850			—			912			—
43			850			—			910			—
44			847			—			905			—
45	864	814	842	780	828	—	924	871	902	818	869	—
46			838			—			900			—
47			833			—			898			—
48			830	773		—			893	818		—
49			826			—			890			—
50		802	821	773	814	—		864	888	811	859	—
51			816			—			883			—
52			811	766		—			881	811		—
53			806			—			878			—
54			802			—			876			—
55	840	790		766→	799	—	900	850	871	811→	845	—

(continued)

TABLE A1. Standards of basal metabolic rate in infants, children, and adults in relation to surface area[a] (kcal/m²/day) (continued)

	Males						Female					
Age (y)	Sherman (13)	Fleish (11)	Robertson, Reid[b] (3)	Boothby et al.[b] (4)	Dubois (56)[c]	Aub, Dubois (10)	Sherman (13)	Fleish (11)	Robertson, Reid[b] (3)	Boothby et al.[b] (4)	Dubois (56)[c]	Aub, Dubois (10)
56	—	—		869	—		—	—		799	—	
57	—	—	802	866	—		—	—	758	797	—	
58	—	—		864	—		—	—		794	—	
59	—	—		859	—		—	—		790	—	
60	—	838	794	857	835		—	785	751	787	778	
61	—	—		854	—		—	—		787	—	
62	—	—		852	—		—	—		785	—	
63	—	—		850	—		—	—		782	—	
64	—	—		847	—	876	—	—		780	—	816
65	—	826	785	842[d]	816		—	773	744	778	763	
66	—	—		840[d]	—		—	—		775	—	
67	—	—		838[d]	—		—	—		775	—	
68	—	—		835[d]	—		—	—		773	—	
69	—	—		833[d]	—		—	—		773	—	
70	—	811	778	828[d]	794		—	761	737	770[d]	751	
71	—	—		826[d]	—		—	—		770[d]	—	
72	—	—		818[d]	—		—	—		770[d]	—	
73	—	—		814[d]	—		—	—		768[d]	—	
74	—	—		809[d]	—	852	—	—		768[d]	—	792
75	—	797	768	802[d]	763		—	751	—		746	
76	—	—		—			—	—	—	—	—	
77	—	—		—			—	—	—	—	—	
78	—	—		—			—	—	—	—	—	
79	—	792		—			—	—	—	—	—	
80	—	792		—			—	742	—	—	—	

[a] The values in kcal/day are calculated to the nearest kcal from the original tables, which tabulated the results in kcal/hour. Surface area is calculated using the formula of Dubois and Dubois (18) (see Table 1).
[b] These authors also give values for the standard error of the estimate (not shown).
[c] The standards of Dubois (56) are based on three sets of data: Boothby et al. (4); Robertson and Reid (3); and Harris and Benedict (5).
[d] Extrapolated values.

50

TABLE A2. *Standards of basal metabolic rate (BMR) in children*

BMR kcal/24 hours

Weight (kg)	Boys Benedict, Talbot[a] (14)	Talbot (54)	Girls Benedict, Talbot[a] (14)	Talbot (54)
3	150	150	150	136
4	210	210	220	205
5	270	270	285	274
6	330	330	350	336
7	390	390	405	395
8	445	445	460	448
9	495	495	500	496
10	545	545	540	541
11	590	590	580	582
12	625	625	610	620
13	660	665	640	655
14	695	700	665	687
15	725	725	690	718
16	755	750	710	747
17	780	780	735	775
18	805	810	760	802
19	830	840	780	827
20	860	870	805	852
21	885	—	830	—
22	910	910	855	898
23	940	—	880	—
24	965	980	900	942
25	990	—	930	—
26	1020	1070	950	984
27	1045	—	975	—
28	1070	1100	1000	1025
29	1090	—	1020	—
30	1115	1140	1045	1063
31	1140	—	1070	—
32	1160	1190	1090	1101
33	1180	—	—	—
34	1200	1230	—	1137
35	1220	—	—	—
36	1240	1270	—	1173
37	1255	—	—	—
38	1275	1305	—	1207
40	—	1340	—	1241
42	—	1370	—	1274
44	—	1400	—	1306
46	—	1430	—	1388
48	—	1460	—	1369
50	—	1485	—	1399
52	—	1505	—	1429
54	—	1555	—	1458
56	—	1580	—	1487
58	—	1600	—	1516

(*continued*)

TABLE A2. *Standards of basal metabolic rate (BMR) in children (continued)*

BMR kcal/24 hours

Weight (kg)	Boys Benedict, Talbot[a] (14)	Boys Talbot (54)	Girls Benedict, Talbot[a] (14)	Girls Talbot (54)
60	—	1630	—	1544
62	—	1660	—	1572
64	—	1690	—	1599
66	—	1725	—	1626
68	—	1765	—	1653
70	—	1785	—	1679
72	—	1815	—	1705
74	—	1845	—	1731
76	—	1870	—	1756
78	—	1900	—	1781
80	—	—	—	1805
82	—	—	—	1830
84	—	2000	—	1855

[a] The original table of Benedict and Talbot (14) tabulates values for ½ kg increment.

TABLE A3. *Basal metabolic rate in children—Johnson (95) based on Sargent (58)[a]*

Age 1 week–10 months[b] Weight (kg)	Boys and girls (kcal/24h)	Age 11–38 months[b] Weight (kg)	Boys (kcal/24h)	Girls (kcal/24h)	Age 3–16 years Weight (kg)	Boys (kcal/24h)	Girls (kcal/24h)
3.5	202	9.0	528	509	15	859	799
4.0	228	9.5	547	528	20	953	898
4.5	252	10.0	566	547	25	1046	996
5.0	278	10.5	586	566	30	1140	1092
5.5	305	11.0	605	586	35	1231	1190
6.0	331	11.5	624	605	40	1325	1289
6.5	358	12.0	643	624	45	1418	1387
7.0	384	12.5	662	646	50	1512	1486
7.5	410	13.0	682	665	55	1606	1584
8.0	437	13.5	701	684	60	1699	1680
8.5	463	14.0	720	703	65	1793	1776
9.0	490	14.5	739	722	70	1886	1874
9.5	514	15.0	758	742	75	1980	1973
10.0	540	15.5	778	761			
10.5	566	16.0	797	782			
11.0	593	16.5	816	802			

[a] The results (kcal/24h) are calculated to the nearest kcal using the original values, which were expressed in kcal/hour. All data are for normal weight-for-height subjects—defined as within ±10% of average weight. Average weight is derived from the following equations: under 11 months, wt = $0.323e^{0.047\,ht}$; over 11 months, weight = $2.6e^{0.018\,ht}$ (e = 2.718, the basis of natural logarithm; height is in cm; and weight in kg). For infants (1 week–10 months) in slender classification, 80–90% of weight for age, add 24 kcal/day (95). BMR prediction for <80% and for obese children >140% is less certain (58).
[b] The values for infants less than 38 months old are derived from measurements made during sleep and include diet-induced thermogenesis.

TABLE A4. *Basal metabolic rate in children (55)[a]*

	kcal/kg/24 hours	
Age	Boys	Girls
1	55.92	55.92
2	54.96	54.96
3	51.12	48.00
4	47.04	43.92
5	45.12	42.00
6	42.96	40.08
7	41.04	39.12
8	40.08	37.92
9	37.92	36.96
10	36.96	36.00
11	35.04	34.08
12	34.08	31.92
13	40.08	30.96
14	41.04	36.96
15	36.00	31.92
16	33.12	30.00
17	30.00	28.08
18	30.00	25.92

[a] The results (kcal/kg/24h) are calculated from the original results, which are expressed in kcal/kg/h.

TABLE A5. *Equations for estimating metabolic rate from weight (W) in males (M) and females (F)[a]*

		kcal/day	MJ/day	n	SEE: kcal(MJ)
Schofield (6)					
<3 y	M	BMR = 59.512W − 30.4	BMR = 0.249W − 0.127	162	69.9 (0.2925)
	F	BMR = 58.317W − 31.1	BMR = 0.244W − 0.130	137	58.7 (0.2456)
3–10 y	M	BMR = 22.706W + 504.3	BMR = 0.095W + 2.110	338	67.0 (0.2803)
	F	BMR = 20.315W + 485.9	BMR = 0.085W + 2.033	413	69.9 (0.2924)
10–18 y	M	BMR = 17.686W + 658.2	BMR = 0.074W + 2.754	734	105.3 (0.4406)
	F	BMR = 13.384W + 692.6	BMR = 0.056W + 2.898	575	111.4 (0.4661)
18–30 y	M	BMR = 15.057W + 692.2	BMR = 0.063W + 2.896	2879	153.1 (0.6407)
	F	BMR = 14.818W + 486.6	BMR = 0.062W + 2.036	829	118.7 (0.4967)
30–60 y	M	BMR = 11.472W + 873.1	BMR = 0.048W + 3.653	646	167.2 (0.6997)
	F	BMR = 8.126W + 845.6	BMR = 0.034W + 3.538	372	111.2 (0.4653)
>65 y	M	BMR = 11.711W + 587.7	BMR = 0.049W + 2.459	50	164.1 (0.6865)
	F	BMR = 9.082W + 658.5	BMR = 0.038W + 2.755	38	107.8 (0.4511)
Owen et al. (29, 31)					
Adults	M	BMR = 10.2W + 879	BMR = 0.0427W + 3.678	60	—
	F	BMR = 7.18W + 795	BMR = 0.0300W + 3.326	36	—
Mifflin et al. (28)					
Adults	M	BMR = 12.3W + 704	BMR = 0.0515W + 2.946	251	—
	F	BMR = 10.9W + 568	BMR = 0.0461W + 2.377	248	—
Brody et al. (20)[b]		BMR = 70.5W^{0.734}	BMR = 0.295W^{0.734}	—	—
Johnson (95)[c]					
1 week–10 mo	M[c]	BMR = 52.32W + 17.688	BMR = 0.2189W + 0.0740		38.4 (0.1607)
	F[c]	BMR = 52.32W + 17.688	BMR = 0.2189W + 0.0740		38.4 (0.1607)
11–38 mo	M	BMR = 38.16W + 185.76	BMR = 0.1597W + 0.7772		52.8 (0.2209)
	F	BMR = 39.12W + 155.52	BMR = 0.1637W + 0.6507		45.6 (0.1908)
3–16 y	M	BMR = 18.672W + 578.64	BMR = 0.0781W + 2.4210		57.6 (0.2410)
	F	BMR = 19.56W + 506.16	BMR = 0.0818W + 2.1177		52.8 (0.2209)

[a] Weight is in kg. Sample size is given as *n* and standard error of the estimate as SEE.
[b] This equation was derived from analysis of data from various species.
[c] These equations form the basis of Table A3. They are applicable to children that are normal weight for height (see legend to Table A3 for further details).

TABLE A6. Equations for estimating basal metabolic rate from weight (W) and height (H) in males (M) and females (F)[a]

	kcal/day	MJ/day	n	SEE: kcal(MJ)
Harris and Benedict (5)				
Adults				
M	$BMR = 13.7516W + 500.33H - 6.775A + 66.473$	$BMR = 0.05754W + 2.0934H - 0.0283A + 0.2781$	136	103.2 (0.4317)[b]
F	$BMR = 9.5634W + 184.96H - 4.6756A + 655.0955$	$BMR = 0.04001W + 0.7739H - 0.0196A + 2.7409$	103	108.0 (0.4519)[b]
Kleiber (12, 96)[c]				
Adults				
M	$BMR = 71.2 \times W^{3/4}[1 + 0.004(30 - A) + 0.010(100H/W^{1/3} - 43.4)]$	$BMR = 0.2979 \times W^{3/4}[1 + 0.004(30 - A) + 0.010(100H/W^{1/3} - 43.4)]$	136	102.0 (0.427)[b]
F	$BMR = 65.8 \times W^{3/4}[1 + 0.004(30 - A) + 0.018(100H/W^{1/3} - 42.1)]$	$BMR = 0.2753 \times W^{3/4}[1 + 0.004(30 - A) + 0.018(100H/W^{1/3} - 42.1)]$	103	110.6 (0.463)[b]
Schofield (6)				
<3 y				
M	$BMR = 0.1673W + 1517.4H - 617.6$	$BMR = 0.0007W + 6.349H - 2.584$	162	58.0 (0.2425)
F	$BMR = 16.252W + 1023.2H - 413.5$	$BMR = 0.068W + 4.281H - 1.730$	137	51.6 (0.2160)
3−10 y				
M	$BMR = 19.598W + 130.3H + 414.9$	$BMR = 0.082W + 0.545H + 1.736$	338	66.8 (0.2795)
F	$BMR = 16.969W + 161.8H + 371.2$	$BMR = 0.071W + 0.677H + 1.553$	413	69.4 (0.2904)
10−18 y				
M	$BMR = 16.252W + 137.2H + 515.5$	$BMR = 0.068W + 0.574H + 2.157$	734	105.0 (0.4394)
F	$BMR = 8.365W + 465.6H + 200.0$	$BMR = 0.035W + 1.948H + 0.837$	575	108.2 (0.4525)
18−30 y				
M	$BMR = 15.057W - 10.04H + 705.8$	$BMR = 0.063W - 0.042H + 2.953$	2879	153.2 (0.6408)
F	$BMR = 13.623W + 283.0H + 98.2$	$BMR = 0.057W + 1.184H + 0.411$	829	117.7 (0.4925)
30−60 y				
M	$BMR = 11.472W - 2.63H + 877.2$	$BMR = 0.048W - 0.011H + 3.670$	646	167.4 (0.7002)
F	$BMR = 8.126W + 1.43H + 843.7$	$BMR = 0.034W + 0.006H + 3.530$	372	111.4 (0.4660)
>60 y				
M	$BMR = 9.082W + 972.3H - 834.4$	$BMR = 0.038W + 4.068H - 3.491$	50	157.7 (0.6600)
F	$BMR = 7.887W + 458.2H + 17.7$	$BMR = 0.033W + 1.917H + 0.074$	38	102.5 (0.4289)
Mifflin et al. (28)				
Adults				
M	$BMR = 10W + 625H - 5A + 5$	$BMR = 0.0418W + 2.615H - 0.0209A + 0.0209$	251	—
F	$BMR = 10W + 625H - 5A - 161$	$BMR = 0.0418W + 2.615H - 0.0209A - 0.6736$	247	—

[a] Weight is shown in kilograms; height is shown in meters; age (A) is shown in years. Sample size is n, and standard error of the estimate is SEE.
[b] Calculated by M. Elia using the data of Harris and Benedict (5) and Kleiber (96).
[c] These equations are based on an analysis of the Harris and Benedict data (5).

TABLE A7. Equations of Quenouille et al. (27) for estimating basal metabolic rate from weight (W), height (H), and surface area (S) in males (M) and females (F)[a]

Quenouille et al., 1951		kcal/day	MJ/day	n
U.S. and N. Europeans	M	BMR = 8.9W + 297.5H + 111.7S + 293.8	BMR = 0.0372W + 1.2447H + 0.4674S + 1.2293	457
	F	BMR = 0.875(8.9W + 297.5H + 111.7S + 293.8) + 29.7	BMR = 0.875(0.0372W + 1.2447H + 0.4674S + 1.2293) + 0.1243	565
Italians	M	BMR = 8.9W + 297.5H + 111.7S + 423.7	BMR = 0.0372W + 1.2447H + 0.4674S + 1.7728	1372
	F	BMR = 0.875(8.9W + 297.5H + 111.7S + 423.7) + 12.5	BMR = 0.875(0.0372W + 1.2447H + 0.4674S + 1.7728) + 0.0523	289
Indians, Chinese, Japanese	M	BMR = 5.02W + 307.5H + 556.6S + 771.6	BMR = 0.0210W − 1.2866H + 2.3288S + 3.2284	332
	F	BMR = 0.875(5.02W − 307.5H + 556.6S + 771.6) − 4.3	BMR = 0.875(0.0210W − 1.2866H + 2.3288S + 3.2284) − 0.0180	329
Residual Mixed Group	M	BMR = 5.02W − 307.5H + 556.6S + 828.2	BMR = 0.0210W − 1.2866H + 2.3288S + 3.4652	413
	F	BMR = 0.875(5.02W − 307.5H + 556.6S + 828.2) − 13.7	BMR = 0.875(0.0210W − 1.2866H + 2.3288S + 3.4652) − 0.0573	115

[a] Weight is in kg, height is in meters, and surface area is in square meters. Sample size (adults) is given as n and refers only to adults >20 years. Quenouille et al. (27) considered the results of ≥8,600 subjects (grouped plus individual data), of which 3,500 were <17 years old. The equations can also be applied to children ≥3 y old, although the predictions for Asian children are not good. Age adjustments are necessary (see Table A8). Further adjustment for temperature and humidity are also required (27). The standard equations shown here refer to 75% humidity and 70°F.

51. Radsma W, Streef GM. On the metabolism during rest and protein consumption in Europeans living in the tropics. *Arch Neerl Phys* 1932;17:97–123.
52. MacCleod G, Crofts EE, Benedict FG. The basal metabolism of some orientals. *Am J Physiol* 1925;73:449–62.
53. Brody S, Proctor RC, Ashworth US. Basal metabolism, endogenous nitrogen, creatinine and neutral sulphur excretions as functions of body weight. *Mo Res Bull* 1934; no. 220.
54. Talbot FB. Basal metabolism standards for children. *Am J Dis Child* 1938;55:455–9.
55. Sherman HC. *Chemistry of food and nutrition*, 8th ed. New York: Macmillan, 1952.
56. Dubois EF. *Basal energy metabolism at various ages: man*. In: Altman PL, Dittmer DS, eds. *Metabolism*. Bethesda, MD: Federation of American Societies for Experimental Biology, 1968;235.
57. Keys A, Taylor HL, Grande F. Basal metabolism and age of adult men. *Metabolism* 1973;22:579–89.
58. Sargent DW. An evaluation of basal metabolic data for children and youths in the United States. Home Economic Report. US Dept Agriculture, Washington, D.C.
59. Hobson FG. A comparative study of basal metabolism in normal men. *Quart J Med* 1923;16:363–89.
60. Thompson EM, Staley MG, Knight MA, Mayfield ME. The effect of high environmental temperature on basal metabolism and serum ascorbic acid concentration in women. *J Nutr* 1959;68:35–47.
61. Banerjee S, Battacharya AK. Basal metabolic rate of boys and young adults of Rajasthan. *Ind J Med Res* 1964;52:1167–72.
62. Elia M, Livesey G. Energy expenditure and fuel selection in biological systems: the theory and practice of calculations based on indirect calorimetry and tracer methods. *Int Rev Nutr and Diet* (in press).
63. Henri CJK, Rees DG. Basal metabolic rate and race. In: Blaxten K, Macdonald I, eds. *Comparative nutrition*. Paris: John Libbey, 1988;149–61.
64. Webb P. Energy expenditure and fat free mass in men and women. *Am J Clin Nutr* 1981;34:1816–26.
65. Grande F, Keys A. Body weight, body composition and calorie status. In: Goodhart RS, Shils ME, eds. *Modern nutrition in health and disease*. Philadelphia: Leo and Febiger, 1980;3–34.
66. Cunningham JJ. Body composition and resting metabolic rate: the myth of feminine metabolism. *Am J Clin Nutr* 1982;36:721–6.
67. Ljuggren H. Sex difference in body composition. In: Brozek J, ed. *Human body composition*. Oxford: Pergamon Press, 1965;129–37.
68. Cunningham JJ. A reanalysis of the factors influencing basal metabolic rate in normal adults. *Am J Clin Nutr* 1980;33:2372–4.
69. McNeill G, Rivers G, Payne GPW, de Britto JJ, Abel R. Basal metabolic rate of Indian men: no evidence of metabolic adaptation to a low plane of nutrition. *Hum Nutr Clin Nutr* 1987;41C:473–84.
70. Heymsfield SB, Hoff RD, Gray TF, Galloway J, Casper K. Heart diseases. In: Kinney JM, Jeejeebhoy KN, Hill GL, Owen OE, eds. *Nutrition and metabolism in patient care*. Philadelphia: WB Saunders, 1988;477–530.
71. Ravussin E, Bogardus C. Relationship of genetics, age and physical fitness to daily energy expenditure. *Am J Clin Nutr* 1989;49:968–75.
72. Ravussin E, Burnand B, Schutz Y, Jéquier E. Twenty four hour energy expenditure and resting metabolic rate in obese, moderately obese and control subjects. *Am J Clin Nutr* 1982;35:566–73.
73. Jensen MD, Braun JS, Vetter RJ, Marsh HM. Measurements of body potassium with a whole body counter: relationship between lean body mass and resting energy expenditure. *Mayo Clin Proc* 1988;63:864–68.
74. Garby L, Garrow JS, Jorgensen B, et al. Relation between energy expenditure and body composition in man: specific energy expenditure in vivo of fat and fat free tissue. *Eur J Clin Nutr* 1988;42:301–5.
75. Bernstein RS, Thornton JC, Young MU, et al. Prediction of resting metabolic rate in obese patients. *Am J Clin Nutr* 1983;37:595–602.
76. Katch VL, Marks CC, Becque MD, Moorehead C, Rocchini A. Basal metabolism of obese adolescents: evidence for energy conservation compared to normal and lean adolescents. *Am J Hum Biol* 1990;2:543–51.
77. Nakamura M, Abe K. *Heat production rates from lean body mass and fat free mass in basal metabolism*. Xth International Congress of Nutrition, Kyoto, Japan. Abstract 1975;1102.
78. Moore FK, Olesen J, McMurray J, Parker V, Ball M, Boyden C. *The body cell mass and its supporting environment*. Philadelphia: W.B. Saunders, 1963;166.

79. Elia M, Parkinson SA, Diaz E. Evaluation of near infrared interactance as a method for predicting body composition. *Eur J Clin Nutr* 1990;44:113–21.
80. Fuller NJ, Elia M. Potential use of bioelectrical impedance of the "whole body" and body segments for the assessment of body composition: comparison with densitometry and anthropometry. *Eur J Clin Nutr* 1989;43:779–91.
81. Pullicino E, Coward WA, Stubbs J, Elia M. Bedside and field methods for assessing body composition: comparison with deuterium dilution. *Eur J Clin Nutr* 1990;44:753–62.
82. Webster JD, Hesp R, Garrow JS. The composition of excess weight in obese women estimated by body density, total body water and total body potassium. *Hum Nutr Clin Nutr* 1984;38C:299–306.
83. Fuller NJ, Cole TJ, Jebb SA, et al. Inter-observer differences in measurement of body composition. *Eur J Clin Nutr* 1991;45:43–9.
84. Schutte JE, Townsend EJ, Hugg J, Shoup RF, Malina RM, Blomquist CG. Density of lean body mass is greater in blacks than whites. *J Appl Physiol* 1984;56:1647–9.
85. Fuller NJ, Elia M. Calculation of body fat in obese by Siri's formula. *Eur J Clin Nutr* 1990;44:165–6.
86. Pierson RN, Wang J, Colt EW, Newmann P. Body composition measurements in normal man: the potassium, sodium, sulphate and tritium spaces in 58 adults. *J Clin Dis* 1982;35:419–28.
87. Bruce A, Andersson M, Arvidsson B, Isaksson B. Body composition. Prediction of normal body potassium, body water and body fat in adults on the basis of body height, body weight and age. *Scand J Clin Lab Inv* 1980;40:461–73.
88. Fukagawa NK, Bandini LG, Young JB. Effect of age on body composition and resting metabolic rate. *Am J Physiol* 1990;259:E233–8.
89. Bloesch D, Schutz Y, Breitenstein E, Jéquier E, Felber JP. Thermogenic response to oral glucose load in man: comparison between young and elderly subjects. *Am J Coll Nutr* 1988;7:471–83.
90. Golay A, Schutz Y, Broquet C, Moeri R, Felber JP, et al. Decreased thermogenic response to an oral glucose load in older subjects. *J Am Geriatr Soc* 1983;31:144–8.
91. Morgan JB, York DA. Thermic effect of feeding in relation to energy balance in elderly men. *Ann Nutr Metab* 1983;27:71–7.
92. Calloway DH, Zanni E. Energy requirements and energy expenditure of elderly men. *Am J Clin Nutr* 1980;33:2088–92.
93. Poehlman ET, Horton ES. Regulation of energy expenditure in aging humans. *Ann Rev Nutr* 1990;10:255–75.
94. Schwartz RS, Jaeger LF, Veith RC. The importance of body composition to the increase in plasma nor-epinephrine appearance rate on elderly men. *J Gerontol* 1987;42:546–51.
95. Johnson HL. Energy metabolism of various weights: man. In: Altman PL, Dittmer DS, eds. *Metabolism.* Bethesda, MD: Federation of American Societies for Experimental Biology, 1968.
96. Kleiber M. Body size and metabolism. *Hilgardia* 1932;6:315–52.

blood flow (6) obtained directly by the xenon clearance technique have been found to be considerably lower than those obtained simultaneously using limb plethysmography. The majority of the resting energy expenditure of the body (~60%) arises from organs such as liver, kidney, heart, and brain, which account for only about 5% to 6% of body weight (Table 1). These tissues have a metabolic rate that is 15–40 times greater than an equivalent weight of muscle (using the more traditional value for the metabolic rate of muscle) and 50–100 times greater than adipose tissue (the variability is smaller when expressed in relation to the protein content of tissues (1). The lungs have not been included in Table 1 because of the lack of adequate data concerned with their oxygen consumption *in vivo*. Holliday et al. (12) estimated that the lungs contribute up to about 20% of the O_2 consumption of the body, which would imply that the five major organs in combination (heart, lung, kidneys, brain, and liver) contribute up to about 80% of the total energy expenditure of the body. However, the estimate of lung metabolic rate should be regarded as tentative, because it appears to have been based on the rate of O_2 consumption of slices of lung *in vitro*. This rate of O_2 consumption is considerably greater than that of lung tissue in a perfusion system (14).

The metabolic rate per gram of each organ appears to change little during growth and development (13). For example, Kennedy and Sokoloff (15) found no change in O_2 consumption/100 g brain/min between children aged 3 to 11 years. The values were also similar (although slightly higher) to those of adults. The higher metabolic rate of infants and children compared to adults (expressed in relation to body weight or fat-free mass or surface area) can therefore be largely explained by the presence of a larger proportion of metabolically active tissues in younger individuals (Table 2). The brain, which accounts for almost one-half of the total energy expenditure of the infant, decreases in proportion to body weight during growth and development so that in the adult it is responsible for only 20% of total energy expenditure. In contrast, skeletal muscle, which is metabolically less active than the brain and other organs, increases in proportion to body weight during growth and development. The contributions of different tissues to body weight and to total energy expenditure in the reference male and female and in a 7.5 kg infant are shown in Table 1.

Table 1 also illustrates that although the reference female has a lower metabolic rate per kg body weight, the discrepancy largely disappears when metabolic rate is expressed in relation to fat-free mass (see table footnote). The lower contribution of muscle to total energy expenditure in females is largely balanced by a greater contribution of other organs.

Using the changing patterns of organ size during growth and development (Table 2), it is possible to construct a figure which readily illustrates the contributions of different organs to total energy expenditure (Fig. 1). Interestingly, if no assumptions are made about organ metabolic rates, it can be shown that BMR per kg organ weights (sum of liver, kidney, brain, and heart) remains remarkably stable during growth and development, in contrast to the changes in metabolic rate per kg body weight or per square meter (Fig. 2).

TABLE 1. Contribution of different organs and tissues to body weight and basal metabolic rate in the reference male, reference female, and a child

	Tissue or organ weight (kg)[a]			Tissue or organ weight (% body weight)			Organ metabolic rate (kcal/kg/day)	Metabolic rate (% total)[b]		
	Reference male	Reference female	Child (0.5 y)	Reference male	Reference female	Child (0.5 y)		Reference male	Reference female	Child (0.5 y)
Liver[c]	1.8	1.4	0.263	2.57	2.41	3.51	200	21	21	14
Brain	1.4	1.2	0.713	2.00	2.07	9.51	240	20	21	44
Heart	0.33	0.24	0.040	0.47	0.41	0.53	440	9	8	4
Kidneys	0.31	0.275	0.053	0.44	0.47	0.71	440	8	9	6
Muscle	28.00	17.00	1.875	40.00	29.31	25.00	13	22	16	6
Adipose tissue	15.00	19.00	1.50	21.43	32.75	20.00	4.5	4	6	2
Miscellaneous tissues by difference (e.g., bone, skin, intestines, glands)	23.16	18.885	3.056	33.09	32.58	40.74	12	16	19	24
Total	70.00	58	7.5	100	100	100		100 (1680 kcal/day)	100 (1340 kcal/day)	100 (390 kcal/day)

[a] Tissue and organ weights for the reference male and reference female were taken from reference 2. Those for the 0.5-year-old child are consistent with results given by various authors (2, 7–9).

[b] The metabolic rates for the reference male (1,680 kcal/day) and reference female (1,340 kcal/day) are close to the mean values obtained by various standards for 30-year-old adults with a body mass index of 22.5 kg/m². The metabolic rate for the 0.5-year-old child (390 kcal/day) is close to the mean value timed by various standards for a male child with a weight of 7.5 kg and height of 0.65 m. If metabolic rate is expressed in relation to body weight, the values are 24.0, 23.3, and 52.0 kcal/day for reference male, reference female, and child, respectively. If metabolic rate is expressed in relation to fat-free mass (56.5 kg for the reference male, 42.0 kg for reference female—see reference man, ref. 2—and 6.1 kg for child) the values are 29.7, 31.9, and 63.9 kcal/kg fat-free mass/day, respectively.

[c] Several workers have estimated that the "liver" is responsible for 25–32% of adult BMR (see 10–13). These values are probably overestimates, since they were usually calculated from the O₂ consumption of liver plus portal drained viscera.

TABLE 2. *Percentage contribution of various organs to the body weight of man*[a]

Age (y)	Brain	Liver	Kidneys	Heart	Brain, Liver, Kidneys, Heart	Muscle
Birth	12.2	4.53	0.82	0.68	18.2	21.3
1–5	8.3	3.45	0.54	0.56	12.9	—
6–10	6.7	3.05	0.54	0.60	10.9	—
11–15	3.7	2.63	0.45	0.51	7.3	36.2
16–20	2.6	2.55	0.46	0.54	6.2	—
21–30	2.2	2.54	0.45	0.54	5.7	45.2
31–40	2.2	2.48	0.46	0.54	5.7	41.8
41–50	2.3	2.56	0.45	0.58	5.9	40.2
51–60	2.4	2.42	0.47	0.56	5.9	—
61–70	2.7	2.14	0.41	0.63	5.9	33.9
>70	2.3	2.03	0.41	0.60	5.3	27.0

[a] Based on Korenchevsky (8). All the measurements were made in subjects who died of accidents, with the exception of the studies concerned with muscle, which included hospitalized patients. The values for muscle agree closely with those reported for normal growth and development by the other workers (2).

Because the organs of the body are so important in determining its metabolic rate, it is pertinent to consider whether variations in their size could explain differences in energy expenditure observed in pathophysiologic circumstances or even differences in energy expenditure between species.

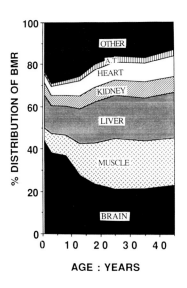

FIG. 1. The contribution of various organs and tissues to body weight and basal metabolic rate of a male during growth and development (0.5–45 years of age). The values for organ (tissue) weights for subjects between 3 and 45 years old are taken from Korenchevsky (1961) (Table 2) and for a 0.5-year-old baby (7.5 kg) from Table 1. Organ (tissue) metabolic rate is calculated from the product of organ (tissue) weight and organ/tissue metabolic rate. The adults were assumed to have a body mass index of 22.5 kg/m^2, height of 1.70 m, and weight of 65 kg. The children (0.5, 3, 8, 13 years old) were assumed to have heights (0.65, 0.97, 1.18, and 1.54 meters, respectively) and weights (7.5, 15, 22, and 45 kg, respectively) close to the 50th percentiles of the NCHS standards and those given by Frisancho (16). The basal metabolic rates for males aged 0.5, 3, 5, 8, 13, 18, 25, 35, and 45 years were taken to be 390, 780, 960, 1440, 1,700, 1,520, 1,590, and 1,550 kcal/day. For adults (18–45 years) the values are close to the mean values obtained from the various reference standards. For children (0.5–13 years) the values are also close to the mean values obtained from various reference standards (although not all standards cover the entire age range).

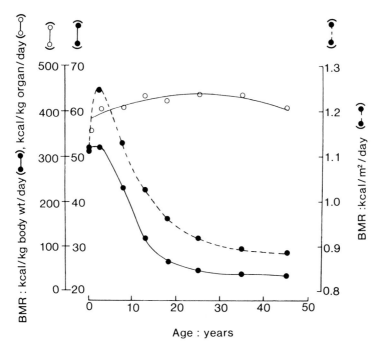

FIG. 2. Change in basal metabolic rate (BMR) during growth and development (0.5 to 45 years). BMR is expressed in relation to body weight (●——●), organ weight (○——○), and surface area (●---●). The graph was constructed from (A) the mean values of BMR, which were obtained using several standards; (B) organ weights, which were calculated using data from Korenchevsky (8) (Table 2) and from the values given in Table 1 for a 0.5-year-old child; and (C) surface area, which was calculated using the formula of Dubois and Dubois (Table 1 in Elia, Energy Expenditure in the Whole Body). The transient rise in BMR/m² between 0.5 and 3.5 years of age is not an artifact but a well-known developmental change.

ORGAN SIZE IN MAN AND OTHER MAMMALS

The metabolic rate/kg body weight of mammals decreases as the animal gets bigger. In this respect, mice have a metabolic rate that is five times greater than that of humans and ten times greater than that of elephants (17). Over a wide range of mammalian species a number of workers have found that resting energy expenditure is proportional to weight$^{0.75}$ (i.e., for every percent increase in weight, there is approximately 0.75% increase in metabolic rate). The mouse, the elephant, and many other mammals conform approximately to this general relationship.

It is possible that the lower metabolic rate per kg body weight of larger animals is due largely to the relatively smaller size of metabolically active tissues (i.e., organ size). If the metabolic rate per gram of individual organs varied little among different mammals, then organ size would be directly related to the metabolic rate of the mammal and to body weight$^{0.75}$.

I have attempted to examine such relationships using values of organ weights

TABLE 3. *Relation of organ weight to body weight (organ weight = K × body weight^x) in approximately mature mammals[a]*

	Live weight (g)	Liver (g)	Kidneys (g)	Brain (g)	Heart (g)	Lung (g)	All 5 organs (g)	All organs minus lung (g)
Elephant	6,650,000	6,300	1,200	5,700	2,200	(6,650)	22,050	15,400
Steer	700,000	5,000	1,000	500	2,300	3,900	12,700	8,800
Horse	600,000	6,700	1,600	670	4,250	5,400	13,220	18,620
Dairy cow	488,000	6,460	1,160	400	1,880	3,600	13,440	9,840
Hog	125,000	1,600	260	120	350	1,300	3,530	2,230
Human	60,000	1,700	250	1,300	320	1,000	4,570	3,570
Sheep	52,000	960	160	106	280	710	2,216	1,506
Dog	10,000	420	70	75	85	120	770	650
Monkey	4,500	110	21	42	23	30	226	196
Guinea pig	800	27	5.6	4.7	2.3	5.0	44.6	39.6
Rat	250	12	2.1	2.0	0.94	1.3	18.34	17.04
KW^{x}[b]		$0.39W^{0.70}$	$0.066W^{0.71}$	$0.76W^{0.71}$	$0.03W^{0.88}$	$0.016W^{0.92}$	$0.406W^{0.77}$	$0.448W^{0.74}$
Correlation coefficient		0.97	0.97	0.94	0.96	0.97	0.97	0.97

[a] Calculated using data from Brody (17).
[b] *K*, constant; W, body weight in grams; *x*, exponent.

provided by Brody (17) (Table 3). A less complete analysis has been undertaken previously (10,12). For abdominal organs (liver and kidney) and brain it would appear that organ size is approximately proportional to body weight$^{0.75}$, but for the thoracic organs (heart and lung), the exponent is higher. The weight of all the major organs combined (liver, kidney, lung, brain, and heart) is proportional to body weight$^{0.77}$, which implies that the overall differences in metabolic rate between the mammals examined can be largely explained by a change in organ size. However, it should be noted that Brody (17) also examined the relationship between metabolic rate and body weight in an unknown number and type of mature mammalian species and obtained generally higher exponents (kidney, 0.846; liver, 0.867; brain, 0.697; and heart, 0.984) than those indicated in Table 3. These other exponents imply that as mammals get bigger, there is not only a smaller contribution of organ weight to body weight but also a reduction in metabolic rate per gram of organ.

There is also some uncertainty as to whether the metabolic rate per unit organ weight *in vivo* is fixed among different mammals. Schmidt et al. (18) found that when the brain metabolic rate is expressed in ml O_2/g brain/min, the values for small spider and rhesus monkeys weighing 2.8 kg to 5.8 kg are similar to that of the human brain (see also ref. 19). Approximately similar values have also been found for rabbit and dog brain (cited in ref. 18). On the other hand, more recent work (20) suggests that the metabolic rate of the rat cerebral tissue is two times greater than that of the human, and it was suggested that this might be due to the presence of a much smaller proportion of supporting glial cells (presumably lower metabolic rate) in the rat brain than in the human brain. Discrepancies can also be found in the metabolic rates of other mammalian organs in vivo, but these are probably at least partly due to the use of different techniques for assessing blood flow in animals under different conditions (e.g., fed or fasted) and the assumptions used to calculate oxygen consumption per gram of tissue (e.g., uncertainties about tissue or organ size in animals that are not sacrificed and uncertainties about the estimated blood flow and the supply of blood in tissues that have dual sources). The work in vitro is also conflicting (e.g., see refs. 14,21,22), and the measurements often do not reflect those in vivo in any systematic way (18). Indeed, the metabolic rate of tissues in vitro can be altered by changing the composition of the medium in which they are immersed. Nevertheless, there is no doubt that differences in organ size between species, with or without some variation in metabolic activity, can go a long way toward explaining the differences in metabolic rates between different mammals.

One other observation that may be of interest to human energy metabolism concerns the ratio of organ weights to body weights in mature mammals of the same species. This ratio appears to get smaller with larger animals (17). If the same is also the case in humans, it could provide an explanation for the observation of several workers that larger individuals have a lower metabolic rate per kg body weight (or per kg fat-free mass) than smaller individuals (see chapter by Elia, *Energy Expenditure in the Whole Body*).

CHANGES IN ORGAN SIZE AND METABOLIC RATE IN PATHOPHYSIOLOGIC STATES

Koong and colleagues (23,24) measured organ weights and metabolic rate in groups of pigs with different nutritional backgrounds. One group lost weight initially and then compensated by rapid weight gain, another achieved rapid weight gain initially and lost weight later, and a third gained weight steadily. At the end of 10 weeks the three groups of animals had achieved similar weights, but their metabolic rate differed by 40%. The animals that had the most recent weight gain had the highest fasting metabolic rate and heaviest weight of liver, kidney, pancreas, and intestine. These weights were 25% to 50% greater than in the animals that had lost weight recently and had the lowest metabolic rate. Similar observations were made in lambs. Unfortunately, it is not possible to assess from these reports whether there were differences in muscle mass, degree of adiposity, or metabolic rate per kg fat-free mass.

Other experiments (25) confirmed that the splanchnic tissues of lambs account for approximately one-half the whole body O_2 consumption, as in cattle (26), and went on to show that in lambs given a maintenance diet, the contribution of portal drained viscera to whole body O_2 consumption was reduced by about one-third compared to animals that fed ad lib and gained weight. The contribution of the liver to whole-body O_2 consumption in the lambs given a maintenance diet was reduced by about one-half compared to the control animals, but this was not considered to be associated with a change in blood flow or O_2 consumption per g liver. This suggests that the diet had an effect on the size of the liver but little or no effect on its overall metabolic activity.

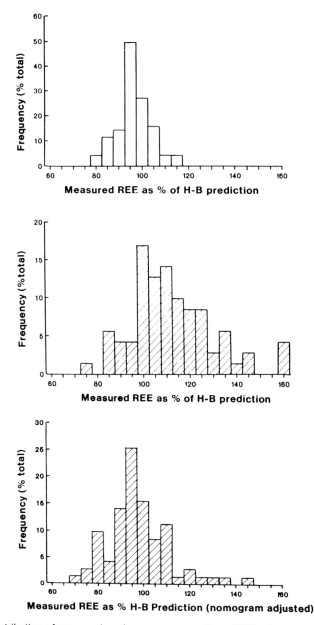

FIG. 3. Distribution of measured resting energy expenditure (REE) when expressed as a percentage of Harris-Benedict (H-B) prediction (normal subjects and patients). **Upper graph**: Normal subjects (n = 92; body mass index, 18–30 kg/m²). **Middle graph**: patients (n = 73) referred for nutritional support (see text). **Lower graph**: Measured REE in the patients shown in the middle graph expressed as a percent of Harris-Benedict prediction after adjustment of metabolic rate according to the nomogram illustrated in Fig. 4.

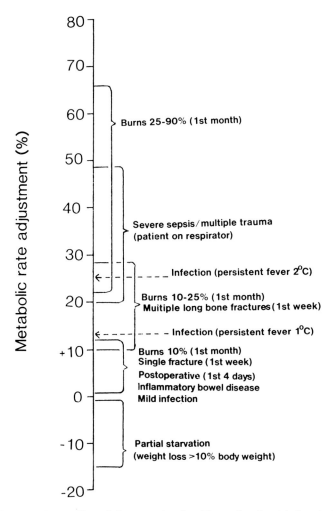

FIG. 4. The approximate effect of disease and malnutrition on basal metabolic rate. The change in metabolic rate is expressed as a percentage change (% adjustment).

diture in the opposite way to the disease. There are also the confounding effects of a variety of drugs and of blood transfusions, which may cause pyrexia and hypermetabolism, and the practice of nursing some patients, such as those in intensive care units, in a near naked state (at variable ambient temperatures) so that important clinical signs can be readily observed. There are also the effects of anxiety, abnormalities in fluid and electrolyte status, which affect body weight, and therefore the prediction of metabolic rate.

Pyrexia has also been used to predict metabolic rate (approximately 13% increase in metabolic rate per °C rise in temperature), but the variability is large, and fluctuations in temperature are also often large and variable.

O₂ CONSUMPTION OF INDIVIDUAL TISSUES IN DISEASE STATES

Although the causes of abnormal energy metabolism in disease states are likely to be multiple, the earlier discussion raises the possibility that abnormality might be due to a change in the proportion of metabolically active tissues (e.g., organs) to less active tissues (e.g., muscle). Such changes may be common in various clinical states, but the available information in humans is scant. It seems unbelievable that there is a substantial change in the size of the brain in acute systemic disease. In some situations it also seem unlikely that an increase in the size of other organs is the major cause of hypermetabolism. For example, major changes in energy expenditure can occur very rapidly in some patients (e.g., post-trauma patients). They can also occur within minutes when hormones such as catecholamines are given either alone or in combination with glucagon and corticosteroids so that they mimic the stress response. It is inconceivable that redistribution of fat-free tissue occurs so rapidly.

Another important consideration is the magnitude of the hypermetabolic response, which may be greater than 50% above normal. If this was due to an increase in organ size without a concomitant increase in energy expenditure per gram tissue, the organs would have to double in size. Such major organomegaly, which is readily detected clinically or on radiologic and scanning investigations, does not normally occur in patients with marked hypermetabolism. Therefore, the cause of hypermetabolism in these types of patients is likely to be due to a greater energy expenditure per g individual organs or tissues (with or without a concomitant small to moderate increase in organ size). This conclusion is consistent with experimental observations in burned patients, which show an apparent increase in O₂ consumption in a wide variety of tissues: peripheral tissues, the size of which can be readily measured, as well as splanchnic tissues, kidneys, and heart (33). The damaged skin is not the major site of increased energy expenditure, although the damage initiates a series of events that leads to increased energy expenditure in a variety of other tissues in the body.

There is very little information about organ metabolic rates in human malnutrition or starvation (i.e., O₂ consumption or energy expenditure per g individual tissues). It is therefore difficult to assess whether adaptation occurs as a result of a disproportionate decrease in the size of metabolically active tissues such as the splanchnic organs or a decrease in metabolic rate per g individual tissue (34). In experimental rats, total starvation for 12 days has been reported to lead to a much greater fractional loss of organs such as liver and kidney than skeletal muscle (35). This could be an important explanation for the reduction in metabolic rate observed in starvation.

ENERGY COST OF SPECIFIC METABOLIC PROCESSES IN HEALTH AND DISEASE

At present there is fragmentary information about the metabolic processes responsible for the energy expenditure of individual tissues or the whole body in health or disease. The energy expenditure associated with protein synthesis; various substrate cycles; Na-K exchange across cell membranes, which alone is estimated to account for about 20% of BMR in a variety of mammals (36); and brown fat activity have all been implicated as being important in normal individuals, although their importance may vary with age (e.g., brown fat activity is probably less important in adults than in infants). Because the activity of several of these processes may be markedly increased in disease states, they may contribute significantly to the hypermetabolism of individual tissues.

One of the complexities of metabolic pathways or cycles is the fact that they may not simply occur in one tissue but span across two or more tissues. For example, glycolytic products such as lactate pyruvate and alanine, which are released by peripheral tissues, may be used by the liver to produce glucose. This may then be reutilized by the peripheral tissues to form more glycolytic products. Similarly, the triglyceride fatty acid cycle involves the hydrolysis of triglyceride in adipose tissue to release fatty acids and glycerol. At the same time, fatty acids may be used to synthesize triglycerides by esterification of glycerophosphate. Because adipose tissue lacks significant activity of glycerokinase, the glycerol released from the hydrolysis of triglyceride cannot be utilized directly. Instead, it is released into the circulation and taken up by the liver, where it is converted to glucose. The glucose finally returns to adipose tissue, where it is used to form glycerophosphate, which allows the triglyceride fatty acid cycle to be completed.

The energy cost of these and other cycles can be estimated using a stoichiometric approach. The ATP required in a substrate cycle (assessed from classic metabolic pathways) is multiplied by the caloric equivalent of ATP. The value for this equivalent may vary somewhat, depending on the degree of coupling of oxidative phosphorylation in the mitochondria and the type of fuel oxidized (37–39). For example, if the combustion of starch yields 679 kcal (2,840 kJ)/glucosyl residue, and its oxidation within the body results in a net gain of about 36.7 ATP/glycosyl residue, the caloric equivalent of ATP is 18.5 kcal/mole ATP (679/36.7). For the same degree of mitochondrial coupling, the corresponding value for fat is close to 18.9/kJ mole ATP. For amino acids (protein) it is about 20.8 kJ/mole ATP, and for glycogen it is 18.0 kJ/mole ATP (37,39). In the calculations used in this chapter, the caloric equivalent of ATP is taken to be 19 kcal/mole (about 80 kJ/mole).

If the activity of a substrate cycle and its ATP requirement are known, then the energy cost of the cycle can be readily estimated and expressed in relation to the energy expenditure of the body. However, the ATP requirement of different cycles varies (e.g., 8 ATP for triglyceride–fatty acid recycling and 1 ATP for glucose-glucose 6-P recycling), and in some cases there is still some uncertainty about the precise requirement. For example, in the protein–amino acid cycle (protein turnover), 2 ATP are required for the activation of amino acids to amino acyl tRNA and a further 2 ATP for elongation (peptide bond synthesis), making a total requirement of 4 ATP per mole amino acid incorporated into protein. However, this requirement assumes that activated amino acids are incorporated into protein with 100% efficiency. If some amino acyl tRNA is hydrolyzed without incorporation of the amino acid into

TABLE 5. *The activity and energy cost of some substrate cycles in normal and burned subjects*

Substrate cycle	Mole ATP used/mole substrate cycled[a]	Normal subjects			Burned subjects				Reference for rates of substrate cycling
		Rate of substrate cycling mole/70 kg/day[a]	Energy cost of cycle		Rate of substrate cycling mole/70 kg/day	Energy cost of cycle		ΔEnergy cost of cycle × 100[d]	
			kcal/d[b]	%BMR[c]		kcal/d	%BMR	ΔBMR	
Protein-amino acid (protein turnover)	(4)	3.1	236	14	6.6	502	15-20	19-32	(43)[e]
Glucose-"lactate"	4	0.42	32	1.9	1.6	122	3.7-4.9	6.5-11	(33)[f]
		0.24	18	1.1	—	—	—	—	(44)
		0.21	16	1.0	—	—	—	—	(45)
Triglyceride-fatty acid	8	0.12	18	0.8	0.53	81	2.9	12	(46)[g]
		0.04	6	0.36	—	—	—	—	(47)
		0.13	20	1.3	—	—	—	—	(48)
Glucose-glucose 1P and	1	0.4	8	0.33	0.96	18	0.65	2	(46)[g]
Fructose 6P-		0.29	6	0.33	—	—	—	—	(49)
Fructose 1-6P		0.69	13	0.85	—	—	—	—	(50)

[a] In the case of the protein-amino acid cycle, this refers to the molar rate of amino acid cycling. For the glucose-lactate cycle the molar rate refers to glucose cycling (not lactate), and for the triglyceride fatty acid cycle it refers to the triglyceride (not fatty acid).

[b] Energy cost (kcal/day) = substrate cycling rate (moles/day) × ATP used/mole substrate cycled × 19 (kcal/mole ATP).

[c] When basal metabolic rate measurements in normal adults were not available, it was assumed that they expended 1,650 kcal/day (70 kg body weight).

[d] Δenergy cost of cycle (kcal) = energy cost of cycling in burned subjects − energy cost of cycling in normal subjects. ΔBMR = BMR of burned patients (70 kg) − BMR of normal subjects (70 kg).

[e] The burned subjects in this study (mean burn size − 65% of total surface area) were studied at 11 ± 4 days. The range in values for %BMR and for Δenergy cost cycle/ΔBMR in the burned subjects were calculated assuming metabolic rate was elevated 50-85% above normal.

[f] The range in values for %BMR and 100 × Δenergy cost cycle/ΔBMR in the burned subjects was calculated assuming metabolic rate was 50-85% above normal. The estimated rate of cycling includes cycling of lactate and other 3-carbon glycolytic products, e.g., alanine (in normal man, glucose-alanine cycling occurs at about one-half the rate of glucose-lactate cycling—ref 45).

[g] Both the control and burned patients in this study were a combination of adults and children. The burned subjects (74 ± 3% surface area burn) were studied 20 ± 5 days after injury when their metabolic rate was found to be 23% above normal (estimated to be ~40 kcal/kg/day compared with ~32.5 kcal/kg/day for the control subjects).

protein, the ATP requirement per peptide bond synthesis will be greater than 4 moles. Furthermore, the ATP required to maintain the turnover of RNA (mRNA, tRNA, rRNA—refs. 40,41) and transport of amino acids is not included in the preceding estimate of ATP requirement for protein synthesis; nor is the one ATP required to initiate protein synthesis and another ATP required to initiate nonlysosomal protein breakdown. Although the energy cost of some of these processes is probably small compared to the energy cost of protein synthesis per se, the value of 4 ATP/mole peptide bond synthesized should be nevertheless regarded as a minimum value (see also ref. 42).

Table 5 illustrates the activity of three cycles: glucose lactate recycling, protein amino acid recycling (protein turnover and triglyceride/fatty acid recycling), and the associated energy expenditure calculated in absolute terms and as a percentage of resting energy expenditure in both normal subjects and those with a severe form of injury (burn injury). Although the majority of basal energy expenditure remains unaccounted for, the increased activity of these three cycles in burned patients accounts for up to one-half of the rise in energy expenditure (Table 5). A further contribution arises from the increased energy cost associated with cardiac output, which may increase more than two times in burned patients. The energy expenditure of the heart may double in burn patients (33), and there may be an increase in the work of breathing, which frequently produces a twofold to fourfold increase in minute ventilation.

REFERENCES

1. Elia M. The inter-organ flux of nutrients in fed and fasted man. *Nutr Res Rev* [in press].
2. Snyder WS, Cook MJ, Nasset ES, Karhausen LR, Howells GP, Tipton IH. *Report of the task group on reference man*. International Commission on radiological protection No. 23. Oxford: Pergamon Press, 1975.
3. Coppack SW, Fisher RM, Gibbons GF, et al. Post-prandial substrate deposition in human forearm and adipose tissue in vivo. *Clin Sci* 1990;79:339–48.
4. Hallgren P, Sjostrom L, Hedlund H, Lundell L, Olbe L. Influence of age, fat cell, weight and obesity on O_2 consumption of human adipose tissue. *Am J Physiol* 1989;256:E467–74.
5. Garby L, Garrow JS, Jorgensen B, et al. Relation between energy expenditure and body composition in man: specific energy expenditure in vivo of fat and fat free tissue. *Eur J Clin Nutr* 1988;42:301–5.
6. Linde B, Hjemdahl P, Freychuss V, Juhlin-Dannfelt A. Adipose tissue and skeletal muscle flow during mental stress. *Am J Physiol* 1989;256:E12–8.
7. Boyd E. *Outline of physical growth and development*. Minneapolis: Burgess Press, 1942.
8. Korenchevsky V. Physiological and pathological aging. New York: Karger, Basel, 1961;38–47.
9. Coppoletta JM, Wolback SB. Body length and organ weights of infants and children; study of body length and normal weights of more important vital organs of body between birth and 12 years of age. *Am J Pathol* 1933;9:55–70.
10. Grande F. Energy expenditure of organs and tissues. In: Kinney JM, ed. Assessment of energy metabolism in health and disease. Columbus, OH: Ross Laboratories, 1989;88–92.
11. Brozek J, Grande F. Body composition and basal metabolism in man: correlation analysis versus physiological approach. *Hum Biol* 1955;27:22–31.
12. Holliday MA, Potter D, Jarrah A, Bearg S. The relation of metabolic rate to organ size. *Paediatr Res* 1967;1:185–95.
13. Holliday MA. Metabolic rate and organ size during growth from infancy to maturity and during late gestation and early infancy. *Paediatrics* 1971;47:169–77.
14. Davies M. On body size and tissue respiration. *J Cell Comp Physiol* 1961;57:135–47.

15. Kennedy C, Sokoloff L. An adaptation of the nitrous oxide method to the study of the cerebral circulation of children: normal values for cerebral blood flow and cerebral metabolic rate in childhood. *J Clin Invest* 1957;36:1130–37.
16. Friscancho R. Anthropometric standards for the assessment of nutritional status. Ann Arbor: The University of Michigan Press, 1990.
17. Brody S. *Bioenergetics of growth*. New York: Reinhold, 1945.
18. Schmidt CF, Ketty S, Pennes HH. The gaseous metabolism of the brain of the monkey. *Am J Physiol* 1945;143:33–52.
19. Kety SS, Schmidt CF. The determination of brain blood flow in man by the use of nitrous oxide at low concentration. *Am J Physiol* 1945;143:53–66.
20. Siesjo BK, Nilsson B. A method for determining blood flow and oxygen consumption in the rat brain. *Acta Physiol Scand* 1976;96:72–82.
21. Kleiber M. *The fire of life*. New York: Krieger Publishing Co. Huntington, 1975.
22. Bertalanffy von L, Pirozynski WJ. Tissue respiration and body size. *Science* 1951;113:559–600.
23. Koong LJ, Ferrell CL, Nienaber. *Effects of plane of nutrition on organ size and fasting heat production in swine and sheep*. Proc 9th Symposium on energy metabolism in farm animals, EAA Publications, Agricultural Institute of Norway 1982;245–8.
24. Koong LJ, Ferrel CL. Effects of short term nutritional manipulation on organ size and fasting meat production. *Eur J Clin Nutr* 1990;44(suppl 1):73–7.
25. Burrin DG, Ferrel CL, Eisemann JH, Britton RA, Nienaber JA. Effect of nutrition on splanchnic blood flow and oxygen consumption in sheep. *Br J Nutr* 1989;62:23–34.
26. Huntington GB. Energy metabolism of the digestive tract and liver of cattle: influence of the physiological state and nutrition. *Reprod Nutr Dev* 1990;30:35–47.
27. Coward WA, Whitehead RG, Lunn PG. Reasons why hypoalbuminaemia may not appear in protein-energy malnutrition. *Br J Nutr* 1977;38:115–26.
28. Lunn PG, Austin S. Differences in nitrogen metabolism between protein-deficient and energy deficient rats with similarly restricted growth rates. *Ann Nutr Metab* 1983;27:242–51.
29. Lunn PG, Whitehead RG, Baker BA, Austin S. The effect of corticosterone acetate on the course of development of experimental protein energy malnutrition in rats. *Br J Nutr* 1976;36:537–50.
30. Wusteman M, Elia M. Protein metabolism after 'injury' with turpentine: a rat model of clinical trauma. *Am J Physiol* 1990;259:E763–9.
31. Heymsfield SB, McManus CB. Tissue components of weight loss in cancer patients. A new method of study and preliminary observations. *Cancer* 1985;55:238–49.
32. Elia M. Artificial nutritional support. *Med Internat* 1990;82:3392–6.
33. Wilmore DW, Aulick LH. Metabolic changes in burned patients. *Surg Clin North Am* 1978;58:1173–87.
34. Montgomery RD. Changes in the basal metabolic rate of the malnourished infant and their relation to body composition. *J Clin Invest* 1962;41:1653–63.
35. Addis T, Poo LJ, Lew W. The quantities of protein lost by the various organs and tissues of the body during a fast. *J Biol Chem* 1936;115:111–16.
36. Kelly JM, McBride BW. The sodium pump and other mechanisms of thermogenesis in selected tissues. *Proc Nutr Soc* 1990;49:185–202.
37. Elia M, Livesey G. Energy expenditure and fuel selection in biological systems: the theory and practice of calculations based on indirect calorimetry and tracer methods [Submitted for publication].
38. Livesey G. The energy equivalents of ATP and the energy values of food proteins and fats. *Br J Nutr* 1984;51:15–28.
39. Elia M, Livesey G. Theory and validity of indirect calorimetry during net lipid synthesis. *Am J Clin Nutr* 1988;47:591–607.
40. Sander G, Hulsemann J, Topp H, Heller-Schöch G. Protein and RNA turnover in pre-term infants and adults; a comparison based on urinary excretion of 3-methyl histidine and a modified one-way RNA catabolite. *Am Nutr Metab* 1986;30:137.
41. Sander G, Topp H, Weiland J, Heller-Schöch G, Schöch G. Possible use of urinary modified RNA metabolites in the measurement of RNA turnover in the human body. *Hum Nutr Clin Nutr* 1986;40C:103–18.
42. Waterlow JC, Millward DJ. The energy cost of turnover of protein and other cellular constituents. In: Wieser W, Graiger E, eds. *Energy transformations in cells and organisms*. Stutgart: Thiem Verlag, 1989;277–82.
43. Jahoor F, Shangraw RE, Miyoshi H, Wallfish H, Herndon DN, Wolfe RR. Role of insulin and glucose oxidation in mediating the protein catabolism of burns and sepsis. *Am J Physiol* 1989;257:E323–31.

44. Reichard GA, Moury NF, Hochella NJ, Patterson AL, Weinhouse S. Quantitative estimation of the Cori cycle in humans. *J Biol Chem* 1963;238:495–501.
45. Consoli A, Nurjan N, Reilly J, Bier DM, Gerich JE. Contribution of liver and skeletal muscle to alanine and lactate metabolism in humans. *Am J Physiol* 1990;259:E677–84.
46. Wolfe RR, Herndon DN, Jahoor F, Miyoshi H, Wolfe M. Effect of severe burn injury on substrate by glucose and fatty acids. *N Engl J Med* 1987;317:403–8.
47. Elia M, Zed C, Neale G, Livesey G. The energy cost of triglyceride-fatty acid recycling in non-obese subjects after an overnight fast and four days of starvation. *Metabolism* 1987;3:251–5.
48. Klein S, Peters EJ, Holland OB, Wolfe RR. Effect of short- and long-term β-adrenergic blockage on lipolysis during fasting in humans. *Am J Physiol* 1989;257:E65–73.
49. Karlander S, Roovete A, Varnic M, Efendic S. Glucose and fructose-6-phosphate cycle in humans. *Am J Physiol* 1986;251:E530–6.
50. Shulman GI, Ladenson PW, Wolfe MA, Ridgeway EC, Wolfe RR. Substrate cycling between gluconeogenesis and glycolysis in leuthyroid, hypothyroid and hyperthyroid man. *J Clin Invest* 1985;76:757–64.

DISCUSSION

Dr. Pi-Sunyer: I'd like to commend Dr. Elia for what I think is a very scholarly and thorough presentation of the problems related to using derived equations for calculating BMR metabolic rate in individuals.

To evaluate whether these derived equations are reasonable or not, we have to ask the question, what are we utilizing the derived equation for? In some cases the derived equation will be perfectly justified and in other conditions will be totally inappropriate.

It seems to me if one is treating a patient in a metabolic ward and trying to feed that patient, the use of an equation from Harris and Benedict to get an estimate of the amount of nutrient that is required, with all the manipulations that have to be done, the derivation of the equation is incredibly inaccurate. However, such equations seem to me perfectly reasonable, because they can be corrected relatively quickly as the metabolic state of the patient is being watched carefully in a metabolic ward.

On the other hand, if one is to derive an equation to diagnose an abnormal metabolic state, the danger of giving an incorrect diagnosis to an individual is rather high.

If the calculations are done for a public health reason, it seems to me since one is going to want to err on the high side anyway, using an equation like the Harris-Benedict equation that might be somewhat high may not necessarily be inappropriate to calculate the public health needs of a population group.

The problems become very great if one is to use an equation to try to characterize a particular population group—for instance, the Pima Indians or the black population of America or the Mexican Indian population—to measure their metabolic rate, compare it to a derived equation, and state, "This particular group is hypometabolic." I think that since we are dealing with uncertainty, it depends a great deal how we're to utilize the result of that calculation: for an individual or for a group of individuals.

Dr. Elia comments on the utilization of surface areas versus the utilization of fat-free mass. He seems rather unhappy with the use of surface area, feeling that it is a rather inaccurate way of trying to derive whether an individual is hypometabolic or hypermetabolic.

It's my impression that surface area is likely to be more accurate than many ways that are being utilized for trying to derive fat-free mass of individuals. We have an enormous number of commercial companies and individuals selling machines that are supposed to measure lean body mass accurately and actually do a rather inaccurate job of it. And yet those derived fat-free mass figures are being used as denominators for calculating metabolic rate in individuals. It seems likely that the surface area calculations may be more accurate than the FF fat-free mass calculations that are being done.

Dr. Elia mentioned the use of weight or BMI as potentially a denominator for expressing metabolic rate. And I have great reservations about either of those measurements because, as the weight increases, the proportion of fat as related to lean body mass changes greatly. Therefore I think weight and BMI are likely to be unhelpful as denominators for the metabolic rate.

The problem of aging is an interesting one. It's interesting that there seems to be a real difference between studies. Maybe part of the problem relates to most of these studies being cross-sectional studies and also possibly to the inability to measure body composition in these aging people. As they age, they change their basal body composition and become fatter and have less lean body mass. I think we need good longitudinal studies in which body composition is measured very accurately in these aging individuals over time to be able to document exactly the nature of the fall in metabolic rate with age.

Dr. Elia mentioned technology as a possible variable in the measurement of metabolic rate and its errors. It's my impression, at least in our hands, that whether one uses a canopy or a mask or a mouthpiece, it really makes very little difference in the accuracy of the method and thus is not really a problem in the right hands. It's much more likely that the problem is related to preparation of the patient, calibration of the instrument, and so on.

The question of different racial groups is an interesting but difficult one. One cannot just lump members of an ethnic group together and use standard tables for that particular ethnic group without any change in relation to what their diet is, what their energy expenditure is, what the prevailing temperature is, and the individual areas. Deriving race-specific equations is fraught with enormous problems.

However, we have to recognize that there is evidence that different racial groups, at least in certain countries of the world, have different body composition. For instance, it's clear that the black population in the United States at the moment has a higher mineral density proportionally than do the Caucasians and that the Asians in the United States have a lower mineral density than Caucasians. This is important if you're going to derive their metabolic rate in relation to their fat-free mass, because how you calculate their fat-free mass will change as to whether you take into account this change in their mineral density. So it is a problem. And it's a problem that needs to be resolved.

I think Dr. Elia is to be commended for talking about this whole area of organ size and trying to begin to derive data relating to size and activity of different organs. I think this will be a great step forward. And I think it requires a great deal of research in the future to try to see whether we can come up with ways. I think the methodology at present is really not available. The technique, the technology, is not available to date to try to do that. But it would certainly be a step, a great step forward if we could move to partitioning metabolic rate better between the different organs of the body.

I would like to comment on the effect of diet on the metabolic rate. Dr. Elia didn't say anything about that. But it seems to me that when we generally take the metabolic rate we're asking individuals generally to fast about 12 hours and then come into the laboratory. And we assume that this is the resting metabolic rate.

I remember an old diagram that J.P. Flat had in a book some years ago, showing the continuing downward trend of the metabolic rate, not only at 12 hours but if you went on down 48 hours and 72 hours. And in fact, when we're measuring the metabolic rate, the resting metabolic rate of an individual at 12 hours of fasting, we are actually including in that a significant component from the previous diet. And therefore, the previous diet is probably significantly important in that component and we don't really deal with that at all. And I think in the future we should begin to deal with that.

Finally, I just want to say something about hypometabolism, per se—the question of what is an abnormal BMR in terms of a downward or a hypometabolic BMR. It's become quite important today when we're dealing with questions of metabolic efficiency in individuals or groups of individuals.

If we measure a group of individuals, when can we say that they're truly abnormal and say they have a genetic lesion or there is something really abnormally wrong with this individual, this group of individuals in relation to their metabolic rate? I think it was a difficult enough question to ask when we were measuring BMR as a single value that was derived from equations, but now we need to normalize for fat-free mass. The calculation and the measurement of fat-free mass is also a problem, so we can get into a double problem of the actual measurement and then the derivation of the fat-free mass, by which we tend to normalize the metabolic rate.

I think we have to ask the question, if we do a measurement and then we control for the age of the individual, we control for the fat-free mass of the individual, we control possibly for the gender of the individual, and then we come up with a figure that's slightly low, can we say that that individual has a metabolic defect? In other words, can we say that this person really has something wrong with them genetically in relation to their energy expenditure?

Or do we have to say that possibly the problem is not there at all, in the energy expenditure, but the problem is in the failure of regulation of that energy expenditure to energy intake? Are we, in a sense, losing sight of the question by saying that the problem is at the expenditure side? Could it not just as easily be that the problem is at the regulation of intake side?

In other words, we know that all of us have different metabolic rates, and we may have a variability within a normal group that's significantly high, 20–25% range, even in what we call normal groups. And yet we all regulate at our particular metabolic rate. We regulate our intake to maintain our body weight reasonably well. And therefore, if there's such a variability within normality, can we say that somebody who has a slightly lower metabolic rate, that the problem is in the energy expenditure set up or is it possible that the problem is related to an inability of whatever it is that regulates food intake to detect that difference and regulate it appropriately?

Energy Metabolism: Tissue Determinants and
Cellular Corollaries, edited by J. M. Kinney
and H. N. Tucker. Raven Press. Ltd..
New York © 1992.

Daily Energy Expenditure in Humans: Measurements in a Respiratory Chamber and by Doubly Labeled Water

Eric Ravussin and Russell Rising

Clinical Diabetes and Nutrition Section, National Institute of Diabetes and Digestive and Kidney Diseases, National Institutes of Health, Phoenix, Arizona 85016

The prevalence of obesity is increasing dramatically throughout the world in parallel with the industrialization of countries. In the United States, obesity affects approximately 34 million adults aged 20 to 74 (1), a slightly higher prevalence than that observed in England, Canada, or Australia (2,3). Obesity represents one of the important public health problems of the latter half of this century. As pointed out in the Surgeon General's Report on Nutrition and Health (4), obesity is clearly a risk factor for the development of non–insulin-dependent diabetes mellitus, hypertension, hyperlipidemia, coronary heart disease and stroke, gallbladder disease, and some types of cancer. Therefore, in the quest to reduce these "modern" diseases, much attention has been focused on the potentially reversible condition of obesity. However, the causes of obesity are not fully understood, and this, not surprisingly, makes its long-term treatment or prevention very difficult.

Obesity is a common familial disorder that is expressed in genetically predisposed individuals when exposed to aggravating environmental conditions (5–8). The familial occurrence of obesity could result from similarities among family members in either an excessive calorie intake, a deficit in energy expenditure, or both. However, family members share not only genes but also diet, cultural background, and many other aspects of lifestyle. One therefore has to separate the familial origins of obesity into its genetic and/or the environmental determinants. Recent adoption and twin studies (7,9,10) have attempted to dissociate the genetic from the environmental influences and clearly have shown the importance of genetics independent of environment in the development of obesity.

The mechanism of the genetic influences have remained unknown, but over the past 10 or 15 years, there has been renewed interest in uncovering differences in energy expenditure between lean and obese subjects (8,11,12). The suggestion has been raised that the obese may be more energy efficient, that is, they require fewer calories per unit of metabolically active tissue than lean individuals (13,14). However, it was clearly stated some time ago that overweight subjects have higher metabolic rates in absolute values (15). There is still great controversy in the literature regarding whether the obese have a lower metabolic rate than their lean counterparts when differences in body weight and body composition are taken into account. One of the major causes of this controversy is the manner of comparing energy expenditure in people of different sizes, i.e., the way of normalizing the data to an estimate of metabolic body size. Since fat-free mass is the major determinant of resting metabolic rate, investigators have tended to divide the measured metabolic rate by the fat-free mass. However, the linear relationship between resting metabolic rate and fat-free mass does not have a zero intercept, so simply dividing by the fat-free mass results in an overestimation of the metabolic rate in individuals with a smaller fat-free mass (16). Because obesity is not a single disorder but represents a heterogenous group of disorders (5,8), the controversy is also the result of a small number of poorly characterized subjects used in many studies. Another confounding factor in the interpretation of the results is that, in many cases, the comparisons of obese versus lean subjects does not allow one to reach conclusions about the causes and effects of the obese state. A physiologic factor playing a role in the pathogenesis of obesity might not be seen in the obese or might even be reversed. For example, obese subjects have a normal, if not high, metabolic rate for their body size and composition when compared to lean subjects; this does not exclude that these same obese subjects had a low metabolic rate before gaining weight. Only longitudinal studies can, therefore, lead to a clear answer on the role of low energy metabolism in the pathogenesis of obesity.

COMPONENTS OF SEDENTARY 24-HOUR ENERGY EXPENDITURE

Durnin et al. (17) suggested that energy expenditure be measured over periods of days or at least over 24-hour periods to determine energy requirements better in humans. To perform these measurements, respiratory chambers have been built around the world to perform further studies of energy metabolism in humans in sedentary conditions or with the addition of exercise (18–22).

The respiratory chamber at the Clinical Diabetes and Nutrition Section of the National Institute of Diabetes and Digestive and Kidney Diseases, National Institutes of Health, in Phoenix was modeled after the chamber built in the late 1970s by Professor Jéquier and colleagues in Lausanne, Switzerland (19) (Fig. 1). The chamber itself is an "environmental walk-in room" 3.33 m long, 2.45 m wide, and 2.39 m high representing a total volume of 19,500 L, with a 19,000 L net volume when the furniture is taken into account. Thanks to the good mixing of the gas in the respiratory chamber, the response time for the respiratory chamber measured during carbon dioxide dilution was 3 minutes for 93% of the total response and 4 minutes for 99% of the total response. We therefore allowed a 3-minute delay for the respiratory chamber exchange measurements compared with the instantaneous measurement of spontaneous physical activity measured using a radar system (MICD 930, Honeywell, Minneapolis, MN). Measurements in the respiratory chamber are performed con-

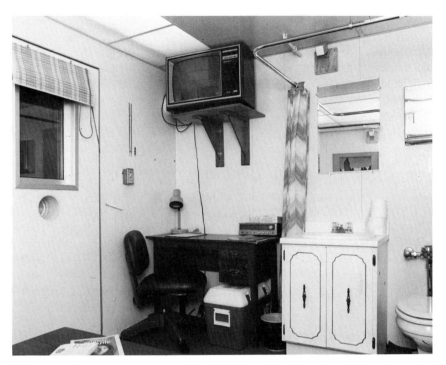

FIG. 1. The Phoenix respiratory chamber (19,000 liters) based on the principle of open-circuit indirect calorimetry. Note the radar system located above the mirror.

tinuously for 23 hours from 0800 to 0700 hours the following day and then extrapolated to 24 hours. In most protocols, no vigorous exercise is allowed in the chamber and spontaneous physical activity is estimated by the radar system mounted on two walls of the chamber. In these conditions, after at least 4 days on a weight-maintaining diet, the intra-individual variability of 24-hour energy expenditure is very small compared to the variance among individuals (21). Most of the intra-individual variance can be accounted for in the variance in the measurements, which was assessed by propane combustion over periods of 6 to 24 hours.

Sleeping metabolic rate is defined as the average energy expenditure of all 15-minute periods between 2330 and 0500 hours, during which time the activity measured by the radar was less than or equal to 1.5%, which means that motion was detected for less than 1.5% of the time. At 0700 hours on the following morning, 11 hours after an evening snack, the chamber is opened. While the volunteer is still lying on the bed, a plastic, transparent ventilated hood is placed over his or her head for approximately 35 minutes. After 10 to 15 minutes of adaptation to the hood, the time during which the analyzers are calibrated, the basal metabolic rate is measured for another 9 to 12 minutes by connecting the hood system to the analyzing equipment of the chamber.

Therefore, using such a chamber, all the components of daily sedentary physical

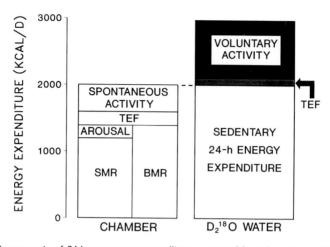

FIG. 2. Components of 24-hour energy expenditure measured in sedentary conditions in a respiratory chamber (left) and in free-living conditions using the doubly labeled water technique (right). The energy cost of voluntary physical activity can be calculated as the difference between the two measurements corrected for the thermic effect of food of the extra energy intake. SMR, sleeping metabolic rate; BMR, basal metabolic rate; TEF, thermic effect of food.

activity can be assessed: the sleeping metabolic rate, the basal metabolic rate, the energy cost of arousal (basal metabolic rate minus sleeping metabolic rate), the thermic effect of the meals, and the energy cost of spontaneous physical activity (Fig. 2).

DETERMINANTS AND VARIABILITY OF ENERGY EXPENDITURE

We selected for analysis all of the healthy, nondiabetic subjects measured for 24 hours in our respiratory chamber after at least three days on a balanced, weight-maintaining diet. Body composition was estimated by hydrostatic weighing. The physical characteristics and energy expenditure of these 597 subjects are presented in Table 1. Analysis of covariance and single and multiple regression analyses were performed using the general linear models of the Statistical Analysis Systems Institute (SAS, Cary, NC) to assess the different determinants of energy expenditure. The results of these analyses and the variance explained by the different determinants are presented in Table 2. Most of the variance in energy expenditure over 24 hours or in the basal or sleeping state is related to differences in fat-free mass (Fig. 3). However, fat mass also explains, to a smaller degree, additional variance in each of the three states. Spontaneous physical activity in the chamber was also a significant determinant of 24-hour energy expenditure.

The variability of 24-hour energy expenditure can best be represented as the frequency distribution of the ratio between 24-hour energy expenditure and the sleeping metabolic rate (Fig. 4). As recently reported, basal metabolic rate was lower in older

TABLE 1. *Physical characteristics and energy expenditure in 597 healthy subjects measured for 24 hours in a respiratory chamber after at least 3 days on a weight maintenance diet*[a]

	Males $N = 327$	Females $N = 270$
Age (y)	32 (18–81)	34 (18–85)
Body weight (kg)	93.2 (50.6–209.9)	88.3 (41.3–215.2)
Body fat (%)	25 (3–49)	36 (9–53)
24-h energy expenditure (kcal/d)	2,418 (1,584–4,225)	2,049 (1,259–3,723)
Basal metabolic rate (kcal/d)	1,903 (1,191–3,797)	1,618 (904–2,889)
Sleeping metabolic rate (kcal/d)	1,732 (1,096–3,728)	1,499 (876–3,096)

[a] Means are presented with the ranges in parentheses.

people, whereas sleeping metabolic rate was not related to age (23). Independent of differences in fat-free mass, fat mass, age, and spontaneous physical activity, females had lower metabolic rates than males, averaging approximately 200 kcal/d. This observation deserves further investigation. In either sex, metabolic rate was not related to the distribution of body fat as assessed by waist or thigh circumference ratio.

POSSIBLE MECHANISMS OF THE VARIABILITY IN METABOLIC RATE

The resting metabolic rate, as well as the 24-hour sedentary energy expenditure, are familial traits independent of fat-free mass, fat mass, age, and sex (Fig. 5) (24,25). This familial trait suggests, but does not prove, that metabolic rate is genetically determined. Bouchard et al. (26) have recently shown in monozygotic and dizygotic twins that the more genes are shared, the more similar the metabolic rate, indepen-

TABLE 2. *Major determinants of energy expenditure by single or multiple regression analyses in healthy subjects (327 males/270 females) measured for 24 hours in a respiratory chamber after at least 3 days on a weight-maintenance diet*[a]

24-hour energy expenditure (24EE)
24EE = 459 + 28.9 FFM $r^2 = 0.82$
24EE = 538 + 25.1 FFM + 5.5 FM $r^2 = 0.85$
24EE = 618 + 18.1 FFM + 10.0 FM − 1.4 age + 17 SPA + 204 (males) $r^2 = 0.89$
Basal metabolic rate (BMR)
BMR = 429 + 21.7 FFM $r^2 = 0.65$
BMR = 465 + 19.9 FFM + 2.6 FM $r^2 = 0.66$
BMR = 773 + 14.3 FFM + 6.0 FM − 4.3 age + 141 (males) $r^2 = 0.68$
Sleeping metabolic rate (SMR)
SMR = 297 + 21.4 FFM $r^2 = 0.76$
SMR = 371 + 17.8 FFM + 5.2 FM $r^2 = 0.80$
SMR = 473 + 14.6 FFM + 7.3 FM − 0.6 age + 99 (males) $r^2 = 0.81$

[a] Energy expenditure values are expressed in kcal/d. FFM, fat-free mass in kg; FM, fat mass in kg; SPA, spontaneous physical activity in percent of the 24-hours during which the subject was moving (21). All variables are significant determinants of energy expenditure at $p < 0.0001$ level except for age for 24EE ($p < 0.01$) and age for SMR (NS).

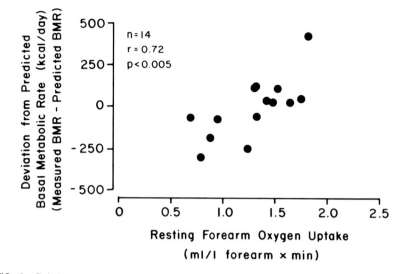

FIG. 6. Relationship between the deviation of the measured basal metabolic rate (BMR) (kcal/d) from the predicted BMR and forearm oxygen uptake expressed per liter of forearm tissue (ml/[liters × min]). Correlation coefficients were 0.80 and 0.75 for males and females, respectively. The predicted BMR was calculated accounting for subjects' FFM, fat mass (FM), age, and sex based on measurements in 138 nondiabetic Caucasians.

conditions in Pima Indians and Caucasians (33). Two approaches were used. In the first study, the relationship between 24-hour energy expenditure and 24-hour urinary norepinephrine excretion was measured in 36 Caucasians and 33 nondiabetic Pima Indian males. After adjusting for differences in fat-free mass, fat mass, and age, 24-hour energy expenditure was strongly correlated with 24-hour urinary norepinephrine in Caucasians but not in Pima Indians. In the second study, the change in resting metabolic rate with beta-adrenergic blockade (propranolol infusion) was measured in 36 Caucasians and 32 nondiabetic Pima Indian males. Resting metabolic rate measured after a 12-hour fast decreased significantly after propranolol infusion in Caucasians but not in Pima Indians. This decrease correlated significantly with resting metabolic rate (adjusted for fat-free mass, fat mass, and age) before propranolol infusion in Caucasians but not in Pimas. These two studies provide one of the first pieces of evidence for an ethnic difference in SNS activity between Caucasian and Pima Indian males under fasting eucaloric conditions. The blunted effectiveness of SNS activity on energy expenditure in Pima Indians might play a role in this population, which has one of the highest prevalence rates of obesity in the world (34). More studies are presently underway to characterize better the impact of SNS activity on energy metabolism as well as the relationship between body temperature and energy metabolism.

In summary, low skeletal muscle metabolism or low SNS-mediated energy expenditure can be at least partially responsible for low metabolic rate in subjects predisposed to weight gain (25).

VALIDATION OF THE DOUBLY LABELED WATER TECHNIQUE

Respiratory chambers provide data only under very sedentary conditions. However, one of the major components of the daily energy expenditure, and certainly the most variable, is the energy expenditure associated with motion and physical activity. Much earlier this century, Widdowson showed that both food intake and energy expenditure is quite variable from one day to the next (35). The day-to-day variability in energy expenditure is most likely to be related to changes in physical activity. For that reason, the energy expenditure in free-living conditions has been estimated from calorimetric determination of different activities and from estimates of the time spans for each of these activities (36). These techniques are tedious, not very sensitive, and not reproducible.

The doubly labeled water method to measure energy expenditure in totally free-living conditions was used for the first time in humans less than 10 years ago (37). Since then, the doubly labeled water technique has been validated by comparison with respiratory gas analysis in different laboratories under sedentary conditions (38–41) as well as during sustained heavy exercise (42). Owing to the high cost of the isotope, most validation studies have been conducted with normal weight volunteers. There is, however, a large interest and need for performing studies in obese volunteers to try to understand better the etiologic factors involved in the development of obesity (25). We therefore performed a validation study with a group of 12 male volunteers covering a wide range of body weight and body composition measured for 7 consecutive days in the respiratory chamber in sedentary conditions (43). Like previous studies, results show that the doubly labeled water method is a suitable technique to assess energy expenditure in free-living conditions with an accuracy of -2.5% and a precision of $\pm 5.8\%$ (Fig. 7). However, larger underestimates were found in heavier and fatter subjects.

Because multiple samples were collected after dosing with the heavy water, we also used the data to compare the accuracy and precision of the method using all the isotopic enrichments: multi-point approach (39), three enrichments (3-point calculation), and only two enrichments (2-point calculation) as proposed initially by Schoeller and van Santen (37). Results were very similar when using all of the points, three points, or two points to calculate the carbon dioxide production. However, it should be pointed out that in the conditions of a respiratory chamber, two of the key assumptions for the methods are very close to being met: (A) the amount of body water is constant throughout the study and (B) the water and carbon dioxide turnover rates are constant throughout the study (45,46). This is far from true in free-living conditions, in which no attempt is made to maintain a constant body weight and in which water and carbon dioxide turnovers are very likely to vary on a day-to-day basis. It might therefore be difficult to fit a single mono-exponential line when turnovers (water and/or CO_2) change over time. The two-point method measures the total flux between two points several days apart, whereas the multipoint method provides a mean value for flux/day over the same interval. The two-point method will therefore not be influenced by changes in flux, which can occur earlier

will help to investigate the role of physical activity in the pathogenesis of obesity and type II diabetes mellitus (48).

In conclusion, we believe that the combination of respiratory chamber and doubly labeled water measurements will help us to understand better the risk factors for the development of obesity.

ACKNOWLEDGMENTS

We thank Dr. Clifton Bogardus for his constant help and encouragement. We are indebted to Dr. Laurent Christin, Dr. Daniel Freymond, Dr. Robert Ferraro, Dr. Anne Marie Fontvieille, Dr. Leslie Schulz, Thomas Anderson, and Karen Larson, who conducted most of the 24-hour energy expenditure measurements in the respiratory chamber. Also, we express our sincere gratitude to Inge Harper, who performed all of the mass spectrometry isotopic enrichment determinations. Our thanks also go to Mrs. Carol Lamkin and the nursing staff, to Vicky Boyce and the dietary staff, and to Susan Elson for her help in preparing the manuscript. Finally, we thank all of the volunteers who have made this study possible.

REFERENCES

1. National Center for Health Statistics. *Health, United States 1986*. DHHS publication no. (PHS) 87–1232. Hyattsville: National Center for Health Statistics, 1986.
2. Bray GA. Obesity: definition, diagnosis and disadvantages. *Med J Australia* 1985;142:S2–8.
3. Millar WJ, Stephens T. The prevalence of overweight and obesity in Britain, Canada, and the United States. *Am J Public Health* 1987;77:38–41.
4. U.S. Department of Health & Human Services, Public Health Service, DHHS. *The Surgeon General's report on nutrition and health*. GPO Stock No. 017-001-00465-1. Washington, D.C.: U.S. Government Printing Office, 1988.
5. Foch TT, McCleark GE. Genetics, body weight and obesity. In: Stunkard AJ, ed. *Obesity*. Philadelphia: WB Saunders, 1980;48–71.
6. Mueller WH. The genetics of human fatness. *Yearb Phys Anthropol* 1983;26:215–30.
7. Stunkard AJ, Sorensen TIA, Hanis C, et al. An adoption study of human obesity. *N Engl J Med* 1986;314:193–8.
8. Garrow JS. *Energy balance and obesity in man*, 2nd ed. Amsterdam: Elsevier/North Holland, 1978.
9. Stunkard AJ, Harris JR, Pedersen NL, McCleark GE. The body-mass index of twins who have been reared apart. *N Engl J Med* 1990;322:1483–7.
10. Bouchard C, Tremblay A, Després J-P, et al. The response to long-term overfeeding in identical twins. *N Engl J Med* 1990;322:1477–82.
11. Sims EA. Energy balance in human beings: the problems of plenitude. *Vitam Horm* 1986;43:1–101.
12. Sims EA, Danforth E Jr. Expenditure and storage of energy in man. *J Clin Invest* 1987;79:1019–25.
13. James WPT, Trayhurn P. An integrated view of the metabolic and genetic basis for obesity. *Lancet* 1976;2:770–3.
14. Miller DS, Parsonage S. Resistance to slimming: adaptation or illusion? *Lancet* 1975;1:773–5.
15. James WPT, Davies HL, Bailes J, Dauncey MJ. Elevated metabolic rates in obesity. *Lancet* 1978;1:1122–5.
16. Ravussin E, Bogardus C. Relationship of genetics, age, and physical fitness to daily energy expenditure and fuel utilization. *Am J Clin Nutr* 1989;49:968–75.
17. Durnin JVGA, Edholm OG, Miller DS, Waterlow J. How much food does man require? *Nature* 1973;242:418.
18. Dauncey MJ, Murgatroyd PR, Cole TJ. A human calorimeter for the direct and indirect measurement of 24 h energy expenditure. *Br J Nutr* 1978;39:557–66.

19. Jéquier E. Long-term measurement of energy expenditure in man: direct or indirect calorimetry. In: Björntorp P, Cairella M, Howard A, eds. *Recent advances in obesity research*, volume III. London: John Libbey, 1981;130–5.
20. Schoffelen PFM, Saris WHM, Westerterp KR, Ten Hoor F. Evaluation of an automated indirect calorimeter for measurement of energy balance in man. In: van Es AJH, ed. *Human energy metabolism: physical activity and energy expenditure measurements in epidemiological research based upon direct and indirect calorimetry*. Wageningen: Stichting Nederlands Instituut voor de Voeding (Eur Nutr Rep 5), 1984;51–4.
21. Ravussin E, Lillioja S, Anderson TE, Christin L, Bogardus C. Determinants of 24-hour energy expenditure in man: methods and results using a respiratory chamber. *J Clin Invest* 1986;78:1568–78.
22. Rumpler WV, Seale JL, Conway JM, Moe PW. Repeatability of 24-h energy expenditure measurements in humans by indirect calorimetry. *Am J Clin Nutr* 1990;51:147–52.
23. Vaughan L, Zurlo F, Ravussin E. Effect of age on energy expenditure. *Am J Clin Nutr* 1991:53:821–5.
24. Bogardus C, Lilloja S, Ravussin E, et al. Familial dependence of resting metabolic rate. *N Engl J Med* 1986;315:96–100.
25. Ravussin E, Lilloja S, Knowler WC, et al. Reduced rate of energy expenditure as a risk factor for body weight gain. *N Engl J Med* 1988;318:467–72.
26. Bouchard C, Tremblay A, Nadeau A, et al. Genetic effect in resting and exercise metabolic rates. *Metabolism* 1989;38:364–70.
27. Astrup A, Simonsen L, Bulow J, Christensen NJ. Measurement of forearm oxygen consumption: role of heating the contralateral hand. *Am J Physiol* 1988;255:E572–8.
28. Wade AJ, Marbut MM, Round JM. Muscle fiber type and aetiology of obesity. *Lancet* 1990;335:805–8.
29. Zurlo F, Larson K, Bogardus C, Ravussin E. Skeletal muscle metabolism is a major determinant of resting energy expenditure. *J Clin Invest* 1990;86:1423–7.
30. Kirkwood SP, Zurlo F, Larson K, Ravussin E. Muscle mitochondrial morphology, body composition and energy expenditure in sedentary individuals. *Am J Physiol* 1991;260:E89–94.
31. Astrup AL, Simonsen L, Bullow J, Madsen J, Christensen NJ. Epinephrine mediates facultative carbohydrate-induced thermogenesis in human skeletal muscle. *Am J Physiol* 1989;257:E340–5.
32. Emorine LJ, Marullo S, Briend-Sutren M-M, et al. Molecular characterization of the human β_3-adrenergic receptor. *Science* 1989;245:1118–21.
33. Saad MF, Alger SA, Zurlo F, Young JB, Bogardus C, Ravussin E. Ethnic differences in the sympathetically-mediated energy expenditure. *Am J Physiol* 1991 [In press].
34. Knowler WC, Pettitt DJ, Savage PJ, Bennett PH. Diabetes incidence in Pima Indians: contributions of obesity and parental diabetes. *Am J Epidemiol* 1981;113:114–56.
35. Widdowson EM, Edholm OG, McCance RA. The food intake and energy expenditure of cadets in training. *Br J Nutr* 1954;8:147–55.
36. Durnin JVGA. *Energy, work and leisure*. London: Heinemann Educational Books, 1967.
37. Schoeller DA, van Santen E. Measurement of energy expenditure in humans by doubly-labeled water method. *J Appl Physiol* 1982;53:955–9.
38. Coward WA, Prentice AM, Murgatroyd PR, et al. Measurement of CO_2 and water production rates in man using ^2H, ^{18}O-labeled H_2O; comparisons between calorimeter and isotope values. In: van Es AJH, ed. *Human energy metabolism: physical activity and energy expenditure measurements in epidemiological research based upon direct and indirect calorimetry*. Wageningen: Stichting Nederlands Institut voor de Voeding (Eur Nutr Rep 5), 1984;126–8.
39. Klein PD, James WPT, Wong WW. Calorimetric validation of the doubly-labelled water method for determination of energy expenditure in man. *Hum Nutr Clin Nutr* 1984;38C:95–106.
40. Schoeller DA, Webb P. Five-day comparison of the doubly labeled water method with respiratory gas exchange. *Am J Clin Nutr* 1984;40:153–8.
41. Schoeller DA, Ravussin E, Schutz Y, Acheson KJ, Baertschi P, Jéquier E. Energy expenditure by doubly-labeled water: validation in humans and proposed calculation. *Am J Physiol* 1986;250:R1–8.
42. Westerterp KR, Brouns F, Saris WHM, Ten Hoor F. Comparison of doubly labeled water with respirometry at low- and high-activity levels. *J Appl Physiol* 1988;65:53–6.
43. Ravussin E, Harper I, Rising R, Bogardus C. Energy expenditure by doubly labeled water: validation in lean and obese subjects. *Am J Physiol* 1991;E402–9.
44. Lifson N, McClintock R. Theory of the turnover rate of body water for measuring energy and material balance. *J Theor Biol* 1966;12:46–74.
45. Nagy KA. CO_2 production in animals: analysis of potential errors in the doubly labeled water method. *Am J Physiol* 1990;238:R466–73.

production, and others have taken the beginning and end of the period of measurement, using the two-point method. These do not necessarily give the same results. The multipoint method gives better precision than the two-point method. But when there is sustained deviation of the points on the log plot, as may occur as a result of sustained increase in CO_2 production during the period of study, the CO_2 output may not remain constant during the period of study. It might remain sustained or may have a sustained increase or decrease during a few days—when that happens, the two-point method may in fact be more accurate. It's reassuring that in this study the two-point method and the multipoint method gave similar results.

To reaffirm the points made by Dr. Ravussin, chamber studies and doubly labeled water studies do not indicate the same thing. But they can be complementary. In free-living situations one tries to get an indication of what is happening while an individual is undertaking normal activities. In a chamber one has the potential for studying properly controlled physiologic measurements under properly controlled conditions with individual changes. The two can be complementary and have been used as such in some of the studies that Dr. Ravussin has described.

Energy Metabolism: Tissue Determinants and Cellular Corollaries, edited by J. M. Kinney and H. N. Tucker. Raven Press, Ltd., New York © 1992.

Energy Metabolism: Tissue Determinants and Cellular Corollaries

J. V. G. A. Durnin

Institute of Physiology, University of Glasgow, Glasgow, G12 8QQ, United Kingdom

In this paper calorimetry will be considered as indirect and not direct, because the latter has only very limited applicability to field studies. And as indirect, methods involving both oxygen consumption and (mentioned very briefly) CO_2 production will be included. The techniques therefore are those which measure oxygen consumption by the traditional Douglas Bag method, by various respirometers, which essentially do the same but for longer periods of time, and by the management of CO_2 production using the stable isotopes of O^{18} and deuterium.

TYPES OF FIELD STUDY

The measurement of energy expenditure in the field may be undertaken for several purposes, some of which are listed as follows.

1. It can provide a *baseline for subsequent interpretation* to measure, for example, the energy expenditure of coal-face workers, forestry workers, some military personnel, or other individuals engaged in severe physical work. Such measurements provide a standard against which other less strenuous occupations may be compared. They might also indicate excessive levels of energy expenditure requiring intervention in order to allow work to be continued without the development of undue fatigue.

2. Measurements may be used to obtain an *estimate of the energy requirements* of different types of population. In both developed and developing countries, there is a great dearth of up-to-date information on the energy—and therefore the food—requirements of various groups of people. These requirements vary for different age groups: as an example, adolescents and elderly people might be particularly important. In the former age group, in many industrialized societies the level of total daily energy expenditure might be low enough to give rise to concern in relation to the subsequent development of degenerative cardiovascular disease. Indirect calorimetric studies, because they provide a breakdown of the energy cost and duration of the various activities of a normal day, have a special importance. In the elderly, we have lamentably little knowledge of the significance of the various factors that can affect levels of energy expenditure, such as whether the individual is institu-

tionalized, the effects of minor or major disability, and the degree to which the progressive diminution of physical activity in a normal, relatively mobile elderly person is simply a reflection of a slow and gradual deterioration. The nutritional importance of having more knowledge about total daily energy expenditures in the elderly lies in the fact that physical activity, by increasing energy expenditure, has probably the greatest influence on the amount of food eaten and will therefore considerably affect the intake of components of the diet such as protein, minerals, and vitamins. Activity also improves appetite, maintains mobility, increases social contacts, and produces a general increase in the feeling of well being.

Many other population groups are also important from the point of view of energy requirements. In the investigation of populations in developing countries it can be argued that when energy requirements are being assessed, the preferred method is to measure energy expenditure. Food in adequate quantities may not be available, and if only food (and therefore energy) intake is being measured, the real energy requirements may not be assessed; energy expenditure measurements will provide much fuller and more pertinent information. However, for the large majority of people in developing countries, the economic returns from work are critical for maintaining living standards. Thus, although sufficient energy may be expended to produce the necessary work output (for example, for a subsistence farmer, a paid laborer, or a female household carer), there may not be enough extra energy for leisure pursuits. In such cases, if we examine only *total* daily energy expenditure, this will not necessarily provide much better information than measuring total daily energy intake in food: both will represent a quantity less than the desirable energy needs for that group. On the other hand, if we subdivide the total daily expenditure so that we have a separate measure for the energy expended at work, this will allow the calculation of an additional amount to cover an acceptable quantity of energy for nonoccupational and leisure activities.

3. Some field studies have been done on specific populations *to obtain estimates of the habitual energy expenditure incurred by their way of life.* These have sometimes been people who were malnourished and in whom levels of energy expenditure would be expected to be low (1,2). However, other populations would not necessarily be undernourished, but the environmental and cultural circumstances might be sufficiently unusual to justify the measurements. Examples are the studies by Norgan, Ferro-Luzzi, and Durnin in New Guinea (3) and by Brun and his colleagues (4) in Iran. Much of the information that can be learned from the results of careful studies on populations in exotic environments has relevance to our basic biologic understanding of human energy metabolism.

Another example of the usefulness of measuring energy expenditure in marginally nourished or malnourished populations relates to the ways in which people adapt when food supplies are periodically inadequate. In many parts of the world, food supplies become progressively diminished in the preharvest period, whereas they may be quite satisfactory post-harvest. One of the ways in which people may adapt to this periodic nutritional stress is to reduce the level of voluntary physical activity. They may also adapt by a lowering of the basal metabolic rate (BMR). Measuring energy expenditure will assist us in determining whether such adaptations have occurred.

4. Measuring energy expenditure may be useful *for special populations* for whom food has to be supplied, such as military personnel, prisoners, or people on long-duration expeditions.

5. Measurement may help *to assess the benefits of a food supplementation program on work output*, either as it might affect total energy expenditure at work or in the ability to expend more effort in specific activities. An example is subsistence farming, where the improvement might be measurable in relation to areas of ground tilled or planted or to actual production. The energy expended in single activities such as ploughing or carrying loads might also be increased.

6. A rather esoteric and specialized use of indirect calorimetry in field studies is illustrated by measurements made by Durnin (5) on the *oxygen consumption of mountain climbing*. This was done to obtain an estimate of the quantity of auxiliary oxygen, carried as compressed gas in cylinders, required during the final stages of the first ascent of Mount Everest. Durnin took measurements on a small group of men climbing at an altitude of about 1,000 m and then at 3,500 m, and extrapolated to the situation at 6,000 m upwards.

7. Field studies of energy expenditure in *various forms of sporting activities* have also been undertaken. Sometimes the purpose has been simply to obtain values of the energy expended in games like soccer, or cricket, with no obvious practical objective except for the intrinsic interest. Other times the measurements have been used to assess the efficiency of different types of muscular activity and the effect of training in competitive athletics. Again, certain extremely active sports such as cross-country skiing have been studied to evaluate the maximal or near-maximal levels of energy capable of being expended by very fit individuals.

Often field measurements of oxygen consumption or energy expenditure have been made on large numbers of individuals in standard exercise tests to determine their physical fitness.

Although unrelated to sport, the energy expended at different rates of walking and while carrying loads of various weights has been of interest in assessing physiologic stress in the military and, for load carriage alone, in the construction industry.

8. Last, studies on *basal metabolic rate* (BMR), although usually carried out in laboratory situations, are frequently done in certain field studies. The BMR provides a baseline for determining total daily energy expenditure and is a most important measure of variability between individuals and groups—perhaps differing in body size, body composition, and ethnicity. BMR is also capable of adaptation, either to high energy intakes or to conditions of chronic energy deficiency. A low BMR in an individual may represent little more than a genetic endowment, but low BMRs in a community usually indicate energy insufficiency.

PHYSICAL ACTIVITY, ENERGY EXPENDITURE, AND PHYSICAL FITNESS

Mention has been made of the fact that some field studies on energy expenditure are concerned with assessing the general levels of physical fitness in individuals and in populations. The most important determinant of total energy expenditure is the amount of voluntary or obligatory physical activity once the maintenance requirements of BMR, dietary-induced thermogenesis (DIT), and the minimal essential amount of movement necessary to maintain life are accounted for. Although it is sometimes treated as controversial, the intensity and the duration of physical activity in large part determines the level of daily energy expenditure and is thus responsible for classifying an individual as relatively inactive, moderately active, or very active. With the very large increase in interest and participation in regular physical exercise, because of its widely accepted importance for general health, levels of total energy expenditure for many people might seem to be on the increase. There is also perhaps almost an obsession with fitness; many people equate health with physical fitness, and physical fitness, of course, is highly related to physical activity. However, the relationships between physical activity, physical fitness, and energy expenditure are sometimes complex, and the amount of physical activity required to cause a significant improvement in physical fitness, and to maintain this state, need occupy perhaps no more than 30 minutes per day if the exercise is sufficiently intense. An increase of this order does not, therefore, necessarily have a large influence on levels of total daily energy expenditure. An illustration of this from an industrial context concerns the energy expenditure of men who were engaged in very heavy labor in a steel mill (6) where the extremely arduous work had a total duration of less than 1 hour per day. Because of the particular nature of the work (which required gravel to be shoveled into the steel furnace at high speed), the men had to be big, muscular, strong, and fit. However, because the duration of this activity was quite limited, and because of the fact that for the remainder of the shift the levels of work were quite low, the total energy expenditure of these steel workers was no higher than that of men working continuously at very modest levels of activity in a conveyor belt factory.

Some industrial jobs necessitate fairly continuous physical activity at moderate intensity, and the energy expended may be relatively high even though the individuals need not be particularly fit.

METHODOLOGY IN FIELD SITUATIONS

Only the actual measurement of energy expenditure by indirect calorimetry will be considered in any detail, and no more than passing reference will be made to other even more indirect approaches such as the recording of heart rate and its subsequent extrapolation to energy expenditure, which is an attractive technique to many field workers because it avoids the necessity to measure oxygen consumption. It is also possible to estimate energy expenditure by assessing physical activity (such as by questionnaire or use of pedometers, actometers, or video cameras) and combining this with BMR measurements or using published values of the energy cost of various activities. Physical activity can be assessed by several methods, which have been described in some detail by Durnin (7,8).

TABLE 1. Mean daily energy expenditure of a middle-aged male office worker
(ht. 175 cm; wt. 85 kg)

Activity	Duration (min)	Metabolic cost (kcal/min)	Total (kcal)
Bed	460	1.12	515
Washing, dressing, etc.	85	2.30	195
Sitting	628	1.79	1,124
Standing	147	2.07	304
Moving around in office	60	3.81	229
Walking	50	3.94	197
Kitchen work	10	2.07	21
Total			2,585

Measuring total daily energy expenditure in field situations, or simply estimating the energy expended in work, requires two sets of information. The *first* is a breakdown of the pattern of daily life by means of a timed-diary record of all the day's normal activities. The collected data should be representative of the habitual lifestyle. The *second* set of information is an acceptable estimate of the actual energy expended in each of the important activities of a normal day. Again, this measurement should be done so that the energy value of each activity is representative. The combination of the duration and the energy cost of the activities of the average day allow calculation of energy expenditure, either as a total for the day or for any subdivision of the day (e.g., time spent at work). Tables 1 and 2 show examples of this.

FIELD STUDIES

Miners and Clerks

One of the earliest descriptions of the combination in a field study of the timed-diary record and measurements of energy expenditure of daily activities was written by Durnin in the monograph by Garry et al., "The Expenditure of Energy and Consumption of Food by Miners and Clerks, Fife, Scotland, 1952" (9). This report was a study of a group of men—coal-face miners—who were considered to represent one of the few remaining occupations requiring hard physical labor. As a contrasting group, simultaneous measurements were made of a group of men who worked in the offices of the coal mine. This investigation, as well as being the earliest of its kind, was also somewhat difficult from the aspect of the work situation. The miners started their work shift at about 5:45 A.M. and finished at about 2:00 P.M. They were wound down in a cage to the bottom of the mine shaft at about 600 m below sea level and then had to walk and crawl for about 1 hour to reach the coal face, which was about 200 m lower. The thickness of the coal seam was between 1 and 1.5 m,

TABLE 2. *Mean duration (percent of total) of various types of activities and their contribution to total mean daily energy expediture (ee) of two New Guinean populations*

	Coastal village				Highland village			
	Males		Females		Males		Females	
	% time	% e.e.	% time	% e.e.	% time	% e.e.	% time	% e.e.
Bed	34.4	20.7	35.7	22.8	37.3	20.9	37.2	20.3
Sitting	36.9	27.8	33.4	27.7	26.7	20.2	29.2	23.1
Standing	4.8	3.9	3.1	2.9	6.9	5.6	3.7	3.1
Strolling	2.2	3.3	2.1	2.9	—	—	—	—
All other walking	7.7	19.4	6.5	17.1	10.9	27.3	9.8	25.4
Gardening	1.2	2.2	2.8	5.3	1.8	4.0	6.4	12.2
Fence making	—	—	—	—	2.5	4.9	0.1	0.1
Cash cropping	0.8	2.6	0.2	0.3	1.5	2.1	0.9	1.2
House building	1.8	4.4	0.1	0.2	0.6	1.0	0.3	0.4
Hunting and gathering	1.5	2.3	—	—	0.4	0.7	—	—
Paid employment	2.1	3.8	—	—	1.3	2.0	0.3	0.6
Handicrafts	0.5	0.6	2.0	2.0	0.7	0.7	2.9	2.5
Food preparation	0.3	0.3	5.5	6.4	1.8	1.4	3.0	2.5
Sitting and standing activities	1.5	2.3	2.4	3.7	2.4	3.4	2.8	4.5
Conspicuous leisure	0.9	1.7	0.2	0.4	2.3	2.2	1.2	1.5
Miscellaneous	3.4	4.6	6.0	8.3	2.9	3.6	1.9	2.7
Total	100.0	99.9	100.0	100.0	100.0	100.0	100.0	100.0

so the work had to be done mostly while kneeling. The atmosphere was hot (27–29°C) and humid (about 95% humidity), the air was dusty, and there was continuous noise from the working of the conveyor belts onto which the coal had to be shoveled. The work was intermittent because of frequent brief breakdowns of the conveyor belts, which had to operate at some distance from the power source. The work itself was arduous, consisting of using a pick axe to bring down the coal from the face, shoveling the coal onto the conveyor belt, and then putting up timbers to support the roof above the area from which the coal had been removed.

Conditions for the observers were difficult because they had to record all of the separate activities of the miners in detail and make measurements by means of Max-Planck respirometers (10) of the actual energy being expended in the important activities. Each miner was studied for a total of 7 consecutive days.

Great care was taken to ensure that the actual measurements were both representative of the normal work situation and accurately carried out. Because each observer spent the complete working week with each miner, it was soon very clear whether any measurement was being consciously altered to impress the observer. Moreover, the fact that the observer was continuously present soon led to a form of rapport with the miner, and within a matter of hours a fairly natural state prevailed.

In any case, it would have been difficult for the manner in which the miner worked to be artificially affected because the pattern and intensity of the work was dictated by the amount of coal that had to be cut and the operation of the conveyor belts. However, it is certainly an area of concern that constant observation might have influenced the work pattern.

The measurement of energy expenditure was carried out by obtaining the volume of the expired air during the period of the measurement (which, in this case, was recorded on a counter in the respirometer in liters) together with the oxygen and CO_2 percentage in the expired air. By Weir's formula (11), energy expenditure was calculated from these values.

As far as the actual measurements of energy expenditure, accuracy was maintained by frequent calibration of the precision of the volumetric readings of the respirometer and by accurate analyses of the oxygen and carbon dioxide contents of the expired air. A sample of the expired air was collected in a bladder attached to a tap on the respirometer and was immediately transferred to a glass container, where it could remain until it was taken to the laboratory for analyses without any alteration resulting from diffusion of gases between the container and the atmosphere.

Essentially the same technique was used to study the office clerks. They also had observers assigned to them to record the time spent in the various activities at work—which mostly consisted of sitting, writing, and moving around the office—and to make measurements of the energy expenditure of these components of work. Observation of the clerks was much simpler than that of the miners, and the variety of work activities was also less.

Timed-Diary Record

Both groups of men used the timed diary for the remainder of the day when they were not at work. Various forms of activity diaries have been used by different investigators; the one employed in this particular study and which we have used with almost no modification for 40 years, involves trying to record, to the nearest minute, each activity in a specially designed notebook. Each page in the notebook is subdivided into 120 small squares, one square representing one minute. Thus, each page covered 2 hours (e.g., 10:00 A.M. to noon). There was a separate notebook for each day. Activities were designated by simple code letters—"S" for sitting, "ST" for standing, "D" for washing and dressing, and so on. An observer visited the subject each day and scrutinized the diary record to elucidate any apparently unusual recording, to ask general questions about the pattern of activities, and to ensure that as precise an indication as possible was obtained about how the nonworking day had been spent.

Self-Recording of Activities

One of the problems with self-recording, which applies particularly to sporting activities, concerns the actual duration of the active part of such activities and the proportion of time when a comparatively low level of energy is being expended. For example, a game of football might be recorded as lasting for 1.5 hours or a period of swimming for 40 minutes. However, during these periods, a considerable proportion might have been spent by moving rather gently or even by standing relatively quietly. The classic study by Mayer and his colleagues (12) demonstrated the difference between obese and nonobese adolescent girls while apparently swimming or playing volleyball or tennis. The obese girls spent between 55% and 80% of the time being inactive, whereas the values for the nonobese girls were between 20% and 50%.

Some allowance must therefore be made in order to translate an appropriate value for the energy expenditure of a sport in such a way that it becomes relevant for a particular individual. This is difficult without actual observation or without a measurement of the energy expended in the activity that continues for long enough to represent an average value. Measurement of energy expenditure in sporting activities is also difficult.

Housewives and Adult Working Daughters

A field study on a different population was described by Durnin, Blake, and Brockway (13). In this study food intake and total daily energy expenditure were measured on a group of middle-aged housewives and were contrasted with similar measurements on their adult working daughters. The routine included a self-recorded timed-diary record and energy expenditure measurements of the various tasks involved in housework, again using the Max-Planck respirometer. The daughters all worked in a large department store—selling clothes or cosmetics or doing hair-dressing—in the city of Glasgow.

It is interesting that this study, which took place with the usual requirements of self-recording of activities and the measurement of energy expenditure by use of the respirometer in all the routine important activities of the work day, was feasible even though this was a busy store with the public being present most of the day, occasionally in moderately large numbers.

New Guinean Villagers

An example of another type of field study, on this occasion in a developing country, is provided by ''Energy and Nutrient Intake and the Energy Expenditure of 204 New Guinean Adults,'' a study done by Norgan, Ferro-Luzzi, and Durnin (3). This investigation was much more complex than the previous two studies, particularly in relation to its duration (2 years) and the living conditions for the research team. Two villages were the loci of the study, one being a coastal village on the edge of a moderately open jungle and the other a highland village where the gardens were situated on steep hillsides. The research workers lived for approximately one year in each village in native-built huts and had to set up a field laboratory equipped with a portable generator. The climate in both villages was hot (30–35°C), although nights in the highland village were often quite cool. The work done by both groups of villagers consisted mainly of subsistence farming and walking, since the gardens were usually several kilometers away.

The experimental routine required a timed diary and measurements of energy expenditure, again using the Max-Planck respirometer. However, in this study the whole of the waking day was observed. The duration varied from 5 to 7 consecutive days on each individual. Continuous observation was possible because it was carried out mostly by local assistants, young men and women who had had some elementary school education. Some of them spoke English, but the usual mode of communication was Pidgin English.

The routine of how energy expenditure was measured varied a little. "Lying" and "sitting" were measured using Douglas Bags; other measurements were done with the respirometer. Because of the difficult climatic conditions of heat and humidity, the paramagnetic O_2 and infrared CO_2 analyzers often did not operate accurately and were frequently unusable. O_2 and CO_2 analyses were therefore made using an apparatus that depended on chemical absorption of the gases (in this case, a Lloyd-Haldane apparatus, although the micro-Scholander would also have been suitable). Field studies in such circumstances provide some advantages over similar studies in a more sophisticated environment: Direct observation covering the whole waking day is possible at relatively little expense by using local helpers. The assistants are usually, as was the case in New Guinea, acquainted with the individuals being studied, and indeed were often related to them, so that they could undertake the observation without influencing the habitual behavior of the subjects. A similar example of this technique was the study of Gambian pregnant women by Lawrence, Lawrence, and Whitehead (14) and Gambian children by Lawrence, Lawrence, Durnin, and Whitehead (15). It is also important that the research workers themselves undertake periods of observation and partake in the general activities of the community, such as walking to and from the gardens; from this experience, checks can be made on the accuracy of the observational data collected by the local helpers. Participation also allows a better impression of whether individual subjects are more or less energetic in the manner in which they lead their daily existence.

OTHER FIELD STUDIES

The preceding three field studies have been described in some detail as illustrations of very different types of investigation using similar techniques. Comparable studies have been undertaken by Edholm, Fletcher, Widdowson, and McCance (16) on military cadets; by Spurr (17) on Colombian sugar-cane loaders, by Spurr and Reina (2) on Colombian children; by Brun and his colleagues (4) on Iranian farmers; by Bleiberg, Brun, Goihman, and Lippman (18) on farmers in the Upper Volta; by Torun and Viteri (19) and Torun, Chew, and Mendoza (20) on Guatemalan children; by de Guzman (21) on men working in various occupations in the Phillipines; and by Durnin, McKillop, Grant, and Fitzgerald (22) on pregnant women in Glasgow. A variant of the technique has been used by McNeil (23) in studies in India. Instead of using the Max-Planck respirometer—which is not a very convenient instrument, being cumbersome, unsophisticated, and generally out-dated although still usable—she has made use of the Oxylog (24) for the measurement of energy expenditure. This is a smaller and slightly lighter (2.6 kg) portable instrument that measures pulmonary ventilation and oxygen consumption. The volume of inspired air is measured by a small turbine flow meter, and a sample of expired air is analyzed in a mixing chamber by two compact polarographic sensors (Beckman 672393). This is potentially a more satisfactory instrument except that its design is somewhat complex and, in difficult field conditions, problems of accuracy may arise. McNeil seems to have been satisfied by the performance of her two instruments during her studies in India, but our own experience does not, unfortunately, match this. We have used several Oxylogs and have never found them very reliable. Their calibration for both volumetric measures and oxygen consumption has demonstrated considerable variation. The situation is further complicated in that often the results obtained by the Oxylog appear quite sensible although they may, in fact, be erroneous, so that there may be no obvious signs that the instrument is not performing satisfactorily. The sad conclusion one must come to is that, even in these days of extreme and minuscule instrumentation capable of performing most complex analyses, there is no satisfactory equipment capable of accurately and consistently measuring energy expenditure in field conditions. This conclusion clearly influences the nature of any particular field study and will have a direct bearing on the type and frequency of measurements of everyday activities. It is rather pathetic that we still occasionally have to rely on using the Douglas Bag, the first description of which was given by C. G. Douglas 80 years ago! (25). Indeed, it is salutary to remember the impressive and complete description of the advantages, disadvantages, problems, and errors involved in measuring energy expenditure by several different techniques given in the excellent monograph by Thorne Carpenter in 1915 (26).

VARIATIONS IN TIMED-DIARY RECORDING

Variations in the procedure for either observation or self-recording have been used. One example is the use of regular episodic notes of the activity instead of recordings of the exact time at which activities change. For example, in the study on the pattern of activity of Gambian infants (15), the children were observed each 2.5 minutes by a field worker who wore a watch that gave a bleep sound at these intervals. A detailed description of the infant's activity at the moment of observation was noted using the specific categories of lying, sitting, standing, crawling, walking, or running. Overall, if the various techniques of obtaining data on the duration and nature of the different activities of normal daily life are employed diligently, any discrepancies in the results are probably of minor importance when we take account of intra-individual and interindividual variability.

PROBLEMS AND SOURCES OF ERROR

Timed-Diary Record Inaccuracies

The reliability of self-recording is a reflection of several factors: first, there must be a genuine desire to cooperate. This will be very much influenced by the skill and personality of the research worker and the rapport formed between researcher and subject. Second, a full description of the aims of the study needs to be given with an adequate explanation of what exactly is required. Third, the subject must be visited several times during the 5 or 7 days that are usually needed for the study to be representative. "It would be idle to claim that the measurement of daily energy expenditure is an easy task. A *co-operative* subject with some intelligence is essential. A staff of observers is also required. Observers must have *plenty of common sense* and the ability to *distinguish important from trivial changes in activity*. They must be conscientious and willing to work long and irregular hours, if necessary. A *good sense of humour is invaluable, but little scientific training is necessary*" (27). It is impossible to generalize on how many observers will be required in a given survey. This depends on whether the subjects are employed in a common place of work and engaged in similar activities, how far apart their homes are, and the nature of their recreations.

It is our opinion that to organize and execute measurement of daily energy expenditure presents difficulties comparable to those in surveys of daily energy intake in the food by the weighed individual inventory technique.

A study by Brockett et al. (28) found no significant differences between the data obtained by self-recording and those obtained by observation of selected varied activities during a 2-week period. Most of the other information on this is anecdotal. However, it ill becomes people who have little or unsatisfactory experience of field work to be dogmatic about the reliability of this type of information.

Measurement of Energy Expenditure in Activities

Other aspects of such studies, including the methodology of measuring energy expenditure in the field and the frequency with which measurements are made, are perhaps more open to dispassionate analysis. It is essential that there be proper and repeated calibration of the equipment. It is also essential that the primary purpose of the study be kept in mind when decisions are made about what is to be measured and when. If only a reasonably precise impression is desired about the life-style, particularly that related to the nature and intensity of physical work, the approach may obviously differ from one where detailed data on the exact pattern of life-style and total daily energy expenditure is the objective.

Weir's Equation

A fairly full description of the sources of error and of ways by which these can be minimized when measurements by indirect calorimetry are done in the field is given by Durnin and Brockway (29). One aspect of this technique that was not mentioned and which is either ignored or inadequately appreciated concerns the use of Weir's (11) equation to calculate energy expenditure. Weir's technique does not require the measurement of CO_2, so no data are obtained by this method of calculating the respiratory quotient (RQ). RQs are notoriously unreliable if measurements of energy expenditure are being made with a duration of only 10 to 15 minutes—which is probably the usual practice—because of the possible confusing influence of hyperventilation or hypoventilation. However, on the assumption that RQs can be obtained with reasonable validity, it can be calculated that appreciable error may arise from the use of Weir's formula. Although it is not obvious from the formula, it is in fact sensitive to changes in RQ. Rosenberg (30) has shown that for a range of RQs greater than 0.72 and less than 1.00 (the range expected from pure fat to pure carbohydrate oxidation), the energy expenditure can vary by between 6% and 7% for the same oxygen consumption. Unless, therefore, RQ is actually measured, and unless it truly represents the metabolic mixture being oxidized, there is a built-in possible error of sizeable proportions. Although the errors may be self-canceling, there must be some concern about this in situations requiring high precision.

Use of Published Values of Energy Output

For certain kinds of field study, it may be unnecessary to carry out measurements on all of the varied activities of a normal day because it is possible to utilize values from the published literature. Probably the most convenient table of energy expenditures in a great variety of activities appears in the FAO/WHO/UNU 1985 monograph (31) on energy and protein requirements. There are also some very useful values quoted in an extensive review by Torun on energy expenditure in children (32). The use of such tables, of course, introduces unknown errors, but if the tables are used intelligently by experienced, knowledgeable research workers, they may be adequate for certain purposes—for example, for moderate or strenuous activities of relatively short duration. For many of the important activities that take up much of a normal day—such as sitting or standing activities—there is no proper substitute for actual measurement.

In the investigation of certain populations groups, such as children, accurate and practicable techniques are not available, and it is probably impossible at present to obtain reliable data in such cases.

BMR as a Basis for Calculating Total Energy

In some field studies of energy requirements, the ability to undertake extensive investigations may be restricted, and a different approach may be attempted by measuring only basal metabolic rates (BMR) and then applying one of the following factors: (A) $1.4 \times BMR$ for relatively inactive population groups; (B) $1.7 \times BMR$ for moderately active people: (C) $2.0 \times$ BMR for very active individuals. These factors may be deduced from general information on the group or. more desirably. from data obtained from observational studies. This kind of information will clearly be inadequate to assess energy expenditures for individuals but may provide useful data that can be utilized on a group basis.

Heart Rates as a Basis for Calculating Total Energy

It has previously been suggested that an even more indirect measurement than indirect calorimetry might involve measuring the heart rates of individual subjects and extrapolating these to energy expenditures. Except in difficult circumstances. this procedure seems fraught with problems and large errors. It is certainly possible to record accurately the total heart rate over almost any length of time. from a few minutes up to several days. and to have this broken down so that the pattern of heart rate throughout the day can be assessed. For this information to be transferred to energy expenditure. some attempt at measuring the relationship of heart rate to energy expenditure in a variety of activities must be attempted. There will usually be quite good correlations at moderately high exercise levels. However. with low-intensity activities. there are many extraneous influences on the heart rate—relationships to meals. effects of smoking or drinking coffee or alcohol. emotion. movements involving large or small muscle groups. environmental temperature—that have little influence on energy expenditure. On basic physiologic grounds it is therefore difficult to envisage this technique as being other than very imprecise. In our own experience. when using regression lines derived from the individual's own energy expenditures and heart rates at differing levels of activity. errors varying from 20% to 50% of the actual value have been found. Because much of an average day consists of relative inactivity for many population groups. these errors are maximal because extraneous factors are likely to operate most obviously on the heart rate and not on energy expenditure. The use of heart rate recording has limited validity other than perhaps to subdivide individuals into very general groupings in relation to physical activity. On the other hand. a different experience is described by Spurr in his studies on Colombian children (33): he appears to be satisfied with the usefulness of this method for certain types of group study.

A different form of indirect calorimetry has been introduced where total CO_2 output is used to calculate energy expenditure instead of oxygen consumption. This needs to be done during a continuous period of several days using the stable isotopes of deuterium and O^{18}. The exact technique will not be discussed here. However. though this method can produce data of considerable value on total energy expenditure that may accurately reflect the mean daily output over many days. it tells us nothing about the breakdown of this energy into all the varied activities of work and nonwork situations that comprise a normal day or about important variations in energy metabolism. such as in BMR. It therefore has an important but limited place in field studies of energy expenditure. Detecting significant differences in physical activity—in its form, frequency, and intensity, which may be most important components of a field study—requires different techniques.

CONCLUSION

A certain attitude seems to have arisen in the recent past concerning the measurement of energy expenditure in the field, which may not be in the best interests of expanding our nutritional knowledge. The implication of this attitude is that modern techniques are automatically more informative than traditional ones. In this context, the suggestion is implicit that the only sensible method of measuring energy expenditure in the field is to use the stable isotopes of deuterium and O^{18} to assess CO_2 output. Valuable though this information is when it can be obtained (because of the problems concerned with expense and unreliable analyzing equipment), the extra knowledge gathered is quite limited. A great deal of extra data of considerable value is generated by the traditional techniques. These data are of physiologic, sociologic, and nutritional interest and are of incomparably more use than simply a mean total daily energy expenditure. They tell us about life-style, the pattern of physical activity, and the physiologic stress to the individual.

Therefore, there is still a place—and a very important one—for measuring energy expenditure by indirect calorimetry in the field. The real problem facing research workers planning this form of investigation is the poor and inadequate equipment. A serious effort needs to be made to persuade a manufacturer to construct a small, light-weight, reliable, and accurate instrument to measure oxygen consumption. There is nothing exceptionally complicated about the development of such a piece of apparatus: the basic elements are more-or-less currently available. A convenient instrument would open up opportunities to expand markedly our information on energy expenditure in field situations.

REFERENCES

1. Viteri F, Torun B, Immink M, Flores R. Marginal malnutrition and working capacity. In: Harper AE, Davis GK, eds. *Nutrition in health and disease.* New York: Alan R. Liss, 1981.
2. Spurr GB, Reina JC. Patterns of daily energy expenditure in normal and marginally undernourished school-aged Colombian children. *Eur J Clin Nutr* 1988;42:819–34.
3. Norgan NG, Ferro-Luzzi A, Durnin JVGA. The energy and nutrient intake and the energy expenditure of 204 New Guinean adults. *Phil Trans R Soc Lond B* 1974;268:309–48.
4. Brun TA, Geissler CA, Mirbagheri I, Hormozdiary H, Bastani J, Hedayat H. The energy expenditure of Iranian agricultural workers. *Am J Clin Nutr* 1979;32:2154–61.
5. Durnin JVGA. The oxygen consumption, energy expenditure, and efficiency of climbing with loads at low altitude. *J Physiol* 1955;128:294–309.
6. Durnin JVGA, Blake EC, Allan MK, et al. The food intake and energy expenditure of some elderly men working in heavy and light engineering. *Br J Nutr* 1961;15:587–91.
7. Durnin JVGA. Assessment of physical activity during leisure and work. In: Bouchard C, Shephard RJ, Stephens T, Sutton JR, McPherson BD, eds. *Exercise, fitness and health.* Champaign, IL: Human Kinetics Books, 1990;63–70.
8. Durnin JVGA. Methods to assess physical activity and the energy expended for it by infants and

children. In: Schurch B. Scrimshaw NS, eds. *Activity, energy expenditure and energy requirements of infants and children*. Lausanne: Nestle Foundation, 1990;45–55.

9. Durnin JVGA. Measuring the expenditure of energy: details of technique. In: Garry RC, Passmore R, Warnock GM, Durnin JVGA. *Expenditure of energy and the consumption of food by miners and clerks, Fife, Scotland, 1952*. Med. Res. Coun. Spec. Rep. Ser. No. 289. London: HMSO, 1955;52–4.

10. Müller EA, Franz H. Energieverbrauchsmessungen bei beruflicher Arbeit mit einer verbesserten Respirations - Gasuhr. *Arbeitsphysiologie* 1952;14:499–504.

11. Weir JB de V. New methods for calculating metabolic rate with special reference to protein metabolism. *J Physiol* 1949;109:1–9.

12. Bullen BA, Reed RB, Mayer J. Physical activity of obese and nonobese adolescent girls. Appraisal by motion picture samples. *Am J Clin Nutr* 1964;14:211–23.

13. Durnin JVGA, Blake EC, Brockway JM. The energy expenditure and food intake of middle-aged Glasgow housewives and their adult daughters. *Br J Nutr* 1957;11:85–94.

14. Lawrence M, Lawrence F, Coward WA, Cole TJ, Whitehead RG. Energy requirements of pregnancy in the Gambia. *Lancet* 1987;2:1072–6.

15. Lawrence M, Lawrence F, Durnin JVGA, Whitehead RG. A comparison of physical activity in Gambian and UK children aged 6–18 months. *Eur J Clin Nutr* 1991. [In press].

16. Edholm OG, Fletcher JG, Widdowson EM, McCance RA. The energy expenditure and food intake of individual men. *Br J Nutr* 1955;9:286–300.

17. Spurr GB, Maksud MG, Barac-Nieto M. Energy expenditure, productivity, and physical work capacity of sugarcane loaders. *Am J Clin Nutr* 1977;30:1740–6.

18. Bleiberg F, Brun TA, Goihman S, Lippman D. Food intake and energy expenditure of male and female farmers from Upper Volta. *Br J Nutr* 1981;45:505–515.

19. Torun B, Viteri FE. Energy requirements of pre-school children and effects of varying energy intakes on protein metabolism. *UNU Food Nutr Bull Supp* 1981;5:229–41.

20. Torun B, Chew F, Mendoza RD. Energy cost of activities of pre-school children. *Nutr Res* 1983; 3:401–6.

21. de Guzman PE. Energy allowances for the Philippine population. In: Parizkova J, ed. *Energy expenditure under field conditions*. Prague: Charles University, 1984:23–38.

22. Durnin JVGA, McKillop FM, Grant S, Fitzgerald G. Energy requirements of pregnancy in Scotland. *Lancet* 1987;2:897–900.

23. McNeil G. Patterns of adult energy nutrition in a South Indian village. Ph.D. Thesis: University of London 1986;165–9, 249–57.

24. Humphrey SJE, Wolff HS. The Oxylog. *J Physiol* 1977;267:12.

25. Douglas CG. A method of determining the total respiratory exchange in man. *J Physiol* 1911;42:17.

26. Carpenter TM. A comparison of methods for determining the respiratory exchange of man. *Carnegie Inst Wash* Report No. 216, 1915.

27. Durnin JVGA, Passmore R. *Energy, work and leisure*. London: Heinemann Education Books, 1967.

28. Brockett JE, Konishi F, Brophy EM, et al. The energy expenditure of soldiers in a training company. *US Army Med Nutr Lab* Rep. No. 212, 1957.

29. Durnin JVGA, Brockway JM. Determination of the total daily energy expenditure in man by indirect calorimetry: assessment of the accuracy of a modern technique. *Br J Nutr* 1959;13:41–53.

30. Rosenberg KA. Studies on energy metabolism in man. The calculation of metabolic rate by Weir's formula. PhD thesis: University of Glasgow, 1978:121–33.

31. FAO/WHO/UNU. *Energy and protein requirements*. WHO Tech. Rep. Ser. 724. Geneva: World Health Organization, 1985.

32. Torun B. Energy cost of various physical activities in healthy children. In: Schurch B, Scrimshaw NS, eds. *Activity, energy expenditure and energy requirements of infants and children*. Lausanne: Nestle Foundation, 1990;139–83.

33. Spurr GB, Reina JC. Estimation and validation of energy expenditure obtained by the minute-by-minute measurement of heart rate. In: Schurch B, Scrimshaw NS, eds. *Activity, energy expenditure and energy requirements of infants and children*. Lausanne: Nestle Foundation, 1990;57–69.

Energy Metabolism: Tissue Determinants and
Cellular Corollaries, edited by J. M. Kinney
and H. N. Tucker. Raven Press, Ltd.,
New York © 1992.

Overview: Indirect Calorimetry: Theory and Practice

John M. Kinney

The Rockefeller University, New York, New York 10021 and St. Luke's/Roosevelt Hospital Center, New York, New York 10025

The purpose of this chapter is to provide an overview of the preceding five chapters to identify common themes and to offer a personal perspective on the development of these themes and how they may influence clinical nutrition in the future. Four such themes have been discussed in several of these chapters: measurement techniques, metabolic body size, variability of metabolic rate, and the combination of other measurements with calorimetry.

COMPARISON OF MEASUREMENT TECHNIQUES

Gas measurements for indirect calorimetry are most commonly performed by measuring gas movement in and out of the upper airway. However, this approach depends on understanding the principles and assumptions involved in the movement of O_2 and CO_2 between the mass of body cells and the airway. Fick proposed in 1870 that O_2 consumption could be measured by knowing the cardiac output and arterial-mixed venous difference of O_2. This type of measurement continues to be of interest when monitoring certain patients in the intensive care unit when catheters are in place for following cardiovascular function. When calorimetry by the Fick principle is compared with measurements of pulmonary gas exchange, it is important to be aware that the two methods agree well for energy expenditure. This is true because energy expenditure depends mainly on O_2 consumption, which is estimated with similar precision by both methods. The CO_2 output is less by the Fick principle, so the respiratory quotient is not reliable.

Ferrannini has examined the assumptions of indirect calorimetry starting with the application of input-output analysis to gas exchange, considering the body as a single compartment containing all living cells. The relatively large body gas stores of CO_2 compared with those of O_2 mean that small changes in cellular CO_2 output are not promptly reflected in expired CO_2, whereas small changes in O_2 uptake are readily followed in the pulmonary gas exchange. Thus, measurements of gas exchange are

113

preferred over the Fick principle for measuring energy expenditure, even in the intensive care setting.

Clinical measurements of energy expenditure are usually performed by obtaining relatively short measurements of gas exchange of patients at variable times during the day. This provides a resting metabolic rate in contrast to a conventional basal metabolic rate. However, the results are often reported as a percentage of one of the normal basal metabolic rate standards developed between 1915 and 1952. The appropriateness of using such standards depends on (A) how completely at rest the patient is, (B) whether any significant thermic effect of food (TEF) is present, and (C) whether the ambient temperature is within the thermoneutral zone for that individual. In the hospital setting the subject is considered at rest if he or she has been lying quietly for a short period such as 30 minutes, the TEF is considered insignificant, and the ambient temperature is routinely ignored. In addition to these considerations, there is the difficulty of choosing which of the many standards to use for establishing the normal basal metabolic rate.

The obvious inadequacy of estimating total energy expenditure from brief measurements of resting gas exchange has led to growing interest in 24-hour measurements obtained in a respiration chamber. The dimensions of a respiration chamber usually allow the extent of activity that is possible in a small bedroom, whereas direct calorimeters usually need to be much smaller. A respiration chamber capable of measuring heat loss directly has recently been described (1). The ability to combine prolonged measurements of direct with indirect calorimetry opens the way to exploring the time course of changes in food oxidation versus the subsequent changes in heat loss, as well as the influence of disease and injury on thermoregulation.

Ravussin and Rising have reviewed many aspects of conducting experiments in a respiration chamber. This method offers accuracy and precision and allows comparative measurements during sleep, at rest, before and after meals, and during controlled periods of exercise. It has become apparent from chamber measurements that some previous reports of postprandial thermogenesis have been incorrect because the effects extended beyond the time period measured after the meal. Although measurements in a respiration chamber yield extensive information, the subject is still not under free-living conditions.

The use of doubly labeled water has provided a technique whereby the total energy expenditure can be measured in a free-living individual over 1 to 2 weeks. This method has provided important new data, but certain important assumptions are reviewed by Ravussin and Rising as well as by Elia. It is particularly important that the metabolic and nutritional status of the individual not undergo significant change during the period of measurement.

The need for measuring energy expenditure in the field continues to be a challenge. Such field studies are most often directed toward understanding the energy expenditure associated with various forms of physical activity and learning how such activity influences the total energy expenditure per day. Durnin has reviewed the factors involved in estimating the energy expenditure of workers in various activities, from office work to coal mining. He notes that a low BMR in any individual may represent little more than genetic variation, whereas a low BMR in a community usually indicates insufficient energy intake.

The use of doubly labeled water has considerable appeal for field studies, but there are limitations beyond the expense and availability of isotope analysis. This method provides an average value for CO_2 production over a period of a week or more, so the energy requirements of specific activities cannot be identified. There is a continuing need for reliable measurements of gas exchange in the field. The miniaturization of modern analytic equipment together with advanced data processing should allow the development of new light-weight equipment for field studies. Such improvements in equipment could also contribute to finding less expensive equipment for bedside measurements and perhaps to streamlining the analytic requirements for respiratory chambers.

EXPRESSING THE METABOLIC BODY SIZE

The search for a suitable reference for energy expenditure between animals of varying sizes and subsequently between human beings of different size, age, and sex began with Rubner and Voit in the late 1800s (2). Their experimental data supported the concept that surface area determines heat loss, which then determines heat production, an idea that had a certain intuitive appeal. The concept of surface area had a profound influence on the investigators who sought to establish standards for normality in human energy metabolism. Elia has provided an incisive review of this extensive field.

Kleiber (3) presented a spirited defense against the various explanations that had been advanced for using the surface area as a reference for metabolic rate. Brody and Proctor (4) and Kleiber (5) had published observations in 1932 that showed a remarkably good correlation between metabolic rate and weight to the 0.75 power for mammals from the mouse to the elephant. The experimental evidence for this approach has been reviewed by Heusner (6).

Elia noted in his chapter Energy Expenditure in the Whole Body that over the past century there has been a progressive change in perspective with regard to the determinants of metabolic rate. Attention has moved from heat loss (surface area) to heat production, to the sites of heat production, and finally to mechanisms of heat production in health and disease. Blaxter (7) has extended this change in perspective by suggesting an alternate view of the metabolic size. His concept is summarized in the following paragraph.

"To maintain stability of body temperature, heat production is set at such a level that heat loss can be facilitated and metabolic acceleration, through the Arrhenius–van't Hoff relationship, avoided. This suggests that the metabolic rates of different species (that collectively lead to the Brody-Kleiber relationship) represent the end results of a series of different solutions to the problem of maintaining temperature stability in a physical environment which, during evolution, has probably been fairly constant in terms of its effects on avenues of heat loss. It should be appreciated that the temperature and radiation limits for sustained plant and animal life are really quite small. Different anatomical and physiological strategies, some of which are dictated by dimensional constraints, have been adopted by different species in reaching such solutions. *The real question is perhaps not so much why metabolic rate should appear to vary with $Wt^{0.75}$, but why central temperature should be set within such relatively narrow limits"*(7).

The concept of the lean body mass (LBM) was developed by Behnke (8) and later replaced by the fat-free mass (FFM) of Grande and Keys (9). Much of the utility of the FFM depends on the reliability of the methods for assessing the FFM. Elia has critically analyzed these methods and emphasized that none of the methods are free of uncertain assumptions and potential errors. Owen et al. (10) reported in their studies that body weight alone was as good a reference as any of the customary approaches to metabolic body size that has been proposed.

There has been a growing uncertainty as to whether age is a factor in predicting resting energy expenditure when FFM is used as a reference. The estimate of FFM from measuring total body water usually assumes a hydration of 0.73. A recent report on elderly subjects has found that the hydration of the FFM varied from 0.69 to 0.80 (11). Such variation is perhaps related to variable expansion of the extracellular phase and emphasizes the need to develop better methods for assessing extracellular as well as total body water.

Ravussin and Rising have presented 24-hour energy expenditure data, expressed per unit of FFM. However, they find that the fat mass of an individual, as well as the FFM, contributes to a small but definite degree in the variation in energy expenditure between normal individuals, whether for the total 24 hours, for the basal, or the sleeping, state. They note that skeletal muscle has often been neglected when seeking to explain interindividual differences in resting energy expenditure. Because skeletal muscle comprises approximately 40% of body weight in nonobese subjects, this tissue can account for 20% to 30% of the total resting oxygen uptake. The resting oxygen uptake of the forearm muscle was found to account for part of the variance in resting metabolic rate among normal subjects.

Miller and Blyth (12) have suggested that the rate of basal metabolism reflects the sum of the contribution of individual organs, which should be related to the "active body mass." Moore et al. (13) used the measurement of total exchangeable potassium to reflect the "body cell mass," which they defined as the sum of the tissues that oxidized substrate, performed work, and yielded heat. The application of neutron activation has offered the possibility of measuring body nitrogen stores. To date this has not served as a useful reference for energy expenditure, although the combined measurement of body potassium and body nitrogen has allowed Burkinshaw et al. (14) and Cohn et al. (15) to make calculations of muscle mass in the body. Jeejeebhoy (16) has emphasized that total body potassium may change independently of body nitrogen, particularly in states of malnutrition.

Grande (17) assessed the contribution made by different organs to overall oxygen consumption. This can be done by measuring blood flow and AV differences in oxygen content as well as by considering organ weight and data for in vitro oxygen consumption. Grande reported, as have others, that such assessments do not add up to the total measured oxygen consumption of the whole body. Differences in organ size between species, with or without some variation in metabolic activity, appear to explain many of the differences in metabolic rate between different mammals. Elia has assembled information that presents the contribution of the major organs to the BMR from birth to the age of 45 years. The metabolic rate per gram of each appears to change little during growth and development. Therefore, the higher metabolic rate of infants and children compared to adults can largely be explained by the presence of a larger proportion of metabolically active tissues in younger individuals. The brain, which accounts for almost one-half of the total energy expenditure of the infant, decreases in proportion to body weight during growth and development so that in the adult it is responsible for only 20% of the BMR. At the same time, skeletal muscle, which is less metabolically active than the brain and other organs, increases in proportion to body weight during growth and development. The sum of metabolic rate per kg of organ weight for the total of liver, kidney, brain, and heat remains remarkably stable during growth and development in contrast to the changes in metabolic rate per kg of body weight or per square meter. In animals of the same species, the ratio of organ weights to body weights appears to get smaller with increasing size of the individual. This is consistent with various observations in humans, in which larger individuals have a lower metabolic rate per kg of body weight or per kg of FFM than smaller individuals.

THE VARIABILITY OF NORMAL METABOLIC RATE

A significant difficulty remains after measuring the basal, or resting, energy expenditure and expressing the results in terms of some reference for metabolic body size. This difficulty involves the decision as to which set of standard values to use for defining normality. Elia has presented a comprehensive review of the various standards for metabolic rate and noted how most of the standards that were introduced between 1917 and 1952 provided empirical relationships between surface area (calculated from height and weight) and basal metabolic rate. Harris and Benedict published their prediction equations in 1919 but refused to involve any calculation of surface area. Their equations are widely used in clinical practice today, although several reports have indicated that these equations tend to overestimate the energy expenditure by 5% to 10%.

Elia has reviewed the discrepancies that become apparent upon comparison of the various standards for metabolic rate. Some of the variability relates to the number of individuals included in a given series despite mild obesity. However, significant differences are still evident when comparing individuals of the same body mass index. The various standards imply different effects of age on metabolic rate. The Harris-Benedict equations predict a decrease of 15% to 21% in the BMR of males and 11% to 16% in females between 25 and 65 years of age. Owen et al. (10) found that the correlation between age and metabolic rate was so low that age was excluded from

fatty acid emphasizes the metabolic events that are not in equilibrium with a substrate entering the blood stream.

Thorburn et al. (22) have recently reported errors in substrate oxidation when the hyperinsulinemic clamp procedure is combined with indirect calorimetry. During the clamp procedure, urinary nitrogen was found to increase by an amount that introduced significant errors in the calculation of glucose and fat oxidation, though causing no change in the estimation of energy expenditure.

The measurement or estimation of energy expenditure cannot be avoided by anyone interested in the nutritional aspects of energy balance. Indeed, much of the resurgence of interest in clinical measurements of energy expenditure has arisen from the stimulus of nutritional support for the ill or depleted patient. The reviews of indirect calorimetry in the preceding chapters, however, emphasize the importance of further development in the methodology for measuring gas exchange and point out the need for a convenient approach to measuring the metabolic body size.

The brief bedside measurements of gas exchange that are common in the hospital setting leave uncertainties when extrapolating to a 24-hour energy expenditure for calculating the appropriate caloric intake. Studies of many hours' duration are possible in a respiration chamber for certain relatively stable clinical conditions. Chamber studies in the future are needed to examine the reliability of daily energy expenditure when estimated from brief bedside measurements.

A different type of clinical validation is available on a research basis, namely, the doubly labeled water technique. The method provides an estimation of the average CO_2 production over a period of a week or more. This approach may be of great importance to measure total energy expenditure in certain relatively stable clinical conditions, but the results would be difficult to interpret when energy expenditure, or nutritional intake, is changing as convalescence progresses.

At the present time, the resting energy expenditure of any particular diagnostic group of patients can be expressed only as a fairly wide range of values. This fact is often obscured by expressing the mean value for that diagnostic group as a percentage above or below the mean for some historic standard of normal values. Future efforts to narrow the ranges for groups of patients will require a better and more convenient definition of the metabolic body size.

The resting energy expenditure of a patient is a balance between catabolic stimuli, which increase the energy expenditure, and tissue depletion, which decreases the energy expenditure. It seems reasonable to expect that in the future, independent evidence beyond gas exchange will be sought to indicate the magnitude of each of these two opposing forces that together result in any deviation from the normal resting energy expenditure.

REFERENCES

1. Seale JL, Rumpler WV, Conway JM, et al. Comparison of doubly labeled water, intake-balance, and direct-indirect calorimetry methods for measuring energy expenditure in adult men. *Am J Clin Nutr* 1990;52:66–71.

2. Kinney JM. Food as fuel: the development of concepts. In: Shils ME, Young VR, eds. *Modern nutrition in health and disease*. Philadelphia: Lea and Febiger, 1980;516–32.
3. Kleiber M. *The fire of life: an introduction to animal energetics*. Huntington, NY: Robert E. Krieger, 1975;179–222.
4. Brody S, Proctor RC. Growth and development with special reference to domestic animals: further investigations of surface area in energy metabolism. *University of Missouri Agricultural Experiment Station Research Bulletin*, No. 116.
5. Kleiber M. Body size and energy metabolism. *Hilgardia* 1932;6:315–53.
6. Heusner AA. Body size and energy metabolism. *Ann Rev Nutr* 1985;5.
7. Blaxter K. *Energy metabolism in animals and man*. Cambridge: Cambridge University Press, 1989;146.
8. Behnke J. *Human body composition*. Oxford: Pergamon Press, 1965.
9. Grande F, Keys A. Body weight, body composition and calorie status. In: Goodhart RS, Shils ME, eds. *Modern nutrition in health and disease*. Philadelphia: Lea and Febiger, 1980;3–34.
10. Owen OE, Holup JL, D'Alessio A, et al. A reappraisal of the caloric requirement of men. *Am Clin Nutr* 1987;46:8765–85.
11. Baumgarten RN, Heymsfield SB, Lichtman S, Wang J, Pierson RN Jr. Body composition in elderly people: effect of criterion estimates on predictive equations 1–3. *Am J Clin Nutr* 1991;53:1345–53.
12. Miller AT, Blyth CS. Lean body mass as a metabolic reference standard. *J Appl Physiol* 1953;5:311–16.
13. Moore FD, Olesen KH, McMurrey JD, et al. *The body cell mass and its supporting environment: body composition in health and disease*. Philadelphia: WB Saunders, 1963.
14. Burkinshaw L, Hill GL, Morgan DB. Assessment of the distribution of protein in the human body by in vivo neutron activation analysis. *IAEA-SM* 1979;39:787–98.
15. Cohn SH, Vaswani AN, Yasumura S, et al. Assessment of cellular mass and lean body mass by non-invasive nuclear techniques. *J Lab Clin Med* 1985;105:305–10.
16. Jeejeebhoy KN. Mechanism of reduction of total body potassium in malnutrition. In: Yasumura S, Harrison JE, McNeill KG, et al., eds. *In vivo body composition studies: recent advances*. New York: Plenum Press, 1990;143–8.
17. Grande F. Energy expenditure of organs and tissue. In: Kinney JM, ed. *Assessment of energy metabolism in health and disease*. Columbus, OH: Ross Laboratories, 1980;88–92.
18. Keys A, Taylor HI, Grande F. Basal metabolism and age of adult men. *Metabolism* 1973;22:579–89.
19. Schofield. Predicting basal metabolic rate, new standards and review of previous work. *Hum Nutr Clin Nutr* 1985;39C:5–91.
20. Quenouille MH, Boyne AW, Fisher WB, et al. *Statistical studies of recorded energy expenditure in man. Part I. Basal metabolism related to sex, stature, age, climate and race*. Commonwealth Bureau of Animal Nutrition. Technical communication, No. 17.
21. Simonson DC, DeFronzo RA. Indirect calorimetry: methodological and interpretative problems. *Am J Physiol* 1990;258:E399–E412.
22. Thorburn AW, Gumbiner B, Flynn T, Henry RR. Substrate oxidation errors during combined indirect calorimetry–hyperinsulinemic glucose clamp studies. *Metabolism* 1991;40:391–8.

Energy Metabolism: Tissue Determinants and Cellular Corollaries, edited by J. M. Kinney and H. N. Tucker. Raven Press, Ltd., New York © 1992.

Calorie Balance Versus Nutrient Balance

Eric Jéquier

Institute of Physiology, University of Lausanne, Lausanne 1005, Switzerland

The mechanisms involved in the regulation of body weight are complex and poorly understood. It is clear that the maintenance of a stable body weight results from a precise balance of energy intake and energy expenditure. It is interesting to mention that if metabolizable energy (which is the food energy available for metabolic processes after subtraction of fecal and urinary losses from energy intake) was every day greater by 5% than energy expenditure, a weight gain of about 5 kg would be observed within one year. This suggests that the mechanisms that adapt energy intake to the level of energy expenditure, or the mechanisms involved in the control of energy expenditure, are efficient in most individuals. Another consequence of this reasoning is the fact that obesity can develop with a very small difference between energy intake and energy expenditure when the energy balance is chronically positive. This is the main reason that it is very difficult to assess the etiology of obesity in most patients.

This chapter presents a summary of recent data obtained in human subjects dealing with investigations on energy and nutrient balances. The first question is to know whether metabolic wastage can be demonstrated in humans or, in other words, whether an excess energy consumption can appear as heat, a concept called "luxus-consumption." It is germane to limit this presentation to human studies, because experiments in animals, such as rats or dogs, are difficult to interpret owing to the difficulty in assessing the influence of physical activity on energy expenditure.

Energy expenditure can be divided into three major components: basal metabolic rate, thermic effect of food, and thermic effect of exercise. Basal metabolic rate is the energy expended for homeostatic processes and is measured in a resting post-absorptive subject in the morning. It represents 60% to 70% of the total energy expended by most sedentary individuals, and it is related to the size of the fat-free mass of the individuals (1–3). It is important to mention that obese subjects are characterized not only by an excessive fat mass but by a concomitant enlargement of the fat-free mass. Thus, obese individuals expend more energy in the basal state than lean subjects.

The thermic effect of food represents the increase in energy expenditure following meal ingestion; it includes two components, which have been called "obligatory" and "facultative" thermogenesis (4). Obligatory thermogenesis results from the energy expended for absorbing, processing, and storing the nutrients. For instance, the cost of converting glucose to glycogen corresponds to about 5% of the glucose energy content, whereas it amounts to 24% of the energetic content of glucose if this compound is converted into lipids (5). Digestion, absorption, and storage of ingested fat is an economical process because it amounts to about 4% of the fat energy being stored. By contrast, protein ingestion induces the largest "obligatory" metabolic response, corresponding to about 25% of the protein energy owing to the high cost of protein synthesis, gluconeogenesis, and ureogenesis (5).

The facultative component of thermogenesis involves the activation of the sympathetic nervous system (6). Carbohydrate overfeeding induces a sustained rise of urinary norepinephrine (7), and infusions of glucose and insulin cause an increase in norepinephrine plasma levels (8). An additional proof of the activation of the sympathetic nervous system after carbohydrate infusion is the reduction of the glucose-induced thermogenic response by β-adrenergic blockade with propranolol (9,10). Figure 1 illustrates the energy cost to store glucose and glycogen in a human; it shows that the biochemical cost of glycogen synthesis of about 0.8 kJ/g (third column) is identical to the measured cost (second column) obtained in man during a euglycemic insulin clamp carried out with a concomitant infusion of propranolol to block β-adrenergic receptors. By contrast, the first column (1.5 kJ/g) shows the real increase in energy expenditure to store 1 g glucose in the absence of β-adrenergic receptors blockade. The difference between the first and second columns represents the facultative thermogenesis, which is a component of energy expenditure that depends on the stimulation of the sympathetic nervous system. The magnitude of the facultative component of the thermic effect of food is, however, limited in humans.

Summarizing the results of human studies under conditions of overfeeding, one can conclude that approximately one-fourth of the excess in energy intake above

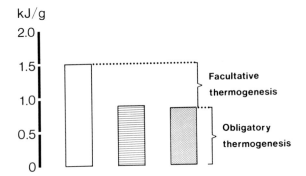

FIG. 1.   Energy cost (kJ/g) to store glucose in man. The first column (open column) represents the energy cost to store glucose measured during intravenous glucose infusions with insulin (euglycemic insulin clamp). The second column (hatched column) represents the energy cost to store glucose after β-receptor blockade with propranolol. The third column (dotted column) illustrates the calculated obligatory cost to store glucose. The difference between the first and the third column represents facultative thermogenesis. The middle column shows that facultative thermogenesis is suppressed by β-receptor blockade (data from ref. 9).

maintenance requirements can be dissipated as heat. This means that about three-fourths of an excess of food energy is stored in the body, mainly as lipid in adipose tissue (11). The thermogenic capacity of the human body toward an excessive food intake is limited. Therefore, since energy expenditure is not much affected by the amount of energy intake, it is likely that the control of energy expenditure plays a smaller role in body weight regulation than the control of food intake.

Studies on calorie balance in humans have shown that the facultative thermogenesis is a small component of the total energy expended (4). Therefore, it is doubtful that changes in the magnitude of the thermic effect of food play a major role in body weight regulation. The third component of total energy expenditure is the thermic effect of exercise. It is clear that the level of spontaneous physical activity varies among individuals and that considerable differences in the amount of energy expended can be accounted for by the duration and the intensity of physical activity. In addition, obese individuals expend more energy in body weight–bearing activities than lean subjects for the same task. When considering the three components of energy expenditure—namely, basal metabolic rate, thermic effect of food, and thermic effect of exercise—it appears that obese individuals expend more energy than lean sedentary subjects, mainly because of their elevated basal metabolic rate (expressed in absolute values) (2,3). These studies (1,2,3) have therefore shown that the concept of obese individuals who claim to be "small eaters" is certainly erroneous.

THE CONCEPT OF NUTRIENT BALANCE

The study of body weight regulation is generally limited to the concept of energy balance. People eat not "energy" but nutrients. Energy is a physical concept, and the body has no receptors to measure energy. It is therefore appropriate to consider the mechanisms responsible for nutrient balance. There are large differences between the balances of the three macronutrients: proteins, carbohydrates, and fats, and this may play an important role in body weight regulation (12).

The ability to achieve protein balance over a wide range of intakes is well documented in humans. Studies on nitrogen balance can be relatively easily carried out, and within a certain range of protein intakes, the maintenance of a constant protein content is observed. Thus, the regulation of body weight is not primarily dependent on protein balance. Before studying how the body maintains carbohydrate and lipid balances, one should know whether de novo synthesis of fatty acids from glucose is an active pathway in humans. If carbohydrate intake could be converted to fat to a great extent, the concept of carbohydrate and lipid balances would be of little interest (12).

DIETARY CARBOHYDRATES DO NOT INCREASE THE FAT MASS BY DE NOVO LIPOGENESIS

It is often assumed that excess carbohydrates are readily transformed into fat in humans (13). Liver and adipose tissue contain the enzymes necessary for the con-rate of net de novo lipogenesis in humans, because a carbohydrate intake of 1 kg per day is an experimental load that is never consumed in everyday life.

This study also showed that glycogen stores must increase by about 500 g before appreciable de novo lipogenesis begins. When the glycogen stores become saturated, the only way of disposing of additional excess carbohydrate is fat synthesis in addition to maximal glucose oxidation for energy generation. These findings also indicate that the body's glycogen stores are not completely filled under normal ad libitum conditions of food intake. Therefore, one can conclude that net de novo lipogenesis from carbohydrates is a quantitatively insignificant pathway in the whole human organism.

EFFECT OF THE FAT CONTENT OF A MEAL ON SUBSTRATE OXIDATION

The ingestion of a mixed meal containing nutrients in the same proportion as the mixture oxidized before food intake (15%, 35%, and 50% for protein, carbohydrate, and fat energy, respectively) induces a stimulation of carbohydrate oxidation and a decrease in fat oxidation (21). This response is due to the carbohydrate content of the meal, because reducing the fat content of the meal (and maintaining the same amount of protein and carbohydrates) induces the same stimulation of carbohydrate oxidation as the 50% fat meal. It is likely that the increase in insulin secretion after the meal plays a major role in stimulating glucose uptake in muscles and glucose oxidation in the whole body. It is interesting to emphasize that part of the stimulation of glucose metabolism by insulin following meal ingestion is related to the inhibitory effect of insulin on lipolysis and to the subsequent decline in plasma FFA levels. The decrease in the availability of free fatty acids favors glucose uptake and its further metabolism in muscles. This is a consequence of the glucose–fatty acid cycle described by Randle et al. (22).

Flatt has shown in our laboratory that the fat content of a mixed meal influences neither the glycemic nor the insulinemic postprandial responses (21). In addition, the time course of the changes in the respiratory quotient following a meal is not affected by its fat content, indicating that the mixture of nutrients oxidized after the meal is independent of the amount of fat intake. Fat intake does not promote fat oxidation over a period of 9 hours following a meal (21), indicating that fat balance is poorly controlled.

The possibility remained that a more delayed effect of fat intake on metabolic fuel oxidation could occur later. To study this question, we carried out a study in which an additional amount of 106 ± 6 g fat was added to a mixed maintenance 24-hour diet given to seven young men. The oxidation rate of nutrients was measured over 24 hours with a respiration chamber (23). The fat supplement did not alter 24-hour energy expenditure and failed to promote the use of fat as a metabolic fuel. Figure 3 shows the results of this study; it is worth emphasizing that the whole fat supplement was stored because there was no evidence of fat malabsorption. Thus, a met-

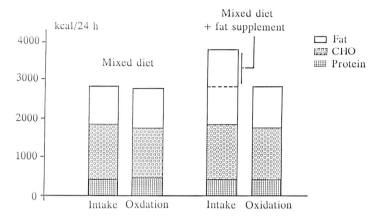

FIG. 3. Effect of a fat supplement on nutrient oxidation. On the first day (mixed diet), seven subjects received three meals—breakfast, lunch, and dinner—with 15%, 50%, and 35% of energy as protein, carbohydrates, and fat, respectively. The first column shows the nutrient intake, and the second column, the nutrient oxidation. The subjects were in energy and nutrient balance. On the second day (third column), the subjects received a 106 g fat supplement above the same nutrient intake as the preceding day. The fourth column shows that the nutrient oxidation rates were identical to the rates measured on the first day.

abolic response serving to increase fat oxidation in the face of an increased fat intake is lacking. The regulation of fat balance differs markedly from the regulation of the carbohydrate balance; only the latter is adjusted by an increased oxidation rate of carbohydrates after meal ingestion, whereas no stimulation of fat oxidation occurs.

In everyday life, gains or losses of fat are small in comparison with the body's fat content. It is therefore difficult to imagine feedback signals from the small changes in adipose tissue fat stores serving to modulate food intake. By contrast, significant deviations from the carbohydrate balance can occur with changes in the everyday intake of carbohydrates, considering the body's relatively small glycogen reserves. Thus, changes in glycogen stores are much more likely to influence subsequent food intake than small changes in the adipose tissue mass. It will therefore be necessary to study separately the mechanisms involved in stabilizing the body's glycogen reserves and its fat stores. In addition, recent investigations have shown how cumulated changes in fat stores from adipose tissue may ultimately contribute to enhanced fat oxidation.

OBESITY MAY RESULT FROM A CHRONICALLY POSITIVE FAT BALANCE

The increased incidence of obesity during this century could be the result of a change in food habits favoring a high percentage of lipids in the diet (24). Since fat intake does not promote fat oxidation, any excess of fat in the everyday diet is stored and contributes to increase the adipose tissue mass. Stability of body weight is achieved when the composition of the fuel mix oxidized is equal on the average to the composition of the diet. According to Flatt (25,26), when the percentage of fat in the everyday diet is high, body weight increases until fat-cell hypertrophy and hyperplasia is such that the overall rate of lipolysis in adipose tissue provides an increased amount of free fatty acids, which stimulate fat oxidation. Thus, stimulation of fat oxidation occurs only when the adipose tissue mass is enlarged. Figure 4 illustrates the rate of lipid glucose oxidation in a group of control subjects, a group of obese patients, and a group of obese patients with impaired glucose tolerance during an oral glucose tolerance test and a euglycemic glucose clamp. Note that the obese groups are characterized by an increased lipid oxidation rate (27). Another mechanism to increase fat oxidation would be an enhancement of physical activity, but this is rarely successful in obese subjects.

The association between diet composition and body fatness was studied recently. As expected, high-fat consumers displayed greater fat mass and percent body fat than did low-fat consumers (28). These results suggest that the fat content of the habitual diet may have a large influence on the steady state of weight maintenance in adult individuals. The important question is to know whether individuals who consume high-fat diets have an elevated energy intake. Lissner et al. (29) showed that a high-fat diet (45–50% energy as fat) induced an increase in energy intake by 15% as compared to a medium-fat diet in 24 women who consumed each diet during a 2-week period. By contrast, a low-fat diet (15–20% energy as fat) induced a decrease in energy intake by 11% during a two-week period. The stimulation of a high-fat diet on energy intake is usually attributable to the high-energy density of fat-rich foods

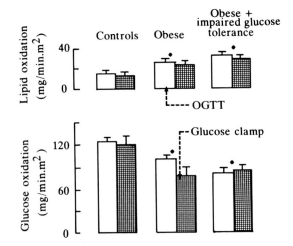

FIG. 4. Rates of lipid and glucose oxidation in a group of control subjects, a group of obese patients, and a group of obese patients with impaired glucose tolerance after glucose ingestion (100 g oral glucose) (open bars) and during a euglycemic insulin clamp (hatched bars). *p < 0.05 vs. Controls. Note the enhanced lipid oxidation rates in the two obese groups and the concomitant lowered glucose oxidation rates (data from ref. 27).

and to the small stomach distension induced by the ingestion of such foods. However, it is also possible that the regulation of food intake depends in part on the carbohydrate needs of the individuals. Because several tissues, such as the brain, have an obligatory requirement of glucose, one should eat more food to ingest a minimal amount of carbohydrates when the diet has a low-carbohydrate, high-fat content. This hypothesis was confirmed by Tremblay et al. (28), who showed that a low-carbohydrate, high-fat diet induced a short-term increase in food intake in young male subjects.

COMPARISON BETWEEN THE FOOD QUOTIENT AND THE RESPIRATORY QUOTIENT

Body weight stability is achieved when the composition of the fuel oxidized is equal on average to the composition of the diet. Flatt has defined the food quotient (FQ) as the ratio of CO_2 produced to O_2 consumed, when a representative sample of the diet consumed is oxidized in a bomb calorimeter (12). When energy balance over 24 hours is achieved, FQ is equal to the mean respiratory quotient (RQ) of the subject. Conditions of positive energy balance are characterized by an RQ/FQ value greater than 1.0 (Fig. 5), indicating that the amount of lipid oxidized is less than that

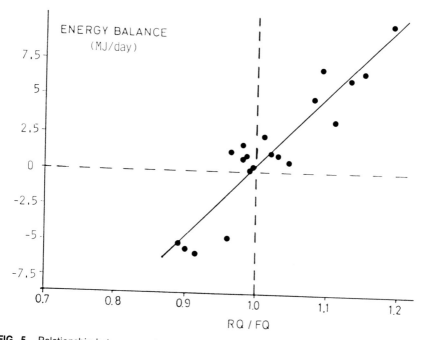

FIG. 5. Relationship between respiratory quotient (RQ)/food quotient (FQ) ratio and the energy balance in humans. Each point represents the values for a given subject measured over a 24-hour period.

ingested (i.e., fat accumulation). By contrast, an RQ/FQ value lower than 1.0 indicates that the amount of lipid oxidized exceeds that ingested (i.e., endogenous fat oxidation) (Fig. 5).

Figure 5 shows a linear relationship between RQ/FQ values and energy balance. This implies that measurements of the RQ/FQ ratio over 24 hours permits an indirect assessment of the subject's energy balance. The figure indicates that when the mean 24-hour RQ is maintained below the FQ (RQ/FQ ratio <1.0), the subject is in negative energy balance. Thus, conditions of negative energy balance imply that the fuel mix oxidized contains more fat than the mixture supplied by the diet. In other words, oxidation of endogenous lipids must occur. This also shows that the storage of carbohydrates is very small in comparison with the lipid storage and that an energy deficit cannot be compensated for by endogenous carbohydrate utilization.

Conditions of positive energy balance are characterized by an average RQ that exceeds the FQ (RQ/FQ ratio >1.0). This means that the fuel mix oxidized contains less fat than the mixture supplied by the diet. This implies a net fat storage of dietary fat into adipose tissue, a condition that may lead to obesity. A second possibility to explain an RQ/FQ ratio >1.0 is a fuel mix oxidized that contains more carbohydrates than the mixture supplied by the diet; this can occur acutely, but this phenomenon must lead to a compensatory increase in food intake in order to maintain carbohydrate balance. Therefore, this mechanism leads to a positive energy balance and to the storage of a fraction of the ingested fat. A third explanation for an RQ/FQ ratio >1.0 could be the occurrence of net lipogenesis, a condition that increases the nonprotein RQ above 1.0. As discussed before, this metabolic process does not occur under normal conditions of food intake and is operating only under conditions of carbohydrate overfeeding and total parenteral nutrition with excess glucose administration.

Energy balance studies are difficult to perform in humans because of the need to measure energy expenditure. The methods of measuring RQs frequently during 24 hours and the calculation of the RQ/FQ ratio is of potential interest to assess the state of energy balance indirectly in patients who need a nutritional support. The strategy of body weight control should aim to maintain an RQ/FQ value lower than 1.0 or equal to 1.0. This is best achieved by lowering the fat content of the everyday diet and by favoring the conditions that increase fat oxidation, such as aerobic exercise of low intensity and long duration. A period with an RQ/FQ ratio lower than 1.0 therefore demonstrates a loss of body fat, a necessary condition for weight loss in an obese patient. This concept also shows that it is easier to maintain the average RQ below the FQ when the diet has a high-carbohydrate, low-fat content (high FQ).

IMPLICATIONS OF THESE CONCEPTS FOR THE TREATMENT OF OBESITY

Regulation of food intake is of primary importance in achieving energy balance because energy expenditure is little affected by the amount of food intake. Spontaneous adjustments of food intake are more likely to be dependent on carbohydrate than on lipid balance. Therefore, a high-carbohydrate, low-fat diet should be a logical approach for weight maintenance. Recent studies provide additional support to this concept by showing that a low caloric density of the diet causes spontaneous caloric deficits (30–33). These studies indicate that reducing fat intake may be a more effective strategy for weight loss than consuming artificially sweetened foods. Advice aiming at the reduction of habitual fat intake without imposing limitation on the quantity of low-fat food consumption, appears to be a promising approach to avoid relapse of body weight regain after a hypocaloric treatment in "postobese" individuals.

Prospective studies are needed to assess whether a small spontaneous caloric deficit induced by a high carbohydrate, low-fat diet can be maintained for prolonged periods. The choice of the carbohydrates in the everyday diet is probably important; starchy foods that are digested slowly and produce low blood glucose and insulin responses (34) may be of interest in appetite control of patients who must chronically restrict their energy intake (35).

REFERENCES

1. Halliday D, Hesp R, Stalley SF, Warwick P, Altman DG, Garrow JS. Resting metabolic rate, weight, surface area and body composition in obese women. *Int J Obes* 1979;3:1–6.
2. Ravussin E, Burnand B, Schutz Y, Jéquier E. Twenty-four-hour energy expenditure and resting metabolic rate in obese, moderately obese, and control subjects. *Am J Clin Nutr* 1982;35:566–73.
3. Ravussin E, Lillioja S, Anderson TE, Christin L, Bogardus C. Determinants of 24-hour energy expenditure in man; methods and results using a respiration chamber. *J Clin Invest* 1986;78:1568–78.
4. Jéquier E, Schutz Y. Energy expenditure in obesity and diabetes. *Diabetes Metab Rev* 1988;4:583–93.
5. Flatt JP. The biochemistry of energy expenditure. In: Bray GA, ed. *Recent advances in obesity research*, vol. II. London: Newman Publishing, 1978;211–28.
6. Welle S, Lilavivat U, Campbell RG. Thermic effect of feeding in man: increased norepinephrine levels following glucose but not protein or fat consumption. *Metabolism* 1981;30:953–8.
7. Schutz Y, Acheson KJ, Jéquier E. Twenty-four-hour energy expenditure and thermogenesis: response to progressive carbohydrate overfeeding in man. *Int J Obes* 1985;9:111–4.
8. Rowe JW, Young JB, Minaker KL, Stevens AL, Pallotta J, Landsberg L. Effect of insulin and glucose infusions on sympathetic nervous system activity in normal man. *Diabetes* 1981;30:219–25.
9. Acheson K, Jéquier E, Wahren J. Influence of beta-adrenergic blockade on glucose-induced thermogenesis in man. *J Clin Invest* 1983;72:981–6.
10. Acheson K, Ravussin E, Wahren J, Jéquier E. Thermic effect of glucose in man. Obligatory and facultative thermogenesis. *J Clin Invest* 1984;74:1572–80.
11. Ravussin E, Schutz Y, Acheson KJ, Dusmet M, Bourqin L, Jéquier E. Short-term, mixed-diet overfeeding in man: no evidence for "luxuskonsumption." *Am J Physiol* 1985;249:E470–7.
12. Flatt JP. Importance of nutrient balance in body weight regulation. *Diabetes Metab Rev* 1988;4:571–81.
13. Masoro EJ. Biochemical mechanisms related to the homeostatic regulation of lipogenesis in animals. *J Lip Res* 1962;3:149–64.
14. Assimacopoulos-Jeannet F, Jeanrenaud B. The hormonal and metabolic basis of experimental obesity. *Clin Endocrinol Metab* 1976;5:337–65.
15. Sjöström L. Adult human adipose tissue cellularity and metabolism. *Acta Med Scand Suppl* 1972;544:1–52.
16. Elwyn DH, Gump FE, Munro HN, et al. Changes in nitrogen balance of depleted patients with increasing infusions of glucose. *Am J Clin Nutr* 1979;32:1597–1611.

17. McGill DB, Jeejeebhoy KN. Long-term total parenteral nutrition. *Gastroenterology* 1974;67:195–7.
18. Hill R, Linazasoro JM, Chevallier F, et al. Regulation of hepatic lipogenesis: the influence of dietary fats. *J Biol Chem* 1958;233:305–10.
19. Acheson KJ, Flatt JP, Jéquier E. Glycogen synthesis versus lipogenesis after a 500 g carbohydrate meal in man. *Metabolism* 1982;31:1234–40.
20. Acheson KJ, Schutz Y, Bessard T, Anantharaman K, Flatt JP, Jéquier E. Glycogen storage capacity and de novo lipogenesis during massive carbohydrate overfeeding in man. *Am J Clin Nutr* 1988;48:240–7.
21. Flatt JP, Ravussin E, Acheson KJ, Jéquier E. Effects of dietary fat on postprandial substrate oxidation and on carbohydrate and fat balances. *J Clin Invest* 1985;76:1019–24.
22. Randle PJ, Garland PB, Newsholme EA, Holes CN. The glucose fatty acid cycle. Its role in insulin sensitivity and the metabolic disturbances of diabetes mellitus. *Lancet* 1963;1:785–9.
23. Schutz Y, Flatt JP, Jéquier E. Failure of dietary fat intake to promote fat oxidation: a factor favoring the development of obesity. *Am J Clin Nutr* 1989;50:307–14.
24. Danforth E. Diet and obesity. *Am J Clin Nutr* 1987;41:1132–45.
25. Flatt JP. Dietary fat, carbohydrate balance, and weight maintenance: effects of exercise. *Am J Clin Nutr* 1987;45:296–306.
26. Flatt JP. The difference in the storage capacities for carbohydrate and for fat, and its implications in the regulation of body weight. *Ann NY Acad Sci* 1987;499:104–23.
27. Felber JP, Ferrannini E, Golay A, et al. Role of lipid oxidation in pathogenesis of insulin resistance of obesity and type II diabetes. *Diabetes* 1987;36:1341–50.
28. Tremblay A, Plourde G, Despres JP, Bouchard C. Impact of dietary fat content and fat oxidation on energy intake in humans. *Am J Clin Nutr* 1989;49:799–805.
29. Lissner L, Levitsky DA, Strupp BJ, Kalkwarf HJ, Roe DA. Dietary fat and the regulation of energy intake in human subjects. *Am J Clin Nutr* 1987;46:866–92.
30. Porikos KP, Booth G, Van Itallie TB. Effects of covert nutritive dilution on the spontaneous food intake of obese individuals: a pilot study. *Am J Clin Nutr* 1977;30:1638–44.
31. Porikos KP, Hesser MF, Van Itallie TB. Caloric regulation in normal-weight men maintained on a palatable diet of conventional foods. *Physiol Behav* 1982;28:293–300.
32. Glueck CJ, Hastings MM, Allen RD, et al. Sucrose polyester and covert caloric dilution. *Am J Clin Nutr* 1982;35:1352–8.
33. Duncan KH, Bacon JA, Weinsier RL. The effects of high and low energy density diets on satiety, energy intake, and eating time of obese and non-obese subjects. *Am J Clin Nutr* 1983;37:763–7.
34. Würsch P, Acheson K, Koellreuter B, Jéquier E. Metabolic effects of instant bean and potato over 6 hours. *Am J Clin Nutr* 1988;48:1418–23.
35. Leathwood P, Pollet P. Effects of slow release carbohydrates in the form of bean flakes on the evolution of hunger and satiety in man. *Appetite* 1988;10:1–11.

DISCUSSION

Dr. W. P. T. James: Eric Jéquier's clear exposition of his group's research highlights the very substantial advances made in our understanding of energy and nutrient balance in humans over the last 10 to 15 years. The advances have come from conducting meticulous studies on volunteers held under precise feeding conditions. These reveal the surprising precision of metabolic control; simple standardization of procedures allows replicate measurements on the basal or 24-hour metabolic rates to within ±2% (c.v.) over a period of days, weeks, or months. In normal circumstances shifts in energy expenditure are modest, but this could reflect substantial changes in a metabolic process that contributes perhaps 5–10% to total energy expenditure. Thus, the detailed study of thermogenic control may come from the more precise measurement of those flexible components of energy expenditure that we originally called "regulatory" (1) but which Jéquier has more properly called "facultative" thermogenesis. Jéquier, drawing on Flatt's calculations, which are readily understandable by reference to McGilverey's long-standing estimates of the net effects of different metabolic pathways (2), highlights the distinction between carbohydrate and fat metabolism and the energetic significance of different pathways. The results and inferences drawn are widely accepted, but we may need to re-examine the explanations for observed thermogenic responses. Thus, it seems reasonable to infer that in humans, carbohydrate-to-fat synthesis is unimportant because adipose tissue lipogenic enzymes are low and the RQ rarely rises above 1.0 except, for example, on intense carbohydrate overfeeding, as shown by Schutz et al. (3). We now have increasing evidence casting doubt on the validity of inferences drawn from in vitro estimates of enzyme activities. Crabtree et al. (4) has highlighted this by showing that the actual flux rates around an acetyl CoA-acetate substrate shuttle or "futile cycle" in liver and muscle are very different from the rates expected from enzyme activity. The problem is then how to best monitor the true flux down a metabolic pathway; rigorous analyses of the critical steps in the interchange of substrates within these pathways can now be undertaken (5), but much depends on being satisfied that the appropriate label and precursor pool is chosen. Clearly all our studies concentrate on net RQ changes, so the calorimetric assignment of X grams to carbohydrate oxidation in practice signifies the equivalent conversion of glucose to fatty acids and the oxidation of a comparable amount of fat. The thermogenic effects of these two options is, however, markedly different.

This issue of metabolic processing following a meal is relevant to the present discussion because Garlick and his colleagues have now found that our earlier and widely used technique of 1-C–labeled leucine for monitoring protein balances after feeding is fundamentally flawed because of label recycling during 6- to 8-hour infusions (6). Thus, instead of accepting our earlier studies on the marked protein synthetic response to meals and amino acid input, derived from rat studies (7), he now finds that the dominant effect on protein balance after a meal is a reduction in protein breakdown rates rather than a surge in synthesis. This in turn means that the energetic significance of postprandial processing of amino acids into protein synthesis has been exaggerated. Without a surge in synthesis and with a fall in the energy-requiring steps of protein breakdown, one might question why amino acid inflow leads to such a marked metabolic response.

The remarkable control of specific metabolic processes came home to us when we first studied dietary fatty acid oxidation in whole-body calorimeters using oral ^{14}C-labeled oleic acid. Although we expected fluctuating results in individuals, we found an astonishing individual replication of $^{14}CO_2$ output over 24 hours, but wide interindividual differences. Thus, some individuals evolved, for example, 15% of the dose, whereas others repeatedly oxidized twice as much. Providing carbohydrate-rich meals consistently reduced ^{14}oleic acid oxidation with the calorimetric responses, suggesting rapid induction of carbohydrate oxidation in keeping with the Randall cycle hypothesis (8). Flatt's reasonable calculations can be used to explain the high thermogenic response to carbohydrates if the unlikely assumption is made of substantial fat synthesis. With fat overfeeding, however, the stoichiometry does not explain the thermogenesis (9,10). This is why we concentrated originally on the idea that dietary fat induced unknown thermogenic mechanisms, which might explain the proposed undue sensitivity of pre-obese individuals to high-fat diets (11). The potential for gene-nutrient interactions in differential sensitivity of individuals to specific dietary substrates remains to be explored.

We also have to assess the nutritional significance of studies that test the human's response to maximum substrate loading. Thus, the glucose insulin clamp technique, which has proved to be readily applicable, often involves infusions at well above the expected inflow rate after a meal. The metabolic processing in the intestinal mucosa and the preferential uptake by the liver may all effect different responses from intravenous loading. Nevertheless, autonomic responses to meals are apparent, and in our own unpublished studies, Kurpad has shown rapid changes in deuterated noradrenaline turnover after carbohydrate-rich meals as well as differences between obese and lean subjects. With our earlier studies, which implied that carbohydrate overfeeding induced positive energy balance by preferential sequestration of dietary fat to stores (12), we still need to question how much the thermogenic response to carbohydrate overfeeding reflects a genuine fat synthetic response. If sympathetic activity does occur, this can be expected to enhance free fatty acid efflux. Jéquier infers a free fatty acid induction of metabolism, which we found to be modest in humans (13), so I suspect that the adrenergic stimulus is more directly involved in enhancing ionic gradients or substrate shuttles than in inducing thermogenesis via a stimulated lipolytic rate. Our own emphasis on noradrenergic infusion (14) attempted to mimic physiologic effects; this modest stimulus does affect amino acid exchange from plasma to tissues and perhaps protein turnover with rapid adjustments in noradrenergic responses and adrenergic receptor reactivity (Kurpad, unpublished data).

If postprandial thermogenesis does depend on heat sensing either at the hepatic or central level with reactive peripheral modulation of metabolism, then we may need to re-evaluate our concepts of appetite control. Jéquier's proposal that appetite control is based on carbohydrate balance harks back to the original theories on glucose-mediated hypothalamic control and in a modern context re-emphasizes the new work of Campfield on glucose transport and the seemingly controlled rapid decline in peripheral glucose concentrations (15) that precedes the onset of feeding. Whether this is central or peripherally mediated remains unclear, and it is still possible that hepatic glucose stores or metabolism are in some way monitored, perhaps via vagal afferents dependent on glucose-mediated transmembrane changes in the potential difference of liver cells (14).

Whatever the mechanism of appetite control, the concept that obesity is best avoided by maintaining the food FQ above the body's RQ is an intriguing way of emphasizing the energetic advantages of a carbohydrate-rich, low-fat diet in a society concerned with obesity (15). Because the modulation of RQ will also depend on the state of energy balance, it is unclear whether the manipulation of diet, independent of its energy value, is the key to modulating energy balance itself.

REFERENCES

1. Jung RT, James WPT. Is obesity metabolic? *Br J Hosp Med* 1980;24:503–9.
2. McGilvery RW. *Biochemistry—a functional approach.* Philadelphia: WB Saunders, 1970.
3. Schutz Y, Acheson KJ, Jéquier E. Twenty-four hour energy expenditure and thermogenesis: Response to progressive carbohydrate overfeeding in man. *Int J Obes* 1985;9:111–4.
4. Crabtree B, Marr SA, Anderson SE, MacRae JC. Measurement of the rate of substrate cycling between acetate and acetyl-CoA in sheep muscle in vivo. Effects of infusion of acetate. *Biochem J* 1987;243:821–7.
5. Crabtree B, Newsholme EA. A systematic approach to describing and analysing metabolic control systems. *Trends Biochem Sci* 1987;12:4–12.
6. Melville S, McNurlan MA, McHardy KC, et al. The role of degradation in the acute control of protein balance in man: failure of feeding to stimulate protein synthesis as assessed by L-[1-^{13}C] leucine infusion. *Metabolism* 1989;38:248–55.
7. Garlick PJ, Millward DJ, James WPT, Waterlow JC. The effect of protein deprivation and starvation on the rate of protein synthesis in tissues of the rat. *Biochim Biophys Acta* 1975;414:71–84.
8. Lean MEJ, James WPT. Metabolic effects of isoenergetic nutrient exchange over 24 hours in relation to obesity in women. *Int J Obes* 1988;12:15–27.
9. Dallosso HM, James WPT. Whole body calorimetry studies in adult men. 1. The effect of fat overfeeding on 24 h energy expenditure. *Br J Nutr* 1984;52:49–64.

10. James WPT. Appetite control and other mechanisms of weight homeostasis. In: Blaxter Sir Kenneth, Waterlow JC, eds. *Nutritional adaptation in man.* London: John Libbey, 1984;141–54.
11. James WPT, Trayhurn P. Thermogenesis and obesity. *Br Med Bull* 1981;37:43–8.
12. Bisdee JT, James WPT. Carbohydrate induced thermogenesis in man. *Proc Nutr Soc* 1984;43:149A.
13. Jung RT, Shetty PS, James WPT. Heparin, free fatty acids and an increased metabolic demand for oxygen. *Postgrad Med J* 1980;56:330–2.
14. Jung RT, Shetty PS, James WPT, Barrand MA, Callingham BA. Reduced thermogenesis in obesity. *Nature* 1979;279:322–3.
15. Campfield LA, Smith FJ. Transient declines in blood glucose signal meal initiation. *Int J Obes* 1990;14(Suppl14):15–33.

Energy Metabolism: Tissue Determinants and
Cellular Corollaries, edited by J. M. Kinney
and H. N. Tucker. Raven Press, Ltd.,
New York © 1992.

Whole Body Energy and Nitrogen (Protein) Relationships

*†Vernon R. Young, †Yong-Ming Yu, and ‡Naomi K. Fukagawa

*School of Science and Clinical Research Center, Massachusetts Institute of
Technology, Cambridge, Massachusetts 02139; †Shriners Burns Institute, Boston,
Massachusetts 02114; and ‡Department of Pediatrics and Medicine, Beth Israel
Hospital and Harvard Medical School, Boston, Massachusetts 02215

There is an extensive body of literature on various aspects of the interrelationships between proteins (and their constituent amino acids), nitrogen utilization, and the other major energy yielding substrates (glucose, triglycerides, fatty acids, ketone bodies) in metabolism and in relation to nutrition (1–5). Indeed, the sensitivity of body nitrogen balance to both energy and protein intake has been recognized for years. Many of the earlier, basic observations in this context were reviewed by Munro in 1951 (6) and a few years later by Calloway and Spector (7). These thoughtful, and now classical, contributions to the literature gave a particular emphasis to the impact of energy and protein on body nitrogen balance and they will serve as a springboard for our particular examination of the relationships between energy and nitrogen (protein).

Because of the potentially broad area of biology involved, we have chosen to limit our survey, giving some consideration to both the metabolic basis of these interactions as well as to their nutritional significance, initially with respect to the healthy subject. Because one of the stated major objectives of this volume is to highlight areas which hold special promise for advancing nutritional support in patient care, we will also consider the interrelationships in disease states. Although our attention is channeled mainly toward human subjects, we include a brief overview of selected associations between protein and energy metabolism among various mammalian species. Our objective is to establish that some of the relationships are broadly similar among these species and, in a general sense, apply to human beings. From this we will also ascertain to what extent protein metabolism contributes to body energy expenditure and how disease might affect this. The range of energy and nitrogen metabolism within which we might explore these various aspects is also quite broad (Table 1); the lower end might be that represented by the basal metabolic rate (BMR) and obligatory level of nitrogen losses, amounting to about 50 mg N $kg^{-1}day^{-1}$ in the healthy adult (8). Parenthetically, when cell mass is used as a basis for comparison, BMR seems not to be reduced in patients with anorexia nervosa, relative

TABLE 1. *Relevant boundaries between which energy-nitrogen relations might be considered*

Metabolic condition		Value	Reference
Low end of range			
Energy	Basal metabolic rate (BMR) for adult	~25 kcal·kg^{-1}·day^{-1}	FAO/WHO/UNU (8)
Nitrogen	Obligatory nitrogen loss (ONL) for adult	~50 mg N·kg^{-1}·day^{-1}	FAO/WHO/UNU (8)
Upper end of range			
Energy	Severe burn injury	1.5–2 × BMR	Bursztein et al. (5)
	Sustained metabolic rate	<5 × BMR	Peterson et al. (10)
	Maximal, acute, exertion	~100 × BMR	Bartholomew (11)
Nitrogen	Multiple trauma with sepsis	7–10 × ONL	Moore (12)
			Schiller et al. (13)

to normal subjects (9). The upper end of the range for energy expenditure could be represented by the considerably higher BMR in burn injury (5) or the maximum level of the so-called sustained metabolic rate, which is usually less than about 5 times BMR (10), or it might extend to as high as 100 times resting expenditure, when exerted for a few seconds (11). The upper extreme of nitrogen excretion might occur in highly catabolic states, such as following bilateral, compound femoral fracture with overwhelming sepsis and in major burn trauma, where it may exceed the obligatory nitrogen losses by about seven to ten times (12,13). However, our attention is going to be within a narrower range of energy expenditure and nitrogen output, particularly because there is little information on the details of the interrelationships at the extreme upper end of the range.

We end with a few thoughts about directions for future research in this area, particularly in relation to the parenteral/enteral nutritional support of hospitalized and sick patients (see chapter by Young et al., *Energy and Protein Turnover*).

ENERGY DEPENDENCY OF PROTEIN AND AMINO ACID METABOLISM

It is worthwhile to consider, briefly, those major processes that require energy, in the form of high energy phosphate bonds, and that are intimately involved in the utilization of nitrogen and amino acids. This energy allows the formation of polypeptides and their further assembly within or outside the cell and, ultimately, in the breakdown and removal of proteins and the catabolism of amino acids. Table 2 provides a list of some of the major processes known to require either ATP or GTP. While these, and other processes not included here, are energy-dependent, it is uncertain as to how much food energy is required to drive them *in vivo* (14). Therefore, it is not possible to assign the quantitative proportion of body energy flux due to them, nor even that related to the substrate cycles, some of which are identified at

TABLE 2. *Some energy-dependent processes associated with protein turnover and amino acid homeostasis*

1. Protein turnover
   Formation of initiation complex
   Peptide bond synthesis
   Protein degradation
   Ubiquitin-dependent
   Ubiquitin-independent
   Autophagic degradation (sequestration, lysosomal proton pump)
2. RNA Turnover
   rRNA; tRNA
   Pre-mRNA splicing (spliceosome) and mRNA
3. Amino acid transport
4. Regulation and integrity
   Reversible phosphorylation; enzymes, factors, GTP-GDP exchange proteins (signal transduction)
   Second messengers (phosphatidylinositol system)
   Ion pumps and channels
   ATP-dependent heat shock proteins (folding)
   Protein translocation
5. Nitrogen metabolism
   Glutamate/glutamine cycle
   Glucose-alanine cycle
   Urea synthesis

the bottom of this list, which confer on the host a mechanism for metabolic control (15).

In the past five years the mechanisms responsible for the regulation of cellular processes, such as protein folding and aggregation (16), intracellular traffic of newly synthesized proteins (17), and transport of proteins across membranes (18), including the import of proteins into mitochondria (19), the organelle of oxidative phosphorylation, and the transduction of signals from outside of cells to their appropriate intracellular sites (20,21) and culminating in physiologic responses, have been identified and are being further clarified. Most of these involve the participation of energy in the form of ATP or GTP or their derivatives (cAMP; cGMP). Indeed, there is a bewildering array of proteins, such as the heterotrimeric G proteins and monomeric GTP-binding proteins, that are turned on when bound to GTP and turned off by hydrolyzing GTP to GDP (22). These appear to be involved in controlling a diverse set of essential cellular functions, including growth, differentiation, intracellular vesicle transport, and secretion, to name just a few (23). However, it is these various processes, including transcription of DNA, followed by splicing of pre-mRNA (24,25), peptide chain initiation (26), the attachment of an amino acid to its cognate tRNA and then chain elongation (27), together with the energy required for protein degradation, via various ATP-dependent and GTP-dependent mechanisms (28,29), which account for the molecular and cellular basis of the interactions between protein, nitrogen, and energy metabolism.

The level of energy intake and the status of body energy balance may affect these various processes in different ways and to a different extent, depending upon the particular set of nutritional and host conditions involved. Thus, a further understanding of the interrelations between nitrogen, protein, amino acid, and energy metabolism might well assist us in better defining nutritional requirements and improve current diagnostic approaches for the objective assessment of nutritional status in man. Furthermore, it is also to be expected that the level, and possibly source, of protein intake and status of protein nutriture would influence energy metabolism (30–32), promoted by alterations in the functioning and activity of the endocrine system (33–35). This emphasizes why it is worthwhile for us to explore the interactions between energy and nitrogen, so as to appreciate the pathophysiology of the various forms of protein-energy malnutrition, the extremes of these being marasmus and kwashiorkor (36), and thus promote the development of more effective approaches for preventing significant tissue and organ protein depletion and for replenishing tissue and organ proteins in the stressed or cachectic patient (37–39).

ENERGY-NITROGEN RELATIONSHIPS EVALUATED FROM N BALANCE MEASUREMENTS

Body protein or nitrogen balance in the healthy, mature human is maintained within relatively narrow limits, indicating a regulation that is achieved by varying the rate of N excretion in relation to changes in nitrogen intake and the individual's metabolic state. The responsiveness of nitrogen excretion to altered dietary conditions, especially nitrogen intake, was demonstrated many years ago and this was, perhaps, the first significant example of the impact of nutrition on a major metabolic pathway (urea synthesis) in the mammalian organism.

At the beginning of this century, Otto Folin (40,41), Professor of Biological Chemistry at Harvard and working at the McLean Hospital for the Insane in Massachusetts, studied the effect of both generous and low nitrogen intakes on the chemical composition of urine. As depicted in Fig. 1, he observed, with himself as the experimental subject in this case, that there was a dramatic effect of reducing nitrogen intake on urea output but there was little influence of this dietary change on other urine constituents, such as creatinine, neutral sulfur, and uric acid. From these observations Folin developed his theory of protein metabolism (41), which he separated into endogenous and exogenous components, a postulate that was later invalidated by the isotopic tracer studies of Schoenheimer (42). However, a number of useful points can be drawn from the data shown in Fig. 1 that are relevant to our further discussion of energy-nitrogen relations. First, there is a certain lag-time associated with changes in N excretion following an alteration in N intake. We do not know exactly the quantitative contribution of the various metabolic processes that account for this temporal pattern beyond a contraction of the size of the body urea pool, and a combination of alterations in amino acid oxidation, tissue enzyme changes, and

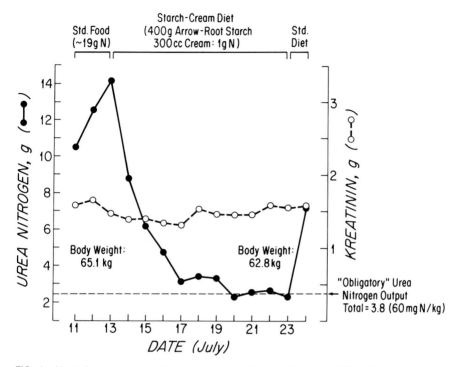

FIG. 1. Urea nitrogen and creatine output via urine in an adult subject (OF) while consuming a high (19 g N/d) and low (1 g N/d) protein diet. (Drawn from the data of Folin, ref. 40.)

tissue and organ protein turnover (synthesis and breakdown). The lag-time in the adjustment of N balance to a dietary or metabolic perturbation (43,44) should be considered in the design and critical interpretation of N balance data, especially where the experimental conditions might not be ideal or difficult to control fully, as often is the case in studies on N balance–energy relationships in hospitalized patients. This has been a consideration in some meticulous N balance investigations (45) but not necessarily so in many, making it rather difficult to draw a completely comprehensive and quantitatively precise picture of energy-N balance relations, especially in reference to various disease states.

A second point is that the new, lower rate of urinary nitrogen output achieved by this subject (Fig. 1) amounted to about 60 mg N $kg^{-1}day^{-1}$. This rate of excretion exceeds that of about 37 mg N $kg^{-1}day^{-1}$ (8) when adult subjects consume a very low or protein-free, but otherwise adequate, diet with energy sufficient to balance total energy expenditure. This latter rate of N output is defined as the "obligatory urinary N loss" (46), which is a major determinant of the total nitrogen requirement for body protein maintenance in both young (46) and adult subjects (47). Thus, it is likely that the relatively high rate of N loss in subject 0.F. (Fig. 1), following adjustment to the low N diet, was due to an inadequate energy intake. This is supported by the fact that a significant loss of body weight was experienced by this subject during the experimental period (Fig. 1). Indeed, N losses of this order are observed after about a 5 week total fast in obese subjects (48) although a higher N excretion occurs in subjects with partial restriction of normal caloric intake while maintaining a normal N intake (49,50). The level of both energy intake and body energy status determines the N balance of the individual.

There are a number of reviews on the effects of N and of energy intake on N balance (1,2,4,6,7) and, in summary, the available data reveal that these effects are not entirely independent of one another and their interactions can be complex. As pointed out by Calloway and Spector (7) the level of caloric intake, whether above or below requirements, determines the change in N balance that can be achieved by an increase in N intake. Furthermore, the level of N intake determines the effect of a change in energy intake on N balance. Munro (1) captured this complexity quite clearly in his summary picture, which is reproduced for reference in Fig. 2.

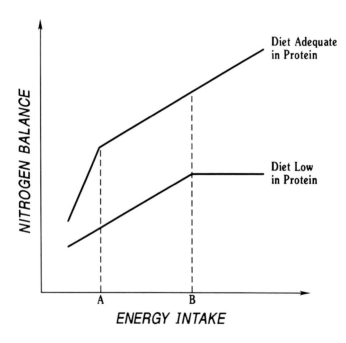

FIG. 2. Relationship of N balance and energy intake with diets of differing protein levels. Between energy intake A (low) and B (higher) the two lines are parallel. (From Munro, ref. 1, with permission.)

TABLE 3. *A selected survey of studies on the responses of N balance in adults to changes in energy intake (E) at adequate or excessive levels of energy*

Subjects	Dietary conditions	N balance response	Reference
Young men	Protein intake varied 0.28–0.76 g/kg/day	~2 mg N/kcal	Inoue *et al.* (51)
Six young men	Protein intake 5–7% of dietary energy, 12 day periods, at low E and excess E	1.74 mg N/kcal at low E; 1.12 mg N/kcal at high E	Calloway (52)
Four young men	Protein intake 0.6 g/kg, 3–4 week diet periods	1.74 mg N/kcal	Garza *et al.* (53)
Four young men	Protein intake 0.6 g/kg plus dispensable amino acids (~0.23 g protein/kg)	~3 mg N/kcal	Garza *et al.* (54)
Young men (46 total)	Variable energy and protein intake among groups	~3 mg N/kcal	Kishi *et al.* (55)
Six young men	Protein intake 1.2 g/kg/ day E 1.15 and 1.3 × maintenance	1.4–2.4 mg N/kcal	Chiang and Huang (56)
Depleted patients	Intravenous glucose, N intake 173 mg/kg	1.7 mg N/kcal	Elwyn *et al.* (45)

The information in Table 3 indicates that an excess energy intake at adequate levels of N intake causes a retention of approximately 1–2 mg N per kcal in healthy subjects (51–56), but at limiting N intakes this response is attenuated or does not occur. Based on the N balance, glucose-infusion studies by Elwyn and coworkers at Columbia University (45) it is apparent that depleted, septic patients show a similar dose-related response to that observed for normal adults, but with some important qualifications, as discussed later.

At lower energy intakes, within the submaintenance range, the impact of changes in energy intake on N balance are greater than those listed in Table 3. The summary presented by Calloway and Spector (7) for normal young men reveals that at a very low energy intake the relationship between energy and N balance changes and is approximately 8 mg N kcal^{-1} with this relationship breaking at a total energy intake of about 1,400 kcal. Again, this also appears to be the case in depleted patients, since Elwyn and coworkers (57,58) report a value of 7.5 mg N/kcal for energy intakes up to about 15 kcal/kg body weight (Fig. 3). These differences in the effects of changes in energy intake on N balance, depending upon the intake range within which alterations in energy intake occur, have been taken to reflect the possibility that a replenishment or maintenance of lean body mass is the process of importance within the low energy range, whereas the extra N retained at generous energy intakes is that needed to support the extra energy retained as fat (57,58). Whether this is an

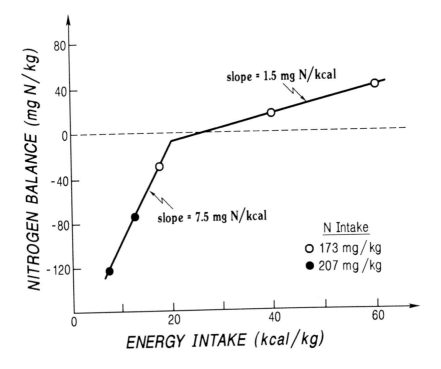

FIG. 3. Relationship between N balance and energy intake in post-absorptive and depleted patients. (Redrawn from Elwyn, ref. 58, based on data in refs. 45 and 57.)

adequate explanation requires, in part, a much deeper search into body and organ compositional changes under these varying conditions, the analytical requirements of which exceed the limits of many of the currently available procedures (59,60). Also, to further complicate our summary is the work by Todd et al. (61) showing that the impact of a negative energy balance on N balance is less when the energy deficit is generated by an increase in physical activity than when it derives from reduced intake. However, a metabolic, rather than tissue composition, focus may be more instructive, since it is worth pointing out that the "break-point" in the energy intake–retention relationship (Fig. 3) occurs at an energy intake level equivalent to a glucose supply of approximately 3 mg $kg^{-1}min^{-1}$. This corresponds to about the level that maximally suppresses endogenous glucose production in the adult (62) and, therefore, presumably a minimum rate of conversion of gluconeogenic precursors, especially amino acids, for maintenance of glucose homeostasis.

DYNAMIC ASPECTS OF NITROGEN/PROTEIN METABOLISM IN RELATION TO ENERGY

Comment on Methods

Although the preceding discussion, concerning N balance and energy intake, provides some useful insight into energy-nitrogen relations, we should focus on the dynamics of body protein, amino acid, and nitrogen metabolism. Our reason is that we have probably gained about as much physiological, mechanistically-based, knowledge regarding protein-energy interactions as we can from nitrogen (N) balance data alone. While such studies have been valuable, chemical balance measurements alone do not indicate either the sensitivity of body and organ protein turnover to alterations in energy (or nitrogen) intake or the mechanism whereby overall body N balance is changed (i.e., whether changes in protein synthesis, protein breakdown, and/or amino acid catabolism and nitrogen interchange and transport are responsible (63). Indeed, a quote attributed to Claude Bernard (1813–1878), the famous physiologist, emphasizes this point very well, when he characterized the limitation of the balance technique as "trying to tell what happens inside a house by watching what goes in by the door and what comes out of the chimney." The therapeutic/nutritional implications, as well as the relations of N to energy metabolism, might well be different depending upon whether the "catabolic loss" of body nitrogen is due to alterations in protein synthesis or breakdown or to specific changes in the regulation of pathways of amino acid metabolism and catabolism. Also, Waterlow (64) has pointed out that changes in N excretion and balance due to changes in energy intake are relatively small when considered in relation to total body nitrogen (protein) turnover. Thus, it is important to consider protein-energy relations with regard to various aspects of protein and amino acid turnover and metabolism.

A further reason why we should go beyond simply energy intake–N balance considerations comes from the study by Elwyn et al. (45), referred to earlier. These investigators showed while the relationship between the change in N balance for a change in energy intake, within the adequate energy intake range, was similar for depleted or septic patients and healthy adults the mean nitrogen intake required to achieve zero N balance at zero energy balance in the sick patient was 150 mg N/kg or significantly more than is needed by normal adults (8). Although the investigations by Elwyn and coworkers (45) involved giving intravenous L-amino acids and glucose whereas the estimates of N intakes required for balance in normal adults have been based on oral feeding with intact proteins and mixed energy sources, we accept the suggestion that the discrepancy between the N intakes required for maintenance of satisfactory body protein balance by normal and septic patients is due largely to their different metabolic characteristics and not to differences in the specific dietary conditions. Furthermore, septic patients may require a higher rate of glucose infusion to achieve the same absolute nitrogen sparing as compared with healthy controls (65), despite the possible similarity in the ratio of the change in N balance with energy intake. The higher nitrogen requirement by the depleted or septic patients leads us to a consideration of the dynamics of nitrogen and amino acid metabolism, as a potentially more informative basis for enhancing our understanding of the relations between nitrogen and energy nutrition/metabolism in healthy and disease states.

A variety of *in vivo* approaches have been used to explore dynamic aspects of protein and amino acid metabolism and the possible mechanisms that account for the changes in body N balance occurring in various pathophysiological states. Most of these approaches recognize the central role played by free amino acids in tissue and organ protein metabolism. Indeed, a consideration of the transport and fate of these substrates for protein synthesis, and for formation of other physiologically important nitrogen-containing compounds, is relevant for any detailed account of the relations between energy and nitrogen metabolism, and their implications for the nutritional treatment of patients.

From various investigations, involving such diverse experimental approaches as measurement of arteriovenous amino acid balances across organs, studies of using isolated organs, or intact tissue preparations as well as evaluation of *in vitro* enzyme activities of different cells, a general picture has now emerged that reveals a co-operative participation of the intestines, liver, muscle, and kidney in the *in vivo* metabolism of most amino acids, whether derived immediately from exogenous or endogenous sources. Thus, a number of the major physiologic pathways of amino acid flow, in relation to whole body amino acid homeostasis, can be presented as shown in Fig. 4 (66) and this also suggests that glutamine and alanine, including their interrelationships with the branched-chain amino acids, are poised to play a key role in the economy of whole body and organ nitrogen metabolism (67,68).

Measurement *in vivo* of the interorgan and whole body transport and fate of nitrogen and of individual amino acids may be based on tracer approaches. These have been reviewed and discussed, in detail, by Waterlow et al. (69,70) by ourselves (71,72), and others (73,74). In Table 4 (75) a selected list of approaches used to study the kinetics of body proteins, their constituent amino acids, and of nitrogen, is given

TABLE 4. *Major methods using stable isotopes to measure amino acid and protein kinetics*

---

1. End-product methods
   ^{15}N-amino acid tracers
   Urea and ammonia ^{15}N excretion

2. Plasma or precursor methods
   Stable isotope labeled amino acid
   Plasma isotope enrichment (with expired air)
   Primed, continuous intravenous administration (alternatives: bolus; "flooding" dose; in-traintestine)

3. Data analysis
   Compartmental
   Stochastic

Based largely on Bier, ref. 75.

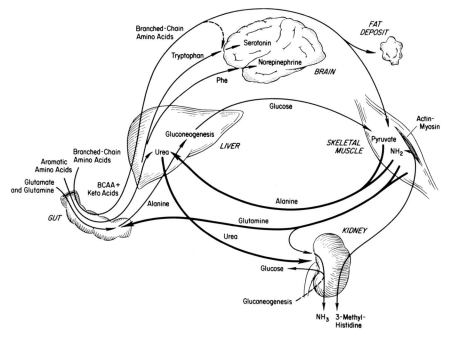

FIG. 4. Major pathways of the transport and fate of various amino acids among the different organs. (Slight modification of Munro, ref. 66.)

for summary purposes. Our own research (71,76) has exploited largely the stochastic measurement of plasma interorgan amino acid and nitrogen transport, utilizing stable isotope probes. The latter offer a number of major advantages for study of *in vivo* kinetics of amino acid metabolism in the human subject (77–81), as well as other aspects of nutrition and substrate metabolism (78), including energy expenditure (82,83).

Interspecies Aspects and Importance of Protein (Nitrogen) Metabolism in Energy Expenditure

As shown in Table 5 (84), rates of protein synthesis, expressed per unit body weight, are high in the smaller mammalian species when compared to rates in the larger ones. However, when expressed to the three-quarter power of body weight ($kg^{0.75}$) there is a relative constancy among the various species listed here. This indicates that protein synthesis is correlated with basal energy metabolism (BM), since the 0.75 power of body weight (in kg; "metabolic body size") is the weight function that approximately equalizes body energy expenditure across the different mammalian species (85,86). Therefore, based on Waterlow (70) it can be seen in Table 6 that the change in the intensity of body protein turnover parallels that for differences in their metabolic rates (kJ); expressed as kJ metabolic rate per g protein

TABLE 5. *Some estimates of protein synthesis in adults of various mammalian species*

Species	Body wt. (kg)	Daily protein synthesis	
		$(g \cdot kg^{-1})$	$(g \cdot kg^{-0.75})$
Rat	0.35	22	16.9
Rabbit	3.6	9.2	12.6
Pig	32	8.1	18.9
Sheep	63	5.6	15.7
Man	71	4.6	13.4
Cow	575	3.0	14.8

Partial summary from Reeds and Harris, ref. 84.

turnover the values shown in Table 6 range from 11–23, with a mean of about 15. From these data it appears that, on average, about 15 kJ of basal energy expenditure are "connected" with each g protein synthesis. Assuming therefore that about 3 kJ are expended, minimally, in the formation of peptide bonds (14), this implies that approximately 20% of basal metabolism is due to the process of polypeptide bond synthesis.

It would be of interest to learn whether these same quantitative associations between whole body protein and energy metabolism continue to hold for the larger land animals. These could include the largest elephants, whose weight may be somewhat under 10,000 kg, or those that could in theory weight between 10^5 and 10^6 kg but have not yet appeared (87).

An example of the second approach for estimating the relationship between protein turnover and energy expenditure is offered by the study of Welle and Nair (88) who examined the variation of leucine flux and its relationship with metabolic rate in a

TABLE 6. *Whole body protein turnover in relation to resting metabolic rate (MR) in adults of mammalian species*

Species	Wt. (kg)	Protein turnover $(g/kg^{-1} \cdot day^{-1})$ A	MR $(kJ/kg^{11} \cdot day^{-1})$ B	Ratio B/A
Mouse	0.04	43.5	760	11
Rat	0.35	22.0	364	17
Rabbit	3.6	9.2	192	20
Sheep	63	5.6	96	17
Man	70	4.6	107	23
Cow	575	3.0	60	20

MR $(kJ \cdot day^{-1}) = 240W^{0.74}$; $r = 0.999$.
Protein turnover $(g \cdot day^{-1}) = 15.8W^{0.72}$; $r = 0.998$.
From Waterlow, ref. 70.

population of 26 adult men and 21 women. These investigators observed a high correlation between leucine flux and resting metabolic rate (RMR). From their regression analysis it was concluded that the contribution of protein turnover to RMR was about 20% in an average subject. This is similar to the value presented above, as derived from the interspecies comparison, but lower than that reported previously by Nair and Halliday (89) in human subjects, possibly because in this earlier study insufficient consideration was given to the influence of effects of differences in body composition on the statistical relationships studied, as has been pointed out by Welle and Nair (88). Additionally, from a study of the thermic effects of food, Robinson et al. (90) have concluded that the thermic response to feeding is due importantly to the stimulation of protein synthesis. They estimate that this process accounts for as much as 68% of the change in energy expenditure between the fasting and fed state when subjects receive a high protein meal.

These relationships between total body protein turnover and energy metabolism also appear to hold for the turnover of tRNA and rRNA. This is demonstrated in the novel studies of Schöch et al. (91) who measured modified RNA catabolites in urine as an index of the turnover of individual classes of RNA. They applied, therefore, a concept which had been earlier proposed for measurement of muscle protein turnover *in vivo*, based on estimates of the urinary excretion of the derived amino acid, N^τ-methylhistidine (92). Thus, tRNA and rRNA turnover among the various but limited, number of mammalian species examined by Schöch et al. (91) was found to be related to the 0.78 and 0.69 power of body weight, respectively, or to a similar body weight function relating protein turnover among these different species (Table 6). The intriguing and challenging question emerging from this and similar work is the nature of the causal or mechanistic link between the energy flux and the turnover of these macromolecules. Schöch et al. (91) hypothesize that the irreversible denaturation of macromolecules is basically a function of the energy flux per unit body mass and that there is a compensatory resynthesis of these macromolecules in order to maintain a steady state. As we learn more about (a) the mechanism of protein degradation, which might well be promoted by oxidative damage or modification of specific amino acid residues (93,94), due, in part, to formation of protein adducts coming from oxidant by products arising from normal metabolism, and (b) the link between protein degradation and protein synthesis, including mRNA translation for example, which conceivably might involve the co-ordinated activity of multifunctional enzyme complexes, such as the proteasome (95–98), we might be in a better position to explain the metabolic basis for the whole body–energy protein relationships just discussed.

Protein-Energy Metabolism and Interrelations Within Man

The relative constancy of the relationship, shown above, between rates of protein synthesis and energy expenditure among the various mammalian species raises the question as to whether a similar relationship might apply throughout the growth and

ENERGY INTAKE AND DYNAMICS OF NITROGEN METABOLISM

To better define the metabolic basis for altered N excretion with changes in energy intake, it is also important to know what happens to protein turnover with energy restriction, especially because the latter results in a reduction in MR (119,120), which over a short period is due mainly to a decrease in the metabolic activity of tissues, whereas in the longer-term it appears to be due to the loss of body tissue. Thus, there have been various studies on the effects of energy restriction and excess on whole body protein dynamics (e.g., see for review 2,3) but two recent studies (121,122), as summarized in Table 9, might be used to make a few major points. Brief starvation in healthy subjects results in an increase in protein turnover despite the fall in MR. Hence, there is a mismatch between the changes in energy flux and turnover of proteins under these conditions of acute energy restriction. In obese subjects, on the other hand, who were fasted for 3 weeks, there is a significant decline in leucine flux (121) which appears to parallel the decline in metabolic rate (123,124). Hence, the effect of reduced energy intake on protein-energy interrelationships is complex and depends upon the nutritional status of the individual and degree and length of the dietary restriction. It is also modulated by the level of protein supplied by the energy restricted diet, since protein turnover may not be reduced if the protein intake, despite a severe limitation in energy intake, is maintained close to a level that permits maintenance of nitrogen balance (125–127).

The effects of an excess intake of energy on protein turnover have also been investigated, but in a limited number of studies. We (128) found that leucine flux and oxidation was not different in the postabsorptive (fasted) state following a period of moderate excess intake but whole body synthesis was higher and leucine oxidation lower during the fed period when energy intake was excessive. On the other hand, Welle et al. (129) found that a substantial, excess intake of carbohydrate in healthy men amounting to 1,600 extra kcal/day stimulated postabsorptive proteolysis and protein synthesis. Thus, in spite of the well-known impact of altered energy intake on N balance, we still do not know in any detail how the source and level of energy intake affects the metabolic and organ fate of specific dietary amino acids. For ex-

TABLE 9. *Leucine kinetics in healthy and obese subjects in relation to a fast*

	Healthy[a]	Obese[b]
Days of fast	3	21
Leucine kinetics		
Flux (proteolysis)	↑ 31%	↓ 31%
Oxidation	↑ 46%	No change
Synthesis	↑ 28%	↓ 38%
3-Methylhistidine excretion	—	↓ 28%

[a] From Nair et al., ref. 121.
[b] From Hoffer and Forse, ref. 122.
Values are % change (↑, increase; ↓, decrease) from value before fast began.

TABLE 10. *Effect of an amino acid meal, with and without carbohydrate (CHO), on leucine kinetics studied with 1-^{13}C-leucine given i.g. and ^{2}H$_3$-leucine given i.v. in young men*

Measurement	Amino acids alone	Amino acids + CHO
Leucine flux (i.g. tracer)	188[a]	158[b]
Leucine oxidation	43[a]	36[b]
Leucine splanchnic removal (%)	29	20[b]
Leucine release from protein	130	100[b]
Net leucine balance	+14	+20[b]

[a] Values are μmol·kg^{-1}·h^{-1}.
[b] Different from amino acids alone; $p < 0.05$.
From M. Krempf et al., *unpublished results.*

ample, it would be worthwhile knowing whether the fate of absorbed amino acids, such as leucine, during their passage through the splanchnic region differs according to the level and source of carbohydrate and/or lipid in meals. Indeed, a detailed exploration of the metabolism of individual amino acids following their absorption represents an area of potentially fruitful investigation. This might be undertaken, in part, by exploiting multiple stable isotope tracer protocols, with simultaneous intravenous and intragastric administration, to quantify so-called "first pass" effects (130).

In a recent study (131) we applied this intravenous-intragastric-tracer approach to explore the metabolic fate of dietary leucine, when the tracer was incorporated into a balanced amino acid mixture which was consumed in the presence or absence of carbohydrate (as glucose). As summarized in Table 10, inclusion of the energy substrate in the experimental meal reduced the "first-pass" disappearance of leucine and this response was associated with a lower rate of whole-body leucine oxidation. Hence, the addition of glucose appeared to promote a greater passage of dietary leucine to peripheral tissues where it was, presumably, used to an increased extent for protein anabolic purposes. This response, however, was not observed for labeled phenylalanine disappearance which reveals, perhaps, that the specific effect of glucose addition will depend upon the test amino acid and its peculiar organ-metabolic structure. Although preliminary, these results indicate the need to probe further, with the aid of tracer techniques, the metabolic basis for changes in nitrogen balance due to alterations in the dietary energy supply. From this brief discussion it is fair to conclude at this point in our analysis that we still have little appreciation for the detailed metabolic events that account for many of the energy-nitrogen relations reviewed above. Protein turnover, oxidative metabolism, and nitrogen (amino acid) utilization will be discussed in detail in our chapter (Young et al., Energy and Protein Turnover) later in this volume.

ACKNOWLEDGMENTS

The senior author's unpublished studies were supported by NIH grants DK15856 and DK42101. Studies were conducted at the general Clinical Research Center at the Massachusetts Institute of Technology funded by a grant (MO1-44-00088) from the National Center of Research Resources—NIH.

REFERENCES

1. Munro HN. General aspects of the regulation of protein metabolism by diet and by hormones. In: Munro HN, Allison JB, eds. *Mammalian protein metabolism*. New York: Academic Press, 1964;381–481.
2. Young VR, Robert JJ, Motil KJ, Matthews DE, Bier DM. Protein and energy intake in relation to protein turnover in man. In: Waterlow JC, Stephen JML, eds. *Nitrogen metabolism in man*. Essex, England: Applied Science Publishers, 1981;417–47.
3. Young VR, Munro HN, Matthews DE, Bier DM. Relationship of energy metabolism to protein metabolism. In: Kleinberger G, Deutsch E, eds. *New aspects of clinical nutrition*. Basel: Karger, 1983;47–73.
4. Edens NK, Gil KM, Elwyn DH. The effects of varying energy and nitrogen intake on nitrogen balance, body composition and metabolic rate. *Clin Chest Med* 1986;7:3–17.
5. Bursztein S, Elwyn DH, Askanazi J, Kinney JM. *Energy metabolism, indirect calorimetry and nutrition*. Baltimore: Williams & Wilkins, 1989;85–118.
6. Munro HN. Carbohydrate and fat as factors in protein utilization. *Physiol Rev* 1951;32:449–88.
7. Calloway DH, Spector H. Nitrogen balance as related to caloric and protein intake in active young men. *Am J Clin Nutr* 1954;2:405–12.
8. FAO/WHO/UNU. Energy and protein requirements. Report of a joint FAO/WHO/UNU Consultation. *Technology report series no 724*. Geneva: World Health Organization, 1985.
9. Ljunggren H, Ikkos D, Luft R. Basal metabolism in women with obesity and anorexia nervosa. *Br J Nutr* 1961;15:21–34.
10. Peterson CC, Nagy KA, Diamond J. Sustained metabolic scope. *Proc Natl Acad Sci (USA)* 1990;87:2324–8.
11. Bartholomew GA. Energy metabolism. In: Gordon MS, ed. *Animal physiology: principles and adaptations*, 4th ed. New York: Macmillan, 1982;46–93.
12. Moore FD. Homeostasis: bodily changes in trauma and surgery. The responses to injury in man as the basis for clinical management. In: Sabiston DC Jr, ed. *Davis-Christopher textbook of surgery. The biological basis of modern surgical practice*, 11th ed. Philadelphia: WB Saunders, 1977;27–64.
13. Schiller WR, Long CL, Blakemore WS. Creatinine and nitrogen excretion in seriously ill and injured patients. *Surg Gynecol Obstet* 1979;149:561–6.
14. Waterlow JC, Millward DJ. Energy cost of turnover of protein and other cellular constituents. In: Wieser W, Gnaiger E, eds. *Energy transformations in cells and organisms*. Stuttgart: Georg Thieme Verlag, 1990;277–82.
15. Newsholme EA, Stanley JC. Substrate cycles: their role in control of metabolism with specific references to the liver. *Diabetes Metab Rev* 1987;3:295–305.
16. Beckmann RP, Mizzen LA, Welch WJ. Interaction of Hsp70 with newly synthesized proteins: implications for protein folding and assembly. *Science* 1990;248:850–4.
17. Lingappa YR. Intracellular traffic of newly synthesized proteins. Current understanding and future prospects. *J Clin Invest* 1989;83:739–51.
18. Rapoport TA. Protein transport across the ER membrane. *Trends Biochem Sci* 1990;15:355–58.
19. Baker KP, Schatz G. Mitochondrial proteins essential for viability mediate protein import into yeast mitochondria. *Nature* 1991;349:205–8.
20. Berridge MJ. Inositol triphosphate and diacylglycerol: two interacting second messengers. *Annu Rev Biochem* 1987;56:159–93.
21. Berridge MJ, Mitchell RH, eds. *Inositol lipids and transmembrane signalling*. London: The Royal Society, 1988.
22. Bourne HR, Sanders DA, McCormick F. The GTPase super family: conserved structure and molecular mechanism. *Nature* 1991;349:117–27.
23. Hall A. The cellular functions of small GTP-binding proteins. *Science* 1990;249:635–40.
24. Company M, Arenas J, Abelson J. Requirement of the RNA helicase-like protein PRP22 for release of messenger RNA from spliceosomes. *Nature* 1991;349:487–93.

25. Schwer B, Guthrie C. PRP16 is an RNA-dependent ATPase that interacts transiently with the spliceosome. *Nature* 1991;349:494–99.
26. Gupta NK. Regulation of eIF-2 activity and peptide chain initiation in animal cells. *Trends Biochem Sci* 1987;12:15–8.
27. Moldave K. Eukaryotic protein synthesis. *Annu Rev Biochem* 1985;54:1109–49.
28. Rechsteiner M. Ubiquitin-mediated pathways for intracellular proteolysis. *Annu Rev Cell Biol* 1987;3:1–30.
29. Plomp PJAM, Wolvetang EJ, Groen AK, Meijer AJ, Gordon PB, Seglen PO. Energy dependence of autophagic protein degradation in isolated hepatocytes. *Eur J Biochem* 1987;164:197–203.
30. Samonds KW, Hegsted DM. Protein deficiency and energy restriction in young cebrus monkeys. *Proc Natl Acad Sci (USA)* 1978;75:1600–4.
31. Coyer PA, Rivers JPW, Millward DJ. The effect of dietary protein and energy restriction on heat production and growth costs in the young rat. *Br J Nutr* 1987;58:73–85.
32. Ausman LM, Gallini DL, Hegsted DM. Protein-calorie malnutrition in squirrel monkeys: adaptive response to calorie deficiency. *Am J Clin Nutr* 1989;50:19–29.
33. Millward DJ. The hormonal control of protein turnover. *Clin Nutr* 1990;9:115–26.
34. Young VR, Marchini JS. Mechanisms and nutritional significance of metabolic responses to altered intakes of protein and amino acids, with reference to nutritional adaptation in humans. *Am J Clin Nutr* 1990;51:270–89.
35. Long CL, Lowry SF. Hormonal regulation of protein metabolism. *J Parenter Enteral Nutr* 1990;14:555–68.
36. Coward WA, Lunn PG. The biochemistry and physiology of kwashiorkor and marasmus. *Br Med Bull* 1987;37:19–24.
37. Costa G. Cachexia, the metabolic component of neoplastic disease. *Cancer Res* 1977;37:2327–35.
38. DeWys WD. Pathophysiology of cancer cachexia: current understanding and areas for future research. *Cancer Res* 1982;42:S721–26.
39. Pisters PWT, Brennan MF. Amino acid metabolism in human cancer cachexia. *Annu Rev Nutr* 1990;10:107–32.
40. Folin O. Laws governing the chemical composition of wine. *Am J Physiol* 1905;13:66–115.
41. Folin O. A theory of protein metabolism. *Am J Physiol* 1905;13:117–38.
42. Schoenheimer R. The dynamic state of body constituents. Cambridge, MA: Harvard University Press, 1942.
43. Rand WM, Young VR, Scrimshaw NS. Change of urinary nitrogen excretion in response to low protein diets in adults. *Am J Clin Nutr* 1975;29:639.
44. Rand WM, Scrimshaw NS, Young VR. Conventional ("long-term") nitrogen balance studies for protein quality evaluation in adults. Rationale and limitations. In: Bodwell CE, Adkins JS, Hopkins DT, eds. *Protein quality in humans: assessment and in vitro estimation.* Westport, CT: AVI Publishing, 1981;61–94.
45. Elwyn DH, Gump FE, Munro HN, Iles M, Kinney JM. Changes in nitrogen balance of depleted patients with increasing infusions of glucose. *Am J Clin Nutr* 1979;32:1597–611.
46. FAO/WHO. Energy and protein requirements. Report of a joint FAO/WHO Ad Hoc Expert Committee. *WHO technical report series no 522.* Geneva: World Health Organization, 1973.
47. Calloway DH, Margen S. Variation in endogenous nitrogen excretion and dietary nitrogen utilization as determinants of human protein requirement. *J Nutr* 1971;101:205–16.
48. Cahill GF Jr. Starvation in Man. *J Clin Endocrinal Metab* 1976;5:397–415.
49. Marliss EB, Murray FT, Narhooda AF. The metabolic response to hypocaloric protein diets in obese man. *J Clin Invest* 1978;62:468–79.
50. Larivere F, Wagner DA, Krupranycz D, Hoffer LJ. Prolonged fasting as conditioned prior protein depletion: effect on urinary nitrogen excretion and whole body protein turnover. *Metabolism* 1990;39:1270–77.
51. Inoue G, Fujita Y, Nijyama Y. Studies on protein requirements of young men fed egg protein and rice protein with excess and maintenance energy intakes. *J Nutr* 1973;103:1673–87.
52. Calloway DH. Nitrogen balance of men with marginal intakes of protein energy. *J Nutr* 1975;105:914–23.
53. Garza C, Scrimshaw NS, Young VR. Human protein requirements: the effect of variations in energy intake within the maintenance range. *Am J Clin Nutr* 1976;29:280–7.
54. Garza C, Scrimshaw NS, Young VR. Human protein requirements: interrelationships between energy intake and nitrogen balance in young men consuming the 1973 FAO/WHO safe level of egg protein, with added non-essential amino acids. *J Nutr* 1978;108:90–6.

55. Kishi Y, Miyatani S, Inoue G. Requirement and utilization of egg protein by Japanese young men with marginal intake of energy. *J Nutr* 1978;108:658–69.
56. Chiang A-N, Huang P-C. Excess energy and nitrogen balance at protein intakes above the requirement level in young men. *Am J Clin Nutr* 1988;48:1015–22.
57. Elwyn DH, Gump FE, Iles M, Long CL, Kinney JM. Protein and energy sparing of glucose added in hypocaloric amounts to peripheral infusions of amino acids. *Metabolism* 1988;27:325–31.
58. Elwyn DH. Nutritional requirements of adult surgical patients. *Crit Care Med* 1980;8:9–20.
59. Lukaski HC. Methods for assessment of human body composition: traditional and new. *Am J Clin Nutr* 1987;46:537–56.
60. Whitehead RG, Prentice A, eds. *New techniques in nutritional research*. San Diego: Academic Press, 1991;433.
61. Todd KS, Butterfield GE, Calloway DH. Nitrogen balance and deficient energy intake at three levels of work. *J Nutr* 1984;114:2107–18.
62. Robert JJ, Cummins JC, Wolfe RR, et al.: Quantitative aspects of glucose production and metabolism in healthy elderly subjects. *Diabetes* 1982;31:203–11.
63. Young VR. Tracer studies of amino acid kinetics: a basis for improving nutritional therapy. In: Tanaka T, Okada A, eds. *Nutritional support in organ failure*. Amsterdam: Excerpta Medica, 1990;3–34.
64. Waterlow JC. Opening remarks. In: Garrow JS, Halliday D, eds. *Substrate and energy metabolism in man*. London: John Libbey, 1985;1–6.
65. Shaw JHF, Klein S, Wolfe RR. Assessment of alanine, urea, and glucose interrelationships in normal subjects and in patients with sepsis with stable isotopic tracers. *Surgery* 1985;97:557–67.
66. Munro HN. Metabolism basis of nutritional care in liver and kidney disease. In: Winters RW, Greene HL, eds. *Nutritional support of the seriously ill patient*. New York: Academic Press, 1983;93–105.
67. Souba WW, Smith RJ, Wilmore DW. Glutamine metabolism by the intestinal tract. *J Parenter Enteral Nutr* 1985;9:608–17.
68. Souba WW. Interorgan ammonia metabolism in health and disease; A surgeon's view. *J Parenter Enteral Nutr* 1987;11:569–79.
69. Waterlow JC, Garlick PJ, Millward DJ. Protein turnover in mammalian tissues and in the whole body. 1978; Amsterdam: North Holland Publishing Co.
70. Waterlow JC. Protein turnover with special reference to man. *Q J Exp Physiol* 1984;69:409–38.
71. Young VR, Yu Y-M, Krempf M. Protein and amino acid turnover using stable isotopes ^{15}N, ^{13}C and ^{2}H as probes. In: Whitehead RG, Prentice A, eds. *New techniques in nutritional research*. San Diego: Academic Press, 1991;17–72.
72. Bier DM, Matthews DE, Young VR. Interpretation of amino acid kinetic studies in the context of whole-body protein metabolism. In: Garrow JS, Halliday D, eds. *Substrate and energy metabolism in man*. London: John Libbey, 1985;27–36.
73. Garrow JS, Halliday D, eds. Substrate and energy metabolism in man. London: John Libbey, 1985;1–250.
74. Millward DJ, Price GM, Pacy PJH, Halliday D. Whole body protein and amino acid turnover in man: what can we measure with confidence? *Proc Nutr Soc* 1991;50:197–216.
75. Bier DM. Intrinsically difficult problems: the kinetics of body proteins and amino acids in man. *Diabetes Metab Rev* 1989;5:111–32.
76. Young VR. 1987 McCollum award lecture: kinetics of human amino acid metabolism: nutritional implications and some lessons. *Am J Clin Nutr* 1987;46:709–25.
77. Bier DM. Stable isotope methods for nutritional diagnosis and research. *Nutr Rev* 1982;40:129–34.
78. Bier DM, Matthews DE. Stable isotope tracer methods for in vivo investigations. *Fed Prod* 1982;41:2679–85.
79. Matthews DE, Bier DM. Stable isotope methods for nutritional investigations. *Annu Rev Nutr* 1983;3:309–39.
80. Rennie MJ, Halliday D. The use of stable isotope tracers as metabolic probes of whole body and limb metabolism. *Proc Nutr Soc* 1984;43:189–96.
81. Schmelz E, Schmidt H-L. Stable isotope-labelled molecules: indispensable tools in clinical diagnosis, pharmacology and nutritional sciences. *Pharmacy Intl* 1983;4:1153–57.
82. Lifson N, Little WS, Levitt DG, Henderson RM. $D_2{}^{18}O$ method for CO_2 output in small animals and economic feasibility in man. *J Appl Physiol* 1975;39:657–63.
83. Prentice AM, ed. *The doubly-labelled water method for measuring energy expenditure. Technical recommendations for use in humans*. A consensus report by the IDECG working group. Vienna: International Atomic Energy Agency, NAHRES-4, 1990;301p.
84. Reeds PJ, Harris CI. Protein turnover in animals: man in his context. In: Waterlow JC, Stephen JML, eds. *Nitrogen metabolism in man*. London: Applied Science Publishers, 1981;391–408.

85. Kleiber M. Body size and metabolic rate. *Physiol Rev* 1947;27:511–41.
86. Blaxter K. Energy metabolism in animals and man. Cambridge: Cambridge University Press, 1989;336p.
87. Hokkanen JEI. The size of the largest land animal. *J Theor Biol* 1986;118:491–99.
88. Welle S, Nair KS. Relationship of resting metabolic rate to body composition and protein turnover. *Am J Physiol* 1990;258:E990–8.
89. Nair KS, Halliday D. Energy and protein metabolism in diabetes and obesity. In: Garrow JS, Halliday D, eds. *Substrate and energy metabolism in man*. London: John Libbey, 1985;195–202.
90. Robinson SM, Jaccard C, Persaud C, Jackson AA, Jéquier E, Schutz Y. Protein turnover and thermogenesis in response to high-protein and high-carbohydrate feeding in men. *Am J Clin Nutr* 1990;52:72–80.
91. Schöch G, Topp H, Held A, et al. Interrelation between whole-body turnover rates of RNA and protein. *Eur J Clin Nutr* 1990;44:647–58.
92. Young VR, Munro HN. N$^\tau$-methylhistidine (3-methylhistidine) and muscle protein turnover: an overview. *Fed Proc* 1978;37:2291–300.
93. Stadtman ER. Protein modification in aging. *J Gerontol* 1988;43:B112–20.
94. Dean RT. A mechanism for accelerated degradation of intracellular proteins after limited damage by free radicals. *FEBS Lett* 1987;220:278–82.
95. Matthews W, Tanaka K, Driscoll J, Ichihara A, Goldberg AL. Involvement of the proteasome in various degradative processes in mammalian cells. *Proc Natl Acad Sci (USA)* 1989;86:2597–601.
96. Driscoll J, Goldberg AL. The proteasome (multi-carbohydrate protease) is a component of the 1500-kDa proteolytic complex which degrades ubiquitin-conjugated proteins. *J Biol Chem* 1990;265:4789–92.
97. Horsch A, Martins de Sa C, Dineva B, Spindler E, Schmid H-P. Proteasomes discriminate between mRNA of adenovirus-infected and uninfected HeLa cells. *FEBS Lett* 1989;246:131–36.
98. Kumatori A, Tanaka K, Inamura N, et al. Abnormally high expression of proteasomes in human leukemic cells. *Proc Natl Acad Sci (USA)* 1990;87:7071–5.
99. Denne SC, Kalhan SC. Leucine metabolism in human newborns. *Am J Physiol* 1987;253:E608–E615.
100. Young VR, Steffee WP, Pencharz PD, Winterer JC, Scrimshaw NS. Total human body protein synthesis in relation to protein requirements at various ages. *Nature* 1975;253:192–4.
101. Beaufrere B, Putet G, Padchiauadi C, Salle B. Whole body protein turnover measured with ^{13}C-leucine and energy expenditure in preterm infants. *Pediatr Res* 1990;28:147–52.
102. Kien CL, Camitta BM. Close association of accelerated rates of whole body protein turnover (synthesis and breakdown) and energy expenditure in children with newly diagnosed acute lymphocytic leukemia. *J Parenter Enteral Nutr* 1987;11:129–34.
103. Kien CL, Rohrbaugh DK, Burke JF, Young VR. Whole body protein synthesis in relation to basal energy expenditure in healthy children and in children recovering from burn injury. *Pediatr Res* 1978;12:211–16.
104. Fearon KCH, Hansell DT, Preston T, et al. Influence of whole body protein turnover rate on resting energy expenditure in patients with cancer. *Cancer Res* 1988;48:2590–5.
105. Winthrop AL, Wesson DE, Pencharz PB, Jacobs DG, Heim T, Filer RM. Injury severity, whole body protein turnover, and energy expenditure in pediatric trauma. *Metabolism* 1987;22:534–7.
106. Melville S, McNurlan MA, Calder AG, Garlick PJ. Increase protein turnover despite normal energy metabolism and responses to feeding in patients with lung cancer. *Cancer Res* 1990;50:1125–31.
107. Edén E, Ekman L, Bennegard K, Lindmark L, Lundholm K. Whole-body tyrosine flux in relation to energy expenditure in weight-losing cancer patients. *Metabolism* 1984;33:1020–7.
108. Duke JH, Jorgensen SB, Broell JR, Long CL, Kinney JM. Contribution of protein to caloric expenditure following injury. *Surgery* 1970;68:168–74.
109. Tzankoff SP, Norris AH. Effect of muscle mass decrease on age-related BMR changes. *J Appl Physiol: Respir Environ Exercise Physiol* 1977;46:1001–6.
110. Young VR. Amino acids and proteins in relation to the nutrition of elderly people. *Age Aging* 1990;19:S10–24.
111. Young VR, Gersovitz M, Munro HN. Human aging: protein and amino acid metabolism and implications for nutritional requirements. In: Moment GM, ed. *Nutritional approaches to aging research*. Boca Raton, FL: CRC Press, 1982;47–81.
112. Nair KS, Halliday D, Griggs RC. Leucine incorporation into mixed skeletal muscle proteins in humans. *Am J Physiol* 1988;254:E208–13.

113. Long CL, Birkharn RH, Geiger JW, Blakemore WS. Contribution of skeletal muscle protein in elevated rates of whole body protein catabolism in trauma. *Am J Clin Nutr* 1981;34:1087–93.
114. Zurlo F, Larson K, Bogardus C, Ravussin E. Skeletal muscle metabolism is a major determinant of resting energy expenditure. *J Clin Invest* 1990;86:1423–7.
115. Fukagawa NK, Bandini LG, Young JB. Effect of age on body composition and resting metabolic rate. *Am J Physiol* 1990;259:E233–8.
116. Gill M, France J, Summers M, McBridge BW, Milligan LP. Simulation of the energy costs associated with protein turnover and Na^+, K^+-transport in growing lambs. *J Nutr* 1989;119:1287–99.
117. McBride BW, Early RJ. Energy expenditure associated with sodium/potassium transport and protein synthesis in skeletal muscle and isolated hepatocytes from hyperthyroid sheep. *Br J Nutr* 1989;62:673–82.
118. Skou JC. The energy coupled exchange of Na^+ for K^+ across the cell membrane. The Na^+, K^+-pump. *FEBS Lett* 1990;268:314–24.
119. Shetty PS. Physiological mechanisms in the adaptive response of metabolic rates to energy restriction. *Nutr Res Rev* 1990;3:49–74.
120. Waterlow JC. Metabolic adaptation to low intakes of energy and protein. *Annu Rev Nutr* 1986;6:495–526.
121. Nair S, Woolf PD, Welle SL, Matthews DE. Leucine, glucose and energy metabolism after 3 days of fasting in healthy human subjects. *Am J Clin Nutr* 1987;46:557–62.
122. Hoffer LJ, Forse RA. Protein metabolic effects of a prolonged fast and hypocaloric refeeding. *Am J Physiol* 1990;258:E832–40.
123. Apfelbaum M, Bostsarran J, Locatis D. Effect of caloric restriction and excessive caloric intake on energy expenditure. *Am J Clin Nutr* 1971;24:1405–9.
124. Heshka S, Yang M-U, Wang J, Burt P, Pi-Sunyer FX. Weight loss and change in resting metabolic rate. *Am J Clin Nutr* 1990;52:981–86.
125. Garlick PJ, Clugston GA, Waterlow JC. Influence of low-energy diets on whole-body protein turnover in obese subjects. *Am J Physiol* 1980;238:E235–44.
126. Pencharz PB, Motil KJ, Parsons HG, Duffy BJ. The effect of an energy restricted diet on the protein metabolism of obese adolescents: nitrogen-balance and whole body nitrogen turnover. *Clin Sci* 1980;59:13–18.
127. Hoffer LJ, Bistrian BR, Young VR, Blackburn GL, Matthews DE. Metabolic effects of very low calorie weight reduction diets. *J Clin Invest* 1984;73:750–58.
128. Motil KJ, Bier DM, Matthews DE, Burke JF, Young VR. Whole body leucine and lysine metabolism studied with [1-^{13}C]leucine and [α-^{15}N]lysine: response in healthy young men given excess energy intake. *Metabolism* 1981;30:783–91.
129. Welle S, Matthews DE, Campbell RG, Nair KS. Stimulation of protein turnover by carbohydrate overfeeding in men. *Am J Physiol* 1989;257:E413–7.
130. Hoerr RA, Matthews DE, Bier DM, Young VR. Leucine kinetics from [^{2}H$_3$]- and [^{13}C] leucine infused simultaneously by gut and vein. *Am J Physiol* 1991;260:E111–7.
131. Krempf M, Hoerr RA, Pelletier VA, Marks LA, Gleason R, Young VR. An isotopic study of the effect of dietary carbohydrate on splanchnic uptake of dietary leucine and phenylalanine. 1991; [*in preparation*].

DISCUSSION (this discussion also applies to the chapter by Young et al., *Energy and Protein Turnover*)

Dr. Milligan: The authors addressed a topic formidable in both its volume and breadth. They successfully managed to bring forward a number of substantial issues, some controversial, that will certainly guide future research and future nutritional approaches.

The starting point of the chapter is a useful reminder that the interrelation of energy and nitrogen is complex because it is an interaction: protein synthesis, and thus the use of amino acids, entails substantial energy, while simultaneously amino acids are also substrates for oxidation and energy metabolism. An additional and welcome reminder is the admonition that nitrogen balance measurements, in and of themselves, are the result of so many variables that they do not provide insight into metabolic mechanisms. It is essential to be able to integrate the entire set of components of nitrogen metabolism and from that arrive at balances. In this respect, it is evident that most of the information currently available on protein and amino acid metabolism in humans is, understandably, highly aggregated across a variety of components. Thus, although a measure of whole-body protein synthesis is a great deal more informative than one of nitrogen balance, we cannot lose sight of the need for identification of the tissue, cell, and indeed molecular components of the aggregated synthesis. The chapter nicely incorporates results from techniques that are currently at the forefront although, as noted elsewhere in the conference, there must be emphasis on going further. Indeed, the topic of peptide use and reuse requires serious attention (1).

Results have been assembled to further confirm a high frequency of positive correlations between whole-body protein synthesis, turnover, and resting metabolic rate in adult mammals. Recently, this has also been measured for chickens (2). Even though the numeric magnitude of association is such that the energetic costs for synthesis of peptide bonds are only a fraction of total resting energy expenditure, it is possible, perhaps, that protein synthesis and its associated metabolism actually establishes resting metabolic rate as has been suggested for animals (3). This holds considerable biological fascination and is yet unresolved. Indeed, the authors of the present chapter take care to bring forward possible causes for the lack of positive correlation. Furthermore, the concept that whole-body protein synthesis and turnover establishes resting metabolic rate would seem, in principle, to be excluded by the authors argument that amino acid requirements are actually determined by the extent to which amino acids are oxidized. In this latter proposal, amino acid oxidation is quite clearly stated to take metabolic precedence over utilization of amino acids for synthesis. That is, oxidative metabolism is considered to be the controller. Alternately, as noted by the authors, there are views (4) for a rather greater role of protein synthesis and its regulation through the anabolic drive of amino acids in the determination of amino acid requirements. In this circumstance, protein synthesis and a regulatory role of amino acids of some as yet undefined breadth could be envisaged to play a more directive role in total energy expenditure.

The authors very effectively show that there are nearly no definitive answers for the whole-body effect of dietary substitution of energy nutrients on protein metabolism. This appears to result in substantive part from the numerous variables that may influence response including state of health, endocrine influences, secondary physiological effects, amount and composition of intake, protein contribution, and possible specific influences on alanine and glutamine metabolism. As noted by the authors, there will, in the future, need to be greater attention given to the effects of specific dietary lipids on protein metabolism. Certainly, omega-3 fatty acids and trans fatty acids do not have equivalent biological effects. Therefore, we cannot simply expect that they can validly be considered only as lipids in their interaction with protein synthesis.

An immediate major practical point in this chapter is the indication that currently accepted amino acid requirements of adults should be revised because of the influence of an energy/protein interaction in the studies underlying the standards.

REFERENCES

1. Furst P, Albers S, Stehle P. Symposium on ''new substrates in clinical nutrition.'' Dipeptides in clinical nutrition. *Proc Nutr Soc* 1990;49:343–59.
2. Aoyagi Y, Tasaki I, Okumura JI, Muramatsu T. Energy costs of whole-body protein synthesis measured *in vivo* in chicks. *Comp Biochem Physiol*, [A] 1988;91:765–8.
3. Webster AJF. Energetics and maintenance and growth. In: Giarardier L, Stock MJ, eds. *Mammalian thermogenesis*. New York: Chapman & Hill, 1983;178–207.
4. Millward DJ, Price GM, Pacy PJH, Halliday D. Symposium on ''protein requirements.'' Maintenance protein requirements: the need for conceptual reevaluation. *Proc Nutr Soc* 1990;49:473–87.

*Energy Metabolism: Tissue Determinants and
Cellular Corollaries*, edited by J. M. Kinney
and H. N. Tucker. Raven Press, Ltd.,
New York © 1992.

From SDA to DIT to TEF

W. P. T. James

The Rowett Research Institute, Aberdeen, AB2 9SB, United Kingdom

It is nearly 90 years since Rubner (1) first coined the term "specific dynamic action" and for subsequent decades there has been intense interest in determining the basis for the increase in oxygen consumption following a meal. The different terms used for this phenomenon are not synonyms but reflect a desire by different investigators to move away from the assumptions implicit in Rubner's hypothesis and terminology. Underlying the whole debate, however, is the drive to identify and quantitate the variety of mechanisms responsive to feeding. Those involved in this area include both human and animal nutritionists and it is to the latter that we must turn for rigorous studies, many of which have been summarized by Blaxter in both his original and recent books (2,3).

Rubner's terminology was developed because he thought that the increased oxygen uptake after a meal was specifically in response to the protein ingested. The "dynamic" component of his term signified his rejection of Voit's concept that normal cellular metabolism was unstimulated by the protein and the word "action" may have reflected his belief that the effect was a direct stimulus of oxygen uptake as those amino acids not used for glucose synthesis were oxidized.

Within 2–3 decades Lusk and others (4) had shown that the effect was not exclusively dependent on dietary protein and that glucose generation was not a key to explaining the observations. The effects of different amino acids such as glycine and phenylalanine on metabolism did show, however, that direct stimulation was involved even if its nature remained obscure. This was also the time when the term "luxuskonsumption" was being coined (5) and two parallel interests were eventually to emerge—the link between the immediate effects of a meal, which was Rubner's chief concern, and the body's capacity to dissipate its energy on prolonged overfeeding. It is little wonder, therefore, that eventually a new term developed and "dietary induced thermogenesis" (DIT) became the favored nomenclature (6). Again an active process was inferred, but no longer was protein the exclusive issue. Thermogenesis dealt with heat generation but this was usually assessed from measurements of oxygen uptake. Human direct calorimetry had lapsed but oxygen uptake studies were still being used. However, the concept of monitoring the longer-term effects of overfeeding was dominated by two investigators' claim that their own weight remained stable on widely different intakes (5,7). The use of the Douglas bag

later). Nevertheless it is clear that the plane of nutrition has to be taken carefully into account if the response to meals is to be understood.

Nutrient Imbalances: A Low Protein Diet

One of the most dramatic claims relating to Mitchell's concept (27) that the balance of nutrients is important in determining the efficiency of utilization came with Miller and Payne's study on the metabolic efficiency achieved by feeding either a low or a normal protein diet in growing pigs (29). In practice, only a single pig was used for each diet and all their conclusions were based on the weight changes of the two animals fed first one and then the other diet. It was suggested that since the low protein diet led to weight maintenance, despite a high energy intake, then there must be a marked metabolic response to the low protein diet. No measurements of either oxygen uptake or body composition were made, however.

Miller later suggested (9) that there was a mechanism in the body which allowed the ready dissipation of heat after a meal as unnecessary nutrients were combusted; an animal could retain the critical mix of nutrients required for its own needs. This theory is little different from that of Voit last century except that Miller was inferring that the mechanism was one which had developed on an evolutionary basis because of its general biological advantage. Miller backed up the conclusions from the pig experiments, however, with a series of studies in human volunteers fed different nutrient mixes at a high plane of nutrition (30,31). Those students overfed a low protein diet had a much smaller rate of weight gain than those fed more protein. Thus Miller considered the "luxuskonsumption" to be very dependent on the protein intakes of the diet. Unfortunately, both the single pig study and the human work were based essentially on the dietary effects of these intakes on weight changes alone.

When Gurr and his colleagues (32) repeated the studies they also found that a high protein intake required only 4.3 MJ daily to maintain body weight compared with an intake of 14 MJ daily if a low protein diet was fed. Gurr went on, however, to measure the energy retained in the carcasses of the pigs and showed that there was a loss of body energy on the high protein diet but a marked accumulation on the low protein regime. Similar results were obtained by McCracken and McAllister (33) and by Fuller (34). One may conclude that the weight changes seen by Miller and Payne (29) had a different basis on the two diets; protein and water were being lost on the low protein diet, but weight was being maintained by the deposition of energy dense fat. These studies provided no experimental back-up for Miller's volunteer studies which were conducted over only a 3-week period of overfeeding and without measures of any change in body composition and only summary data on oxygen uptake (31).

Alcohol

Although the response to carbohydrate, fat, and protein has received intense study, far less research has been undertaken on the effects of alcohol on PPT. Never-

*Energy Metabolism: Tissue Determinants and
Cellular Corollaries*, edited by J. M. Kinney
and H. N. Tucker. Raven Press, Ltd.,
New York © 1992.

From SDA to DIT to TEF

W. P. T. James

The Rowett Research Institute, Aberdeen, AB2 9SB, United Kingdom

It is nearly 90 years since Rubner (1) first coined the term "specific dynamic action" and for subsequent decades there has been intense interest in determining the basis for the increase in oxygen consumption following a meal. The different terms used for this phenomenon are not synonyms but reflect a desire by different investigators to move away from the assumptions implicit in Rubner's hypothesis and terminology. Underlying the whole debate, however, is the drive to identify and quantitate the variety of mechanisms responsive to feeding. Those involved in this area include both human and animal nutritionists and it is to the latter that we must turn for rigorous studies, many of which have been summarized by Blaxter in both his original and recent books (2,3).

Rubner's terminology was developed because he thought that the increased oxygen uptake after a meal was specifically in response to the protein ingested. The "dynamic" component of his term signified his rejection of Voit's concept that normal cellular metabolism was unstimulated by the protein and the word "action" may have reflected his belief that the effect was a direct stimulus of oxygen uptake as those amino acids not used for glucose synthesis were oxidized.

Within 2–3 decades Lusk and others (4) had shown that the effect was not exclusively dependent on dietary protein and that glucose generation was not a key to explaining the observations. The effects of different amino acids such as glycine and phenylalanine on metabolism did show, however, that direct stimulation was involved even if its nature remained obscure. This was also the time when the term "luxuskonsumption" was being coined (5) and two parallel interests were eventually to emerge—the link between the immediate effects of a meal, which was Rubner's chief concern, and the body's capacity to dissipate its energy on prolonged overfeeding. It is little wonder, therefore, that eventually a new term developed and "dietary induced thermogenesis" (DIT) became the favored nomenclature (6). Again an active process was inferred, but no longer was protein the exclusive issue. Thermogenesis dealt with heat generation but this was usually assessed from measurements of oxygen uptake. Human direct calorimetry had lapsed but oxygen uptake studies were still being used. However, the concept of monitoring the longer-term effects of overfeeding was dominated by two investigators' claim that their own weight remained stable on widely different intakes (5,7). The use of the Douglas bag and Kofranyi-Michaelis system shifted to the domain of exercise physiologists with Passmore and Durnin dominating the field as they continued the classic studies of Garry on the energy costs of work (8). For 30 or more years from the 1940s onwards, their studies of the energy cost of work were the principal interests with the exception of the maverick nutritionist Miller (9) who sought to demonstrate that DIT was the fundamental regulatory process controlling energy balance in man. The two opposing camps of Miller and Passmore (10) fought over the basis for the control of energy balance, with neither group producing the definitive studies which would convince the world at large of the validity of their case.

With post-war human studies on DIT in the doldrums, animal nutritionists had begun from scratch to build calorimeters and to assess animal responses to feeding. Blaxter in his AFRC unit at the Hannah Research Institute went back to first principles (2) simulating in ruminant animal experiments the approaches to energetics displayed so vividly by Atwater. Given the apparent complexity of intestinal fermentation, the issue of how best to distinguish bacterial from mammalian metabolism and how to assess the short- and long-term responses of different types and forms of diet for use in growth studies it is little wonder that animal calorimetricians returned to first principles and simply discussed the "thermic effect of feeding," the heat being measured directly in gradient layer or in heat sink calorimeters. We thus see parallel investigations on human and farm animal physiology which are only now being brought together so that those involved in medical aspects of nutritional support can talk in the same language with those who grapple with the basis for the relative inefficiency of forage feeding of sheep, dairy cows, or other ruminant species. More recently we have chosen to distinguish the short- and long-term effects of food by referring to "postprandial thermogenesis" (PPT) when dealing with the response over a few hours to a meal (11), this to be distinguished from the longer-term component of DIT induced by sustained overfeeding where changes in the basal metabolic rate also occur. There have therefore been twin track developments which have brought us to the point where once more we can develop a coherent approach to unraveling the perturbations in the mammalian's physiological and biochemical responses to food ingestion.

It is intriguing to note that whereas human studies still concentrate on demonstrating the magnitude of the responses, animal nutritionists, with their extensive data from experimental observations, have been more concerned with explaining the basis of thermogenesis and assessing whether diets can be changed to alter the efficiency of use of dietary energy and nutrients. It is perhaps helpful to separate these two issues, i.e., the magnitude and the nature of the response, although the two aspects of dietary thermogenesis have been interwoven in discussions throughout this century.

THE SPECIFIC DYNAMIC ACTION OF PROTEINS

The fascination for studying the specific effects of food goes back more than a century and has been beautifully set out by Lusk in his classic textbook on nutrition

(4). He ascribes to Bidder and Schmidt the first studies showing that a food-deprived cat, given unlimited quantities of meat, responded with a marked increase in oxygen uptake and carbon dioxide output. Von Mering and Zuntz believed that the increase in metabolism reflected the response of the intestinal tract to the ingested protein but by 1881 Voit had experimented on dogs and considered the response far too great to be attributed to gut activity. Voit claimed somewhat surprisingly that the magnitude of the response was equivalent to that seen during hard exercise and according to Lusk concluded that "the inherent power of the cells to metabolize was augmented by the presence of increased quantities of foodstuffs."

It was Rubner (1), with his classic work in Voit's laboratory at the turn of the century, who began the systematic studies which led to a clear distinction being made between the energy used by a fasting animal over a 24 h period in an environment free from the thermal influence of cold and the energy being used after food ingestion. Rubner held trained dogs in calorimeters at 33°C under fasting conditions for more than 24 hours. When the equivalent to 100% of their basal energy requirement was then provided as fat free meat protein, he found a 30.9% increase in metabolism. Feeding the basal requirement as fat, however, stimulated metabolism by 12.7%, whereas sugar only led to a 5.8% increase. He concluded that the "specific dynamic action" or SDA of food should be considered as a specific form of energy which was evolved in amounts in excess of the basal requirement of the fasting animal. Rubner claimed that this effect was exclusively dependent on protein and could not be considered in Voit's terms. Voit had favored the early splitting of the N from protein with conservation of the carbon skeleton with most of the protein's energy being stored as either glycogen or fat, this energy being "gradually doled out to the tissues as the need required" (4). It is this concept that gave rise to Voit's "theory of plethora" when explaining the metabolic response to food. Rubner, however, proposed that the cell's inherent metabolism did not change but the extra oxygen uptake simply reflected the extra heat being formed by those intermediate cleavage products of protein metabolism which were *not* being converted to glucose. The low response to glucose led him to believe that this substance was the fundamental cellular fuel to which other nutrients could or could not be converted.

Lusk and his colleagues did not agree with Rubner's glucose theory in part because Lusk in 1912 (12) found a 4.9 calorie stimulus on providing a 100 calories of glucose whereas the response to fat was only 4.1 cal/100 calories dietary fat (13). Furthermore, meticulous studies in dogs of the effects of different proteins and selected amino acids (14) although confirming Rubner's 30% figure for protein, led to a clear distinction between the value of an amino acid in generating glucose and the immediate stimulus to metabolism of this amino acid. Thus alanine, known to be fully convertible to glucose in the diabetic state, should have had no SDA effect, whereas glutamic acid, with only three of its five carbon atoms considered convertible, should have had a clearly greater SDA effect. Lusk found the reverse (4).

It seemed true that the SDA from a wide range of proteins. e.g., beef, chicken, codfish, gliadin, or even gelatin, fed in amounts sufficient to provide a constant nitrogen intake led to similar SDA responses (15). Rapport and Beard (16) also discovered that phenylalanine provided the greatest stimulus to an animal's metabolism, but the effects of selective amino acids on testing in detail did not provide clear evidence of a link between the failure to generate glucose and the amino acid's SDA *in vivo*. The gluconeogenic potential of the amino acid was at that stage assessed in separate experiments on dogs made diabetic with phlorhizine and/or estimated from a wide variety of *in vitro* and *in vivo* studies (4). Those of us who have a combination of surgical and physiological skills and consider organ perfusion a modern investigative tool, should be reminded that Rapport and Katz by 1927 (17) were reporting that glycine could be added to the perfusion of an isolated hind limb preparation of a dog receiving its blood from a second dog. The glycine had a direct stimulating effect on the oxygen uptake of the perfused hind limb so clearly direct rather than centrally mediated stimuli seemed to be involved in the response.

HUMAN STUDIES

While these sophisticated studies were proceeding, human experiments were not neglected. The SDA of meat protein was measured by Aub and DuBois (18) in a variety of rather extraordinary experiments. Equivalent responses were observed in two unusual conditions, i.e., in an achondroplastic dwarf and in an individual with no legs where the muscle mass was considerably less than in a normal adult. Aub and DuBois concluded (wrongly) that SDA related to the surface area of the individual but this was at a time when physiologists were constantly relating all their basal metabolic rate measurements to surface area.

Since then a huge number of studies have been conducted and, despite Garrow's doubts (19), that protein provides the greatest stimulus to oxygen consumption, it seems clear that this is true both for animals and man. Blaxter (3) has recently summarized a large body of animal and human data which emphasize the need to distinguish between the short-term postprandial responses to food and the effects of sustained feeding with differences in dietary composition at levels below and above the maintenance energy needs. This distinction is important because if the postprandial response to dietary fat is to be examined then a short delay in gastric emptying will lead to an even greater delay in the processing and oxidation of the fat. We have shown, using isotopically labeled fat fed to volunteers in whole body calorimeters, that the evolution of ^{14}C labeled oleic acid in the diet as $^{14}CO_2$ only begins after 4–6 hours, with a peak rate of label production 8–10 hours after the ingestion of the labeled meal (20). Thus it would not be surprising if the immediate metabolic response to a fat meal is unimpressive (21). As Blaxter (3) has pointed out by highlighting Acheson's (22) calorimetry studies, it may take 15 hours or more for the metabolic rate to return to fasting levels, implying that many human studies have been too brief to allow proper conclusions to be drawn.

THE DESIGN OF STUDIES ON POSTPRANDIAL THERMOGENESIS

The foregoing therefore raises several issues. First, whether the PPT of a single meal can vary with both the magnitude of the energy ingested and its nutrient composition. Second, whether the same meal given at different times of day produces different effects and third, whether the sequential provision of standardized meals entrains a different response to the second and subsequent meals because metabolic processes are affected by the earlier inflow of nutrients. Few systematic studies in man have been conducted on these issues and the control of meal ingestion has not been a prominent feature of studies on circadian rhythms (23).

These experiments are not, however, easy to design in man. For example, if the response to a standard meal is sought, one can reasonably specify a protocol where volunteers fast for 24 h in calorimeters, then on another occasion have single meals equivalent to perhaps 50% or 100% of this fasting requirement given at different times of day. The effects of meals with either 50% or 100% of the daily maintenance requirement taken at, for example, 2000 h could be compared with a similar meal given at 0800 h or with meals given at both 0800 h and 2000 h. This protocol neglects the problem of varying times of fasting so additional control studies may be needed. These studies are therefore very tedious to conduct and fraught with problems of interpretation; small errors in design or volunteer response can have a very great impact on what in absolute terms are very small changes.

DIURNAL VARIATION

Westrate et al. (24) have recently assessed the diurnal variation in both the RMR and DIT of volunteers fed a standard liquid diet at either 0800–0900 h or at 1400–1500 h. Unfortunately those receiving the meal in the afternoon were given a Dutch breakfast of 2 MJ so the two conditions were not as comparable as they might have been. The metabolic response was also measured for only 4 hours despite the inclusion of fat in the meal so there could have been more sustained if subtle differences. The authors note, however, that the metabolic response had almost returned to baseline values after 4 hours, this presumably reflecting the modest thermogenic effect of fat under these experimental circumstances. They found the RMR in the afternoons to be slightly but not statistically lower than that observed in the mornings. Similarly, the DIT was not significantly different although the overall response in oxygen consumption was slightly greater in the 4 hour morning period. However, the difference amounted to only about 0.5% of the energy content of the meal so any true differences are likely to be remarkably small. To have any hope of establishing significant differences in this type of study would require a substantial number of volunteers and repeated measurements of PPT because the response is far from reproducible. The timing of the response also seemed to alter at different times of the day with the thermogenic surge occurring later and with a higher RQ after the afternoon meal. Thus studies could be interpreted as showing that the fasted subject presented with a liquid meal in the morning immediately responds by metabolizing the meal's glucose with the rapid storage of glycogen also. An afternoon meal, however, will be presented to a volunteer with a different liver glycogen content.

Westrate and his colleagues note that few studies have been conducted with varying fasting periods and that any rise in metabolic rate has to take account of the increasing "stress" of the fasting condition. Personal experience also suggests that very prolonged fasting, together with the need to lie in a totally relaxed state for hours on end into the afternoon is uncomfortable and boring. It requires substantial mental discipline to maintain total muscular relaxation. Thus to have no rise in metabolic rate is surprising; one may conclude that there is little diurnal variation in basal metabolic rate or in DIT. Nevertheless it is a common experience of human calorimetry to find a nadir in sleeping metabolic rates at about 0300 h so some diurnal variation in energy metabolism occurs (25).

FACTORS INFLUENCING DIT

A number of physiological interactions have been investigated over the years and some will only be touched on since they are dealt with extensively in other chapters.

Single Nutrients and Mixed Meals

By 1944 Forbes and Swift (26) were already highlighting the differences between the response to simple nutrients given alone and as part of a mixed feeding regime. They chose mature male rats fed protein, carbohydrate, or fat in single amounts or in combinations as supplements to a basic and standardized ration. They again observed that protein increased metabolism by 32.3% of the ingested energy, carbohydrate by 20.2%, and fat by 16%. They then showed a small metabolic response if these foods were fed in combination in a fixed regime over several days. Thus combining all these three led to a 22% reduction from the additive effects of protein, carbohydrate, and fat given separately whereas protein plus fat induced a 54% smaller response and carbohydrate plus fat a 35% reduction. They concluded that fat was an important thermogenic stimulus which could only be displayed by chronic feeding studies when the rate of assimilation of dietary fat over the hours of the experiment was not an issue.

It was this type of observation which led Mitchell (27) to observe that "the better balanced a ration is in satisfying an animal's requirements, the smaller will be its heat increment and the greater its net energy value." Later Hamilton (28) showed that increasing the protein content of the diet of growing male rats from 4% to 18% decreased the purported specific dynamic effect of the protein but then the SDA remained constant up to a dietary protein intake of 30% before increasing once more as the dietary protein exceeded 40%. These responses are, of course, tied up with the issue of whether animals are growing or at least laying down energy at levels above their maintenance requirements when tests are being conducted. It is, however, clear that the plane of feeding is important as is the balance of nutrients in the diet.

Plane of Nutrition

Blaxter has collated serially over the years the effect of nutrient intakes on the efficiency of their utilization when fed below and above the maintenance value of the animal. Table 1 provides some of his estimated values. It is clear that whatever the species, the efficiency of utilization, i.e., of energy deposition, is high for either fat or carbohydrate if fed below maintenance, but that even at this plane of feeding, 20–30% of the protein's energy is reflected in an increase in oxygen uptake and heat production. When, however, these foods are given at levels above maintenance the responses are very different with 20–46% of the carbohydrate energy being dissipated as heat, 15–22% of the fat, and 36–55% of the protein. His collation of the effects in different species shows modest differences except when it comes to herbivores, e.g., the horse, ox, and sheep, when the question of fermentation re-emerges (see

TABLE 1. *Heat increments of feeding below and above maintenance for individual nutrients and average diets*

Nutrient	Species or group	Heat increment	
		Below maintenance	Above maintenance
Carbohydrate	Simple-stomached	0.06	0.22
	Ruminants	0.20	0.46
	Other herbivores	0.10	0.36
	Birds	0.05	0.23
Fat	Simple-stomached	0.02	0.15
	Ruminants	?	0.21
	Other herbivores	?	0.21
	Birds	0.05	0.22
Protein	Simple-stomached	0.23	0.36
	Ruminants	0.30	0.55
	Other herbivores	0.24	0.50
	Birds	0.20	0.45
Approximate values for species consuming average diets			
	Man	0.10	0.25
	Rat	0.10	0.25
	Dog	0.15	0.30
	Pig	0.15	0.30
	Rabbit	0.20	0.35
	Horse	0.25	0.40
	Ox	0.30	0.50
	Sheep	0.30	0.50
	Chicken	0.10	0.25

Data extracted from Blaxter, ref. 3.

later). Nevertheless it is clear that the plane of nutrition has to be taken carefully into account if the response to meals is to be understood.

Nutrient Imbalances: A Low Protein Diet

One of the most dramatic claims relating to Mitchell's concept (27) that the balance of nutrients is important in determining the efficiency of utilization came with Miller and Payne's study on the metabolic efficiency achieved by feeding either a low or a normal protein diet in growing pigs (29). In practice, only a single pig was used for each diet and all their conclusions were based on the weight changes of the two animals fed first one and then the other diet. It was suggested that since the low protein diet led to weight maintenance, despite a high energy intake, then there must be a marked metabolic response to the low protein diet. No measurements of either oxygen uptake or body composition were made, however.

Miller later suggested (9) that there was a mechanism in the body which allowed the ready dissipation of heat after a meal as unnecessary nutrients were combusted; an animal could retain the critical mix of nutrients required for its own needs. This theory is little different from that of Voit last century except that Miller was inferring that the mechanism was one which had developed on an evolutionary basis because of its general biological advantage. Miller backed up the conclusions from the pig experiments, however, with a series of studies in human volunteers fed different nutrient mixes at a high plane of nutrition (30,31). Those students overfed a low protein diet had a much smaller rate of weight gain than those fed more protein. Thus Miller considered the "luxuskonsumption" to be very dependent on the protein intakes of the diet. Unfortunately, both the single pig study and the human work were based essentially on the dietary effects of these intakes on weight changes alone.

When Gurr and his colleagues (32) repeated the studies they also found that a high protein intake required only 4.3 MJ daily to maintain body weight compared with an intake of 14 MJ daily if a low protein diet was fed. Gurr went on, however, to measure the energy retained in the carcasses of the pigs and showed that there was a loss of body energy on the high protein diet but a marked accumulation on the low protein regime. Similar results were obtained by McCracken and McAllister (33) and by Fuller (34). One may conclude that the weight changes seen by Miller and Payne (29) had a different basis on the two diets; protein and water were being lost on the low protein diet, but weight was being maintained by the deposition of energy dense fat. These studies provided no experimental back-up for Miller's volunteer studies which were conducted over only a 3-week period of overfeeding and without measures of any change in body composition and only summary data on oxygen uptake (31).

Alcohol

Although the response to carbohydrate, fat, and protein has received intense study, far less research has been undertaken on the effects of alcohol on PPT. Nevertheless sporadic studies on alcohol go back to Atwater and Benedict [see Rosenberg and Durnin for a review (35)]. The Glaswegian investigators noted that many previous studies had failed to find an effect but this may be explained by the surprisingly small amounts of energy ingested as alcohol in the tests employed. Furthermore, there does seem to be an interaction between alcohol and food with a prolongation and amplification of the thermic response from about one hour postprandially onwards. Thus, short-term studies are likely to miss the effect. Substantial individual differences between subjects were apparent in Durnin's data and this might be explained by the degree to which subjects were habituated to alcohol. Physiologists, conversant with the details of basal and postprandial measurements, rarely interact with physicians versed in the problems of alcoholism but Lieber has clearly shown the profound energetic differences of substantial alcohol intakes in adults who are either alcohol naive or habituated to large intakes (36). Alcohol induces marked hepatic changes with microsomal proliferation and an enhanced peroxidation of alcohol so that chronic excess alcohol intakes lead to progressive weight losses whereas smaller intakes in previously unexposed subjects lead to progressive weight gain. These metabolic studies imply a marked thermogenic effect of alcohol in habituated subjects.

Meal Size

There is considerable controversy over the importance of the size of the energy load in determining postprandial thermogenesis (37). Some of this controversy seems to depend on the degree to which the energy load substitutes for the energy derived from tissue stores under basal conditions rather than providing so much energy that the input exceeds the immediate metabolic demand. Under the latter circumstances nutrient storage and perhaps general metabolic stimulation may occur.

Dietary Fiber

Scalfi and his colleagues (38) have recently compared the effects over a 6-hour period of a glucomannan supplemented meal and of a generally high fiber meal with a low fiber test meal of equivalent energy content. They observed a systematically lower rate of thermogenesis with the fiber containing foods and particularly after the high fiber meal. The differences were particularly apparent from 2–6 hours after eating; the PPT on the low fiber diet was 6.9% of the energy ingested, 5.1% after the glucomannan supplemented meal, and 4.5% after the high fiber meal. Both groups fed fiber supplemented meals had significantly different responses from that after the low fiber test. Mechanistic explanations including delays in intestinal glucose absorption seem reasonable and consistent with the observed reduction in both the glucose and insulin responses. Gastrointestinal hormone responses cannot be excluded as an explanation, however.

Nutritional Status and Constitutional Differences in Thermogenesis

A distinction needs to be made between the response in postprandial thermogenesis to a meal in subjects of different nutritional states and the effects of sustained feeding systems which, if given below or above maintenance, will themselves steadily alter nutritional state. Few studies have been conducted in man but in 1927 Mason et al. (39) suggested that postprandial heat production was greater in the undernourished. In studies conducted in the Warsaw ghetto there seemed to be increased responses to large 200 g doses of glucose in malnourished adults and children (40) but the choice of such a large dose may be important and it is difficult to discriminate the issue of nutritional state as such. Keys et al. (41) in their review of the literature noted that PPT in undernutrition was very variable and the interpretation of many of the earlier studies was bedeviled by the method of expressing the response. Thus, Strang and McClugage critically reviewed the earlier literature (42) and pointed out that expressing data as a percentage increment from the baseline reading would lead to a supposed greater percentage response in thin individuals than obese because of their lower resting metabolic rate; the proper mathematical approach was therefore to assess the true thermic effects of a meal in terms of the absolute increment above the baseline. They also emphasized the need for more prolonged studies to assess the true effects of the meal since a third of the effect was observed from 4–8 hours after the meal. Previous studies had often only monitored individuals for one hour after feeding. They concluded that identical meals produced the same total increase in oxygen consumption in normal, thin, and obese individuals, but noted that the same meal would have a different impact on the three groups since they were markedly different in size. More recently Ashworth (43) showed a greater surge in metabolism after a meal in malnourished children but Shetty and his colleagues have recently reported a lower response in malnourished Indian adults (44).

Studies in Obesity

After a gap of many decades, the 1970s saw a resurgence of interest in measurements in man and particularly in the possibility that obese individuals might have reduced postprandial thermogenesis. Much of these earlier data have been reviewed elsewhere (45) and it becomes increasingly clear that only a proportion of obese studied in their obese state have a reduced response (46) with little as yet to discriminate those showing the "defect." Recently physiological studies on the effects of food on hepatic vein temperature and oxygen consumption after a meal suggest that extra abdominal insulation, as in advanced obesity, may be the key issue determining a depressed PPT in obesity (47). If true, this would imply a secondary effect of obesity. Thus those in a "post-obese" state, i.e., with a normal weight after a prolonged slimming program, should have returned their PPT to normal. This would demonstrate that the PPT change was a response to the development of obesity rather than a prime factor in its genesis. In practice where studies have been conducted on post-obese subjects, a reduced thermogenesis has still been observed, implying that the different PPT is not dependent on the weight gain and the development of insulated abdominal obesity. Stordy et al. (48) reported that anorexics who were previously obese had a lower PPT than normal controls, even after they had gained weight.

These reports on obesity are, of course, concerned with a somewhat different concept, i.e., whether there is an intrinsic difference between people of different nutritional state rather than trying to establish whether a change in nutritional state can lead to an alteration in postprandial thermogenesis. To document this would require sustained overfeeding studies on previously normal weight volunteers similar to those conducted by Sims (49). Unfortunately Sims did not report formal studies on PPT before and after weight gain so the issue remains unclear.

Exercise

This issue is dealt with in more detail by Pi-Sunyer (*this volume*) and has received extensive analysis. The interactions of exercise with feeding seem clear in short-term minute by minute studies but seem less evident in 24 h calorimetric studies even when volunteers are overfed in a sustained controlled way with either fat (50), carbohydrate (51), or a mixed meal (52). Purported constitutional differences in the amplitude of the short-term interactions are evident (53) but the effect is very small.

Psychological Stress

Westrate et al. have recently studied psychological stress by monitoring the differential effects of either a horror film or a romantic family type video watched by volunteers fed a standard meal (54). To their surprise, the PPT response was substantially elevated in the group shown the horror film, but the response in the pre-meal resting metabolism rate was negligible. Analyses were made of urinary catecholamine excretion but these were not significantly affected. The differential impact of stress on PPT but not on resting metabolic rate implied that an increase in muscle tone was not responsible. The authors excluded activation of the sympathetic nervous system on the grounds that this is accompanied by a clear rise in urinary catecholamines but this conclusion may prove to be premature. Nevertheless, whatever its metabolic basis, this was the first report of an attempt to assess the interactions of DIT with mental stress.

Pregnancy and Lactation

Many studies have been concerned with the efficiency of utilization of food by the pregnant animal laying down extra fat and protein in the maternal body as well as in the developing fetus. These overall energetics combine the energy demand of new tissues, the energy cost of their expansion, and the intrinsic metabolic costs, changed or unchanged, of the rest of the maternal organs. A very large number of studies, mostly conducted by the Rowett Research Institute, have been summarized by Blaxter (3) who felt unable to draw any general conclusions because of the complexities of the issues. Nevertheless, Illingworth et al. (55) in humans has been able to show a suppression of PPT measured over two hours. This effect, amounting to a reduction of 28% below the normal effect, persists from its first documentation at 12 weeks throughout pregnancy and until the mother stops lactating. These effects clearly parallel the greater efficiency of metabolism, particularly in lactation, in experimental animals where the prime target organ seems to be the suppression of brown adipose tissue (56). In humans the overall energetics of pregnancy have been assessed in a multinational study with some evidence of an adaptive suppression of BMR in food-deprived Gambian women (57). However, detailed studies of DIT have not been conducted as part of this multinational project although calorimetric studies on UK women have (58).

The Interaction with Other Stimuli

Three factors associated with meal eating in man might be expected to interact, *viz.*, the incorporation of spices in the food, coexisting smoking, and the ingestion of coffee as well as food. Henry and Emery (59) have shown a marked increase in PPT (measured over 3 hours) in subjects eating spiced rather than non-spiced identical meals. The chili and mustard powder increased the oxygen uptakes by 53 ± 8% compared with a rise of 28 ± 7% after the blander meals.

Caffeine can also increase the metabolic rate for several hours (60–62) but no clear study has yet been conducted to see if there is genuine synergism between the effects of caffeine and the normal metabolic response to meals.

Smokers, when they give up the habit, usually display a fall in their basal metabolic rates. They also lose the immediate thermogenic response to a cigarette as well as increasing their food intake (63). The overall 24 h energy expenditure of smokers is also increased if they smoke but not immediate effect on BMR is apparent (64) implying that there is a more chronic effect of smoking on BMR.

A common mechanism may underlie the impact of these three stimuli if they affect the sympathetic nervous system and thereby increase 24 h energy expenditure. Some interaction with the thermogenic mechanisms associated with food is likely but a remarkable stimulation of the sympathetic nervous system after caffeine ingestion is displayed in individuals who are not normally exposed to high doses of caffeine. The clear effects of smoking on heart rate and on catecholamine excretion point to the involvement of sympathetic nervous system activation.

Environmental Temperature

In the early part of this century the Japanese conducted a remarkable number of serial studies to show the cyclical seasonal variation in basal metabolic rate (65) but few, if any, studies on the seasonal effects on DIT were reported in the English literature.

Recently, however, Kashiwazaki et al. (66) have reviewed the effects of both room and ambient temperatures on fasting and postprandial metabolism. If studies are conducted at 20°C with volunteers kept at this temperature overnight, then a marked increase in fasting metabolism is evident if the studies are conducted in winter, but not in summer. Thus there seems to be some entraining procedure whereby a cool environment in subjects adapted to the cooler climate of winter can stimulate metabolism. However, although the absolute increment in metabolism is sustained after a meal, inspection of their data provides few grounds for believing that there is an additional increment in PPT in the studies conducted at 20°C rather than 25°C and in winter. Thus acclimatization and metabolic responsiveness seem to be confined to basal rather than postprandial metabolism.

Age

Morgan and York (67) and Schwartz and his colleagues (68) have found a reduction in PPT in older men. Schwartz found that the thermogenesis correlated with norepinephrine turnover, measured with a ^{3}H norepinephrine bolus plus constant infusion technique, in young men. A similar relationship was not, however, found in the older group. Thus they infer that it is the responsiveness to the sympathetic component of facultative thermogenesis which is impaired in old age (see later). Golay et al. in studies with glucose loads also found a reduction in thermogenesis in the elderly (69).

THE BASIS FOR THE THERMIC EFFECT OF FEEDING

Given the long-standing interweaving of interests in both the magnitude and causes for the thermogenic response to food, it is perhaps a little surprising to discover how little is known of the nature of the metabolic responses even in animal studies. The explanation is that whole body physiologists attempt to document the differential oxygen uptake of the intestine, liver, muscle, and other organs, but it is experimentally extremely difficult to develop truly physiological studies and at the same time ensure that the precise state of energy and nutrient balance is set to simulate the *in vivo* situation. If this is achieved, it is unusual to find these skills combined with biochemical expertise in the analysis of nutrient uptake and metabolism while combining these studies with rigorous isotopic methodology so that quantitative analyses are made. Two examples will be given of current controversies, one in human studies and the other in ruminants to show how complex the issues can be. Much of this experimental work has, however, dealt with attempts to manipulate the diet and infer from theoretical analyses what might in practice be happening as heat production rises.

PHYSIOLOGICAL COSTS OF EATING

This is a great issue in animal studies (70) but can readily be overcome in humans by providing the nutrients in a simple liquid form. In this way it is easy to ingest the meal over a 2–3 minute interval and have the subject resting quietly once more. Indeed, some investigators have given the load via a nasogastric tube to overcome even this minimal disturbance. The use of the tube, however, may not simply remove the costs of skeletal, muscular, and pharyngeal contraction: the immediate passage of food into the stomach removes the oral and olfactory stimuli which have themselves been recognized to affect the body's reactions to a meal. Nicolaidis and his colleagues showed that rats displayed a rapid rise in RQ and oxygen uptake immediately after a meal even when this was given to a curarized animal maintained on artificial respiration (71). Furthermore, the effect was seen even if a sucrose solution was applied to the rat's tongue. Nicolaidis also claimed that the effect depended on the sympathetic nervous system because a general β-adrenergic blocking drug such as propranolol could block the immediate surge in metabolism. This anticipatory response preceded what he regarded as the classic SDA of food.

Leblanc has conducted studies in man to establish the role of food palatability on postprandial thermogenesis (72). Providing the meal through an orogastric tube reduced the usual postprandial response observed after normal meal feeding. In further experiments volunteers were asked to simulate eating palatable food and showed only a very small increment in oxygen uptake in keeping with the cost of the movement involved in cutting and moving the food towards the mouth; eating the food caused a rapid increase in O_2 uptake within the first 15 minutes with a slower rise thereafter. Sham feeding (where the food was chewed but not swallowed) led to a much greater increase in oxygen uptake which was associated with a greater rise in plasma norepinephrine concentrations 10–60 minutes after feeding. Whether the somewhat unusual task of chewing and spitting out the food induced anxiety rather than the simulation of major oral and olfactory stimulation is not clear but we did show some years ago a series of acute hormonal changes during the anticipatory phase of a meal which were best explained by a vagal induction of insulin secretion (73). More recently Fletcher et al. (74) have shown similar early responses with differences between lean and post-obese subjects which are consistent with acute alterations in parasympathetic stimulation. More formalized studies on the energetic influence of the autonomic nervous system have been undertaken by Nacht et al. (75) who tested the effects of atropine and propranolol on the thermic response to a meal. They found that acute β-adrenergic blockade did not affect the thermic response to food whereas atropine, the muscarinic receptor blocker, did. Obvious concerns about a delay in gastric emptying after atropine are not readily overcome, but the early responses within a few minutes of feeding are unlikely to depend on gastric emptying. Thus it would appear that the autonomic system does have a postprandial effect but that there is increasing doubt about the role of the sympathetic nervous system in determining the thermic response to food under practical everyday conditions. Clearly this field merits more work so that a distinction can be made

between the activation of the sympathetic nervous system and its effectiveness. The steps of secretion and catecholamine activation of the tissue cannot be differentiated by the use of a β-adrenergic blocking drug such as propranolol which acts on the effector organs rather than on the releasing or clearing systems for catecholamine turnover. Nevertheless a change in response to propranolol signifies a physiological catecholaminergic process is involved. This issue is dealt with in greater detail elsewhere in this volume.

INTESTINAL SECRETION AND MOTILITY CHANGES

These effects are not readily quantitated. Blaxter (3) has calculated that the enthalpy of the enzymatic hydrolysis of lipid, polysaccharides, and proteins in the gut lumen amounts to only 0.1–0.2% of the energy content of the substrates hydrolyzed so this makes a very small contribution to the thermic response of a meal. The energy cost of secreting the preformed enzymes from the pancreas is also probably small and the motor activity of the intestine is likely to be of greater significance. Logically one might infer that one could assess this by comparing the effects of the same nutrients given intravenously rather than orally but this presupposes that any difference is solely the result of obviating the need for enzyme secretion, intestinal contraction and absorption. Furthermore, feeding studies with agar-agar or cathartics which provide metabolizable substrates if any only to the colon stimulate motility but have very modest thermogenic effects indeed.

Similarly the potential input of lower gut fermentation of food is also small. Despite early observations that volatile fatty acids are readily absorbed from the large bowel (76) estimates of the substrate input and energetic loss through fermentation are very small (77). Blaxter (3) also estimates the colonic fermentation effect to be about 1% in man. It would seem then that in man the energetic input of luminal digestion, fermentation, mechanical mixing, and nutrient absorption makes only a very modest contribution to postprandial thermogenesis.

RESPONSES TO PROTEIN: AMINO ACID OXIDATION AND PROTEIN SYNTHESIS

This issue dominated Rubner's considerations (1) and has recently been challenged by Ashworth's early work (43) and her later studies on recovering malnourished children (78). Ashworth showed that the surge in oxygen uptake on feeding malnourished children was modest in the early phase of treatment when substantial metabolic readjustments were being made. However, once the children had passed the first week or two of recovery from their extreme metabolic derangement and had begun on the recovery phase then the increase in oxygen uptake was proportional to the induced growth rate (78). The marked growth rate, which is known to be associated with an increase in both protein synthesis and breakdown (79) tends to be associated, at least in the early phases, with a marked conservation of amino acids as revealed by nitrogen balance studies. Therefore Ashworth observed a thermogenic response when amino acid catabolism was low but protein turnover high. For this reason she questioned not only Rubner's original theory but the analysis advanced by Krebs (80) who calculated the oxygen uptake associated with specific amino acid oxidative pathways and concluded that this was a relatively inefficient process which involved the catabolism of amino acids unassociated with ATP synthesis. Ashworth's work clearly implies that amino acid catabolism is not the dominant issue determining postprandial thermogenesis at all times. Garrow and Hawes (21) have worked on the same problem and found that gelatin, a protein with a limited amino acid composition inappropriate for general protein synthesis, does not induce a particularly high thermogenic response such as one might expect if amino acid catabolism were the dominant response to its feeding. Clearly to explore this issue in more detail requires an accurate analysis of amino acid catabolism and protein synthesis in association with feeding in humans. This would appear to be straightforward but Garlick's recent studies (81) have highlighted the methodological difficulties of monitoring protein synthesis using the standard techniques which were introduced using L-[1-^{13}C] leucine infusions over periods of several hours (82). Although the methods have become standard practice in clinical studies, Garlick in painstaking experiments has shown that prolonged infusions of labeled leucine produces very different results depending on the length of the infusion in relation to meal intake (81). Recycling of isotope from intermediate compounds or from synthesized protein seems to be a particular problem if infusions are prolonged. So the purported surge in protein synthesis after a meal may not in practice occur in man. It should be remembered that in our original studies on rats we showed that liver and muscle respond very differently to feeding (83). Thus, liver modulates its protein mass primarily by changing liver protein breakdown rates whereas muscle responds to food primarily by an increase in protein synthesis. In man, Garlick found no change in whole body protein synthesis on feeding but a fall in whole body protein breakdown rates provided the studies were conducted to limit isotope recycling. In effect this may indicate that in man the short-term response to dietary protein involves a reduction in hepatic protein breakdown rates, this effect predominating over any increase in muscle protein synthesis. In this case any surge in oxygen uptake cannot be ascribed to an increase in protein turnover—the reverse is true. In conditions of growth, however, the surge in protein turnover shown by Golden et al. (79) may explain the correlation between growth rates and postprandial oxygen consumption noted by Brooke and Ashworth (78).

These new measurements of nutrient turnover illustrate a major problem in assessing the basis for postprandial thermogenesis—not only are the processes involved numerous but different thermogenic systems may operate at different times and some effects may change direction under different circumstances. It is therefore a mistake to presume that the postprandial thermogenesis is based on a single constant mechanism, a point recognized many years ago. For example, Reeds and Fuller in collating a series of studies showed that changes in protein balance are achieved in response to altered dietary energy intakes by an alteration in protein synthesis rates, whereas a change in protein intake achieves a greater change in protein balance by altering both protein synthesis and breakdown rates (84). These studies were, of course, conducted with the older but standard prolonged infusion technique.

The energetics of these responses is difficult to interpret. As noted already, the thermogenic response is less if nutrients are provided below maintenance levels. The substitution of endogenous energy sources by dietary nutrients spares the use of endogenous substrates. Thus, the final oxygen demand will vary depending on the relative ratios of the oxygen used per mole ATP of the dietary compared with endogenous nutrients used.

INTRINSIC COSTS OF ENERGY STORAGE

This issue is dealt with extensively by Flatt (*this volume*). It is noteworthy, however, that when estimates are made of the response to carbohydrate overfeeding in man the increment in oxygen uptake can be greater than that expected for the ATP requirements for fat synthesis from carbohydrate (85). Furthermore, there is an unexplained failure of RQ to rise sufficiently above 1.0 to account calorimetrically for a net synthesis of fat from carbohydrate. In theory there could be a high turnover of glucose to fatty acids with RQs held below one if the equivalent amount of fatty acid were oxidized. This would then be manifest as carbohydrate oxidation calorimetrically but with a high oxygen uptake as more carbohydrate energy was used to fuel the substrate cycle. On this basis, as carbohydrate feeding continued, free fatty acid release from lipolysis would continue. But in practice lipolysis is normally suppressed. Thus, another mechanism, perhaps involving sympathetic activation or thyroidal changes, may have to be invoked under conditions of severe overfeeding. As Norgan (86) has noted in commenting on our own studies on fat overfeeding (50,87) the thermogenic response is far higher than can be inferred from the theoretical costs of fat storage. Some form of metabolic stimulus therefore seems to be involved.

METABOLIC STIMULATION

Thyroidal and autonomic stimuli have often been studied (88,89) and in end organ terms could also involve changes in the sodium pump as well as in substrate cycles, protein turnover, etc. (90). If the concept holds that postprandial thermogenesis can be affected by abdominal insulation (47) with a peripheral stimulation of thermogenesis then consideration will need to be given to the theories of Clark and colleagues (91) who suggest that much of the thermogenic response depends on the activation of endothelial cell metabolism in the arteriolar walls, thereby providing a new approach to explaining the link among overfeeding, weight gain, and an increase in blood pressure.

CONCLUSIONS

That such a long list of effector systems and modulating factors of postprandial thermogenesis has to be set out is in itself a sign that we know surprisingly little about the metabolic basis for the responses of man to food. The last 10 years have shown that the extent of adaptation of human energy expenditure under normal everyday conditions is far less than originally suggested. Nevertheless, a sustained change in postprandial thermogenesis could alter energy balance over a prolonged period. Whether our research is into the metabolic basis of obesity, the response to stress, or the efficiency of growth, the range of metabolic processes and their energetic significance still need to be determined. We are, however, in a position to reject the idea that protein has a specific dynamic action, to recognize that dietary input may not induce much thermogenesis if modest amounts are fed or if food is given to a very malnourished person. We are left therefore with the more modest designation of the thermic effect of food as a physiological feature with many regulators and with a variety of biochemical bases.

When several reliable isotopic techniques are combined we will be able to assign different explanations to the same thermogenic responses observed under different circumstances. Then progress will really begin to be made.

REFERENCES

1. Rubner M. *Die Gesetze des Energieverbrauchs bei der Ernährung*. Lepizig: Franz Deuticke, 1902;426.
2. Blaxter KL. *The energy metabolism of ruminants*. London: Hutchinson, 1962.
3. Blaxter KL. *Energy metabolism in animals and man*. Cambridge: Cambridge University Press, 1989.
4. Lusk G. *The science of nutrition*, 4th ed. Philadelphia: WB Saunders, 1928.
5. Neumann RA. Experimentelle Beitrage zur Lehre von dem taglichen Nahrungsbedarf de Menschen unter besonderer Berucksichitigung der notvendigen Eisweissmenge. *Arch Hyg Bakt* 1902;45:1–87.
6. Miller DS, Mumford PM. Luxuskonsumption. In: Apfelbaum M, ed. *Energy balance in man*. Paris:Masson et Cie, 1973;195–207.
7. Gulick A. A study of weight regulation in the adult human body during overnutrition. *Am J Physiol* 1922;60:371–395.
8. Passmore R, Durnin JVGA. *Energy, work and leisure*. London: Heinemann Educational Books, 1967.
9. Miller DS. Thermogenesis in everyday life. In: Jequier E, ed. *Regulation of energy balance in man*. Geneva: Editions Médicine et Hygiène, 1975;198–208.
10. Passmore R. Energy balance in man. *Proc Nutr Soc* 1967;26:97–101.
11. Shetty PS, Jung RT, James WPT, Barrand MA, Callingham BA. Postprandial thermogenesis in obesity. *Clin Sci* 1981;60:519–525.
12. Lusk G. Metabolism after ingestion of dextrose and fat, including the behaviour of water, urea and sodium chloride solutions. *J Biol Chem* 1912;13:27–47.
13. Murlin JR, Lusk G. The influence of the ingestion of fat. *J Biol Chem* 1915;22:15–41.
14. Williams HB, Riche JA, Lusk G. Metabolism of the dog following the ingestion of meat in large quantity. *J Biol Chem* 1912;12:349–376.
15. Rapport D. The relative specific dynamic action of various proteins. *J Biol Chem* 1924;60:497–511.
16. Rapport D, Beard HH. The effects of protein split-products upon metabolism. II. The individual amino acids of fraction I of the butyl alcohol extraction and their relation to the specific dynamic action of protein. *J Biol Chem* 1927;73:299–319.
17. Rapport D, Katz LN. The effect of glycine upon the metabolism of isolated perfused muscle. *Am J Physiol* 1927;80:185–199.
18. Aub JC, DuBois EF. The basal metabolism of dwarfs and legless men with observations in the specific dynamic action of protein. *Arch Intern Med* 1917;19:840–864.

19. Garrow JS. *Energy balance and obesity in man*, 2nd ed. Oxford: Elsevier, 1978.
20. Lean MEJ. *Brown adipose tissue in humans*. [Thesis]. Cambridge: University of Cambridge, 1986.
21. Garrow JS, Hawes SF. The role of amino acid oxidation in causing "specific dynamic action" in man. *Br J Nutr* 1972;27:211–219.
22. Acheson KJ, Schutz Y, Bessard E, Ravussin E, Jéquier E. Nutritional influences in lipogenesis and thermogenesis after a carbohydrate meal. *Am J Physiol* 1984;246:E62–E70.
23. Aschoff J, Pohl H. Rhythmic variations in energy metabolism. *Fed Proc* 1970;29:1541–1552.
24. Westrate JA, Weys PJM, Poortvliet EJ, Deurenberg P, Hautvast JGAJ. Diurnal variation in postabsorptive resting metabolic rates and diet-induced thermogenesis. *Am J Clin Nutr* 1989;50:908–914.
25. Goldberg GR, Prentice AM, Davies HL, Murgatroyd PR. Overnight and basal metabolic rates in men and women. *Eur J Clin Nutr* 1988;42:137–144.
26. Forbes EB, Swift RW. Associative dynamic effects of protein, carbohydrate and fat. *J Nutr* 1944;27:453–468.
27. Mitchell HH. Balanced diets, net energy value and specific dynamic effects. *Science* 1934;80:558–561.
28. Hamilton TS. The heat increments of diets balanced and unbalanced with respect to protein. *J Nutr* 1939;17:583–599.
29. Miller DS, Payne PR. Weight maintenance and food intake. *J Nutr* 1962;78:255–261.
30. Miller DS, Mumford P. Gluttony. I. An experimental study of overeating on low or high protein diets. *Am J Clin Nutr* 1967;20:1212–1222.
31. Miller DS, Mumford P, Stock MJ. Gluttony. II. Thermogenesis in over-eating man. *Am J Clin Nutr* 1967;20:1223–1229.
32. Gurr MI, Mawson R, Rothwell MJ, Stock M. Effects of manipulating dietary protein and energy intake on energy balance and thermogenesis in the pig. *J Nutr* 1980;110:532–542.
33. McCracken KJ, McAllister A. Energy metabolism and body composition of young pigs given low protein diets. *Br J Nutr* 1984;51:225–234.
34. Fuller MF. Energy and nitrogen balances in young pigs maintained at constant weight with diets of differing protein content. *J Nutr* 1983;113:15–20.
35. Rosenberg K, Durnin JVGA. The effect of alcohol on resting metabolic rate. *Br J Nutr* 1978;40:293–298.
36. Lieber C. The influence of alcohol on nutritional status. *Nutr Rev* 1988;46:241–254.
37. Kinabo JL, Durnin JVGA. Thermic effect of food in man: effect of meal composition and energy content. *Br J Nutr* 1990;64:37–44.
38. Scalfi L, Coltorti A, D'Arrigo E, et al. The effect of dietary fibre on postprandial thermogenesis. *Int J Obes* 1987;11(Suppl 1):95–99.
39. Mason EH, Hill E, Charlton D. Abnormal specific dynamic action of protein, glucose, and fat associated with undernutrition. *J Clin Invest* 1927;4:353–387.
40. Fliederbaum J, Heller A, Zweibaum K, Szejnfinkel S, Elbinger R, Ferszt F. Metabolic changes in hunger disease. In: Winick M, ed. *Hunger disease*. New York, Wiley-Interscience, 1979;71–123.
41. Keys A, Brozek J, Henschel A, Mickelsen D, Taylor HC. *Biology of human starvation*. Minneapolis: University of Minnesota Press, 1950.
42. Strang JM, McClugage HB. The specific dynamic action of food in abnormal states of nutrition. *Am J Med Sci* 1931;182:49–81.
43. Ashworth A. Metabolic rates during recovery from protein-calorie malnutrition: the need for a new concept of specific dynamic action. *Nature* 1969;223:407–409.
44. Kurpad AV, Kulkarni RN, Sheela ML, Shetty PS. Thermogenic responses to graded doses of noradrenaline in undernourished Indian male subjects. *Br J Nutr* 1989;61:201–208.
45. James WPT. Is there a thermogenic abnormality in obesity? In: Garrow JS, Halliday D, eds. *Substrate and energy metabolism in man*. London: John Libbey, 1985:108–118.
46. Jéquier E, Schutz Y. New evidence for a thermogenic defect in human obesity. *Int J Obes* 1985;9(Suppl 2):1–7.
47. Brundin T, Wahren J. Thermal insulation of the abdominal wall reduces meal-induced thermogenesis. *Int J Obes* 1989;13(Suppl 1):1.
48. Stordy BJ, Marks V, Kalucy RS, Crisp AH. Weight gain, thermic effect of glucose and resting metabolic rate during recovery from anorexia nervosa. *Am J Clin Nutr* 1977;30:138–146.
49. Sims EAH, Goldman RF, Gluck CM, Horton ES, Kelleher PC, Rowe DW. Experimental obesity in man. *Trans Assoc Am Physicians* 1968;81:153–170.
50. Dallosso HM, James WPT. Whole body calorimetry studies in adult man. I. The effect of fat overfeeding on 24 h energy expenditure. *Br J Nutr* 1984;52:49–64.

51. Bisdee JT, James WPT. Carbohydrate-induced thermogenesis in man. *Proc Nutr Soc* 1984;43:149A.
52. Ravussin E, Schutz Y, Acheson KJ, Dusmet M, Bourquin L, Jéquier E. Short-term, mixed-diet overfeeding in man: no evidence for "Luxuskonsumption". *Am J Physiol* 1985;249:E470–E477.
53. Segal KR, Gutin B, Albu J, Pi-Sunyer X. Thermic effects of food and exercise in lean and obese men of similar lean body mass. *Am J Physiol* 1987;252:E110–E117.
54. Westrate JA, Van Der Kooy K, Deurenberg P, Hautvast JGAJ. Surprisingly large impact of psychological stress on diet-induced thermogenesis but not on resting metabolic rate. In: Westrate JA, ed. *Resting metabolic rate and diet induced thermogenesis.* Wageningen, 1989;131–137.
55. Illingworth PJ, Jung RT, Howie PW, Isles TE. Reduction in postprandial energy expenditure during pregnancy. *Br Med J* 1987;294:1573–1576.
56. Trayhurn P. Thermogenesis and the energetics of pregnancy and lactation. *Can J Physiol Pharmacol* 1989;67:370–375.
57. Durnin JVGA. Energy requirements of pregnancy: an integration of the longitudinal data from the five-country study. *Lancet* 1987;2:1131–1133.
58. Prentice AM, Goldberg GR, Davies HL, Murgatroyd PR, Scott W. Energy sparing adaptation in human pregnancy assessed by whole body calorimetry. *Br J Nutr* 1989;62:5–22.
59. Henry CJK, Emery B. Effect of spiced food on metabolic rate. *Hum Nutr: Clin Nutr* 1985;40C:165–168.
60. Acheson KJ, Zahorska-Markiewicz B, Pittet Ph, Anantharaman K, Jéquier E. Caffeine and coffee: their influence on metabolic rate and substrate utilization in normal weight and obese individuals. *Am J Clin Nutr* 1980;33:989–997.
61. Jung RT, Shetty PS, James WPT, Barrand MA, Callingham BA. Caffeine: its effect on catecholamines and metabolism in lean and obese humans. *Clin Sci* 1981;60:527–535.
62. Dulloo AG, Geissler CA, Orton T, Collins A, Miller DS. Normal caffeine consumption: influence on thermogenesis and daily energy expenditure in lean and post obese human volunteers. *Am J Clin Nutr* 1989;49:44–50.
63. Dallosso HM, James WPT. The role of smoking in the regulation of energy balance. *Int J Obes* 1984;8:365–375.
64. Hofstetter A, Schutz Y, Jéquier E, Wahren J. Increased 24-hour energy expenditure in cigarette smokers. *N Engl J Med* 1986;314:79–82.
65. Osiba S. The seasonal variation in basal metabolism and activity of thyroid gland in man. *Jpn J Physiol* 1957;7:355–365.
66. Kashiwazaki H, Dejima Y, Suzuki T. Influence of upper and lower thermoneutral room temperatures (20°C and 25°C) on fasting and post-prandial resting metabolism under different outdoor temperatures. *Eur J Clin Nutr* 1990;44:405–413.
67. Morgan JB, York DA. Thermic effect of feeding in relation to energy balance in man. *Ann Nutr Metab* 1983;27:71–77.
68. Schwartz RS, Jaeger LF, Veith R. The thermic effect of feeding in older men: the importance of the sympathetic nervous system. *Metabolism* 1990;39:733–737.
69. Golay A, Schutz Y, Broquet C, Moeri R, Felber JP, Jequier E. Decreased thermogenic response to an oral glucose load in older subjects. *J Am Geriatrics* 1983;31:144–148.
70. Adam I, Young BA, Nicol AM, Degen AA. Energy cost of eating in cattle given diet of different forms. *Anim Prod* 1984;38:53–56.
71. Nicolaidis S. Early systematic responses to orogastric stimulation in the regulation of food and water balance: functional and electrophysiological data. *Ann N Y Acad Sci* 1969;157:1176.
72. Leblanc J, Cabanac M, Samson P. Reduced postprandial heat production with gavage as compared with meal feeding in human subjects. *Am J Physiol* 1984;246:E95–E101.
73. Sahakian BJ, Lean MEJ, Robbins TW, James WPT. Salivation and insulin secretion in response to food in non-obese men and women. *Appetite* 1981;2:209–216.
74. Fletcher JM, McNurlan MA, McHardy KC. Residual abnormality of insulin secretion and sensitivity after weight loss by obese women. *Eur J Clin Nutr* 1989;43:539–545.
75. Nacht CA, Christin L, Temler E, Chiolero R, Jéquier E, Acheson KJ. Thermic effect of food: possible implication of parasympathetic nervous system. *Am J Physiol* 1987;253:E481–488.
76. McNeil NI, Cummings JH, James WPT. Rectal absorption of short chain fatty acids in the absence of chloride. *Gut* 1979;20:400–403.
77. McNeil NI. The contribution of the large intestine to energy supplies in man. *Am J Clin Nutr* 1984;39:338–342.
78. Brooke OG, Ashworth A. The influence of malnutrition on the postprandial metabolic rate and respiratory quotient. *Br J Nutr* 1972;27:407–415.

79. Golden MHN, Waterlow JC, Picou D. Protein turnover, synthesis and breakdown before and after recovery from protein-energy malnutrition. *Clin Sci* 1977;53:473–477.
80. Krebs HA. The metabolic fate of amino acids. In: Munro HN, Allison JB, eds. *Mammalian protein metabolism*, vol 1. New York: Academic Press, 1964:125–176.
81. Melville S, McNurlan MA, McHardy KC, et al. The role of degradation in the acute control of protein balance in man: failure of feeding to stimulate protein synthesis as assessed by L-[1-^{13}C] leucine infusion. *Metabolism* 1989;38:248–255.
82. James WPT, Sender PM, Garlick PJ, Waterlow JC. The choice of label and measurement technique in tracer studies of body protein metabolism in man. In: *Dynamic studies with radioisotopes in medicine 1974*, vol 1. Vienna: International Atomic Energy Agency, 1974:461–472.
83. Garlick PJ, Millward DJ, James WPT, Waterlow JC. The effect of protein deprivation and starvation on the rate of protein synthesis in tissues of the rat. *Biochem Biophys Acta* 1975;414:71–84.
84. Reeds PJ, Fuller MF. Nutrient intake and protein turnover. *Proc Nutr Soc* 1983;42:463–471.
85. Schutz Y, Acheson KJ, Jéquier E. Twenty-four-hour energy expenditure and thermogenesis: response to progressive carbohydrate overfeeding in man. *Int J Obes* 1985;9(Suppl 2):111–114.
86. Norgan NG. Thermogenesis above maintenance in humans. *Proc Nutr Soc* 1990;49:217–226.
87. Zed C, James WPT. Dietary thermogenesis in obesity: fat feeding at different energy intakes. *Int J Obes* 1986;10:375–390.
88. Dauncey MJ. Thyroid hormones and thermogenesis. *Proc Nutr Soc* 1990;49:203–215.
89. Landsberg L, Young JB. Autonomic regulation of thermogenesis. In:Girardier L, Stock MJ, eds. *Mammalian thermogenesis*. London: Chapman Hall, 1983;99–140.
90. Kelly JM, McBride BW. The sodium pump and other mechanisms of thermogenesis in selected tissues. *Proc Nutr Soc* 1990;49:185–202.
91. Ye JM, Colquhoun EQ, Hettiarachchi M, Clark MG. Flow-induced oxygen uptake by the perfused rat hindlimb is inhibited by vasocilators and augmented by norepinephrine: a possible role for the microvasculature in hindlimb thermogenesis. *Am J Physiol Pharmacol* 1989;68:119–125.

DISCUSSION

Dr. Jéquier: Professor Philip James presents a very interesting overview of the mechanisms involved in the increase in oxygen consumption following a meal. He concludes his chapter by mentioning "that such a long list of effector systems and modulating factors of postprandial thermogenesis has to be set out is in itself a sign that we know surprisingly little about the metabolic basis for the responses of man to food." The fact that after a century of intensive research in animals and men on this subject, one of the foremost experts in the field reaches this conclusion emphasizes the complexity of the mechanisms involved in the responses to food.

The term "specific dynamic action" coined by Rubner 90 years ago was replaced by "dietary induced thermogenesis" when it was recognized that the stimulation of oxygen consumption following a meal was not exclusively dependent on dietary protein but that carbohydrate and fat intake also produce an increment in heat generation. More recently, dietary induced thermogenesis has been proposed to describe the long-term effect of food intake on energy metabolism, such as the effect of sustained overfeeding which affects both basal metabolic rate and the thermic effect of feeding. It is germane to follow Professor James' advice when he proposes to use "postprandial thermogenesis" when dealing with the short-term effects after food intake (the response being measured over a few hours after a meal), and "dietary induced thermogenesis" for describing the longer component of food intake which depends on the effects of sustained feeding at levels below or above maintenance energy needs. The designation of "thermic effect of food" can be used as a general term to describe the physiological responses which contribute to increased energy expenditure after the ingestion of a meal.

Doctor James emphasizes the need to distinguish between the magnitude and the nature of the postprandial thermogenic response. It is interesting to assess the magnitude of these responses when nutrients are given by the parenteral route, since the effects of sensory stimuli such as taste and olfaction are absent, and there is no influence of chewing on energy expenditure. Although this procedure does not elicit the full postprandial thermogenic response, it is interesting to know the effects of nutrients on energy expenditure after the phases of ingestion, digestion, and absorption.

When glucose is administered by the intravenous route together with insulin in order to maintain euglycemia (hyperinsulinemic glucose clamp) (1), about 85% of the infused glucose is taken up by muscles, and less than 5% by the liver (2). Throughout the physiologic and pharmacologic range of insulinemia, there is a highly significant relationship between the amount of glucose infused and the net increase in energy expenditure over preinfusion baseline values (3). The slope of the regression line gives the glucose-induced thermogenesis (GIT). At physiological plasma insulin concentrations (i.e., below 200 μU/ml), GIT was found to be 6% of the energy content of glucose infused, whereas the supraphysiological concentrations (i.e., > 400 μU/ml) GIT was increased up to 8%.

When infusing glucose + insulin to a patient, it is interesting to know the rate of replenishment of glycogen stores. The combined technique of the glucose clamp (1) with continuous indirect calorimetry allows the determination of the rate of glucose storage. Glucose storage is obtained by subtracting the rate of glucose oxidation from the total rate of glucose infused (4). The energy cost of glucose storage was found to be 0.45 kcal per gram of glucose stored or 12% of the energy content of glucose infused (4). If one compares this value to the cost of glycogen synthesis, which amounts to about 6% of the energy content of the glycosyl residues transformed into glycogen (5), one notes that the measured cost of glycogen storage is higher than the biochemical "obligatory cost" of glycogen synthesis. The reason for this high energy cost is probably due to the stimulation of sympathetic activity, since plasma norepinephrine levels increase following intravenous infusion of glucose + insulin (6), and a concomitant infusion of a β-adrenergic receptors antagonist, propranolol, decreases by half the thermogenic response to glucose + insulin (7). Thus, the concept of an "obligatory thermogenesis" which accounts for the biochemical cost of glucose storage and of a "facultative thermogenesis," which depends on the stimulation of sympathetic activity (6,7) and of substrate cycling (2) is supported by experimental evidence during intravenous infusion of glucose + insulin in man. Whether the sympathetic nervous system determines the thermic response to the ingestion of food under practical conditions is a subject of controversy.

The thermogenic response to fat infusion is smaller than that of glucose since it amounts to about 3% of the energy of the infused lipids (8). By contrast, amino acid infusion elicits a large increase in energy expenditure, which is about 30% of the value of the infused energy (9).

The possibility that obese individuals might have reduced postprandial thermogenesis needs a few comments. It is well established that only a proportion of obese patients studied have a reduced response (10). Glucose- and diet-induced thermogenesis are blunted in obese patients with insulin resistance (11). Insulin resistance is responsible for a decreased rate of tissue glucose uptake after a meal; this is accompanied by a reduced rate of glucose storage as glycogen in muscles with an economy of expended energy since glycogen synthesis is an energy consuming process. After a meal, a greater fraction of absorbed glucose remains in the extracellular space in obese individuals with insulin resistance as compared with subjects having an unaltered insulin sensitivity. This unstored glucose is available for further uptake and oxidation by various tissues without the need of being transformed first into glycogen. This concept is supported by the finding that the thermic effect of insulin/glucose infusion is proportional to the rate of nonoxidative glucose disposal which mainly corresponds to glucose storage as glycogen (12–14). Thus, the reported differences in glucose-induced thermogenesis between obese individuals appear largely to result from differences in rates of non-oxidative glucose disposal.

The question of the energetic cost of nutrient digestion, mechanical mixing of nutrients in the gastrointestinal tract, and of intestinal absorption also needs to be addressed in man. We have compared the thermogenic responses to the administration of a nutrient mixture given either by the intravenous or the intragastric (nasogastric feeding tube) route (15). The thermic effect of the nutrient was similar during intravenous and intragastric administration, the latter being delayed by about 30 minutes. These results confirm the animal studies described by Doctor James; it seems therefore well established that intestinal digestion and absorption of the nutrients make only a very modest contribution to postprandial thermogenesis.

It is true that the extent of adaptation of human energy expenditure under normal conditions is less than originally suggested. However, a small adaptation is observed in individuals of developing countries submitted to seasonal changes in food availability (16). A field which needs to be further studied is the mechanism involved in the reduced postprandial thermogenesis observed in obese patients after weight loss (10). The use of stable isotopic techniques opens new areas of research for the near future.

REFERENCES

1. DeFronzo RA, Tobin JD, Andres R. Glucose clamp technique: a method for quantifying insulin secretion and resistance. *Am J Physiol* 1979;237:E214–E223.
2. DeFronzo RA, Jacot E, Jéquier E, Maeder E, Wahren J, Felber JP. The effect of insulin on the disposal of intravenous glucose: results from indirect calorimetry, hepatic and femoral venous catheterization. *Diabetes* 1981;30:1000–1007.
3. Schutz Y, Thiébaud D, Acheson KJ, Felber JP, DeFronzo RA, Jéquier E. Thermogenesis induced by five different intravenous glucose/insulin infusions in healthy young men. *Clin Nutr* 1983;2:93–96.
4. Thiébaud D, Schutz Y, Acheson K, et al. Energy cost of glucose storage in man during glucose/insulin infusion. *Am J Physiol* 1983;244:E216–E221.
5. Flatt JP. The biochemistry of energy expenditure. In: Bray GA, (ed). *Recent advances in obesity research* II. London: Newman, 1978, 211–218.
6. Rowe JW, Young JB, Minaker KL, Stevens AL, Pallotta L, Landsberg L. Effect of insulin and glucose infusions on sympathetic nervous system activity in normal man. *Diabetes* 1981;30:219–225.
7. Acheson KJ, Jéquier E, Wahren J. Influence of beta adrenergic blockade on glucose-induced thermogenesis in man. *J Clin Invest* 1983;72:981–986.
8. Thiébaud D, Acheson K, Schutz Y, et al. Stimulation of thermogenesis in man following combined glucose long-chain triglyceride infusion. *Am J Clin Nutr* 1983;37:603–611.
9. Shaw SN, Elwyn DH, Askanazi J, Iles M, Schwartz Y, Kinney JM. Effects of increasing nitrogen intake on nitrogen balance and energy expenditure in nutritionally depleted adult patients receiving parenteral nutrition. *Am J Clin Nutr* 1983;37:930–940.
10. Jéquier E, Schutz Y. Energy expenditure in obesity and diabetes. *Diabetes Metab Rev* 1988;4:583–593.
11. Ravussin E, Acheson KJ, Vernet O, Danforth E Jr., Jéquier E. Evidence that insulin resistance is responsible for the decreased thermic effect of glucose in human obesity. *J Clin Invest* 1985;76:1268–1273.

12. Ravussin E, Bogardus C, Schwartz RS, et al. Thermic effect of infused glucose and insulin in man: decreased response with increased insulin resistance in obesity and non-insulin-dependent diabetes mellitus. *J Clin Invest* 1983;72:893–902.
13. Bogardus C, Lillioja S, Mott D, Zawadski J, Young A, Abbot W. Evidence for reduced thermic effect of insulin and glucose infusions in Pima Indians. *J Clin Invest* 1985;75:1264–1269.
14. Golay A, Schutz Y, Felber JP, DeFronzo RA, Jéquier E. Lack of thermogenic response to glucose/insulin infusion in diabetic obese subjects. *Int J Obes* 1986;10:107–116.
15. Vernet O, Christin L, Schutz Y, Danforth E Jr, Jéquier E. Enteral vs parenteral nutrition: comparison of energy metabolism in healthy subjects. *Am J Physiol* 1986;250:E47–E54.
16. Minghelli G, Schutz Y, Whitehead R, Jéquier E. Seasonal changes in 24-h and basal energy expenditures in rural Gambian men as measured in a respiration chamber. *Am J Clin Nutr* 1991;53:14–20.

Energy Metabolism: Tissue Determinants and
Cellular Corollaries, edited by J. M. Kinney
and H. N. Tucker. Raven Press, Ltd.,
New York © 1992.

Relationship of Diet and Exercise

*F. Xavier Pi-Sunyer and †Karen R. Segal

*Department of Medicine, Division of Endocrinology, Diabetes and Nutrition, Obesity
Research Center, Columbia University at St. Luke's/Roosevelt Hospital Center, New
York, New York 10025; and, †Department of Pediatrics, Division of Pediatric
Cardiology, Mount Sinai School of Medicine, New York, New York 10029

Food enhances thermogenesis and so does exercise. In fact, they are the two primary components of human energy expenditure above the resting metabolic rate, and the independent activation of a thermogenic response by each is well known. What the influence of one is on the thermogenic response of the other has been investigated more recently and is somewhat more controversial. It is the latter phenomenon that will be discussed in this chapter with a focus on differences in the differing responses of lean and obese individuals. Much of this material has been discussed by the authors in previous publications (1,2).

THERMIC EFFECT OF FOOD DURING EXERCISE

An early investigation of the effect of exercise on the thermic effect of food (TEF) was that of Miller and Mumford (3). They exercised volunteers after the ingestion of a meal and measured the thermic effect of food. The exercise, bench-stepping, was done for 30 min. They found that the thermic effect of food was almost twice as large with the exercise compared to rest. This study, however, is flawed because the energy cost of the exercise was not subtracted from the total thermogenic response, so it is impossible to know whether the extra thermogenic response is due only to the exercise itself or to an added synergistic component.

We (4) also explored the relation of the effect of exercise on the thermic effect of food. The metabolic rate was measured for 5 min every half hour for 4 h under six conditions: at rest with and without ingesting a 910-kcal mixed meal; during 5 min of cycle ergometer exercise every half hour at a workload of 50 W, with and without eating, and during 5 min of cycling every half hour at a workload just below each woman's anaerobic threshold, with and without the test meal. A total of 40 min of exercise was performed, spread over a 4-h period so that we could study the time course of the interaction between the meal and exercise. While the thermic effect of food was the same for the lean and obese women, the thermic effect of food during exercise was 2.5-fold greater than at rest for the lean women. As can be seen in Fig.

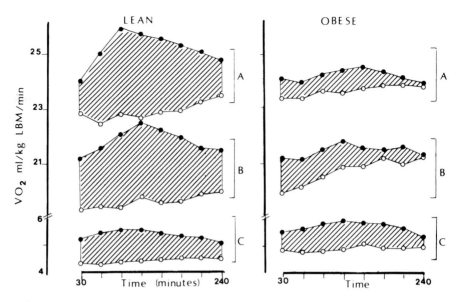

FIG. 1. Effects of exercise and a 910-kcal meal on metabolic rates of lean and obese women. Levels of exercise are (A) anaerobic threshold, (B) 50 W, and (C) rest. Closed circles, postprandial state; open circles, postabsorptive state. Shaded areas represent the thermic effect of food at each level of activity. (From Segal and Gutin, ref. 4, with permission.)

1, exercise did not alter the thermic effect of the meal in the obese women. Thus, in this situation where exercise was done for 5 min every half hour during the whole 240 min postprandial period, exercise potentiated the thermic effect of food for the lean but not the obese women. The energy expended, calculated by adding up the 8 exercise periods of 5 min each, was about 20 kcal greater in the fed condition than the fasted condition in the lean women but we essentially found no difference in the obese. Thus, the potentiating effect of exercise is very small, though statistically significant. Over long periods of time, however, such an effect could become incrementally important.

Studying six normal-weight men, Bray et al. (5) reported results similar to the above. On three mornings, after an overnight fast, the volunteers cycled on an ergometer without having eaten, or after a 1,000 or a 3,000 kcal meal. A greater oxygen consumption was noted when the same exercise was performed in the postprandial than the postabsorptive state.

In the studies cited above, and others not cited, postprandial exercise was performed at only one workload. Therefore, other estimates of efficiency that depend on evaluating the rate of increase in power output which are thought to reflect muscular efficiency (6) could not be calculated and compared to the corresponding fasting values. This measure of efficiency, termed *delta efficiency* by Gaessner and Brooks (6) is reflected in the slope of the regression of energy expended on work performed during graded exercise, such that the steeper the slope is, the lower the efficiency.

We studied this further (7). Graded exercise tests were performed after a 12 h fast and 60 min after the start of a 910 kcal mixed meal, on separate days. The thermic effect of food during exercise was significantly greater for the normal than the obese men at submaximal intensities from unloaded cycling (0 watts to 100 watts). As shown in Fig. 2, the mean slope of the regressions of VO_2 on power output (W), which reflects the rate of increase in energy expended relative to increases in external work performed, did not differ significantly between the fed and fasting conditions for either group, but the mean intercept was significantly higher in the fed than the fasting state for the normal, but not the obese men. The values were 599 ± 53 vs 497 ± 47 ml O_2 per min for the normal men and 819 ± 126 vs 821 ± 145 ml O_2 per min for the obese men. These results indicate that the thermic effect of food during exercise, which was found to be virtually absent in the obese men, did not increase significantly across submaximal power outputs for the normal men and therefore does not reflect a significant reduction in efficiency. That is, there is a fairly constant thermic effect of food during exercise across various levels of submaximal exercise for the normal men. However, there is not a significant thermic effect of food during

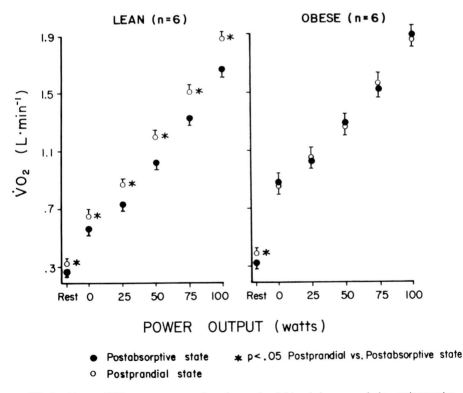

FIG. 2. Mean ±SEM oxygen consumption of normal-weight and obese men during cycle exercise in the postabsorptive and postprandial states. ●, postabsorptive state; ○, postprandial state; * $p <$ .05 postprandial vs postabsorptive state. (From Segal et al., ref. 7, with permission.)

RELATIONSHIP OF DIET AND EXERCISE

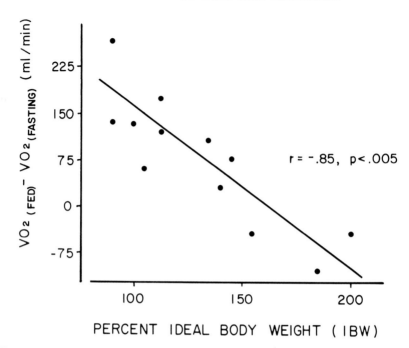

FIG. 3. Relationship between percentage ideal body weight and the thermic effect of food during exercise, which is the postprandial minus postabsorptive VO_2, averaged over workloads from 0 to 100 W. (From Segal et al., ref. 7, with permission.)

exercise for the obese group. The mean thermic effect of food during exercise was significantly negatively related to percentage body fat, total body fat, and percentage ideal body weight (Fig. 3).

The coupling between external or mechanical work and metabolic processes was not significantly altered by the ingestion of a meal. Thus, the thermogenic effect of food during exercise is perhaps related more to processes such as cycling of substrates (8) rather than to a metabolic response within the active skeletal muscles.

No significant thermic effect of food for either the obese or the normal subjects was observed during maximal exercise. This demonstrates that when someone is working at the level of VO_2max, the prior ingestion of a meal does not increase VO_2 further. This seems reasonable since a maximal exercise effort should elicit the maximal energy expenditure from an individual. In effect, a physiological ceiling has been reached on the expenditure of energy by the exercise, and food cannot enhance the effect further.

The thermic effect of food during cycle ergometer exercise was also investigated by Dalloso and James (9). They studied male volunteers while on a weight maintenance diet. They compared the energy cost of exercise performed before and after a meal with the thermic effect of the meal at rest. The energy cost of exercise was greater in the fed than the fasted state, but this added effect of food was not significantly different from the thermic response to the meal at rest. In this study, however, the thermic effect of food was measured for only a short period of time and the fasting and fed conditions were measured on the same day for each activity condition (rest or exercise).

It is important to point out that some of the disagreements of the effect of a meal on exercise thermogenic response may relate to the amount of calories fed in the test meal. For instance, Swindells (10) studying lean women did not find a thermic effect of food during exercise if the test meal contained less than 1,000 kcal. Testing her subjects with a 900 kcal meal followed by 5 hours of rest or preceded and followed by two 30 min exercise bouts on a treadmill at 5.3 km/h, she found the energy increment measured 90 min after the meal to be equivalent to 15 kcal with no exercise and 16 kcal with exercise. Thus, no significant increase in response to the meal as a result of exercise was found.

Zahorska-Markiewicz (11) measured the thermic effect of food at rest and during exercise in 10 lean and 14 obese women. The subjects performed cycle ergometer exercise at 60 watts. The increased thermogenesis from the ingestion of the 4,200 kJ mixed content meal under resting conditions was similar in the two groups,(12–17%). She found, however, that exercise potentiated the thermic effect of the meal in the lean a further 17% but was virtually absent in the obese subjects, who showed a potentiation of only 0.8%. Thus, the energy cost of this exercise after a meal was greater than the sum of the thermic effect of food at rest plus the energy cost of the exercise in the fasted state for the lean but not the obese women.

Warnold et al. (12) studied the effect of adding a meal to exercise thermogenic response in a group of obese volunteers. They tested the effect of cycle ergometer exercise at 65 W with and without a meal of 620 kcal given beforehand. They measured a significant thermic response to the meal at rest, but could find no difference in the energy expended during cycle ergometer exercise at 65 W between the post-absorptive and postprandial states.

EFFECT OF EXERCISE ON POSTPRANDIAL THERMOGENESIS

The studies summarized above focused on determining the effect of the thermic effect of a meal *during* exercise. There have been a number of studies examining the effect of the thermic effect of a meal *after* exercise. These will be summarized below.

Bradfield et al. (13) measured the thermic effect of a meal when subjects walked for 45 min before and after the meal and compared it to a sedentary day. They found that exercise potentiated the thermic effect of the meal. Bielinski et al. (14) conducted a similar study, but the exercise bout was a much more intense 3 hours of treadmill walking. They also found an enhanced thermic effect of food after a previous exercise bout.

A study by Young et al. (15) also measured the effect of prior exercise on the thermic effect of food in lean subjects and, like the above results, showed a potentiation. Zahorska-Markiewicz (11) also documented this.

OBESITY, EXERCISE, AND THERMOGENESIS

We (16) conducted studies of lean and obese subjects, 18 to 35 years of age (Table 1). Both groups were overweight but were similar in body weight and body mass index. We controlled for body weight but deliberately chose them to have extremely different body composition, so that while the lean group of men was 10% fat, the obese group was 30% fat. Body fat accounted for excess weight of the obese group, whereas muscle mass accounted for the excess weight of the lean group. The purpose of this study was to clarify the relationship between body composition and thermogenesis by comparing the responses of men of similar body weight and body mass index but extremely different body composition.

We measured metabolic rate by indirect calorimetry on 4 separate mornings after an overnight fast: (i) 3 h of rest in the postabsorptive state; (ii) 3 h of rest after a 750 kcal mixed meal (14% protein, 31% fat, 55% carbohydrate); (iii) during 30 min of cycling and for 3 h postexercise in the postabsorptive state; and (iv) during 30 min of cycling performed 30 min after the test meal and for 3 h postexercise. The tests were performed in randomized order. Under resting conditions, as can be seen in Fig. 4, the thermic effect of food was greater in the lean compared with the obese group. The exercise treatment consisted of 30 min on a cycle ergometer at a work rate just below each individual's ventilatory threshold performed 30 min after ingestion of the meal. This reflects the highest work rate before the onset of anaerobiosis. There was a significant thermic effect of food during exercise in both groups as indicated by the greater energy expenditure during the 30-min exercise bout in the postprandial than the postabsorptive state (Fig. 5). The thermic effect of food during exercise was significantly greater for the lean than the obese men. During the 30 min exercise bout, the difference in energy expenditure between the postprandial and postabsorptive treatments was 19 ± 3 vs 6 ± 3 kcal for lean vs obese men ($p <$

TABLE 1. *Characteristics of lean and obese men of similar body weight*

Subject characteristics	Obese ($n = 8$)	Lean ($n = 8$)	p
Age (yr)	25.4 ± 1.6	24.6 ± 1.2	NS
Weight (kg)	96.4 ± 4.3	95.0 ± 4.3	NS
Height (cm)	179 ± 2.0	180 ± 3.0	NS
BMI (kg/m^2)	30.0 ± 0.9	29.6 ± 0.6	NS
BSA (m^2)	$2.15 \pm .06$	$2.15 \pm .06$	NS
% Fat	30 ± 2.0	10 ± 1.0	<0.001
Lean body mass (kg)	67.4 ± 2.7	85.0 ± 3.2	<0.001

Values are mean $\pm$ SEM.
From Segal et al., ref. 16, with permission.

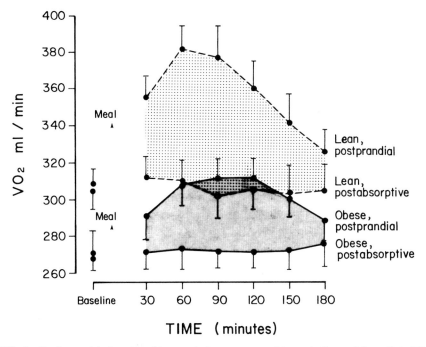

TIME (minutes)

FIG. 4. Resting metabolic rates of lean and obese men over 3 hours in the postabsorptive state and after a 750-kcal mixed meal. The shaded areas represent the thermic effect of food for each group. (From Segal et al., ref. 16, with permission.)

0.05). The thermic effect of food was greater for the lean but not for the obese men during the 30 min exercise bout than during the equivalent 30 min period of rest.

As shown in Fig. 6, in the postexercise condition, the thermic effect of food does not manifest as an increase in metabolic rate, but rather as a reduction in the rate of decline in metabolic rate after exercise. Expressed as the increment in caloric expenditure over 3 h, the thermic effect of food postexercise was 44 ± 7 vs 16 ± 4 kcal for the lean and obese men ($p < 0.05$), respectively. Thus, when the effect of excess weight *per se* is controlled for by use of a lean control group of similar weight, obesity is associated with reduced energy expenditure and a diminished capacity for thermogenesis, both at rest and during exercise. The thermic effect of food was not different between the postexercise and rest conditions for either group.

This study showed that the thermic effect of food at rest, during exercise, and postexercise are significantly greater for lean than obese men of similar height, weight, and degree of overweight, and that body composition is a significant determinant of thermogenesis. The capacity for thermogenesis is blunted in overly fat as compared to overly muscular men.

It is interesting that, in this study (16), as in our previous one (4), percent fat was the best predictor of the thermic effect of food at rest ($r = -0.55$), postexercise

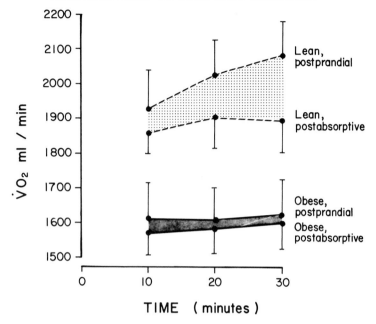

FIG. 5. Metabolic rates of lean and obese men during 30 min of cycle ergometer exercise performed in the postabsorptive state and 30 min after the start of a 750-kcal mixed meal. The shaded areas represent the thermic effect of food during exercise for each group. (From Segal et al., ref. 16, with permission.)

($r = -0.66$) and during exercise ($r = -0.58$). It was a better predictor than lean body mass, body weight, body surface area, and BMI.

We (17) did a second study exploring the interaction of body composition with the effect of food on thermogenic response at rest and during exercise. Two groups of male subjects were chosen who were similar with respect to age, height, and lean body mass, but differed with regard to body fat content and total body weight. Their characteristics are shown in Table 2. Thus, the men were matched with respect to LBM, but differed in percent body fat and total weight. In this study, five, rather than four, experimental treatments were done on each volunteer in randomized order: (i) postabsorptive resting metabolic rate; (ii) postprandial metabolic rate (750 kcal meal of 14% protein, 31.5% fat, and 54.5% carbohydrate); (iii) postabsorptive metabolic rate during and after exercise for 30 min on a cycle ergometer just below the anaerobic threshold; (iv) postprandial metabolic rate during and after exercise, the meal being consumed 30 min prior to the start of exercise; and (v) the 30 min exercise bout was performed in the postabsorptive state and the subjects consumed the test meal within 5 min immediately after the end of exercise.

In this second study, the thermic effect of food at rest was again significantly greater for the lean (53 ± 5 kcal) than for the obese (26 ± 5 kcal). On the exercise

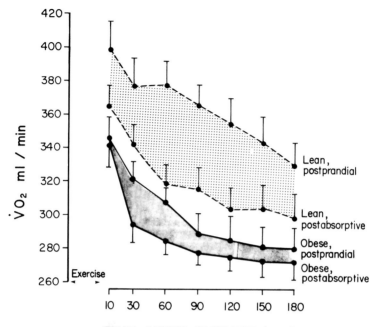

TIME AFTER EXERCISE (min)

FIG. 6. Postexercise metabolic rates of lean and obese men in the postabsorptive and postprandial state. The meal was given 30 min prior to the start of the 30-min exercise bout. The shaded areas represent the postexercise thermic effect of food for each group. (From Segal et al., ref. 16, with permission.)

days, the exercise intensity was adjusted according to each subject's aerobic fitness: the work rate was assigned so that each subject exercised at the highest work rate before the onset of anaerobiosis. The exercise intensity was 53 ± 2% and 54 ± 3% of VO_2max for the obese and lean groups, respectively. The difference in energy expenditure during the exercise between the postprandial and postabsorptive con-

TABLE 2. *Characteristics of lean and obese men of similar body mass*

Subject characteristics	Lean	Obese	p
Age (yr)	24.4 ± 2.1	26.4 ± 1.7	NS
Weight (kg)	74.4 ± 2.2	90.8 ± 3.0	<0.001
Height (cm)	179 ± 3.0	176 ± 3.0	NS
BMI (kg/m^2)	23.2 ± 0.6	29.7 ± 0.6	<0.005
% Fat	12.8 ± 0.7	29.6 ± 1.3	<0.001
Lean body mass (kg)	64.9 ± 2.2	63.8 ± 1.5	NS

Values are mean ± SEM.
From Segal et al., ref. 17, with permission.

ditions was significantly greater for the lean men than the obese men, even though the energy cost of the exercise in the fasted state was similar in the two groups. During the 30 min exercise bout, the difference in energy expenditure between the postprandial and postabsorptive treatments was 24 ± 6 vs 4 ± 2 for the lean and obese men, respectively ($p < 0.05$). In the meal before exercise condition, the effect was again greater for the lean than the obese (67 ± 5) vs (24 ± 6), and the same was true for the meal after exercise condition (57 ± 6) vs (36 ± 7). This study compared the thermic effect of food with two sequences of food and exercise. The effect of the sequence of the meal and exercise on postexercise thermic response to food was significantly different in the lean and obese groups. For the lean men, the thermic effect of food was greater when the meal was eaten before exercise than when the meal followed exercise or when no exercise was performed (Fig. 7). But for the obese men, the thermic effect of food was significantly greater when the meal followed exercise than when the meal preceded exercise or when no exercise was performed, although it was still blunted significantly compared with the lean subjects (Fig. 7). Thus exercise potentiated the thermic effect of a subsequent meal in the obese subjects, raising the thermic response a very significant 50%. This was not so in the lean men.

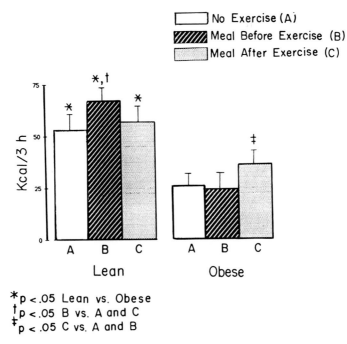

FIG. 7.   Thermic effect of food at rest and postexercise, with two sequences of meal and exercise in lean and obese men. The calculated thermic effect of food is the difference in energy expenditure (kcal per 3 hours) between the postabsorptive and postprandial states. *$p < 0.05$ lean vs obese; †$p < 0.05$ B vs A and C; ‡$p < 0.05$ C vs A and B. (From Segal and Pi-Sunyer, ref. 2, with permission.)

In this second study (17) the correlations between percent fat and thermic response were $r = -0.85$ for thermic effect of food at rest, $r = -0.75$ and -0.61 for the meal before and meal-after exercise conditions, and $r = -0.86$ for the postexercise thermic response.

In conclusion, while some studies have not found an enhancement of the thermic effect of food during exercise (9,18), most have measured a potentiation of postprandial thermogenesis by exercise in lean individuals. The potentiation effect has generally not been found, or found to be less, in obese subjects. While this potentiation effect in energy expenditure is quite small (in the last experiment cited on the order of a difference of 20 kcal for a 30 min exercise bout at 54% VO_2max), it may nevertheless be important in conserving a certain amount of energy daily in obese individuals and thereby incrementally making their obesity even worse.

EFFECTS OF CHRONIC EXERCISE ON THERMOGENESIS

The evaluation of the effects of chronic exercise on energy expenditure is complicated by the difficulty in isolating the effects of physical training from concomitant and possibly confounding changes in energy intake, which by itself can influence energy expenditure and body weight.

The data on the effect of chronic exercise on thermogenesis has been primarily gathered in cross-sectional rather than longitudinal studies. These compare sedentary with highly trained persons. Since there is a great variability in metabolic rate between individuals, longitudinal within subjects studies are actually much superior than the usual between subjects studies. Because longitudinal studies are difficult and expensive to conduct, however, not many of them are available.

Cross-Sectional Studies of Chronic Exercise

There has been controversy as to whether chronic exercise affects resting metabolic rate or food-induced thermogenesis. LeBlanc et al. (19) have reported on the thermic effect of food in three groups of women who differed in their level of habitual exercise and aerobic fitness. They found that resting metabolism was not different among the groups, but the thermic effect of food was smaller in the most highly trained women. However, this study is difficult to interpret because energy expenditure was only measured 120 min postprandially and, since the thermic response to the meal was delayed in the highly trained women, the full thermic response may not have been appropriately measured.

Tremblay et al. (20) gave a 1,636 kcal mixed meal to 8 highly trained (VO_2max of 69.2 ± 2 ml/kg/min) and 8 untrained (VO_2max 47.7 ml/kg/min) men. Again, resting metabolic rate was not found to be different between groups, but the thermic effect of food was significantly smaller in the highly trained as opposed to the sedentary group. Interestingly, the RQ after the meal was lower in the trained men, implying greater fat oxidation, and the RQ correlated with the thermic response to the meal.

Tremblay et al. hypothesized that this smaller thermic response and higher fat oxidation was an adaptation to the heavy program of physical training, allowing carbohydrate to be spared for use during exercise or to replenish glycogen stores.

Hammer et al. (21) studied the effect of 16 weeks of exercise vs no exercise in 2 groups of premenopausal women and found that while VO_2max improved with exercise, there was no effect on RMR. The effect of this on the thermic effect of food was not measured.

Poehlman et al. (22) in a 22-day ergocycle exercise program in which they exercised male monozygotic twins a mean of 166 min/day at a mean intensity of 50% of VO_2max, found no changes in either resting metabolic rate or thermic effect of food with the training.

Poehlman et al. in another study (23) have recently reported on the influence of age and endurance training on metabolic rate in healthy men. They studied four groups, old and young and fit and unfit. They found an RMR (normalized per kg FFM) approximately 6% higher in trained men. This study is in conflict with the four previously mentioned with regard to a training effect on RMR. It is likely that if there is an effect, it is very small, since it cannot be consistently documented. Interestingly, in a third study, Poehlman et al. found the thermic effect of food to be lower in trained than untrained men (24).

Basal metabolic rate and the thermic effect of food were examined in physically well-trained elderly men in comparison with sedentary weight- and age-matched controls by Lundhom et al. (25). BMR was not found to be significantly different but TEF was significantly higher in the physically well-trained men than in the controls. The authors postulated that the elevated TEF might be related to a greater catecholamine sensitivity in the physically trained condition, but this was not actually measured in any manner.

In our studies (16), we have found it difficult to dissect body fatness from physical fitness. We have found an inverse intercorrelation ($r = -0.58$) between the two. We have found that percent fat was the best predictor of the thermic effect of food ($r = --0.55$), postexercise ($r = -0.66$) and during exercise ($r = -0.58$). It was a better predictor than other measures of body composition: lean body mass, body weight, body surface area, or body mass index. The correlation between aerobic fitness (VO_2max) and the thermic effect of food approached but did not reach statistical significance under either the resting ($r = -0.41$) or postexercise ($r = 0.37$) conditions. Since the lean men were more fit than the obese men, it was difficult to separate the effect of aerobic fitness and body composition. We statistically partialed out body fat and found the correlation between aerobic fitness and the thermic effect of food to be essentially zero ($r = 0.04$). We also found that the fasting plasma insulin and the insulin area measured for 2 hours after 75 g oral glucose were related negatively to the thermic effect of food. But we also found that body fat was related to the insulin levels, and when the effect of fat was factored out, the insulin variables were not significantly related to thermogenesis.

Longitudinal Studies of Chronic Exercise

Longitudinal studies in human subjects are harder to conduct and, as a result, fewer are available. We (26) measured resting metabolic rate and the energy cost of five other usual activities during physical training in lean, normal weight women. The exercise periods were 19 days long, and increased the activity of each individual to 10% and 25% above normal expenditure. The exercise was done by treadmill walking at a rapid pace, requiring an average of 96 min per day to raise total 24-hour expenditure by 10% and 240 min per day to raise it 25%. The mean energy cost of activities during a sedentary and the two exercise treatments are shown in Fig. 8. There was no change in either the resting metabolic rate or the cost of various activities. Over this brief period of time, with *ad lib* food intake, lean body mass did not change significantly, but there was a definite training effect, attested to by the continued need to increase the length of time on the treadmill to expend a similar amount of energy. We have done similar studies in obese subjects for 19-day (27) and for 57-day periods (28) with similar results to the above. Thus, this lack of increase in thermogenic response speaks against a thermogenic effect of exercise beyond the energy cost of the exercise itself, or as discussed above, a synergistic effect with a preceding or subsequent meal.

Another longitudinal study was done by Davis et al. (29). They trained three men

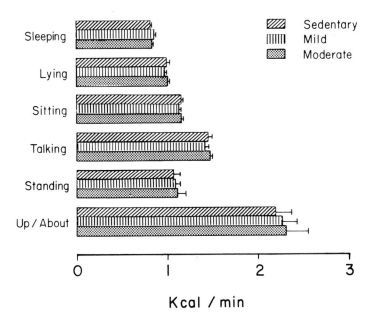

FIG. 8. Mean energy cost of activities during sedentary and two exercise treatments for five women. The mild exercise treatment was 114 ± 4% and the moderate treatment was 129 ± 3% of the sedentary expenditure. (From Woo and Pi-Sunyer, ref. 26, with permission.)

and three women aerobically for 12 weeks. Goal heart rate during training was 150/ min for 30 min and training occurred 3–5 times per week. While VO_2max improved, body composition did not change and resting metabolic rate did not differ before and after training. Also, the same investigators then measured the thermic response to a similar meal in a group of 26 men and women chosen at random (that is, not on a training program) and found that the thermic response to the meal showed a positive relationship to the VO_2max ($r = 0.658$). In addition, the percent fat and the VO_2max were strongly interrelated ($r = -0.727$). It is therefore very difficult to sort out whether the higher thermic response of these individuals is related to their fitness or to their leanness.

EFFECT OF EXERCISE ON SUBSEQUENT METABOLIC RATE

There has been continued controversy as to whether a bout of exercise enhances thermogenesis for an extended period of time. This has been professed by many exercise enthusiasts who maintain that the benefits of exercise derive not only from the energy expended during the exercise period but also for many hours afterwards when the metabolic rate remains elevated.

Studies by Edwards et al. (30), Passmore et al. (31), Margaria et al. (32), and deVries and Gray (33) all described a sustained effect of exercise on subsequent metabolic rate that was variously estimated to last from 7 to 48 hours. Steinhaus (34) and also Karpovich (35) reviewed earlier published data and concluded that no change in subsequent resting metabolism could be demonstrated in response to exercise.

Bielinski et al. (14) reported a 9% increase in metabolic rate for a 4-hour period following a strenuous bout of treadmill exercise and a 4.7% increase in basal metabolic rate on the morning after the exercise. However, this study is complicated by the fact that a greater caloric load was given on the exercise than the control day, confounding the experiment with regard to the 4-hour postexercise period. Also, the exercise bout prescribed was severe (2,100 kcal over 3 hours). During the late postrecovery period, 10 out of 11 metabolic rate values were not significantly different between the rest and exercise trials. It was only the 11th, at 8 A.M., which was elevated by 4.7% on the exercise trial. This amounted to an increase of 0.07 kcal/min and was only present in half the subjects. Thus, this is a problematic study, difficult to interpret. Another study from the same laboratory (36), in which subjects were asked to walk for 1 hour on a treadmill at 4 km/h with a 5% grade, the metabolic rate returned to baseline after the exercise.

We (37) studied thermogenesis after exercise by measuring oxygen consumption in 23 subjects who were classified into 3 groups according to their routine level of physical activity. VO_2 was first measured after a 30-min rest period 4 hours after a standard breakfast. Then each subject either exercised for 20 min at approximately the anaerobic threshold or on a separate non-exercise day remained recumbent. The subject then returned to or remained at rest. We found no significant difference in

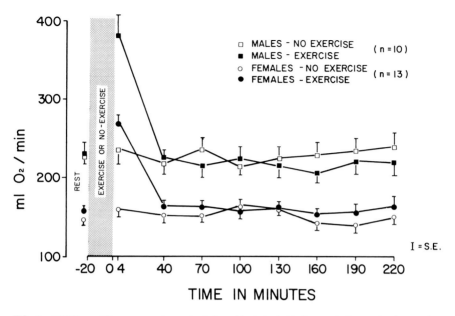

FIG. 9. Milliliters of O_2 consumed per minute by subjects tested before and after moderate exercise or rest. VO_2 values have been collapsed over fitness group since there was no effect of fitness. (From Freedman-Akabas et al., ref. 37, with permission.)

VO_2 from the resting level from 40 min to 3 hours after the exercise, between exercise and non-exercise days in any fitness group. This is shown in Fig. 9. Seven subjects also exercised for a longer period or at a higher intensity. Again, there was no significant difference in the time course of VO_2 from 40 min to 220 min after the exercise, between exercise and non-exercise days. Thus these data do not support claims for sustained increases in metabolic rate after exercise. The difference between this study and others in which a sustained effect of exercise on VO_2 was found may be related to the experimental protocol pursued. A preliminary rest period, a 4-hour interval from the last meal (which was low fat and therefore rapidly absorbed) and a quiet, temperature-controlled room may have allowed for better comparison of the exercise/no-exercise conditions than in the previous studies. The need for such carefully controlled conditions has been stressed by Steinhaus (34).

Blaza and Garrow (38) did a study of heat loss in a direct room calorimeter in lean and obese women which included a 500 W bicycle ergometer bout and they could find no evidence in either group of a measurable long-term increase in metabolism which would increase the energy cost of exercise above that predicted from indirect calorimetry during exercise.

Bingham et al. (39) have also studied this phenomenon in six normal weight volunteers who trained aerobically for 9 weeks. In a room calorimeter, basal metabolic rate, overnight metabolic rate, and sleeping metabolic rate were measured on three occasions: in a baseline control period with minimal physical activity, and at the beginning and end of the training period. These investigators found no changes in any of these three metabolic rate measurements with training. During the peak of training, subjects were running 1 h/day 5 d/wk and VO$_2$max had increased 30%. They concluded that their results do not support the suggestions that there is a sustained increase in BMR following exercise that can usually assist in weight-loss programs beyond the effect of the exercise itself.

Thus, the general consensus is that there is little evidence for a sustained effect of exercise on metabolic rate for long periods after a typical exercise bout.

EFFECT OF UNDERFEEDING

The effect of underfeeding on metabolic rate has been well described. This was first reported by Benedict (40). He placed normal weight volunteers on a hypocaloric diet and showed a fall in metabolic rate. This returned to normal with refeeding and fell again when a restricted diet was reinstituted. Subsequent studies by Keys et al. (41) in normal weight patients showed a similar effect. Bray (42), Apfelbaum (43), and Garrow (44), among others, have shown a similar effect in obese subjects. Because this phenomenon is so well known, it will not be further discussed here.

While there has been some suggestion that exercise may enhance resting metabolic rate during a hypocaloric diet (45) and tend to sustain it closer to the normal level, this has not been borne out in other studies (46). In fact, we have found that resting metabolic rate may actually drop if the diet is too severely restricted and exercise is maintained at a heavy level (47).

EFFECT OF OVERFEEDING

The effect of overfeeding on thermogenesis is the subject of another chapter and will not be discussed here.

MECHANISMS FOR THERMOGENESIS AND THE POSSIBLE LINKS BETWEEN FOOD AND EXERCISE

The thermogenic response to a meal can be divided into two components: obligatory and facultative thermogenesis. The first describes the energy cost of digesting, absorbing, and processing the nutrients and the second defines the energy expended in excess of the obligatory, metabolic demands (48). The mechanisms controlling these two components are not yet clearly worked out. Insulin, catecholamines, glucagon, futile cycles, all may be involved. They also may be involved in exercise effects.

Insulin

The role of insulin in thermogenesis may be best understood by examining the differing response to diet and exercise in lean and obese subjects. In studying the role of insulin in thermogenesis, the nutrient that has been generally used is glucose. It has become clear in the last few years that insulin resistance and impaired insulin-mediated glucose disposal is partly responsible for the blunted thermic response to a glucose load observed in obese people.

Felber et al. (49) showed that the disposal of a 100 g oral glucose load was different in obese subjects with and without glucose intolerance. While the obese subjects without glucose intolerance responded like the lean; the obese subjects with impaired glucose tolerance showed no significant changes in glucose storage and basal oxidation, but a significant decrease in oxidation in response to the load. The subjects with overt diabetes showed both a decrease in glucose oxidation and also a marked reduction in glucose storage. A later important study defining this further was that of Golay et al. (50). These investigators measured the thermic response to oral glucose in lean subjects and in obese subjects with (i) normal glucose tolerance, (ii) impaired glucose tolerance, (iii) type II diabetes with an increased insulin response, and (iv) type II diabetes with a decreased insulin response. They found that the thermic effect of glucose was significantly depressed in the obese compared with normal-weight subjects and that the degree of the reduction in thermogenesis was related to the degree of insulin resistance.

Ravussin et al. (51,52), using the glucose clamp technique, showed that the cost of glucose storage accounted for much of the obligatory component. They suggested that the thermic effect of glucose is the net result of two major components: (a) glucose storage which increases expenditure and (b) suppression of endogenous glucose production which decreases expenditure. Wahren (53) has reported that hepatic glucose production is about 0.8 to 1.0 mmol/min in normal subjects who are postabsorptive. Glycogenolysis accounts for 74–84% of this and gluconeogenesis for the rest (54,55). The more normal the carbohydrate metabolism in an individual, the more is hepatic glucose production suppressed by carbohydrate infusion or a carbohydrate meal.

In their studies Ravussin et al. (52) reported that metabolic rate changes during the glucose clamp correlated well with the rate of glucose storage. In their regression showing the proportion of glucose energy which could be ascribed to glucose storage, they found the slope to be 8.5%, which was greater than the theoretical 5.3% (56). This suggests that other factors must also be important in enhancing energy expenditure produced by glucose disposal. Hormonal thermogenic effects could account for this.

Thiébaud et al. (57) had very similar results. Infusing gradually increasing amounts of insulin in glucose clamp experiments (from 0.5 to 10 mU kg^{-1} min^{-1}) they found that glucose storage accounted for 60–70% of glucose uptake and that there was a significant relationship between the increment in energy expenditure and glucose storage, so that per g of glucose stored, the energy cost was 0.45 kcal. They also found that the energy cost of glucose storage (assuming that all of the glucose was stored as glycogen) only accounted for 45–63% of the increase in energy expenditure. This again suggests that other factors must be important in the increase in energy expenditure accompanying glucose disposal.

Catecholamines

Norepinephrine increases energy expenditure, and it is increased after glucose infusion or ingestion (58–62). Rowe (60) has shown that during the euglycemic insulin clamp plasma norepinephrine may rise by as much as 50% at insulin levels of 154 μU/ml and by 117% at levels of 601 μU/ml. Thus, norepinephrine thermogenic effects may be very important. This is given greater weight by the studies of DeFronzo et al. (63) and Acheson et al. (64) in which the thermic effect of infused glucose was measured before and after β-adrenergic blockade by propanolol during the euglycemic hyperinsulinemic clamp. Both studies reported a greatly reduced (by 50%) thermic response with β-blockade, suggesting a significant role for β-adrenergically mediated sympathetic nervous activity in the thermic response to glucose and insulin. In addition, Welle et al. (62) has shown a significant rise in plasma norepinephrine after a carbohydrate meal.

All of the above observations suggest that the sympathetic nervous system is an important mediator of glucose/insulin-induced thermogenesis and that obese subjects may be resistant to the thermogenic effect of norepinephrine.

OTHER FACTORS AFFECTING THERMOGENESIS

The above discussion has focused on the effect of carbohydrate (in the form of glucose) being stored as glycogen. However, it is possible that some lipid storage may also occur. There is, however, the report by Acheson et al. (65) suggesting that in a mixed meal, little of the carbohydrate is stored as fat. However, if such were to occur, which is unlikely, about 21% of the glucose energy would be required for the conversion (56). It is possible that some energy is utilized in the form of so-called "futile cycles," where substrate is cycled in cells, utilizing ATP but not forming any new net products (8). It is also possible that Na-Ka ATPase is stimulated, enhancing energy expenditure, but little data is available with regard to this phenomenon.

EFFECT OF OTHER NUTRIENTS

The other macronutrients, fat and protein, also have a thermic effect (56). Part of it is again obligatory and part facultative. The phenomenon has been less fully investigated than the carbohydrate effect, but Flatt (56) has discussed the energy cost of this.

EFFECT OF EXERCISE

That exercise *per se* enhances energy expenditure is well known. The energetics of exercise will be discussed by others in this volume and will therefore not be reviewed repetitively here. Suffice it to state that the work of exercise requires energy and this is obtained from the breakdown of creatine phosphate and ATP.

Also, exercise greatly activates the sympathetic nervous system, with an increase in plasma epinephrine and norepinephrine (66). These, as mentioned above, are calorigenic hormones. Also, glucagon is activated, and it also has been reported to enhance energy expenditure (67).

In addition to the obvious direct effect of exercise on thermogenesis, it has been proposed that skeletal muscle may be an important regulatory site for meal-induced thermogenesis (68,69). It is known that the metabolic rate of muscle is much greater than that of fat tissue. The high cost of protein synthesis and turnover may account for much of this (60). In addition, it has been shown that prior exercise enhances the thermic response to the infusion of insulin and glucose in rat skeletal muscle (70).

FITNESS

The effect of physical fitness on thermogenesis has already been discussed. There is controversy about its effects and these effects are confounded by changes in body composition, which themselves have important effects on energy expenditure and thermogenesis (1,2).

COMBINATION OF DIET AND EXERCISE

It seems clear from the literature that exercise enhances the thermic effect of food, although the response is blunted in obese persons. It is likely that the mechanism is due to a number of factors which are activated after a meal is ingested but are further enhanced by the exercise. In response to an acute bout of exercise, peripheral insulin sensitivity is enhanced (71). Thus during and after exercise, glucose uptake is increased and since glycogen has been depleted, the energy-dependent process of glycogen regeneration is activated.

In addition, the increased catecholamine and glucagon levels also abet an enhanced thermogenic response. In addition, Newsholme (8) has speculated that since exercise and ingestion of a meal stimulate substrate cycles individually, the combination of a meal and exercise may lead to an exaggerated greater metabolic response by increasing the rate of substrate cycling.

In summary, the combined stimulus of a meal and exercise may amplify the normal and hormonal responses to the individual stimuli, leading to an overall enhanced thermogenic response (1,2).

CONCLUSION

There are a number of conclusions that we can come to and a number of questions that we need to address.

There is no sustained thermic effect of exercise after mild to moderate intensity exercise, and there is no post-exercise effect of exercise on resting metabolic rate unless the exercise is very prolonged or severe. The quantity of lean body mass is the main determinant of resting metabolic rate.

While in normal weight persons the thermic effect of food is greater during exercise than at rest, in obese persons the potentiating effect of exercise on a meal seems to greatly diminish or disappear. Also, the thermic effect of a meal postexercise is lower in obese compared with lean individuals. In addition, the timing of the meal in relation to exercise and the sequence of the meal and the exercise have important effects. Mechanisms important in the effect of exercise on the thermic response to food include tissue sensitivity to insulin, and increased norepinephrine and glucagon levels. It must be pointed out, however, that the difference between the thermic effect of food during and after exercise, and the thermic effect of food at rest, while consistently statistically significant in our studies, is very small. This makes it rather unimportant in short-term energy balance. However, long-term the difference in expenditure could add up.

The impact of the degree of aerobic fitness and how it relates to thermogenic response is confused because of the intercorrelation of aerobic fitness and body fatness. Body fatness appears to be negatively correlated to the thermic effect of a meal. It is also confusing that while the thermic effect of food is reported to be higher in moderately trained as contrasted to sedentary subjects, in very well-trained subjects the thermic effect of food is decreased.

This paradoxical effect in very fit individuals may be related to a greater reliance on lipid metabolism and a lesser degree of glycogen depletion during exercise. Also, reports of a smaller effect of a meal as well as exercise on sympathetic response in well-trained individuals may be important.

Several questions remain to be answered. What are the specific mechanisms by which exercise enhances the thermic response to a meal? What is the relationship between aerobic fitness and thermogenesis throughout the range of fitness from sedentary to highly conditioned athletes? What are the mechanisms by which physical fitness affects the capacity for thermogenesis?

ACKNOWLEDGMENTS

This project was supported in part by NIH grants DK26687, DK40414, DK37665, and DK37948.

REFERENCES

1. Segal KR, Pi-Sunyer FX. Exercise, resting metabolic rate, and thermogenesis. *Diabetes Metab Rev* 1986;2(1 and 2):29–34.

2. Segal KR, Pi-Sunyer FX. Exercise and obesity. *Med Clin North Am* 1989;73:217–236.
3. Miller DS, Mumford P. Gluttony 2: thermogenesis in overeating man. *Am J Clin Nutr* 1967;20:1223–1229.
4. Segal KR, Gutin B. Thermic effects of food and exercise in lean and obese women. *Metabolism* 1983;32:531–589.
5. Bray GA, Whipp BJ, Koyal SN. The acute effects of food on energy expenditure during cycle ergometry. *Am J Clin Nutr* 1974;27:254–259.
6. Gaesser GA, Brooks GA. Muscular efficiency during steady rate exercise. *J Appl Physiol* 1975;31:1132–1139.
7. Segal KR, Presta E, Gutin B. Thermic effect of food during graded exercise in normal weight and obese men. *Am J Clin Nutr* 1984;40:995–1000.
8. Newsholme EA. A possible metabolic basis for the control of body weight. *N Engl J Med* 1980;302:400–405.
9. Dallosso HM, James WPT. Whole body calorimetry studies in adult men, 2. The interaction of exercise and over-feeding on the thermic effect of a meal. *Br J Nutr* 1984;52:65–72.
10. Swindells YE. The influence of activity and size of meals on caloric response in women. *Br J Nutr* 1972;27:65–73.
11. Zahorska-Markiewicz B: Thermic effect of food and exercise in obesity. *Eur J Appl Physiol* 1980;44:231–235.
12. Warnold I, Carlgren G, Kotkiewski M. Energy expenditure and body composition during weight reduction in hyperplastic obese women. *Am J Clin Nutr* 1978;31:750–763.
13. Bradfield RB, Curtis DE, Margen S. Effect of activity on caloric response of obese women. *Am J Clin Nutr* 1968;21:1208–1210.
14. Bielinski R, Schutz Y, Jéquier E. Energy metabolism during post exercise recovery in man. *Am J Clin Nutr* 1985;42:69–82.
15. Young JC, Treadway JL, Balon TW, Gavras HP, Ruderman NB. Prior exercise potentiates the thermic effect of a carbohydrate load. *Metabolism* 1986;35:1048–1053.
16. Segal KR, Gutin B, Nyman AM, Pi-Sunyer FX. Thermic effect of food at rest, during exercise, and after exercise in lean and obese men of similar body weight. *J Clin Invest* 1985;76:1107–1112.
17. Segal KR, Gutin B, Albu J, Pi-Sunyer FX. Thermic effect of food and exercise in lean and obese men of similar lean body mass. *Am J Physiol* 1987;252E:110–117.
18. Welle S. Metabolic response to a meal during rest and low-intensity exercise. *Am J Clin Nutr* 1984;40:990–994.
19. LeBlanc J, Mercier P, Samson P. Diet-induced thermogenesis with relation to training state in female subjects. *Can J Physiol Pharmacol* 1984;62:334–337.
20. Tremblay A, Côe J, LeBlanc J. Diminished dietary thermogenesis in exercise-trained human subjects. *Eur J Appl Physiol* 1983;52:1–4.
21. Hammer RL, Barrier CA, Roundy ES, Bradford JM, Fisher AG. Calorie-restricted low-fat diet and exercise in obese women. *Am J Clin Nutr* 1988;1:77–85.
22. Poehlman ET, Tremblay A, Nadeau A, Dussault J, Theriault G, Bouchard C. Heredity and changes in hormones and metabolic rates with short-term training. *Am J Physiol* 1986;250:E711–717.
23. Poehlman ET, McAuliffe TL, Van Houten DR, Danforth E Jr. Influence of age and endurance training on metabolic rate and hormones in healthy men. *Am J Physiol* 1990;259:E66–E72.
24. Poehlman ET, Melby CL, Badylak SF. Resting metabolic rate and postprandial thermogenesis in highly trained and untrained males. *Am J Clin Nutr* 1988;48:209–213.
25. Lundholm K, Holm G, Lindmark L, Larsson B, Sjostrom L, Bjorntorp P. Thermogenic effect of food in physically well-trained elderly men. *Eur J Applied Physiol* 1986;55:486–492.
26. Woo R, Pi-Sunyer FX. Effect of increased physical activity on voluntary intake in lean women. *Metabolism* 1985;34:836–841.
27. Woo R, Garrow JS, Pi-Sunyer FX. Effect of exercise on spontaneous calorie intake in obesity. *Am J Clin Nutr* 1982;36:470–477.
28. Woo R, Garrow JS, Pi-Sunyer FX. Voluntary food intake during prolonged exercise in obese women. *Am J Clin Nutr* 1982;36:478–484.
29. Davis JR, Tagliaferro AR, Kertzer R, Gerardo T, Nichols J, Wheeler J. Variations of dietary-induced thermogenesis and body fatness with aerobic capacity. *Eur J Appl Physiol* 1983;509:319–329.
30. Edwards HT, Thorndike A, Dill DB. The energy requirement in strenuous muscular exercise. *N Engl J Med* 1935;213:532–535.
31. Passmore R, Rand RE. Some metabolic changes following prolonged moderate exercise. *Metabolism* 1960;9:452–455.

32. Margaria R, Edwards HT, Dill DB. The possible mechanism of contracting and paying O_2 debt and the role of lactic acid in muscle contraction. *Am J Physiol* 1973;106:689–715.
33. deVries HA, Gray DE. After effects of exercise upon resting metabolic rate. *Res Quart* 1963;34:314–321.
34. Steinhaus AH. Chronic effects of exercise. *Metabolism* 1960;9:452–456.
35. Karpovitch PV. Metabolism and energy used in exercise. *Res Quart* 1941;12:423–431.
36. Schutz Y, Flatt JP, Jéquier E. Failure of dietary fat intake to promote fat oxidation; a factor favoring the development of obesity. *Am J Clin Nutr* 1989;50:307–314.
37. Freedman-Akabas S, Colt E, Kissilleff HR, Pi-Sunyer FX. Lack of sustained increase in VO_2 following exercise in fit and unfit subjects. *Am J Clin Nutr* 1985;41:545–549.
38. Blaza S, Garrow JS. Thermogenic response to temperature, exercise and food stimuli in lean and obese women, studied by 24-hour direct calorimetry. *Br J Nutr* 1983;49:171–180.
39. Bingham SA, Goldberg GR, Coward WA, Prentice AM, Cummings JH. The effect of exercise and improved physical fitness on basal metabolic rate. *Br J Nutr* 1989;61:155–173.
40. Benedict FG, Miles WR, Roth P, Smith M. Carnegie Institution of Washington, publication no 280, 1919;701 p.
41. Keys A, Brozek J, Hanschel A, Mickelson O, Taylor HL. *The biology of human starvation*. Minneapolis: University of Minnesota Press, 1950.
42. Bray GA. The myth of diet in the management of obesity. *Am J Clin Nutr* 1970;23:1141–1148.
43. Apfelbaum M, Bostsarron J, Lacatis D. Effect of caloric restriction and excessive calorie intake on energy expenditure. *Am J Clin Nutr* 1971;24:1405–1409.
44. Garrow JS. Energy balance in man: an overview. *Am J Clin Nutr.* 1987;45:1114–1119.
45. Schultz CK, Bernaver E, Mole PA, et al. Effects of severe caloric restriction and moderate exercise on basal metabolic rate and hormonal status in adult humans. *Fed Proc* 1980;39:783.
46. Krotkiewsky M, Toss L, Bjorntorp P, Holm G. The effect of a very low calorie diet with and without chronic exercise on thyroid and sex hormones, oxygen uptake, insulin and C-peptide concentrations in obese women. *Int J Obesity* 1981;5:287–293.
47. Myerson M, Gutin B, Warren M, et al. Resting metabolic rate and energy balance in amenorrheic and eumenorrheic runners. *Med Sci Sports Exerc* 1991;23:15–22.
48. Trayhurn P, James WPT. Thermogenesis, dietary and non-shivering aspects. In: Cioffi IA, James WPT, Van Itallie TB, eds. *The body weight regulatory system: normal and disturbed mechanisms.* New York: Raven Press, 1981;97–105.
49. Felber JP, Meyer HU, Curchod B, et al. Glucose storage and oxidation in different degrees of human obesity measured by continuous indirect calorimetry. *Diabetologia* 1981;20:39–44.
50. Golay A, Schutz Y, Meyer HU, et al. Glucose induced thermogenesis in nondiabetic and diabetic obese subjects. *Diabetes* 1982;31:1023–1028.
51. Ravussin E, Bogardus C. Thermogenic response to insulin and glucose infusions in man: a model to evaluate the different components of the thermic effect of carbohydrate. *Life Sci* 1982;31:2011–2018.
52. Ravussin E, Bogardus C, Schwartz RS, et al. Thermic effect of glucose and insulin in man; decreased response with increased insulin resistance in obesity and noninsulin-dependent diabetes mellitus. *J Clin Invest* 1983;72:893–902.
53. Wahren J. Glucose turnover during exercise in healthy man and in patients with diabetes mellitus. *Diabetes* 1979;28:82–88.
54. Wahren J, Felig P, Ahlborg G, Jorfeldt L. Glucose metabolism during leg exercise in man. *J Clin Invest* 1971;50:2715–2725.
55. Felig P, Wahren J. Influence of endogenous secretion on splanchnic glucose and amino acid metabolism in man. *J Clin Invest* 1971;50:1702–1711.
56. Flatt JP. The biochemistry of energy expenditure. In: Bray G, ed. *Recent advances in obesity research II.* London: Newman Publishing, 1978;211–238.
57. Thiébaud D, Schutz Y, Acheson K, et al. Energy cost of glucose storage in human subjects during glucose-insulin infusions. *Am J Physiol* 1983;244:E216–E221.
58. Landsberg L, Young JB. The sympathetic nervous system and carbohydrate metabolism. In: Bjorntorp P, Cairella M, Howard AN, eds. *Recent advances in obesity research III.* London: J Libbey, 1981;42–51.
59. Rothwell NJ, Stock MJ. A role for insulin in the diet-induced thermogenesis of cafeteria-fed rats. *Metabolism* 1981;30:673–678.
60. Rowe JW, Young JB, Minaker KL, Stevens AL, Pallotta J, Landsberg L. Effect of insulin and glucose infusions on sympathetic nervous system activity in normal man. *Diabetes* 1981;30:219–225.

61. Stirling JL, Stock MJ. Metabolic origins of thermogenesis by diet. *Nature* 1968;220:801–802.
62. Welle S, Lilavivathana U, Campbell RG. Increased plasma norepinephrine concentrations and metabolic rates following glucose ingestion in man. *Metabolism* 1980;29:806–809.
63. DeFronzo RA, Thorin D, Felber JP, et al. Effect of beta- and alpha-adrenergic blockade on glucose-induced thermogenesis in man. *J Clin Invest* 1984;73:633–639.
64. Acheson KJ, Ravussin E, Wahren J, Jéquier E: Thermic effect of glucose in man: obligatory and facultative thermogenesis. *J Clin Invest* 1984;74:1572–1580.
65. Acheson KJ, Schutz Y, Bessard T, Ravussin E, Jéquier E, Flatt JP. Nutritional influences on lipogenesis and thermogenesis after a carbohydrate meal. *Am J Physiol* 1984;246:E62–E70.
66. Von Euler US. Sympathoadrenal activity in physical exercise. *Med Sci Sports* 1974;6:165–173.
67. Nair KS. Hyperglucagonemia increases resting metabolic rate in man during insulin deficiency. *J Clin Endocrinol Metab* 1987;64:896–900.
68. Himms-Hagen J. Cellular thermogenesis. *Annu Rev Physiol* 1976;38:315–351.
69. Nair KS, Garrow JS, Ford C, Mahler RF, Halliday D. Effect of diabetic control and obesity on whole body protein metabolism in man. *Diabetologia* 1984;27:13–16.
70. Balon TW, Zorzano A, Goodman MN, Ruderman NB. Insulin increases thermogenesis in rat skeletal muscle following exercise. *Am J Physiol* 1985;248:E148–E151.
71. Bogardus C, Thuillez ER, Ravussin E, Vasquez B, Narimiga M, Azhar S: Effect of muscle glycogen depletion on in vivo insulin action in man. *J Clin Invest* 1983;72:1605–1610.

DISCUSSION

Dr. Ravussin: Daily energy expenditure has three major components: the basal metabolic rate (BMR), the thermic effect of food (TEF), and the energy cost of physical activity. In most sedentary adults, RMR accounts for 60–70% of daily energy expenditure (1). The thermic effect of food accounts for only another 10% whereas the contribution of physical activity represents 20–30% of daily energy expenditure.

Since Pittet's study showing a decreased thermic effect of glucose in the obese compared to controls (2), studies of energy expenditure in lean and obese persons have focused predominantly on the thermic effect of food. This seems to have occurred for two reasons. First, it was assumed that BMR was constant for a given body size and therefore an unlikely cause of variability in daily caloric expenditure among individuals. This concept of fixed BMR for a given body size has led to the development of equations now widely used to predict BMR based on height and weight (3,4). Second, studies using crude methods to assess physical activity have failed to demonstrate that obese subjects are consistently less active than lean persons. Thus, the thermic effect of food appeared to be the only component of daily energy expenditure that could cause variation in predisposition to obesity among individuals. Unfortunately, it has also been shown that the thermic effect of food is the most difficult and the least reproducible component to measure (5).

In 1987, eleven years after the original observation by Pittet et al. (2), I was asked to review the literature on the differences in thermogenesis between lean and obese subjects. Among the 34 studies addressing this issue, half of them reported an impaired thermogenesis in obese subjects compared to lean subjects whereas the other half were unable to distinguish any differences. A year later, D'Alessio et al. (6) also reviewed the literature and came up with a similar conclusion. In their elegant studies D'Alessio et al. could not find any relationship between the thermic effect of food and the degree of obesity. However, most of the recent studies conducted by Doctor Pi-Sunyer's group investigating the relationship between the thermic effect of food and obesity have convincingly shown that obese subjects have lower thermic effect of food than lean subjects. These authors have shown that after matching subjects for body weight, or for lean body mass, fatter subjects always showed an impaired thermic effect of food. They also showed that exercise can potentiate the thermic effect of food in lean, but not in obese subjects.

One of the major reasons for the poor reproducibility of the thermic effect of food measurement is that many factors influence the thermic effect of food: the test meal size and composition, the time and duration of the measurement, the technique used for measurement, the palatability of food and the subject's genetic background, age, physical fitness, and sensitivity to insulin. All the above factors might explain the inconsistency and variability of the published data regarding the thermic effect of food in man (7).

Stoichiometric calculations of the energy cost of nutrient absorption, transport, and storage provide numbers that are usually lower than the measured thermic effect of food (8). This has led to the view that the thermic effect of food can be divided into two parts: (a) an *obligatory* component related to the metabolic processing of the macronutrients, and (b) a *facultative* component which seems to have a "cephalic phase" and a "postprandial phase." Whereas the relevance of the cephalic facultative phase of the thermic effect of food has been questioned in man, the postprandial facultative phase is believed to be mediated through activation of the sympathetic nervous system (9,10).

Whether a low thermic effect of food is a risk factor in the development of obesity is not known. Studies in post-obese subjects have led to contradictory results (11,12). More prospective studies are needed to investigate whether the low thermic effect of food reported in the obese is a cause or a consequence of the obese state. Furthermore, larger differences in energy expenditure are more likely to be found in the other components of daily energy expenditure, i.e., the basal metabolic rate and the physical activity component. For these reasons, future studies of the pathogenic mechanisms of obesity should focus on the variability of basal metabolic rate and physical activity.

REFERENCES

1. Jéquier E. Energy expenditure in obesity. In: James WPT, ed. *Clinics in endocrinology and metabolism.* Philadelphia: WB Saunders, 1984;563–580.
2. Pittet P, Chappuis P, Acheson K, de Techtermann F, Jéuqier E. Thermic effect of glucose in obese subjects studied by direct and indirect calorimetry. *Br J Nutr* 1976;35:281–292.
3. Harris JA, Benedict FG. *A biometric study of basal metabolism in man.* Washington, DC: The Carnegie Institute, 1919.
4. Roza AM, Shizgal HM. The Harris-Benedict equation reevaluated: resting energy requirements and the body cell mass. *Am J Clin Nutr* 1984;40:168–182.
5. Ravussin E, Lillioja S, Anderson TE, Christin L, Bogardus C. Determinants of 24-hour energy expenditure in man: methods and results using a respiratory chamber. *J Clin Invest* 1986;78:1568–1578.
6. D'Alessio DA, Kavie EC, Mozzoli MA, et al. Thermic effect of food in lean and obese men. *J Clin Invest* 1988;81:1781–1789.
7. Sims EA. Energy balance in human beings: the problems of plenitude. *Vitam Horm* 1986;43:1–101.
8. Flatt JP. Biochemistry of energy expenditure. In: Bray G, ed. *Recent advances in obesity research II.* London: John Libbey 1978;211.
9. Acheson KJ, Ravussin E, Wahren J, Jéquier E. Obligatory and facultative thermogenesis. *J Clin Invest* 1984;70:1570–1580.
10. Schwartz RS, Jaeger LF, Veith RC. Effect of clonidine on the thermic effect of feeding in humans. *Am J Physiol* 1988;254:R90–R94.
11. Schutz Y, Golay A, Felber JP, Jéquier E. Decreased glucose-induced thermogenesis after weight loss in obese subjects: a predisposing factor for the relapse of obesity? *Am J Clin Nutr* 1984;39:380–387.
12. Thörne A, Näslund I, Wahren J. Meal-induced thermogenesis in previously obese patients. *Clin Physiol* 1990;10:99–109.

Energy Metabolism: Tissue Determinants and
Cellular Corollaries, edited by J. M. Kinney
and H. N. Tucker. Raven Press, Ltd.,
New York © 1992.

Overview: Energy Requirements and Energy Storage

Andrew M. Prentice, R. James Stubbs, Bakary J. Sonko,
Erik Diaz, Gail R. Goldberg, Peter R. Murgatroyd, and
Alison E. Black

MRC Dunn Clinical Nutrition Centre, Cambridge, CB2 1QL, United Kingdom

The section on "Energy Requirements and Energy Storage" contains chapters by four of the most eminent nutritionists currently working in the field of energy metabolism. My brief as chairman is to draw together any common threads which have emerged and to contribute additional data from our own laboratory wherever pertinent.

The topic encompasses a huge field of scientific endeavor, which has been expertly reviewed by Professors Jéquier, Young, James, and Pi-Sunyer. I will make no attempt to summarize their chapters as this could not match the excellence of the originals. Similarly, in order to avoid being superficial, I will confine my comments to just two themes which emerge quite clearly from the four primary chapters.

The first theme is diet-induced thermogenesis (DIT). This warrants a detailed coverage since it features in all four chapters. My aim will be to place DIT into perspective in terms of its significance for man's overall 24-hour energy budget.

The second theme is that of macronutrient balance. This forms the central topic of Jéquier's chapter as well as receiving coverage by Young when he discusses the influence of fat and carbohydrate ingestion on protein balance. It is also an area which currently assumes a very high priority in our own work since we believe that an understanding of the factors regulating macronutrient balance holds the key to understanding the regulation of overall energy balance.

FROM SDA TO DIT TO TEF

It is fitting that James, as the current director of the Rowett Research Institute, should provide us with a comprehensive review of the historical background of both animal and human studies into the component of energy expenditure that human nutritionists now generally term DIT (see chapter by James). This conference occurred within weeks of the untimely death of James' predecessor, Sir Kenneth Blaxter, who has been so influential in developing many of the modern concepts in this field and whose books will remain among the best reference guides to this and related topics (1,2). Both James and Blaxter highlight the value of early studies on SDA and DIT, and implicitly stress the importance of having a thorough grounding in these if we are to avoid the danger of trying to reinvent the wheel.

James's chapter can be recommended both as a starting point for those who wish to embark on the journey back through the literature on energy metabolism, and as a state-of-the-art summary. Unfortunately the state of the art is such that he is left asking as many questions as he answers. His concluding paragraph contains the following rather depressing sentences:

> That such a long list of effector systems and modulating factors of postprandial thermogenesis has to be set out is in itself a sign that we know surprisingly little about the metabolic basis for the responses of man to food. We are left therefore with the modest designation of the thermic effect of food as a physiological feature with many regulators and with a variety of biochemical bases.

I interpret his pessimism in two ways. First, there is disagreement about the quantitative aspects of DIT under different dietary and environmental circumstances, among different individuals, and in various nutritional states. This is often caused not by an absence of data but rather by a plethora of data suggesting different answers due to inadequately controlled experimental protocols. Second, there is a shortage of data relating to the metabolic processes involved in DIT.

The first of these problems is, in theory, immediately correctable and James points out a number of prerequisites including the need for rigorously standardized conditions, for measurements of sufficient duration and for the uniform expression of results. These criteria can be applied prospectively to the design of new studies as well as retrospectively to the selection of studies to which we attach a high level of credibility. In this respect we are fortunate to have contributions within this section from Jéquier (this volume) whose group has published some of the most elegant and robust work on DIT in humans, and from Pi-Sunyer and Segal (this volume) who report on their impeccably controlled studies of the interactions between the thermic effects of food and exercise. If we direct our attention to the results from these two groups alone the pessimism begins to clear, and a relatively clear picture of DIT emerges at least with respect to the areas which they have covered. It seems that Jéquier must concur with this view since he is confident enough to summarize the salient features of DIT, insofar as they impinge on questions of energy balance, in just two paragraphs of his chapter (this volume).

The second problem, which relates to the biochemical and physiological processes involved in DIT, must partly await further technological advances in fields such as magnetic resonance spectroscopy discussed by Gadian later in this volume. However, a number of contributors to this symposium have already furthered our understanding of the mechanisms behind DIT. Jéquier has made important contributions in this area which are only briefly alluded to by James. The significance of Jéquier's work is that it clearly shows that DIT can be divided into an "obligatory" and a so-called "facultative" component (3,4). The obligatory component appears to correspond to the theoretical costs of nutrient handling (see chapter by Flatt and Fig. 1 of chapter by Jéquier) and cannot be blocked. The facultative component involves the action of the sympathetic nervous system and can readily be blocked by administration of propranolol (3). The facultative component [amounting to about 40% of the total response to oral glucose in the experiments reported by Acheson et al. (3,4)] can potentially be viewed as wasted energy. An important corollary of this statement is that the remainder is not wasted energy, but that it is doing useful biochemical work. Many researchers who only have a peripheral interest in DIT tend to forget this fact. Perhaps they have been encouraged to do so by the various studies which have investigated "energy-sparing" reductions in DIT (5) since these imply that DIT is disposable. Jéquier's distinction between "obligatory" and "facultative" thermogenesis represents an important conceptual point, and I would encourage a wider adoption of both the concept and the terminology in future studies.

Other chapters in this volume discuss the biochemical basis for thermogenesis in some detail (see chapters by Flatt, Henriksson, Milligan, Newsholme, and Wolfe), and provide a comprehensive qualitative summary even though they admit that the quantitative significance of many of the different components has yet to be clarified.

ADDITIONAL DATA ON DIET-INDUCED THERMOGENESIS

Before considering the overall significance of DIT as a determinant of energy balance we can contribute new information in two areas which were raised by James (this volume) and Pi-Sunyer and Segal (this volume). The first relates to the effect of alcohol on short-term DIT or postprandial thermogenesis (PPT) which, as James points out, has received far less attention than have the effects of carbohydrate, fat, or protein. The second relates to the putative phenomenon of "luxusconsumption" or adaptive thermogenesis in response to sustained overfeeding.

The Influence of Alcohol on Postprandial Thermogenesis

In many societies alcohol contributes quite significantly as a source of dietary energy. Self-recorded weighed food intakes often indicate average levels as high as 6–8% of dietary energy in man (6) and there is evidence from national production and sales statistics to suggest that consumption is underestimated by many diet surveys.

We believe that social alcohol consumption may be of particular significance in promoting weight gain for the following reasons. First, alcohol energy very often adds to the usual diet rather than replacing other energy sources. Indeed it is frequently consumed simultaneously with a gross excess of energy at a given meal. Second, alcohol differs from the other energy-yielding substrates because there is effectively no storage capacity in the body. It must therefore be oxidized immediately and would be expected to inhibit the oxidation of alternative substrates unless there is a massive energy-dissipating thermic effect. A likely consequence of alcohol's domination of oxidative pathways would be a promotion of excess fat storage in the postprandial period. Furthermore, since alcohol is known to suppress hepatic glucose production it may have a subsequent stimulatory effect on food intake if Flatt's theories concerning the centrality of carbohydrate status to appetite regulation are correct (7,8).

We have recently completed a whole-body calorimetry study of the effects of alcohol ingestion on energy expenditure and substrate disposal (9 and Sonko et al., *unpublished data*). The results concerning the effects of alcohol on PPT will be discussed here, and the substrate disposal results will be discussed in the section on nutrient balance (see chapter by Jéquier). We believe that our study meets many of the experimental criteria set out by James (this volume) particularly with respect to the duration of the postprandial measurements.

Five young males who were regular moderate drinkers were each studied on 3 occasions for 37 hours in a whole-body calorimeter. The calorimeters have been described in full elsewhere (10,11). On Day 0 of the experiment they were fed a normal diet to energy balance and strenuous activity was prohibited. At 2000 h on Day 0 they entered an 11 m^3 indirect calorimeter, slept from 2300–0800 h, had BMR measured from 0800–0900 h, dressed and then sat quietly until a test meal was eaten from 1200–1230 h. The test meal provided 0.5 × MEE where MEE is maintenance energy expenditure estimated as 1.4 × BMR. The composition of the test meals as fat:carbohydrate:protein:alcohol expressed in terms of energy was: *Control* 40: 46: 14:0; Isoenergetic replacement of 50% of carbohydrate 40:23:14:23; Addition of alcohol 34:36:12:18. The amount of alcohol (provided as Calvados since the ^{13}C enrichment matched the subjects' natural background) was the same for each subject in each of the alcohol meals (average 38 g). All test meals contained ^{13}C-labeled palmitic acid in order to differentiate between endogenous and exogenous fat oxidation. Following the test meal the subjects sat quietly until bedtime at 2300 h. They collected hourly breath samples for ^{13}CO$_2$ analysis by isotope ratio mass spectrometry (VG Sira 10), and they measured their own breath alcohol levels (Lion Alcolmeter AE-D3) at 30 min intervals. At 1900 h they received a supper providing 0.33 × MEE in the same dietary proportions as the control meal. Measurements continued until a second BMR period was completed at 0900 h on Day 2.

Breath alcohol levels had returned to baseline within 6 hours from ingestion. This approximated to the time of the next meal. The data are therefore presented for 3 periods: 0–6 h, 6–20.5 h and 0–20.5 h. Table 1 presents the values for energy expenditure. These seem to confirm James's suspicion, based on the study by Rosenburg and Durnin (12) that "there does seem to be an interaction between alcohol and food with a prolongation and amplification of the thermic response from about one hour postprandially onwards" (see chapter by James). In the immediate post-meal period PPT was virtually identical in the two meals providing 0.5 × MEE in spite of the fact that one contained alcohol. The third meal provided 23% more energy and elicited a 7% greater PPT. Although this increase in PPT was significant it was not a pro rata increase. However, after all of the alcohol had been oxidized and after a subsequent meal both of the alcohol-containing meals elicited a delayed increase

TABLE 1. *The effect of alcohol on postprandial thermogenesis*

	Test meals		
	Control	50% CHO replacement by alcohol	Alcohol addition
0–6 hours	2301 ± 74	2333 ± 163	2460[a] ± 84
6–20.5 hours	4426 ± 385	4774[a] ± 350	4729[a] ± 213
0–20.5 hours	6727 ± 443	7107[a] ± 509	7189[a] ± 309

[a] $p < 0.05$ vs control by paired-t test. See text for description of protocol and test meals. All values are kJ (± SD for $n = 5$).
Data from Sonko et al., ref. 9 and Sonko et al., *unpublished data.*

in energy expenditure (8% and 7%, respectively) thus also confirming James's statement that previous short-term studies are likely to have missed this effect (see chapter by James).

The mechanism of this effect is particularly intriguing. As will be presented in the section on nutrient balance (see chapter by Jéquier) the alcohol caused profound changes in substrate fluxes and balance which may be partly responsible. Alternatively the effect may be related to delayed effects of the alcohol on minor physical movements. For this reason we are repeating the study with the alcohol administered with an evening meal so that the subjects will be asleep during the period of interest.

Absence of Adaptive Thermogenesis in Response to Sustained Overfeeding in Lean and Overweight Men

The long-standing controversy as to whether humans possess an inducible mechanism for dissipating excess dietary energy in the form of heat was raised in three of the chapters in this section. Jéquier states that "the thermogenic capacity of the human body towards an excessive food intake is limited" and effectively dismisses the concept (this volume). James also accords the topic remarkably little attention in view of the fact that it has dominated many peoples' thinking about DIT (this volume). In the precirculated version of their chapter (but later deleted) Pi-Sunyer and Segal (this volume) provided a brief summary of 28 studies of experimental overfeeding in humans by citing Garrow's review of 16 studies prior to 1978 (13), Sims' review of 10 studies from 1978 to 1985 (14), and by adding the subsequent studies by Forbes et al. (15) and Ravussin et al. (16). They concluded that 16 studies argue in favor of some unexplained energy loss (i.e., luxusconsumption) and that 12 argue against. However, in spite of this balance in favor of the phenomenon they were heavily influenced by the last two studies and concluded that recent, more careful and more technically sophisticated studies with better measurement of energy expenditure and body composition changes do not confirm the premise that overfeeding in man leads to wasted calories.

James (this volume) points out that in most studies the existence of luxusconsumption has merely been inferred from an apparent failure to gain the expected amount of weight. However, he does not make it explicit that only three studies lasting longer than 10 days made any measurements of heat production. These are the experiments by: Norgan and Durnin (17) who overfed 6 men by 6.2 MJ/day for 42 days and measured energy expenditure by the factorial approach employing actual measurements of BMR and a limited number of activities (but not PPT); Webb and Annis (18) who overfed 8 lean and overweight subjects (some on two occasions) for 30 days by an excess of 4.2 MJ/day on three different diets ranging from high carbohydrate (60% by energy) to high fat (70% by energy), and reported daily metabolic rate assessed over two sedentary periods of 24 hours in a direct/indirect "body suit" calorimeter; and Forbes et al. (15) who overfed 13 women and 2 men by 3.8–7.6 MJ/day over 21 days and only measured BMR.

In view of this remarkable failure to measure the primary outcome variable in question (i.e., heat production over at least 24 hours) we have performed yet another study (19,20). Six lean and three overweight young men were overfed by 50% above their carefully characterized baseline requirement for 42 days. The energy excess averaged 6.3 ± 1.1 MJ/day or a total of 265 ± 45 MJ. The volunteers lived in a long-stay metabolic facility which afforded good control of diet and of full fecal and urinary collections. However they were free to leave the unit at most times and to follow their usual activity patterns except when required for investigative procedures. Energy expenditure was assessed during baseline and at weeks 2, 4, 5, and 6 of overfeeding by 36 hour whole-body calorimetry during which the subjects followed a rigidly standardized protocol in order to exclude behavioral noise and to measure the true physiological response to overfeeding. The calorimeter run at 5 weeks was performed under conditions of cold stress since it had been suggested that the thermogenic response might be suppressed at a high environmental temperature in order to avoid thermal overload. During the last 2 weeks of overfeeding energy expenditure was also assessed by the doubly-labeled water method (21) in order to investigate possible behavioral adaptations in addition to any physiological ones.

The main results are summarized in Table 2. The subjects gained weight in a virtually linear manner to a total of +7.6 ± 1.6 kg. Fat mass increased by 4.6 ± 2.1 kg and fat-free mass by 3.0 ± 0.9 kg. The percentage of new tissue as fat was 61% which accords with predictions for these particular subjects (22). The energy cost of weight gain was 28.7 ± 4.4 MJ/kg which also accords with the predicted costs for gaining tissue of this composition (15).

Basal metabolic rate was increased by overfeeding (0.9 ± 0.4 MJ/day, $p<0.001$), but most of this effect was accounted for by the increase in fat-free mass since the adjusted increment was only 9 ± 10 kJ/kg FFM/day and the significance decreased to $p<0.05$. The fact that the BMR per kg FFM was still slightly raised might be interpreted as some evidence for luxusconsumption, however inspection of the calorimeter traces showed that the expectedly large PPT following the excessive evening meal had probably not completely subsided by the time of the BMR measurement. In other words the classic definition of BMR as being measured 12–13 hours after

TABLE 2. *Summary of the changes induced by overfeeding (OF) compared with baseline (BAS) (means ± SD)*

	BAS	OF	OF-BAS	p^a
Energy intake (MJ/d)	13.3 ± 1.3	19.5 ± 2.0	6.2 ± 1.9	<0.001
Body mass (kg)	73.7 ± 9.5	81.4 ± 9.6^b	7.6 ± 1.6^b	<0.001
Fat free mass (kg)	57.4 ± 4.0	60.7 ± 4.2^b	3.0 ± 0.9^b	<0.001
Fat mass (kg)	16.3 ± 7.0	20.3 ± 7.4^b	4.6 ± 2.1^b	<0.001
CAL EE (MJ/d)	10.6 ± 0.6	12.4 ± 0.6	1.8 ± 0.5	<0.001
CAL EE (kJ/kg/d)	146 ± 17	154 ± 15	9 ± 4	<0.001
CAL A&T (MJ/d)	3.3 ± 0.2	4.2 ± 0.4	0.9 ± 0.4	<0.001
BMR (MJ/d)	7.3 ± 0.5	8.2 ± 0.2	0.9 ± 0.4	<0.001
BMR (kJ/kg FFM/d)	128 ± 9	137 ± 9^b	9 ± 10^b	<0.05
Stepping (kJ/30 min/kg)	7.2 ± 0.5	7.3 ± 0.4	0.1 ± 0.4	NS
Cycling (kJ/30 min/kg)	8.2 ± 1.2	8.2 ± 0.9	0.0 ± 0.5	NS
DLW TEE (MJ/d)	13.2 ± 1.2	14.8 ± 1.6^b	1.4 ± 2.0^b	NS
DLW TEE (kJ/kg/d)	187 ± 35	186 ± 35^b	−1 ± 25^b	NS
DLW A&T (MJ/d)	5.9 ± 1.4	6.5 ± 1.6^b	0.5 ± 1.8^b	NS
TEE/BMR	1.8 ± 0.3	1.8 ± 0.2^b	1.7 ± 0.2^b	NS
Energy/kg gained (MJ/kg)	NA	28.7 ± 4.4^c	NA	

^{a} Significance tested by paired *t*-test. All values are means from $n = 9$ unless indicated otherwise.
^{b} $n = 8$ due to missing data.
^{c} $n = 7$ due to missing data.
Data from Diaz *et al.*, refs. 19 and 20.

the previous meal may not be sufficiently rigorous when the previous meal is excessive.

Twenty-four hour energy expenditure in the calorimeter (CAL EE) was increased both as a consequence of the increase in BMR and due to an increase in DIT (+1.8 ± 0.5 MJ/day, $p<0.001$). When BMR is subtracted from CAL EE in order to compute the amount of energy expended on activity and thermogenesis (A&T) the increase was 0.9 ± 0.4 MJ/day ($p<0.001$). The critical question with respect to luxusconsumption is whether this increase in A&T is any larger than would be expected. We concluded, on the basis of the following calculation, that it is not. Due to the constrained protocol and conditions of the calorimeter, energy expenditure was lower than when free living and the actual energy excess on calorimeter days was therefore 7.1 MJ/day rather than the 6.2 MJ/day quoted above. Even if there was no increase in the activity component of A&T (which is somewhat unlikely since body weight increased) and if all of the 0.9 MJ/day increase in A&T was due to a rise in thermogenesis this would only represent 12.7% of the excess intake. This value is somewhat lower than the computed value based on Flatt's figures for substrate handling (this volume). We therefore concluded that the concept of luxusconsumption is firmly refuted in our study.

With respect to the possible interactions between the thermic effect of food and exercise discussed by Pi-Sunyer and Segal (this volume) we found that the energy cost of weight-dependent and weight-independent exercises was unaffected by overfeeding (Table 2).

The final component of this study which is of interest in the present context is that free-living energy expenditure as assessed by doubly-labeled water increased by slightly less than CAL EE (1.4 ± 2.0 MJ/day, NS). This provides concrete evidence to support our initial supposition that there would be no behavioral mechanism by which energy expenditure would increase in order to counteract an excess energy intake in an analogous manner to the lethargy which spares energy during starvation.

These new results therefore confirm and extend the line taken by the three chapters in this section, and further encourage the view that the thesis of luxusconsumption can now be buried so far as it might relate to man. In fact the whole concept of a high level of metabolic flexibility which may compensate for differing levels of intake in an autoregulatory manner (23) begins to look decidedly fragile and we would concur with Jéquier's statement that "since energy expenditure is not much affected by the amount of energy intake, it is likely that the control of energy expenditure plays a smaller role in body weight regulation than the control of food intake" (this volume).

Thus far we have made little mention of the significance of these findings in clinical situations. However, it should be readily appreciated that Jéquier's fundamental statement quoted above has far-reaching implications in a clinical setting as well as in non-clinical circumstances. For instance, there has been an all too ready tendency in recent years to assume that the wasting associated with conditions such as cancer cachexia or AIDS is due to hypermetabolism and to somewhat ignore the food intake side of the equation. An example of this will be cited later.

PPT IN PERSPECTIVE

It is interesting that PPT has featured so prominently in a session in which only one of the assigned titles required it to do so. James's acronymic title "From SDA to DIT to TEF" (this volume) clearly warranted the full and informative coverage which it received, and Pi-Sunyer and Segal's title "Diet and Exercise" (this volume) also required some coverage of PPT, but it need not have assumed the dominance that it did. Jéquier, who has probably published more in this field than anyone else, has condensed his coverage into just two paragraphs. Finally, Young covers PPT when he discusses the energetic significance of protein turnover (see Young et al., Energy and Nitrogen (Protein) Relationships).

We would promote the view that the topic has received far too much attention over the past decade and that this has been to the detriment of a more balanced perspective on energy balance. One of the reasons for the preponderance of interest in DIT and PPT is that, after BMR, it is seemingly the easiest component of expenditure to measure. (The word "seemingly" must be included since, as pointed out by James (this volume), many very short-term studies of PPT are of dubious value because they do not integrate the total metabolic costs of meal ingestion.) In our view this ease of measurement has generated a level of interest in DIT which

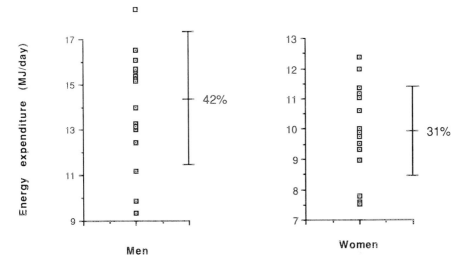

FIG. 1. Variability in total energy expenditure of randomly selected free-living adults. Expenditure was assessed by doubly-labeled water. Variance bars span −1SD to +1SD. (Data from Livingstone et al., ref. 24.)

is disproportionate to its real significance in the overall energy balance question. A few examples will illustrate this point.

Figure 1 illustrates the range of free-living energy expenditure measured by doubly-labeled water in groups of randomly selected men and women studied by Livingstone et al. (24). This data is selected simply as a convenient example and many others could be used. The coefficients of variation were 21% and 16%, respectively. These would yield an average −1 SD to +1 SD range of about 35%. In order to provide a perspective this has been plotted in Fig. 2 on the same scale as the differences in PPT between lean and obese subjects observed in the studies of Segal et al. (25,26). It can be seen that the normal variation in energy requirements is far greater than any defect in PPT.

In the same vein James cites the studies by Illingworth et al. (5,27) into "energy-sparing" decreases in PPT during pregnancy and lactation. These authors describe reductions in PPT during pregnancy and lactation which are highly significant in a statistical sense, but as we have previously pointed out (28) the biological significance is highly questionable since the effect amounts to 0.6% of daily expenditure.

Jéquier has pointed out that if two subjects ate exactly the same amount of food and one of them had a 5% lower energy expenditure then that person would accumulate 5 kg more adipose tissue in the course of a year (this volume). In principle this is perfectly true, but the argument revolves about the operative phrase "if two subjects ate exactly the same amount." We argue that there is no reason to anticipate that they would eat the same amount if their appetite control processes were functioning adequately since these should detect that their energy requirements were different and modulate food intake accordingly (29).

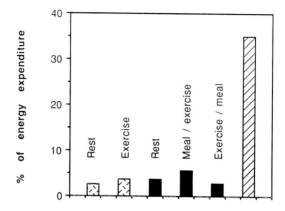

FIG. 2. DIT in perspective. The observed differences in DIT between lean and obese subjects in the studies by Segal et al. (25,26) are plotted against the average variance from Fig. 1.

Our thesis is therefore that appetite control has to operate over a wide range of energy expenditures within any individual as they change their activity pattern, and between individuals with different levels of activity. In most people this process operates efficiently over their whole lifetime and successfully accommodates large changes in energy flux due, for instance, to illness, pregnancy and lactation, or gross changes in lifestyle. Thus, even if we accept the evidence that some pre-obese people may have a slightly lower DIT, it would still not be the primary cause of their obesity. The primary cause would be the failure of their system to recognize that they had a low energy requirement. This conviction has led us to redirect much of our current research toward reaching an understanding of the physiological mechanisms which, together with the many biosocial and psychological influences, contribute to the control of energy intake.

In a similar manner it is pertinent to note that any hypermetabolism associated with illness will not be the primary cause of weight loss. The primary cause will be the organism's failure to increase food intake in order to match the new requirements in the way that occurs, for instance, when women have to meet the additional energy drain of lactation.

CONTROL OF ENERGY BALANCE THROUGH THE CONTROL OF MACRONUTRIENT BALANCE

In introducing the concept of nutrient balance Jéquier (this volume) observed that "the study of weight regulation is generally limited to the concept of energy balance. It is trivial to mention that people do not eat 'energy' but nutrients. Energy is a physical concept, and the body has no receptors to measure energy. It is therefore appropriate to consider the mechanisms responsible for nutrient balance." These comments reflect the current thinking of many research teams at the forefront of energy regulation research.

It is now widely appreciated that the common assumption that the major energy-yielding substrates are easily interconvertible within the body is an oversimplification, and that it is not valid to reduce them all down to the common currency of "energy." Jéquier rehearses many of the arguments leading to this conclusion (this volume). One of the primary arguments is that net de novo fat synthesis from carbohydrate appears to be a rather rare event in human metabolism which only occurs when the system is pushed to its limits. This fact has focused attention on carbohydrate metabolism and on the importance of maintaining carbohydrate balance (7,8). There is an increasing awareness of the fact that carbohydrate plays a preeminent role in regulating the balance of fuel oxidation and that fat oxidation plays a secondary role. Jéquier (this volume) summarizes some of the experiments which have led to this conclusion. The substrate balance results from our alcohol study cited above provide further support for this concept as well as emphasizing a similarly dominant role for alcohol. The data, summarized in Table 3, provide an excellent example of how important it is to study substrate balances rather than simply to measure energy balance.

The alcohol was completely oxidized in the first 6 hours after ingestion. During this period it significantly suppressed fat oxidation and even induced net fat synthesis

TABLE 3. *The effect of alcohol on substrate oxidation*

	Test meals		
	Control	50% CHO replacement by alcohol	Alcohol addition
Alcohol oxidation			
0–6 h	0	1,142[a]	1,135[a]
6–20.5 h	0	0	0
0–20.5 h	0	1,142[a]	1,135[a]
Carbohydrate oxidation			
0–6 h	1,326	817[a,b]	1,112
6–20.5 h	2,372	2,087	2,636
0–20.5 h	3,698	2,904[a]	3,748
Fat oxidation			
0–6 h	619	80[a]	−125[a]
6–20.5 h	1,400	2,010[a,b]	1,345
0–20.5 h	2,019	2,090	1,220[b,c]
Protein oxidation			
0–6 h	355	294	339
6–20.5 h	654	676	748
0–20.5 h	1,009	970	1,087

[a] $p < 0.05$ vs control.
[b] $p < 0.05$ vs alcohol addition.
[c] $p < 0.05$ vs CHO replacement by paired-t test.
See text for description of protocol and test meals. All values are kJ.
Data from Sonko *et al.*, ref. 9 and Sonko *et al.*, *unpublished data.*

after the meal in which the alcohol was added to the control formulation. Note that carbohydrate oxidation was related to the amount of carbohydrate ingested since it was significantly reduced when 50% of the carbohydrate energy had been replaced by alcohol. Thus, alcohol and carbohydrate dominated that oxidative pathways and displaced fat toward storage.

If the study had been terminated at this stage we would have drawn the erroneous conclusion that both alcohol addition and alcohol replacement had induced fat storage when compared to the control meal without alcohol. However, the data from 6 hours onward showed an interesting reversal on the alcohol replacement day. Fat oxidation suddenly switched to become significantly greater than after the control or the alcohol addition to meals. This was presumably caused by the fact that the subjects were effectively carbohydrate deficient which suppressed carbohydrate oxidation and stimulated fat oxidation. The overall consequence of the switch was that total fat oxidation was unaffected when alcohol energy replaced carbohydrate energy, but was significantly reduced when the alcohol energy was added to the control meal. The ^{13}C-palmitate results demonstrated that exogenous fat oxidation mirrored the total fat oxidation results presented in the table.

This study is cited in some detail both because it relates to several issues raised within this section on "Energy Requirements and Energy Storage" and because it illustrates the power of modern techniques to examine substrate balances in the way that has been advocated within this volume. One further example will be given below.

THE IMPORTANCE OF FACTORS REGULATING FOOD INTAKE

Jéquier discusses food intake and considers this side of the nutrient balance equation (this volume). As mentioned above he states that "it is likely that the control of energy expenditure plays a smaller role in body weight regulation than the control of food intake." We have previously reached a similar conclusion (29) and are now directing much of our research toward obtaining an understanding of the metabolic integration of nutrient intake and disposal. This is a complex area in which to work and is full of pitfalls because of the many and diverse factors which influence food intake. Nonetheless, we believe that there is scope for researchers studying whole-body metabolism to identify the underlying physiological drives affecting nutrient intake in man, and to try to dissect these out from the social and psychological factors.

Experimental Approaches

One example of the approach we are taking again involves the use of whole-body calorimeters to assess substrate oxidation rates. By combining the calorimeter measurements with data on nutrient intake it is possible to plot nutrient and energy balance relative to a nominal zero at the start of the experiment. This approach can be used to assess, for instance, Flatt's hypothesis that regulation is driven by the

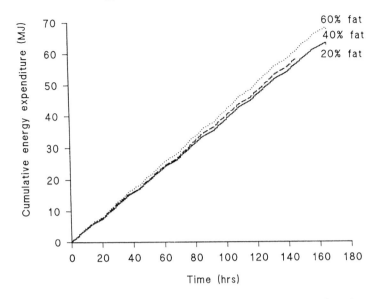

FIG. 3. Effect of covert macronutrient manipulation on energy expenditure. Data from a single subject studied by 7-day whole-body calorimetry on 3 occasions.

need to maintain carbohydrate balance within narrow limits (7,8). As a first attempt to test this we are studying normal-weight young men who each spend 3 periods of 7 days in a whole-body calorimeter on diets containing 20%, 40%, or 60% of energy as fat. The macronutrient manipulations and the intention of the study are covert. The subjects are given ad libitum access to food both in terms of time and quantity. The study is still in progress so only a limited selection of data from a single subject will be used to illustrate the approach. Figure 3 shows that the cumulative energy expenditure is remarkably similar on the 3 diet treatments. This confirms much of the discussion above concerning the relative constancy of energy expenditure, and our view that variations in expenditure are of little significance in maintaining balance. However, Figs. 4 and 5 show that the dietary treatment has a profound influence on energy and fat balance due to very significant changes in food intake. It must be emphasized that these data are intended only to illustrate that it is quite feasible to track substrate balance using noninvasive procedures over quite long periods. These measurements can then be related to changes in appetite, hunger, and satiety, and ultimately to changes in body composition and function. It is our belief that such studies will be much more informative than studies which (a) ignore the question of substrate balance and (b) concentrate on only one side of the energy balance equation.

The Clinical Setting

An earlier study from this laboratory will illustrate the need not to ignore the food intake side of the equation in a clinical setting.

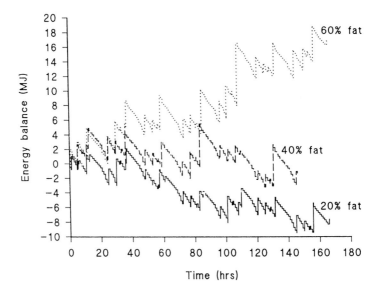

FIG. 4. Effect of covert macronutrient manipulation on energy balance. Data from same subject as in Fig 3.

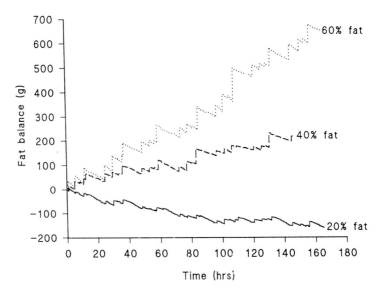

FIG. 5. Effect of covert macronutrient manipulation on fat balance. Data from same subject as in Fig 3.

We were approached by physicians from a long-stay mental hospital for the elderly who were interested in the problem of acute wasting which appeared to be particularly severe in patients with Alzheimer's disease. The patients showed rapid wasting of both fat and lean tissue. The problem was sufficiently severe for some patients to lose over 40% of body weight within two years. Dietary assessments appeared to reveal an adequate food intake and malabsorption was excluded. The obvious hypothesis was that the weight loss must be secondary to hypermetabolism and/or hyperactivity.

We made careful measurements of food intake (continuously observed by a dietitian who recorded all wastage), of sleeping metabolic rate (by ventilated hood), and of total energy expenditure over 21 days (by doubly-labeled water) in 14 subjects with varying diagnoses (30). The results revealed the lowest average energy expenditure values that we have ever recorded in adults. Far from being elevated, their energy requirements averaged only 6.1 MJ/day. At the time of observation their average intake was 6.3 MJ/day indicating that the group as a whole were in energy balance. Indeed there was no evidence of significant energy imbalance in any of the patients. This left the original question concerning the cause of their weight loss unanswered. We concluded that there could be two explanations. The first is that the weight loss may be an episodic phenomenon associated with infections and the consequent inanition. This seems likely to be partly responsible. However, examination of the food intake data revealed a more likely and much more worrying possibility. It emerged that 5 out of the 14 patients ate absolutely all of the food that was offered to them in the week of measurement with no wastage or refusal. It is impossible to believe that the amount of food offered to the patients exactly matched their requirements. The only logical conclusion is that if the patients had been offered more food they would have accepted it, and that they were effectively suffering from institutional starvation. Other evidence leading to this conclusion is presented in the original paper to which the interested reader is referred (31).

The reason for citing this study is that it is frequently assumed that weight loss in many clinical conditions is caused by hypermetabolism. This implies that little can be done about it and is often used to excuse our failure to achieve a higher success rate with programs of nutritional support and rehabilitation. We suspect that a greater emphasis on studying food intake will increasingly reveal that a defective intake is more often the cause of deteriorating nutritional status than a defective expenditure.

PROTEIN, FAT, AND CARBOHYDRATE INTERRELATIONSHIPS

A final issue which is related to the above comments concerning the importance of understanding the processes controlling substrate balance was raised by Young in his excellent and comprehensive chapter in this section (see Young et al., Energy and Nitrogen (Protein) Relationships). He discusses protein-energy interactions in some detail, and then addresses the question of the relative effectiveness of fat and carbohydrate in terms of their nitrogen-sparing capacity and other effects on protein metabolism. The latter field is of considerable practical significance in the development of enteral and parenteral feeds, but remains rather confused. Young et al. (see Young et al., Energy and Nitrogen (Protein) Relationships) failed to reach definitive conclusions on several aspects of this problem, and in reviewing all of the literature cited by them we have failed to improve on their interpretation. We will therefore add no further comments except to stress that this topic stands out as one in need of particular attention.

CONCLUSIONS

A number of prominent researchers in the field of energy metabolism have acknowledged that focusing on diet-induced thermogenesis is unlikely to yield answers to the central questions of how man maintains energy and nutrient homeostasis in health and disease. This in no way implies that such studies have been fruitless, but rather that a broader and more integrated approach which includes attention to food intake control must be adopted in the future. Many studies of the type advocated by us are already underway and it remains to be seen whether they can overcome the inevitable complexities which arise when such multidimensional problems are tackled.

REFERENCES

1. Blaxter KL. *The energy metabolism of ruminants*. London: Hutchinson, 1962.
2. Blaxter KL. *Energy metabolism in animals and man*. Cambridge: Cambridge University Press, 1989.
3. Acheson K, Jéquier E, Wahren J. Influence of beta-adrenergic blockade on glucose-induced thermogenesis in man. *J Clin Invest* 1983;72:981–986.
4. Acheson K, Ravussin E, Wahren J, Jéquier E. Thermic effect of glucose in man. Obligatory and facultative thermogenesis. *J Clin Invest* 1984;74:1572–1580.
5. Illingworth PJ, Jung RT, Howie PW, Isles TE. Reduction in postprandial energy expenditure during pregnancy. *Br Med J* 1987;294:1573–1576.
6. Black AE, Prentice AM, Coward WA. Use of food quotients to predict respiratory quotients for the doubly-labelled water method of measuring energy expenditure. *Human Nutr: Clin Nutr* 1986;40C:381–391.
7. Flatt JP. Dietary fat, carbohydrate balance, and weight maintenance: effects of exercise. *Am J Clin Nutr* 1987;45:296–306.
8. Flatt JP. The difference in the storage capacities for carbohydrate and fat, and its implications in the regulation of body weight. *Ann N Y Acad Sci* 1987;499:104–123.
9. Sonko BJ, Goldberg GR, Murgatroyd PR, Coward WA, Prentice AM. Does consumption of alcohol with a meal promote fat storage? *Proc Nutr Soc* 1991;50:38A.
10. Murgatroyd PR, Davies HL, Prentice AM. Intra-individual variability and measurement noise in estimates of energy expenditure by whole-body indirect calorimetry. *Br J Nutr* 1987;58:347–356.
11. Prentice AM, Goldberg GR, Davies HL, Murgatroyd PR, Scott W. Energy-sparing adaptations in human pregnancy assessed by whole-body calorimetry. *Br J Nutr* 1989;62:5–22.
12. Rosenburg K, Durnin JVGA. The effect of alcohol on resting metabolic rate. *Br J Nutr* 1978;40:293–298.
13. Garrow JS. *Energy balance and obesity in man*, 2nd ed. Amsterdam: Elsevier, 1978.
14. Sims EAH. Energy balance in human beings: the problems of plenitude. *Vitam Horm* 1986;43:1–101.

15. Forbes GB, Brown MR, Welle SL, Lipinski BA. Deliberate overfeeding in women and men: energy cost and composition of weight gain. *Br J Nutr* 1986;56:1–9.
16. Ravussin E, Schutz Y, Acheson KJ, Dusmet M, Bourquin L, Jéquier E. Short-term mixed diet overfeeding in man: evidence for "luxusconsumption." *Am J Physiol* 1985;249:E470–E477.
17. Norgan NG, Durnin JVGA. The effect of 6 weeks of overfeeding on the body composition and energy metabolism of young men. *Am J Clin Nutr* 1980;33:978–988.
18. Webb P, Annis JF. Adaptation to overeating in lean and overweight women. *Hum Nutr: Clin Nutr* 1983;37C:117–131.
19. Diaz E, Prentice AM, Goldberg GR, Murgatroyd PR, Coward WA. Metabolic and behavioural responses to altered energy intake in man. 1. Experimental overfeeding. *Proc Nutr Soc* 1991;50:110A.
20. Diaz E, Prentice AM, Goldberg GR, Murgatroyd PR, Coward WA. Metabolic response to experimental overfeeding in lean and overweight healthy volunteers. *Am J Clin Nutr* 1991 [*in press*].
21. Prentice AM, ed. *The doubly-labelled water method for measuring energy expenditure. Technical recommendations for use in humans.* Vienna: International Dietary Energy Consultancy Group. IDECG/IAEA, NAHRES-4, 1990.
22. Forbes G. Lean body mass-body fat interrelationships in humans. *Nutr Rev* 1987;45:225–231.
23. Sukhatme P, Margen S. Autoregulatory homeostatic nature of energy balance. *Am J Clin Nutr* 1982;35:355–365.
24. Livingstone MBE, Prentice AM, Strain JJ, et al. Accuracy of weighed diet records in studies of diet and health. *Br Med J* 1990;300:708–712.
25. Segal KR, Gutin B, Nyman AM, Pi-Sunyer FX. Thermic effect of food at rest, during exercise, and after exercise in lean and obese men of similar body weight. *J Clin Invest* 1985;76:1107–1112.
26. Segal KR, Gutin B, Albu J, Pi-Sunyer FX. Thermic effect of food and exercise in lean and obese men of similar lean body mass. *Am J Physiol* 1987;252:E110–E117.
27. Illingworth PJ, Jung RT, Howie PW, Leslie P, Isles TE. Diminution in energy expenditure during lactation. *Br Med J* 1986;292:437–441.
28. Prentice AM, Whitehead RG, Coward WA, Goldberg GR, Davies HL, Murgatroyd PR. Reduction in postprandial energy expenditure during pregnancy. *Br Med J* 1987;295:266–267.
29. Prentice AM, Black AE, Murgatroyd PR, Goldberg GR, Coward WA. Metabolism or appetite: questions of energy balance with particular reference to obesity. *J Hum Nutr Diet* 1989;2:95–104.
30. Prentice AM, Leavesley K, Murgatroyd PR, et al. Is severe wasting in elderly mental patients caused by an excessive energy requirement? *Age Ageing* 1989;18:158–167.

Energy Metabolism: Tissue Determinants and
Cellular Corollaries, edited by J. M. Kinney
and H. N. Tucker. Raven Press, Ltd.,
New York © 1992.

Hypothalamus and Thermogenesis

Nancy J. Rothwell

Department of Physiological Sciences, University of Manchester,
M13 9PT, United Kingdom

Metabolic rate in homeotherms is a complex and variable process which is dependent on both obligatory mechanisms such as the heat produced as a by product of basal metabolism, maintenance and repair, and adaptive processes (e.g., diet or non-shivering thermogenesis). A major component of metabolic rate, usually referred to as basal or resting metabolic rate (BMR), is relatively constant under defined conditions for an organism of a given mass. Unfortunately, although this theoretical definition may appear simple, practical estimates of BMR often present difficulties and yield variable results. In many cases it is impossible to distinguish whether changes in total heat production result from alterations in BMR or adaptive processes.

TERMINOLOGY

Further confusion arises from the disconcertingly large number of terms used to describe various aspects of metabolic rate, e.g., heat production, energy expenditure, thermogenesis, luxusconsumption, specific dynamic action, thermic effect of food, heat increment of feeding, and hypermetabolism. This plethora of names, often describing the same components, has arisen partly because interest in metabolism has come from scientists and clinicians with very different backgrounds. In this review, metabolic rate and energy expenditure will be used synonymously, adaptive thermogenesis will be used to describe physiological responses to factors such as environmental temperature and dietary stimuli, while hypermetabolism will refer to increases in metabolic rate associated with stress or illness and injury, since we are still uncertain whether these represent adaptive or inappropriate responses.

PERIPHERAL MECHANISMS

For almost all practical purposes metabolic rate, assessed by indirect calorimetry, is equivalent to heat production (the exception being when heat content varies). At a molecular level, heat is produced as a result of either ATP utilization or reduced efficiency of ATP synthesis (uncoupling of oxidative phosphorylation). Most ex-

TABLE 1. *Possible mechanisms contributing to adaptive thermogenesis*

Increases in:
Protein turnover
Triglyceride turnover
Cori cycle activity
Substrate cycles (e.g., in glycolysis)
Ion pumping (Na-K ATPase)
Uncoupling of oxidative phosphorylation

amples of heat production in mammals are due to the former, e.g., muscular contraction, ion transport, synthetic processes, and the only physiological example in homeotherms of the latter is the uncoupling of oxidative phosphorylation which occurs in brown adipose tissue (BAT).

A detailed description of each of these mechanisms of heat production, and critical discussion of their likely contribution to observed changes in metabolic rate have been published in several reviews (1,2), and will therefore not be considered in detail here. However to briefly summarize the current consensus, it seems that all of the mechanisms described in Table 1 can contribute to physiological or pathological changes in metabolic rate, it is their quantitative significance which is more doubtful. Research in this area has generally focused on animal studies which have revealed brown adipose tissue as a major effector of non-shivering (NST) and diet-induced thermogenesis (DIT). Heat production in BAT, which is under control of the sympathetic nervous system (3), is also increased in animals subjected to peripheral, or brain injury, infection, malignant disease, or treated with bacterial endotoxin, recombinant cytokines (interleukins 1 and 6 and tumor necrosis factor α ([IL-1, IL-6, TNFα)], or inflammatory mediators such as eicosanoids (4–10). The validity of extrapolating these data to humans remains questionable. Functional brown adipose tissue (i.e., possessing the proton conductance pathway responsible for uncoupling of oxidative phosphorylation) is present in adults up to 80 years of age (11). However, it is impossible in man to assess the amount and physiological importance of this tissue, which decreases with increasing body size. In neonates and young children, BAT probably contributes significantly to thermoregulation but no data exist on its possible involvement in energy balance regulation.

Nevertheless BAT activity is markedly increased in children with malignant disease or injury (12,13), observations which correlate with animal studies.

All of the mechanisms of heat production described in Table 1 can be influenced by sympathetic nervous system (SNS) activity, particularly substrate cycling and BAT activity (1,2,14). The evidence for activation of SNS in humans during injury, infection, cold exposure, and overfeeding is much less equivocal than for the effector mechanisms (3,15–19).

METABOLIC RATE DURING INJURY AND INFECTION

A more detailed description of the changes in metabolic rate associated with illness will be presented in accompanying chapters. However before discussing the central nervous system (CNS) control of metabolism, it is worth considering briefly how such metabolic responses may be compared to physiological changes in heat production (i.e., NST and DIT), and the correlations which exist between animal and human studies. This is necessary because the majority of our current understanding of CNS control of metabolism has been derived from research on animals.

For both practical and ethical reasons, it is difficult to closely mimic human illness and injury in animals particularly for chronic studies. Nevertheless the results to date have shown close parallels (9,16). A possible exception to this is the very early response to injury (ebb phase) which is often characterized by a fall in metabolic rate and body temperature in animals, but this is rarely apparent in clinical studies (16). Since NST and DIT in animals clearly depend on activation of the SNS which also contributes to many forms of hypermetabolism in patients (15,16,18), cautious extrapolation of data between studies on the two phenomena seems appropriate.

CENTRAL CONTROL OF METABOLIC RATE

Like most autonomic functions, metabolic rate is largely under central nervous system control. Studies related to this topic have revealed many mechanisms which are common (or at least related) to the central control of metabolic rate, food intake, and body temperature.

BRAIN REGIONS INFLUENCING THERMOGENESIS

The control of autonomic functions, particularly feeding behavior and thermoregulation are primarily controlled by the hypothalamus, and this brain area has been the primary focus for studies on thermogenesis. The ventromedial hypothalamus (VMH) was first implicated in the regulation of body weight and energy balance almost 40 years ago, when destruction of the ventromedial nucleus was shown to result in hyperphagia and obesity. The VMH was subsequently referred to as a "satiety" center, acting reciprocally with the lateral hypothalamus (LH; known as the hunger center) to control food intake (20). Indications that the VMH can also modify energy expenditure arise from the fact that obesity will develop in VMH lesioned animals even if food intake is not increased. Perkins et al. (21) reported marked increases in thermogenesis (implied from measurements of temperature) of brown fat in response to VMH stimulation, which were dependent on the sympathetic nervous system, and several groups have confirmed the involvement of the VMH in the control of BAT thermogenesis (21–24). Stimulation of the VMH raises brown fat temperature in conscious as well as anesthetized animals, causes marked increases in noradrenaline turnover (25), and blood flow (26) to BAT, and increases in whole body resting oxygen consumption.

Indirect evidence for impaired thermogenesis following VMH destruction has been suggested by observations of increased efficiency of weight gain (25), and reduction in the thermogenic responses to food (27), noradrenaline turnover, and thermogenic activity of brown fat (28,29), all of which may contribute to the development of obesity.

The ventral noradrenergic bundle (VNAB) may in fact be responsible for many of the effects ascribed to the VMH, and this pathway runs along the base of the brain and projects to the paraventricular nuclei (PVN), dorsomedial nuclei (DMN), and the preoptic region of the hypothalamus, all of which have been implicated in the control of brown fat thermogenesis. There is some debate over whether the VMH is involved in the control of NST as well as DIT, and this may again relate to differential effects of the ventromedial nucleus and of noradrenergic fibers. Hogan et al. (28) reported impaired DIT, but no deficiency of NST in VMH-lesioned rats, whereas Imai-Matsumura et al. (30) demonstrated that injection of lidocaine into the VMH prevented the increase in BAT temperature in response to cooling of the preoptic area in conscious rats. The preoptic and anterior areas of the hypothalamus have been studied in some detail because of their involvement in temperature regulation, and both can apparently activate a variety of peripheral mechanisms causing increased heat production and conservation. The PVN has been more specifically associated with dietary responses and its destruction results in an obesity which shares some common features with the VMH syndrome (31,32).

Several extra hypothalamic areas have been implicated in the control of thermogenesis but detailed studies are rare. Activation of thermogenesis in response to conditioning (e.g., at the time of darkness) in the laboratory rats and the sight and smell of food (see 1,2) suggests that there is some cortical influence on thermogenesis, presumably via the hypothalamus. Stereotaxic knife cuts or suction decerebration in the cat or the rat have indicated the presence of a tonic inhibitory center in the upper pontine region. Decerebration in the prepontine region produces dramatic increases in body temperature in several species (33,34) which are associated with marked increases in metabolic rate (34). In contrast, premammillary transections prevent or inhibit these responses, indicating that a tonic inhibitory system is located somewhere between the lower midbrain and upper pons which controls sympathetic outflow (34,35).

CENTRAL AMINES

The majority of our current understanding of the involvement of noradrenergic mechanisms in CNS control of metabolism arises from studies on body weight regulation. Sahakian et al. (36) reported that chemical destruction of noradrenergic pathways in the region of the VNAB resulted in inhibition of BAT activity and obesity. In contrast, Shimazu et al. (37) described rapid weight gains in rats following infusion of noradrenaline into the VMH of rats over several weeks, but found no changes in body weight in response to noradrenaline infusion into the PVN or the lateral hypothalamus, and only modest obesity in response to adrenaline infusion into the VMH. Siviy et al. (38) found that infusion of noradrenaline into the PVN inhibited energy expenditure in the rat probably via an α_2 adrenoreceptor action.

These apparently conflicting findings may represent subtle but crucial differences in the site of infusion and the location and type of receptors affected by experimental manipulation. For example, microinjection of noradrenaline into the PVN can elicit feeding via an α-adrenoreceptor mechanism (31), whereas activation of β-adreno-receptors in the lateral hypothalamus may inhibit feeding (39). It is likely that the control of thermogenesis is also dependent on both the site of action and receptor subtype.

More consistent data are available for the actions of serotonergic pathways on thermogenesis. Central or peripheral injections of 5-hydroxytryptamine (5HT), serotonergic agonists, or releasing agents such as a D-fenfluramine all stimulate metabolic rate and BAT thermogenesis by increasing sympathetic outflow (LeFeuvre et al., *unpublished results*; 40) Chemical depletion of 5HT pathways by injection of parachlorophenylalanine (PCPA) inhibits BAT activity (41), and causes hyperphagia and obesity in the rat (42). However, central injection of the slightly more selective neurotoxic agent 5,7-dihydroxytryptamine (5,7-DHT), in combination with desipramine to protect noradrenergic pathways, fails to induce obesity, but greatly enhances the thermogenic effects of D-fenfluramine, presumably because of increased receptor density or enhanced receptor sensitivity (24). The varied effects of PCPA and 5,7-DHT are probably due to selective destruction of 5HT pathways in different brain regions, since not all serotonergic pathways are involved in the control of food intake and body weight regulation (43). We have observed that the thermogenic and anorectic effects of 5HT and 5HT-releasing agents in the rat are dependent on central actions of corticotrophin releasing factor (CRF) since they are markedly attenuated by central injection of neutralizing anti-CRF antibody (LeFeuvre and Rothwell, *unpublished data*).

There are relatively few studies on dopaminergic or cholinergic pathways and thermogenesis, although Shimazu et al. (37) observed no changes in body weight after chronic infusions of acetylcholine into the hypothalamus.

AMINO ACIDS

Peripheral administration of GABA transaminase inhibitors, which increases brain gamma amino acid (GABA) concentrations inhibits the development of genetic obesity (44) and stimulates thermogenesis (45). The use of selective GABA agonists and antagonists, injected centrally (into the VMH or third ventricle) has shown that activation of $GABA_B$ receptors, for example by baclofen, causes very large increases in thermogenesis (46), whereas activation of the $GABA_A$ receptor inhibits metabolic rate and BAT activity (47). Several other amino acids could modify brain function and metabolic rate indirectly as they act as precursors for neurotransmitters (see above). Excitatory amino acids (e.g., glutamate and aspartate) however appear to act directly to influence CNS function, and are released in response to local brain injury. Injection of excitatory amino acids into the VMH stimulates brown fat thermogenesis in the rat (48). A physiological role of these transmitters has not been identified but they are strong candidates as mediators of hypermetabolic responses to brain injury and cerebral ischemia (49).

PEPTIDES

We have identified several peptides which cause dose dependent increases in metabolic rate in conscious animals when injected into the third ventricle of the brain, and in most cases these have been associated with increased BAT activity (17,24,50). Many of these peptides have been demonstrated to exert reciprocal effects on appetite and thermogenesis (51), although the physiological importance of endogenous peptides in appetite control or thermogenesis has not been elucidated.

Insulin has been strongly implicated in the central control of energy balance (52–54 for reviews). When injected peripherally in high doses insulin can cause obesity, but at lower physiological concentrations could have CNS actions which inhibit food intake and stimulate thermogenesis. Central infusion of insulin suppresses body weight gain in the rat, and cerebroventricular injections enhance the thermogenic actions of glucose (see 54 for review).

Thyrotropin releasing factor (TRH) or its chemical analogues are potent stimulators of metabolic rate in the rat (55), and TRH has been suggested as an activator of the increased thermogenesis associated with arousal from hibernation and a mediator of neural thermoregulation and fever (56,57). Lin et al. (58) reported a strong correlation between fever, thermogenesis, and hypothalamic TRH concentrations in rats in response to pyrogenic agents. From these data the authors suggested that TRH mediates fever and interacts with serotonin and prostaglandins.

CRF

Considerable interest has centered on corticotropin releasing factor (CRF), which is now emerging as an important factor in the central control of energy balance and in the metabolic responses to stress, infection, and injury (see 9 for review).

CRF is synthesized mainly in the paraventricular nucleus of the hypothalamus, although many other sites of synthesis within the CNS and the periphery have been identified (see 59,60). CRF is recognized mainly for its effects on the synthesis and release of ACTH and other proopiomelanocortin (POMC) derived peptides from the pituitary. However, CRF can also exert CNS actions which appear to be independent of the pituitary, and it can thus function as a neurotransmitter or neuromodulator. The effects of CRF on thermogenesis, food intake, and the sympathetic nervous system are included in this category.

The earliest suggestion that CRF might be involved in the control of energy balance was implied from studies on the effects of adrenalectomy in genetically obese rodents (see 61,62). Adrenalectomy almost completely normalizes the defective energy balance of genetically obese and aging rats and mice, by both suppressing food intake and stimulating metabolic rate and brown fat activity (63–68). These effects are inhibited by replacement of the animals with either corticosterone or dexamethasone and, in the case of obese animals, only very low doses of replacement are required (63). Hypophysectomy has similar effects on energy balance (69), and this finding led to the suggestion that reduced synthesis, release, or actions of CRF might be responsible for the impaired energy balance regulation and thermogenesis in obese mutants (62,70).

Central injection of CRF causes dose dependent increases in metabolic rate, BAT blood flow, and thermogenic activity which are dependent on the sympathetic nervous system in the rat (71). Brown et al. (72) demonstrated increased sympathetic outflow in response to CRF but in spite of an extensive study, failed to identify its site of action within the brain. Preliminary reports have indicated that the concentration of CRF in specific hypothalamic nuclei of genetically obese Zucker rats (73) are reduced and these mutants may be unable to synthesize and/or release CRF in response to other stimuli (see later), although they can respond normally to exogenous CRF (74). Intracerebroventricular infusion of CRF in lean or obese animals inhibits body weight gain and stimulates BAT (75,76).

Glucocorticoids inhibit thermogenesis, probably by suppressing CRF synthesis, but the thermogenic effects of CRF are not modified by glucocorticoid status and are almost identical in adrenalectomized animals or those treated with high doses of dexamethasone (see 50 for review). This illustrates an important difference between the central (e.g., thermogenic) and pituitary (i.e., ACTH release) effects of CRF. The glucocorticoid antagonist RU-38486 stimulates thermogenesis and this effect is reversed by pretreatment of the animals with a CRF receptor antagonist (77).

The effects of serotonergic agents in thermogenesis, described previously could also be mediated by CRF. 5HT causes release of CRF (78,79), and results obtained in conscious rats, indicate that thermogenic responses to 5HT and its precursors are attenuated by inhibition of CRF release or action (LeFeuvre and Rothwell, *unpublished data*).

CRF has many other central actions in addition to those described above, for example on behavior, sleep, peripheral glucose metabolism, and immune function (see 50 for review). CRF could thus be of considerable importance in the central control of these processes in response to stress, injury, or illness and this possibility is supported by recent reports that CRF also mediates central effects of immune signals, most notably interleukin-1 (see below).

CYTOKINES

The cytokines are now emerging as important mediators of the immune, inflammatory, and metabolic responses to injury and infection. The cytokines most pertinent to this discussion are interleukin-1α and β (IL-1α and IL-1β), tumor necrosis factor α (TNFα), and interleukin 6 (IL-6). IL-1 has been considered the most important endogenous pyrogen (see 80–84).

Administration of recombinant IL-1 to rats, mice, and rabbits induces fever and activation of thermogenesis whether injected peripherally or directly into the cerebroventricular space (5,84). These effects are dependent on the same peripheral effectors as the thermogenic responses to cold and diet, i.e., sympathetic activation of BAT. Genetically obese rodents (fatty Zucker rat and obese ob/ob mice) which show defective dietary activation of thermogenesis but a normal response to cold, also exhibit impaired responses to IL-1 (85). The main site of action for IL-1 appears to be within the brain (see 5,80,85,86), since very low doses (ng range) are required to induce fever compared to peripheral injection. Kuriyama et al. (87) have reported direct effects of IL-1β on the firing rate of glucose-sensitive neurones in the VMH. However, the means by which IL-1 derived from peripheral tissues gains access to hypothalamic sites of action is unknown, and IL-1 is probably unable to cross the blood brain barrier (see 82). Circulating concentrations of IL-1 often fail to correlate with fever in animals (88) or humans (89,90).

It is likely that IL-1 is synthesized within the brain in response to peripherally released pyrogen signals by both neurones and glia (91). We have observed release of IL-1 and IL-6 from hypothalamii *in vitro* (Hopkins and Rothwell, *unpublished data*) and increased synthesis of mRNA for IL-1β in the brain in response to peripheral injection of endotoxin (Bartfai, et al. *unpublished data*). Furthermore central injection of anti IL-1β antibody markedly attenuates the responses to peripheral endotoxin (88).

In contrast to IL-1, IL-6 concentrations in plasma increase dramatically during the development of fever and hypermetabolism (83,88,92). Central injection of IL-6 also causes increases in body temperature and metabolic rate in the rat (93). These data indicate that IL-6 may be a more important circulating pyrogen than IL-1. Nevertheless the involvement of IL-1 in fever and hypermetabolism is supported by the finding that peripheral as well as central administration of antibodies to IL-1β or to the IL-1 receptor attenuate the acute and chronic metabolic responses to endotoxin (83,88,94) or local inflammation induced by injection of turpentine (95). Our preliminary data suggest that central injection of an IL-6 Ab also attenuates endotoxin-induced fever in the rat, indicating that like IL-1, it is also synthesized and acts within the brain (Rothwell, *unpublished data*).

Tumor necrosis factor (TNF)α which has been proposed as a mediator of cancer cachexia and was originally termed "cachectin," induces wasting (96) and also activates thermogenesis when injected centrally or peripherally into rodents (97) although the doses required are rather higher than for other cytokines, questioning its physiological importance. TNFα has, however, been strongly implicated in the control of fever (82) although a recent report has suggested that administration of TNF antibody enhances fever in the rat and that TNF may act as an antipyretic agent (98).

Macrophage inflammatory protein 1 (MIP-1) and IL-8 are both lower molecular weight (8 kDa) cytokines and can also induce fever and hypermetabolism when injected centrally or peripherally in rodents, but unlike the other pyrogenic cytokines, their effects are independent of eicosanoid synthesis (99,100).

In addition to the well-documented effects of cytokines on fever, metabolism, and immune function, they have now been demonstrated to exert a number of actions of neuroendocrine systems. Activation of the pituitary adrenal system by interleukin-1 involves hypothalamic release of CRF (101,102) and this may explain many of the endocrine responses to infection and injury, particularly the observed increases in circulating glucocorticoid concentrations. Glucocorticoids can form an important feedback mechanism by subsequently inhibiting the metabolic and inflammatory effects of infection (102,103) and the synthesis of CRF in the brain. It has now been demonstrated that the central effects of IL-1β on fever and thermogenesis are also dependent on CRF, since they are inhibited by treatment of animals with a CRF receptor antagonist (α-helical CRF 9-41), or monoclonal or polyclonal antibodies to CRF (93,104). The central effects of IL-6 are also dependent on CRF release (*unpublished data*), although the actions of IL-1α and TNFα are independent of CRF. Uehara et al. (105) have reported differential effects of IL-1α and IL-1β on ACTH release in the rat and we have observed that, genetically obese mutants fail to show significant thermogenic responses to IL-1β (106), but they can respond normally to IL-1α (Busbridge et al. *unpublished data*). This observation supports the suggestion that obese mutants have some impairment in the synthesis or release of CRF in response to thermogenic stimuli such as IL-1β, and strongly questions the dogma that IL-1α and IL-1b both act on the same receptor (109).

A recent report has demonstrated that the inhibitory effects of IL-1 on food intake are also dependent on CRF release (107). Thus, inhibition of CRF release or action could be of benefit in the clinical management of cachexia. The precise site of action of cytokines is not known, although *in vitro* effects on hypothalamic slice preparations have been reported (108).

CYTOKINE RECEPTORS IN THE BRAIN

There is current debate over the nature of IL-1 receptors particularly within the CNS. An 80 kDa receptor has been described in detail in many tissues and this shows equal affinity for both IL-1α and IL-1β (109). However, there is now considerable evidence to suggest that IL-1α and IL-1β have different actions within the CNS, (see above and Table 2) a finding which is not consistent with interaction with the classical receptor. Several autoradiographic studies have described IL-1 receptors

TABLE 2. *Evidence for different central actions of interleukins-1α and β*

1. Recombinant preparations of IL-1β are more effective and induce greater maximal responses than IL-1α
2. IL-1α and IL-1β are additive at maximal doses
3. Effects of IL-1β are dependent on CRF release, effects of IL-1α are not
4. Genetically obese rats and mice show impaired responses to IL-1β but respond normally to IL-1α

within the brain (e.g., 110). In contrast Katsuura et al. (111) reported preferential binding of IL-1β to membranes prepared from hypothalamic tissue with a much lower affinity than the 80 kDa receptor. We have been unable to detect expression of mRNA for this receptor by PCR analysis in brain tissue. (Busbridge et al., *unpublished data*). Furthermore our preliminary *in vitro* studies have indicated that the endogenous IL-1 receptor antagonist inhibits fever and hypermetabolism induced by peripheral but not by central administration of rIL-1β in the rat *in vivo* (Rothwell, *unpublished data*). These data strongly support the existence of a different IL-1 receptor in the brain. This proposal, if verified, has important implications for therapeutic modification of centrally mediated effects of IL-1 such as fever and metabolism.

EICOSANOIDS

Eicosanoids are important mediators of fever and the central effects of cytokines. Prostaglandin E_2 (PGE_2) is generally thought to be the main mediator of fever, and therefore of the hypermetabolic responses to pyrogens (112). However a number of other eicosanoids stimulate fever and thermogenesis, and in the rat $PGF_2\alpha$ is slightly more effective than PGE_2 (113). Bernadini et al. (114) have reported that several arachidonic acid metabolites induce release of CRF from hypothalami *in vitro*. $PGF_2\alpha$ and thromboxane A_2 (TXA_2) are both potent releasers of CRF while PGE_2 is ineffective or inhibitory. The *in vivo* thermogenic effects of $PGF_2\alpha$ but not PGE_2 are dependent on CRF (10), suggesting that $PGF_2\alpha$ or TXA_2 rather than PGE_2 mediate the effects of those cytokines which depend on CRF release for their action (i.e., IL-1β and IL-6).

GLUCOCORTICOIDS

Glucocorticoids are potent inhibitors of the inflammatory, pyrogenic, and metabolic responses to injury, and also inhibit diet-induced thermogenesis by central actions (see 62). These effects could be mediated by inhibition of either eicosanoid or CRF synthesis within the CNS. The antiinflammatory actions of steroids have been ascribed to their inhibition of phospholipase A_2 activity, thus causing suppression of eicosanoid synthesis and are thought to depend on release of a second mediator(s) known as lipocortins (see 115). These proteins are synthesized in many tissues and have diverse actions on intracellular calcium, phospholipid binding, and can act as substrates for receptor phosphorylation. Lipocortin-1 has been identified in the CNS (Strijbos et al., *unpublished data*; 116), and central or peripheral injection of a recombinant fragment of lipocortin-1 suppresses the thermogenic effects of cytokines in the rat (117). Conversely, administration of antibody to lipocortin-1 can enhance such responses, particularly in animals with impaired thermogenesis (117). Thus lipocortin may act as an endogenous modulator of the metabolic responses to injury, but the factors controlling its synthesis and action are largely unknown.

SUMMARY AND CONCLUSIONS

Changes in metabolic rate form an important component of the host response to injury and infection. The efferent and central mechanisms responsible for hypermetabolism are in many cases comparable to those involved in other physiological responses (e.g., fever, hyperphagia, and behavior) and all are mediated by the central nervous system. Afferent pathways which have been identified include neural signals relating to pain or local inflammation and circulating cytokines, most notably IL-1, IL-6, and TNFα. These cytokines also act (and are probably synthesized) within the brain. Central mechanisms are numerous and complex, but appear to be integrated within the hypothalamus and are probably dependent on eicosanoid synthesis, aminergic pathways, and release of a number of endogenous peptides (CRF, TRH, opioids, lipocortin).

Our understanding of the central control of metabolism has been increased considerably over the past 2–3 years, opening several possible avenues for therapeutic intervention. However, the benefits of such intervention remain to be fully clarified and may depend on factors such as the type, duration, and severity of illness, current nutritional status, and the general condition of the patient.

REFERENCES

1. Rothwell NJ, Stock MJ. Brown adipose tissue and diet-induced thermogenesis. In: Trayhurn P, Nicholls DG, eds. *Brown adipose tissue*. London: Arnold, 1986;269–298.
2. Rothwell NJ, Stock MJ. Whither brown fat? *Biosci Rep* 1986;6:3–18.
3. Landsberg L, Young JB. Autonomic regulation of thermogenesis. In: Girardier L, Stock MJ, eds. *Mammalian thermogenesis*. London: Chapman & Hall, 1983;99–140.
4. Brooks SL, Neville AM, Rothwell NJ, Stock MJ, Wilson S. Sympathetic activation of brown adipose tissue thermogenesis in cachexia. *Biosci Rep* 1981;1:509–517.
5. Dascombe MJ, Rothwell NJ, Sagay BO, Stock MJ. Pyrogenic and thermogenic effects of interleukin 1β in the rat. *Am J Physiol* 1989;256:E7–E11.
6. Jepson MM, Cox M, Bates PC, Rothwell NJ, Stock MJ, Cady EB, Millward DJ. Regional blood flow and skeletal muscle energy status in endotoxemic rats. *Am J Physiol* 1987;252:E581–E587.
7. Jepson MM, Millward DJ, Rothwell NJ, Stock MJ. Involvement of the sympathetic nervous system and brown fat in endotoxin induced fever in the rat. *Am J Physiol* 1988;255:E617–E623.
8. McCarthy HD, O'Shaughnessy CT, Rothwell NJ. Endogenous mediators of cerebral ischaemia-induced hypermetabolism in the rat. *Br J Pharm* 1990;99:838.
9. Rothwell NJ. Thermogenesis on obesity and cachexia. In: Muller M, ed. *Endocrinology and metabolism—hormones and nutrition in obesity and cachexia*. Heidelberg: Springer, 1990;77–85.
10. Rothwell NJ. Central activation of thermogenesis by prostaglandins, dependence on CRF. *Horm Metab Res* 1991;22:616–618.
11. Lean MEJ, James WPT, Jennings G, Trayhurn P. Brown adipose tissue uncoupling protein content in human infants, children and adults. *Clin Sci* 1986;71:291–297.
12. Bianchi A, Bruce J, Cooper AL, et al. Increased brown adipose tissue activity in children with malignant diseases. *Horm Metab Res* 1989;21:587–642.
13. Bruce J, Childs CC, Cooper AL, Rothwell NJ. Brown adipose tissue activity in children in relation to disease status. *Proc Nutr Soc* 1990;49:189A.
14. Newsholme E, Crabtree B. Substrate cycles in metabolic regulation and in heat generation. *Biochem Soc Symp* 1976;41:61–109.
15. Aulick LH, Wilmore DW. Hypermetabolism in trauma. In: Girardier L, Stock MJ, eds. *Mammalian thermogenesis*. London: Chapman & Hall, 1983;259–304.

16. Little RA. Metabolic rate and thermoregulation after injury. In: Ledingham I, ed. *Recent Advances in Critical Care Medicine.* vol 3, London: Churchill Livingstone, 1988;159–172.
17. Rothwell NJ. Central control of thermogenesis. *Proc Nutr Soc* 1989;48:241–250.
18. Wilmore DW, Long JM, Mason AD, Skreen RW, Pruitt BA. Catecholamines: mediator of the hypermetabolic response to thermal injury. *Ann Surg* 1974;870:653–670.
19. Young JB, Fish S, Landsberg L. Sympathetic nervous system and adrenal medullary responses to ischaemic injury in mice. *Am J Physiol* 1983;245:E67–E73.
20. Stellar E. The physiology of motivation. *Psychol Rev* 1954;61:522–580.
21. Perkins MN, Rothwell NJ, Stock MJ, Stone TW. Activation of brown adipose tissue thermogenesis by the ventromedial hypothalamus. *Nature* 1981;89:401–402.
22. Freeman PH, Wellman PJ. Brown adipose tissue thermogenesis induced by low level electrical stimulation of the hypothalamus in rats. *Brain Res Bull* 1987;18:7–11.
23. Holt S, Wheal H, York DA. Hypothalamic control of BAT in Zucker lean and obese rats; effects of electrical stimulation of the VMH and other hypothalamic nuclei. *Brain Res* 1987;405:227–233.
24. LeFeuvre RA. *The hypothalamic control of thermogenesis* [Thesis.]. London: University of London, 1990.
25. Saito M, Minokoshi Y, Shimanin R. Accelerated norepinephrine turnover in peripheral tissues after ventromedial hypothalamic stimulation in rats. *Brain Res* 1989;481:298–303.
26. Iwai M, Hell NS, Shimazu T. Effects of VMH stimulation on blood flow of BAT in rats. *Pflugers Arch* 1987;410:44–47.
27. Carlisle HJ, Rothwell NJ, Stock MJ. Thermic responses to food in rats with lesions of the ventromedial hypothalamus. *Proc Nutr Soc* 1988;47:24A.
28. Hogan S, Coscina DV, Himms-Hagen J. Brown adipose tissue of rats with obesity inducing ventromedial hypothalamic lesions. *Am J Physiol* 1982;243:E334–E338.
29. Seydoux J, Rohner-Jeanrenaud F, Assimacoupoulos-Jeannet F, Jeanrenaud B, Girardier L. Functional disconnection of brown adipose tissue in hypothalamic obesity in rats. *Pflugers Arch* 1981;390:1–4.
30. Imai-Matsumura K, Matsumura K, Nakayama T. Involvement of the ventromedial hypothalamus in brown adipose tissue thermogenesis induced by preoptic cooling in rats. *Jpn J Physiol* 1984;34:939–943.
31. Leibowitz SF. Brain monoamines and peptides: role in the control of eating behaviour. *Fed Proc* 1986;45:1396–1403.
32. Weingarten HP, Chang P, McDonald TJ. Comparison of the metabolic and behavioural disturbances following PVN and VMH lesions. *Brain Res Bull* 1985;14:551–559.
33. Bignall KE, Heggenness FW, Palmer JE. Effect of neonatal decerebration on thermogenesis during starvation and cold exposure in the rat. *Exp Neurol* 1975;40:174–188.
34. Rothwell NJ, Stock MJ, Thexton AJ. Decerebration activates thermogenesis in the rat. *J Physiol* 1983;342:15–22.
35. Benzi RH, Shibata M, Seydoux J, Girardier L. Prepontine knife cut induced hyperthermia in the rat. *Pflugers Arch* 1988;411:593–599.
36. Sahakian BJ, Trayhurn P, Wallace M, et al. Increased weight gain and reduced activity in brown adipose tissue produced by depletion of hypothalamic noradrenaline. *Neurosci Lett* 1983;39:321–326.
37. Shimazu T, Noma M, Saito M. Chronic infusion of norepinephrine into the VMH induces obesity in rats. *Brain Res* 1986;369:215–223.
38. Siviy SM, Kritikos A, Atrens DM, Shepherd A. Effects of norepinephrine infusion in the paraventricular hypothalamus on energy expenditure in the rat. *Brain Res* 1989;487:79–88.
39. Grossman SP. Direct adrenergic and cholinergic stimulation of hypothalamic mechanisms. *Am J Physiol* 1962;303:782–882.
40. Rothwell NJ, Stock MJ. Effects of diet and fenfluramine on thermogenesis in the rat: possible involvement of serotonergic mechanisms in the rat. *Int J Obes* 1987;11:319–324.
41. Fuller MJ, Stirling DM, Dunnett S, Reynolds GP, Ashwell M. Decreased brown adipose tissue thermogenic activity following a reduction in brain serotonin by intraventricular p-chlorophenylalanine. *Biosci Rep* 1987;7:121–127.
42. Breisch ST, Zemlan FP, Hoebel BG. Hyperphagic obesity following serotonergic depletion by intraventricular p-chlorophenylanine. *Science* 1976;192:382–384.
43. Coscina DV, Madger RJ. Effects of serotonin depleting and brain lesions on the defense of hypothalamic obesity. *Physiol Behav* 1984;33:575–579.

44. Coscina DV, Nobrega JN. Anorectic potency of inhibiting GABA transaminase in brain: studies of hypothalamic dietary and genetic obesities. *Int J Obes* 1984;8:181–200.
45. Horton RW, Rothwell NJ, Stock MJ. Chronic inhibition of GABA transaminase results in activation of thermogenesis and brown fat in the rat. *Gen Pharm* 1989;19:403–406.
46. Addae JI, Rothwell NJ, Stock MJ, Stone TW. Activation of brown fat thermogenesis in rats by baclofen. *Neuropharmacology* 1986;25:627–631.
47. Horton RW, LeFeuvre RA, Rothwell NJ, Stock MJ. Opposing effects of activation of central GABA$_A$ and GABA$_B$ receptors on brown fat thermogenesis in the rat. *Neuropharmacology* 1988;27:363–366.
48. Amir S. Intraventromedial injection of glutamate stimulates BAT thermogenesis. *Brain Res* 1990;571:341–344.
49. Choi DW, Rothman SM. The role of glutamate neurotoxicity in hypoxic ischaemic neuronal death. *Annu Rev Neurosci* 1990;13:171–182.
50. Rothwell NJ. Central effects of CRF on metabolism and energy balance. *Neurosci Biobehav Rev* 1990;14:263–271.
51. Morley JE. Neuropeptide regulation of appetite and weight. *Endocr Rev* 1987;8:256–287.
52. Baskin DG, Porte D, Guest K, Dorsa DM. Insulin in the brain. *Annu Rev Physiol* 1987;49:335–347.
53. Figlewicz DP, Lacour F, Sipols A, Porte D, Woods D. Gastroenteropancreatic peptides and the central nervous system. *Annu Rev Physiol* 1987;49:383–395.
54. Rothwell NJ, Stock MJ. Insulin and thermogenesis. *Int J Obes* 1988;1:93–102.
55. Griffiths EC, Rothwell NJ, Stock MJ. Thermogenic effects of thyrotropin releasing hormone and its analogues in the rat. *Experientia* 1988;44:41–42.
56. Lin MT. Metabolic respiratory, vasomotor and body temperature responses to TRH, angiotensin II, substance P, neurotensin, somatostatin, LH-RH beta endorphin, oxytone and vasopressin in the rat. *Adv Biosci* 1982;38:229–251.
57. Metcalfe G. TRH: a possible mediator of thermoregulation. *Nature* 1974;252:310–311.
58. Lin MT, Wang PS, Chuang J, Fan LJ, Won SJ. Cold stress on a pyrogenic substrate deviates tryptophan releasing hormone levels in rat hypothalamus and induces thermogenic reactions. *Neuroendocrinology* 1989;50:177–181.
59. Emeric-Sauval E. CRF a review. *Psychoneuroendocrinology* 1986;11:277–294.
60. Gillies G, Grossman A. The CRF's and their control: chemistry, physiology and clinical implications. *J Clin Endocrinol Metab* 1985;14:821–845.
61. York DA. Neural activity in hypothalamic and genetic obesity. *Proc Nutr Soc* 1987;46:105–117.
62. York DA. Corticosteroid inhibition of thermogenesis in obese animals. *Proc Nutr Soc* 1989;48:231–235.
63. Holt S, York DA. The effect of adrenalectomy on GDP binding to brown adipose tissue mitochondria of obese rats. *Biochem J* 1982;208:819–822.
64. Marchington D, Rothwell NJ, Stock MJ, York DA. Energy balance diet-induced thermogenesis and brown adipose tissue in lean and obese (fa/fa) Zucker rats after adrenalectomy. *J Nutr* 1983;113:1395–1402.
65. Marchington D, Rothwell NJ, Stock MJ, York DA. Thermogenesis and sympathetic activity in BAT of overfed rats after adrenalectomy. *Am J Physiol* 1986;250:E362–E366.
66. Rothwell NJ, Stock MJ. Sympathetic and adrenocorticoid influences on diet-induced thermogenesis and brown fat activity in the rat. *Comp Biochem Physiol* 1984;79A:575–579.
67. Rothwell NJ, Stock MJ. Influence of adrenalectomy on age-related changes in energy balance thermogenesis and brown fat activity in the rat. *Comp Biochem Physiol* 1988;89A:265–269.
68. Yukimura Y, Bray GA, Wolfsen AR. Some effects of adrenalectomy in the fatty rat. *Endocrinology* 1978;103:1924–1928.
69. King BM, Smith RL. Hypothalamic obesity after hypophysectomy or adrenalectomy: dependence on corticosterone. *Am J Physiol* 1985;249:522–526.
70. Rothwell NJ, Stock MJ. Thermogenesis and BAT activity in hypophysectomized rats with and without corticotrophin replacement. *Am J Physiol* 1985;249:E330–E333.
71. LeFeuvre RA, Rothwell NJ, Stock MJ. Activation of brown fat thermogenesis in response to central injection of CRF in the rat. *Neuropharmacology* 1987;26:1217–1221.
72. Brown M, Fisher LA, Speiss J, Rivier C, Rivier J, Vale W. CRF actions on the sympathetic nervous system and metabolism. *Endocrinology* 1982;111:928–931.
73. Moore BJ, Routh VH. Corticotropin releasing factor (CRF) levels are altered in the brain of the genetically obese fatty Zucker rat. *Fed Proc* 1988;22:5386.

74. Carnie JA, LeFeuvre RA, Linton EA, McCarthy HD, Rothwell NJ. Thermogenic effect of CRF in genetically obese Zucker rats. *Proc Nutr Soc* 1988;47:165A.
75. Arase K, York Da, Shimizu H, Shargill N, Bray GA. Effects of corticotrophin releasing factor on food intake and brown adipose tissue thermogenesis in rats. *Am J Physiol* 1988;255:E255–259.
76. Rohner-Jeanrenaud F, Walker C, Greco Perotto R, Jeanrenaud B. Chronic intracerebroventricular administration of corticotrophin releasing factor (CRF) to genetically obese fa/fa rats arrests the further increase of their body weight. In: Bjorntorp P, Rossner SJ, eds. *Obesity in Europe '88: Proceedings European Congress on Obesity.* London: John Libbey, 1988;253–258.
77. Hardwick AJ, Linton EA, Rothwell NJ. Thermogenic effects of the antiglucocorticoid RU486 in the rat: involvement of corticotropin releasing factor and sympathetic activation of brown adipose tissue. *Endocrinology* 1989;124:1684–1688.
78. Calogero AE, Bernadini R, Margioris AN, et al. Effects of serotonergic agonists and antagonists on CRH secretion by explanted hypothalami. *Peptides* 1989;10:189–200.
79. Gibbs DM, Vale W. Effect of the serotonin uptake inhibitor fluoxetine on corticotropin releasing factor and vasopressin secretion into hypophysial portal blood. *Brain Res* 1983;280:176–179.
80. Blatteis CM. Neural mechanisms in the pyrogenic and acute phase responses to interleukin-1. *Int J Neurosci* 1988;38:223–232.
81. Cooper KE. The neurobiology of fever: thoughts on recent developments. *Annu Rev Neurosci* 1987;10:297–394.
82. Dinarello CA, Cannon JG, Wolff SM. New concepts on the pathogenesis of fever. *Rev Infect Dis* 1988;10:168–187.
83. Kluger MJ. Body temperature changes during inflammation: their mediation and nutritional significance. *Proc Nutr Soc* 1989;48:337–345.
84. Kluger MJ. Fever and sepsis. In: Rothwell NJ, Stock MJ, eds. *Biological Council symposium.* London: Wiley, 1990 [In press].
85. Dascombe MJ, Hardwick A, LeFeuvre RA, Rothwell NJ. Impaired effects of interleukin 1β in fever, thermogenesis and brown fat in genetically obese rats. *Int J Obes* 1989;13:367–374.
86. Sternberg EM. Monokines, lymphokines and the brain. In: Cruse JM, Lewis RE, eds. *The year in immunology* Basel: Karger, 1989;205–217.
87. Kuriyama K, Hon Mori T, Nakashima T. Activities of interferon-α and interleukin-1β on the glucose responsive neurons of the ventromedial hypothalamus. *Brain Res* 1990;24:803–810.
88. Rothwell NJ, Busbridge NJ, Humphray H, Hissey P. Central actions of interleukin-1β on fever and thermogenesis. *Cytokine* 1989;1:153.
89. Childs C, Ratcliffe RJ, Hold I, Hopkins SJ. Relationships between interleukin 1, interleukin 6 and pyrexia in burned children. *Cytokine* 1989;1:36.
90. Horan MA, Gibbons L, Hopkins SJ, Cooper A, Strijbos P, Rothwell NJ, Little RA. Changes in plasma interleukin 6 during experimentally induced fever in normal humans. *Cytokine* 1989;1:138.
91. Breder CD, Dinarello CA, Saper CB. Interleukin-1, immunoreactive innervation of human hypothalamus. *Science* 1988;240:321–324.
92. LeMay LG, Vander A, Kluger M. The effects of psychological stress and anaesthesia on plasma interleukin 6 (1L-6) activity in rat. *Cytokine* 1989;1:123.
93. Busbridge NJ, Dascombe MJ, Tilders FJA, van Oers JWAM, Linton EA, Rothwell NJ. Central activation of thermogenesis and fever by interleukin-1β and interleukin-1α involves different mechanisms. *Biochem Biophys Res Commun* 1989;162:591–596.
94. Wong N, LeMay LG, Otterness I, Kunkel SC, Vander AJ, Kluger MJ. The roles of IL-1α and β, TNF and IL-6 in LPS fever in the rat. In: Dinarello C, et al. eds. *Pathophysiologic and therapeutic roles of cytokines. Progress in leukocyte biology* 1990;10B:313–318.
95. Gershenwald JE, Fong Y, Fahey TJ, et al. Interleukin-1 receptor blockade attenuates the host-inflammatory response. *Proc Nat Acad Sci* 1989;87:4966–4970.
96. Beutler B, Carami A. Cachectin and tumour necrosis factor as two sides of the same biological coin. *Nature* 320:1986;584–588.
97. Rothwell NJ. Central effects of TNFα in the rat. *Biosci Rep* 1988;8:345–352.
98. Long NC, Kunkel SC, Vander AJ, Kluger MJ. Antiserum against tumour necrosis factor enhances lipopoly saccharide fever in rats. *Am J Physiol* 1990;258:R332–R337.
99. Minano FJ, Sancibrian M, Vizciano M, et al. *Brain Res Bull* 1990;24:849–852.
100. Rothwell NJ, Harwick AJ, Lindley I. Central actions of interleukin-8 in the rat are independent of prostaglandins. *Horm Metab Res* 1990;22:595–596.
101. Berkenbosch F, van Oers J, Del Rey A, Tilders F, Besedovsky H. Corticotrophin releasing factor producing neurones in the rat—activation by interleukin 1β. *Science* 238:1987;524–528.

102. Sapolsky RM, Rivier C, Yamamoto G, Plotsky G, Vale W. Interleukin 1 stimulates the secretion of hypothalamic corticotrophin releasing factor. *Science* 238:1987;522–524.
103. Besedovsky H, del Ray A, Sorkin E, Dinarello CA. Immunoregulatory feedback between interleukin-1 and glucocorticoid hormones. *Science* 233:1986;652–654.
104. Rothwell NJ. CRF is involved in the pyrogenic and thermogenic effects of interleukin 1β in the rat. *Am J Physiol* 1989;256:E111–E115.
105. Uehara A, Gottschall PE, Dahl RR, Arimura A. Stimulation of ACTH release by human interleukin-1 beta but not by interleukin-1 alpha in conscious freely moving rats. *Biochem Biophys Res Commun* 1987;146:1286–1290.
106. Busbridge NJ, Carnie JA, Dascombe MJ, Johnston JA, Rothwell NJ. Adrenalectomy reverses the impaired pyrogenic responses to interleukin 1β in obese Zucker rats. *Int J Obes* 1991;14:809–819.
107. Uehara A, Sekuya C, Takasagi Y, Namiki M, Armura A. Anorexia induced by interleukin 1: involvement of corticotropin releasing factor. *Am J Physiol* 1989;257:R613–R617.
108. Tsagakaris S, Gillies G, Rees LH, Bessner M, Grossman A. Interleukin 1 directly stimulates the release of corticotropin releasing factor from rat hypothalamus. *Neuroendocrinology* 1989;49:98–101.
109. Dower SK, Kronheim SR, Hopp TP, et al. The cell surface receptors for interleukin-1α and interleukin-1β are identical. *Nature* 324:1986;266–268.
110. Farrar WL, Kilian PC, Ruff MR, Hill JM, Pert CB. Visualization and characterization of interleukin 1 receptors in brain. *J Immunol* 1987;139:459–463.
111. Katsuura G, Gothenshall PG, Arimera A. Identification of a high affinity receptor for interleukin-1 beta in rat brain. *Biochem Biophys Res Commun* 1988;150:61–67.
112. Dascombe MJ. The pharmacology of fever. *Rev Infect Dis* 1985;6:51–95.
113. Morimoto A, Murakami N, Watanabe T. Is the central arachidonic acid cascade system involved in the development of acute phase response in rabbits? *J Physiol* 1988;397:281–289.
114. Bernadini R, Chiorenza A, Cologero AE, Gold PNN, Chrousos GP. Arachidonic acid metabolites modulate rat hypothalamic corticotrophin-releasing hormone secretion in vitro. *Neuroendocrinology* 1989;50:708–715.
115. Flower RJ. Lipocortin and the mechanisms of action of the glucocorticoids. *Br J Pharmacol* 1988;65:987–1015.
116. Smillie F, Boulton C, Peers S, Flower RJ. Distribution of lipocortins I, II and V in tissues of the rat, mouse and guinea pig. *Br J Pharmacol* 1989;97:P90.
117. Carey F, Forder R, Edge MD, et al. Lipocortin 1 fragment modifies the pyrogenic actions of cytokines in the rat. *Am J Physiol* 1990;259:R266–R269.

DISCUSSION

Dr. Frayn: Alterations of metabolic rate occur in many conditions. The hypermetabolism of trauma and sepsis is the most marked of these, and it seems reasonable to suppose that this condition would be the easiest to understand. The belief that central changes underlie the hypermetabolism of trauma and sepsis has emerged over the past two decades, based in part upon an increased understanding of the important role of the sympatho-adrenal system in this response (1). Along with this belief has risen the hope that it will be possible to understand the central pathways regulating hypermetabolism, and eventually to intervene with centrally-acting drugs. Similar hopes might be advanced for the treatment of obesity, for instance, and indeed appetite suppressant drugs may be an example of this in practice. An understanding of the pathways concerned in the central regulation of metabolic rate is therefore a very desirable clinical goal.

Doctor Rothwell has reviewed our current knowledge of these pathways. This field has expanded rapidly in recent years, thanks at least in part to Doctor Rothwell's own contributions, but also because of increased knowledge of the many possible mediators: cytokines, small peptides such as CRF, excitatory and inhibitory amino acids, and eicosanoids as well as the "classical" catecholamines, glucocorticoids, and acetylcholine. She has brought together information on thermoregulation in obesity, cold adaptation, fever, and trauma/sepsis. Rather than discuss the details of the individual pathways which Doctor Rothwell describes, I will make a few general (and deliberately controversial) points about our understanding of the central control of metabolism.

Corticotrophin-Releasing Factor (CRF): Central and Peripheral Effects

Doctor Rothwell's review of the role of CRF illustrates the problems which I feel make the interpretation of this type of work difficult. There is a view of obesity, summarized by York (2), which holds that excess pituitary ACTH production plays an important role. ACTH is derived from a larger precursor, proopiocortin, which is broken down within the pituitary to yield a number of peptides with potential biological activity, including ACTH and β-endorphin. ACTH may be further cleaved to yield the so-called β-cell tropin ($ACTH_{22-39}$) (3), a peptide which stimulates insulin secretion. Excess glucocorticoids and (peripheral) insulin are, as Doctor Rothwell discusses, well recognized factors in the development of obesity. One could therefore view hypothalamic CRF as "obesogenic." On the other hand, CRF appears to have "non-classical" central effects which are the exact opposite of these, resulting in increased sympathetic outflow and thermogenesis. That one transmitter should have opposing effects depending, presumably, upon the micro-anatomy of where it is produced and what receptors are nearby, is not in itself surprising. To take an example from "peripheral physiology," noradrenaline can cause either vasoconstriction or vasodilation in white adipose tissue. My real point for discussion is this: do we really have any hope of elucidating the details of central control by our present "macroscopic" techniques such as intraventricular injection, or pharmacological blockade, when the effects of any one modulator must be so dependent upon the exact locations at which it is produced and acts?

Simplicity or Complexity?

When Wilmore so convincingly showed the role of catecholamines in the hypermetabolism of trauma (1), a naive biochemist (such as myself) might have expected rapid progress in understanding the central connections responsible. Now, as Doctor Rothwell again so convincingly shows, the picture has become more complicated rather than simpler. A host of neurotransmitters or neuromodulators seem to be involved, and may have opposing actions under different conditions (as with CRF, above). I should like to take an analogy from metabolic regulation. Over recent years the role of insulin in the reciprocal control of glycogen synthesis and breakdown has become more and more complex with the discovery of a variety of phosphatases and inhibitor proteins. There has been an apparent paradox that the initial step in insulin action (binding to the receptor) causes protein kinase activity, and yet most (but not all) cellular effects of insulin involve protein dephosphorylation. Recently, to my mind, the whole tangle has been unraveled at a stroke by the demonstration, by Cohen and colleagues, that an insulin-stimulated protein kinase phosphorylates, and thus activates, the type-1 protein phosphatase that controls glycogen metabolism (4).

The points which follow are these: first, is central control really so complex, or are we being misled by our experimental techniques? (After all, it is not perhaps surprising that many substances affect the brain when administered, but this does not mean that they are involved in physiological changes.) Second, is there any simplification on the horizon which will suddenly enable us to see the wood for the trees? Will we find, for instance, that one particular pathway is of major significance and all the others simply "epiphenomena"?

A Teleological Viewpoint

The concept of central control of metabolic pathways seems to me to presuppose a coordinated response to some change in the environment. It is often useful, in unraveling complex physiological problems, to turn to teleology and ask: what is the body "trying to achieve"? Looked at in this way, I wonder whether it is justified to expect the central regulation of metabolic rate to be common to the diverse situations which Doctor Rothwell discusses.

In the case of obesity, there is a concept of the "thrifty genotype," which suggests that the tendency to accumulate spare calories was, in evolutionary terms, a useful trait. To this extent, processes such as diet-induced thermogenesis are wasteful of precious energy resources. I find it difficult to believe that we, or other mammals, should have evolved mechanisms specifically to dispose of excess calories. Overeating is not usually a problem for wild animals. Might we be deceiving ourselves: is diet-induced thermogenesis simply an "effect of," rather than a true "response to," overeating?

In the case of trauma, it is possible to see many teleological arguments for the hypermetabolic response. None of these, except perhaps fever, is very convincing: in particular, arguments about the body "cannibalizing" its own healthy tissues to provide essential amino acids or glucose for wound repair, resistance to infection, etc. seem to be overthrown by the simple fact that the response is not readily ablated by the provision of these nutrients from outside. In fact, I have argued previously (5) that the flow-phase "response" to trauma and sepsis may not be a response in the true sense; rather, we are now studying conditions which would have been unsurvivable before the advent of modern medicine. In this case, we may again be looking more at "the effects of" rather than "the response to" injury, sepsis etc., and perhaps it is not reasonable to expect to see a centrally coordinated, "purposeful" response.

My point for discussion is this: is there any evidence from the studies of central pathways that we are indeed looking at purposeful, coordinated responses, and to what extent are there common threads between the different states which have been studied?

REFERENCES

1. Wilmore DW, Long JM, Mason AD, Skreen RW, Pruitt BA. Catecholamines: mediator of the hypermetabolic response to thermal injury. *Annu Surg* 1974;180:653–669.
2. York DA. The role of hormone status in the development of excess adiposity in animal models of obesity. In: Cryer A, Van RLR, eds. *New perspectives in adipose tissue*. London: Butterworths, 1985;407–445.
3. Beloff-Chain A, Morton J, Dunmore S, Taylor GW, Morris HR. Evidence that the insulin secretagogue, β-cell-tropin, is $ACTH_{22-39}$. *Nature* 1983;301:255–258.
4. Dent P, Lavoinne A, Nakielny S, Caudwell FB, Watt P, Cohen P. The molecular mechanism by which insulin stimulates glycogen synthesis in mammalian skeletal muscle. *Nature* 1990;348:302–308.
5. Frayn KN. Neuroendocrine control of metabolism acutely after injury: implications for nutritional care. *Nutrition* 1987;3:201–202.

Energy Metabolism: Tissue Determinants and Cellular Corollaries, edited by J. M. Kinney and H. N. Tucker. Raven Press, Ltd., New York © 1992.

Sympathetic Nervous System and Malnutrition

Ian A. Macdonald

Department of Physiology and Pharmacology, Queen's Medical Centre, Nottingham, NG7 2UH, United Kingdom

The sympathetic nervous system (SNS) is one of the principal efferent pathways involved in the maintenance of blood pressure (BP) and regulation of body temperature. The predominant post-ganglionic neurotransmitter is noradrenaline (NA), although in some instances acetylcholine is released into the neuroeffector junction. It is now apparent that in many tissues there is co-release of neuropeptides with the NA (or acetylcholine) and these may modulate the effects of the primary transmitter. In humans, the SNS is involved in regulating both overall cardiac output and its distribution to most organs and tissues—effects which contribute to both BP homeostasis and thermoregulation. The proposition that the SNS is also a primary regulator of thermogenesis in humans is somewhat contentious, but there is no doubt that exogenous catecholamines produce a thermogenic response (1,2) and that β-adrenoceptor antagonists reduce thermogenic responses to some metabolic stimuli.

One of the major difficulties in assessing the role of the SNS in humans concerns the assessment of SNS activity and any related functional alterations. The SNS is a discrete regulatory system, spread diffusely throughout the body. Thus, a single index of SNS activity may be very misleading when considering specific functional events. In addition, alterations in adrenoceptor sensitivity, in the balance between α and β-adrenoceptors (which usually have opposing effects), or in other regulatory systems with opposite effects, can alter the relationship between SNS activity and physiological processes. Thus, when investigating nutritional influences on the SNS, it is essential to also make functional assessments to determine the overall importance of any changes observed.

For the purposes of this review, the term malnutrition will be limited to deviations from normal of either body weight, or energy intake. Thus the opposite clinical conditions of patients who are obese or severely underweight, and the experimental or therapeutic situations of reduced or increased energy intakes will be considered. This review will assess the extent to which these types of malnutrition are associated with alterations in the SNS, and whether such altered SNS activity in malnutrition gives rise to functional changes. The main emphasis will be on studies involving patients and healthy volunteers, but some animal work will also be considered.

247

EXPERIMENTAL STUDIES OF THE SNS AND MALNUTRITION

This section will deal with the various techniques available for assessing SNS activity and the physiological effects of any changes in the SNS during alterations in nutritional status.

Measuring SNS Activity

Interest in the effects of nutritional factors on the SNS has grown substantially since the demonstration by Young and Landsberg (3,4) that fasting reduces, while dietary supplementation with sucrose increases, cardiac NA turnover. Measurements of tissue NA turnover provide an index of the level of SNS activity in specific tissues. Although useful, this technique is restricted to experimental animals and requires other measurements to be made to indicate the functional importance of any observed changes.

Assessing SNS activity in humans involves either measurement of nerve firing rates (using microneurography), or of indices of NA release into plasma from the sympathetic nerve endings. Microneurography has been used extensively to assess SNS firing rates by Wallin and colleagues (5). This technique has not yet been used in nutritional studies. but increases in sympathetic nerve firing rates have been observed during hypoglycemia (6) and after glucose ingestion (7). However, the main limitations of this technique are that it can only be used on superficial nerves (supplying skin or skeletal muscle vasculature) and that changes in nerve firing rate are not always consistent with the observed changes in blood flow because of the influence of other factors.

For many years, plasma NA concentration has been used as an index of SNS activity. This is based on the majority of circulating NA arising from sympathetic nerves, and there is surprisingly good agreement between forearm venous plasma NA and (leg) peroneal nerve SNS firing rates (8). However, the latter simply illustrates that venous plasma NA provides an index of SNS activity in resting, healthy subjects. There are problems in interpreting venous plasma NA values in other conditions, as the concentration is affected by the forearm blood flow, the proportion of arterial NA taken up by the forearm tissue, and the amount of NA spilling over from forearm sympathetic nerve endings. More specific techniques for assessing the spillover of NA into plasma utilize the infusion of tracer amounts of radiolabeled NA and measuring its dilution by endogenous NA, and clearance rate from plasma (9). This approach is preferable to the infusion of unlabeled NA, as this has to be administered in amounts which may have physiological effects. The alternative to measuring NA in plasma is to determine its rate of excretion in urine. There is a reasonable relationship between arterial NA concentration and the rate of urinary NA excretion in animal studies (10), but it is not known to what extent this applies in humans. Furthermore, alterations in the metabolism of catecholamines may change the proportions of free NA, conjugated NA and the methylated or deaminated metabolites which are excreted, thus weakening any relationship between SNS activity and urinary NA excretion.

Effects of Alterations in Nutritional Status

Cardiovascular

O'Dea et al. (11) measured plasma NA turnover, heart rate, and blood pressure changes in response to 10 days of under or overfeeding in healthy subjects. Overall, there were significant increases in NA spillover rate (an index of SNS activity) and NA clearance with increasing energy intake. However, the effect of overfeeding to increase NA spillover was much greater than the reduction in spillover seen with underfeeding, (and even this was due mainly to three of the subjects having a marked response to overfeeding whereas the other three showed little change). In association with the effect on NA spillover, there was a significant rise in systolic blood pressure (SBP) with increasing energy intake. This indicates a link between energy intake, SNS activity and blood pressure consistent with the observation that fasting reduces both SBP and cardiac NA turnover in spontaneously hypertensive rats (12,13).

Schwartz et al. (14) showed that 3 months of restricted feeding (to 6 MJ/day) in moderately obese men was accompanied by a small fall in plasma NA appearance rate, with no change in plasma NA concentration. Resting heart rate fell by 5 beats/min, but there was no change in BP. A preliminary report from Del Rio et al. (15) described a reduction in urinary excretion of NA, with enhanced excretion of adrenaline, in obese men after 14 days of very low energy intake (2 MJ per day) with maintained sodium intake. There have been other studies which have failed to show an effect of underfeeding on NA kinetics or excretion rate, but these have usually failed to maintain sodium intake.

A major problem of studying the effects of starvation and underfeeding is the possible confounding effect of a reduction in body sodium content causing volume depletion leading to activation of the SNS to maintain BP. However, starvation with sodium supplementation for 48 hours in healthy men was accompanied by minor changes in supine BP. When the subjects stood erect for 10 min there was a fall in SBP of 15 mmHg (compared to no change in the non-starved state), despite a greater increase in heart rate, indicating impaired reflex control of BP during starvation (16). Jung et al. (17) showed that underfeeding of obese patients (without sodium depletion) was accompanied by reductions in supine SBP and diastolic blood pressure (DBP), within 3 days in association with substantial reductions in venous plasma NA concentrations and urinary excretion of the catecholamine metabolite, hydroxymethylmandelic acid. Thus, it would appear that starvation and underfeeding have effects on arterial BP and its regulation which are consistent with a fall in SNS activity or effectiveness.

There have been reports that overfeeding carbohydrate in normal weight subjects is accompanied by an enhanced plasma NA response to standing, with no alteration in the BP or heart rate changes (18). This would be consistent with overfeeding having increased SNS activity, but this has little functional importance as there was no effect on the cardiovascular responses.

Thermoregulation and Thermogenesis

The demonstration that fasting reduced SNS activity in rats (3) prompted us to speculate whether such an effect in humans might have functional consequences by influencing thermoregulation. In humans, body core temperature is maintained during cold exposure by a combination of reduced heat loss (due to peripheral vasoconstriction) and increased heat production. The peripheral vasoconstrictor responses are mediated primarily through activation of SNS vasoconstrictor fibers to skin blood vessels. Diabetic patients with autonomic neuropathy have impaired vasoconstrictor responses to cooling and show a fall in core temperature in comparison to control patients without neuropathy (19). Thus, if starvation reduced SNS mediated vasoconstrictor response to cooling, one would expect a fall in core temperature to occur. The heat production responses to cold exposure are due to a combination of shivering and non-shivering thermogenesis. The relative contributions of these mechanisms have not been determined, and there is some debate as to the site of such non-shivering thermogenesis in adult humans. There is insufficient brown adipose tissue to make any quantitatively significant contribution to total heat production in normal adults (20) and it seems likely that the splanchnic bed (21) and skeletal muscle make important contributions. Jessen et al. (22) demonstrated an increase in heat production during cold exposure in patients receiving muscle relaxant therapy (curare), thus indicating that non-shivering thermogenesis occurs in adult humans. However, it has not yet been established whether such thermogenesis is regulated by hormonal factors or by the SNS. Thus, one would predict that any sympathetically mediated stimulation of heat production during cold exposure would be affected by a reduction in SNS activity during starvation.

We tested these possibilities by determining the peripheral blood flow, heat production, and body core temperature responses to cooling in healthy young men in the control state and after 48 hours starvation (23). Cooling was imposed in a graded fashion using a water perfused suit which fitted closely to the skin surface. In the control state progressive cooling was associated with marked reductions in hand blood flow and forearm blood flow, an increase in heat production, and no changes in core temperature. By contrast, after 48 hours starvation core temperature fell progressively during cooling. Although there were reductions in peripheral blood flow during cooling, the absolute level of flow was higher than in the control state. Heat production only increased after core temperature had fallen, and the observed rise was much less than would have been predicted from the fall in core temperature (Fig. 1). Thus, this study provided evidence of impaired thermoregulation during acute starvation. We subsequently confirmed that starvation impaired thermoregulation in healthy young women, in particular reducing the heat production response,

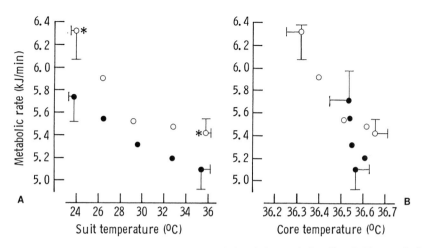

FIG. 1. Effect of 48 hours starvation on thermoregulation during graded cooling. **A.**: The metabolic rate response is shown in relation to the external cold stimulus (suit temperature). **B.**: The response is shown in relation to the internal stimulus (core temperature). Values are mean ± SEM. ●, control; ○, 48 hours starvation. (From Macdonald et al., ref. 23, with permission of the Biochemical Society and Portland Press.)

but 7 days of underfeeding (an intake of 3.2 MJ per day) did not affect the responses to cold exposure (24).

Thus, acute starvation impairs the thermogenic responses to cold exposure, but the studies described above provide no evidence as to whether this is due to the absence of the appropriate efferent stimuli or to the inability to respond at all. However, subsequent investigations into the effect of acute starvation on the control of thermogenesis indicates that any alteration affects the stimulus rather than the ability to respond. When adrenaline is infused into healthy young subjects who have starved for 48 hours (25) or underfed for 7 days (26) the thermogenic response is not reduced compared to the control state (Fig. 2). In fact after 48 hours starvation the thermogenic and heart rate responses to adrenaline are significantly enhanced compared to the control state.

In contrast to the normal or enhanced thermogenic response to adrenaline in acute starvation or underfeeding, the thermogenic responses to the infusion of insulin and glucose are reduced by both types of experimental undernutrition. The technique of infusing insulin at a constant rate, and glucose as required to maintain a desired blood glucose concentration was first described by DeFronzo et al. (27) and is known as the "glucose clamp." If insulin is infused at a rate which produces plasma insulin levels in excess of 120 mU/l (approximately 10–20 times overnight fasting values) then hepatic glucose production is suppressed, and the rate of glucose infusion equals the rate at which glucose disappears from the circulation (glucose uptake). The glucose taken up by the tissues is normally either used as a metabolic fuel, producing CO_2 and water, or is stored. Under normal circumstances the glucose would be stored as glycogen, only while refeeding severely depleted patients is it likely that net li-

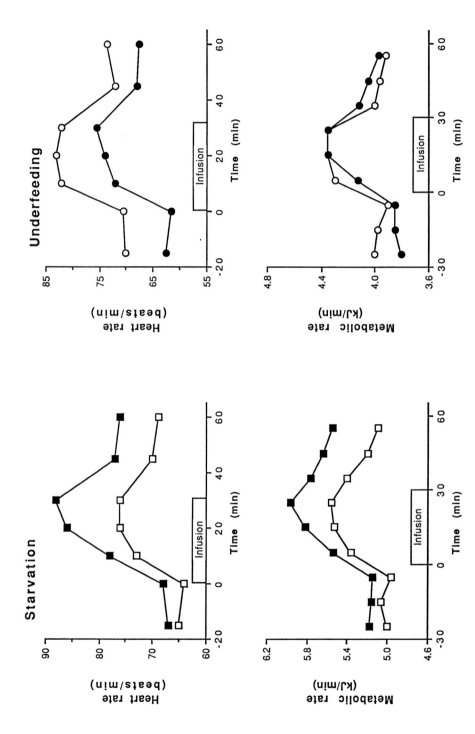

pogenesis would occur. The formation of glycogen from glucose has a predictable energy cost which is equivalent to approximately 5.5% of the energy stored as glycogen (28). However it has been observed that the net increase in thermogenesis observed during a glucose clamp in healthy, normally-nourished subjects is equivalent to approximately 10% of the glucose energy being stored as glycogen (29). This additional component of thermogenesis has been described as facultative, and can be abolished by infusing the β-adrenoceptor antagonist, propranolol, during the glucose clamp (30). This effect of propranolol has led to the suggestion that the facultative component of the thermogenic response to insulin-glucose infusion is mediated by the SNS.

When subjects starve for 48 hours, there is no net thermogenic response to a glucose clamp (31), while underfeeding for 7 days reduces the net thermogenic response significantly below the control values, to a level not significantly different from the theoretical energy cost of glycogen synthesis (32). Thus, the absence of facultative thermogenesis during the glucose clamps in experimental underfeeding would be consistent with a reduction in SNS activity. It is interesting to note that there was no effect on plasma NA concentration of either of these experimental conditions. Thus, the functional changes consistent with altered SNS activity were not reflected in lower plasma NA levels.

The commonest situation in which underfeeding is imposed, either clinically or experimentally, is of course when dealing with obese subjects. The specific problems of obesity and thermogenesis are addressed by Professor Astrup in his chapter. However, some aspects of the link between nutritional status and the SNS in obesity are worthy of mention here. Jung et al. (33) provided evidence of reduced thermogenic responses to NA (compared to non-obese controls) in weight stable obese patients and in a group who had previously been obese. In this paper they comment that the response to NA in two obese women was similar on a weight maintenance diet and after 3 weeks of a low energy intake (25% of maintenance). By contrast Finer et al. (34) reported that the thermogenic response to NA was reduced markedly in seven grossly obese patients after at least 3 months on a very low energy diet (approximately 12% of maintenance), with a trend for the greatest reduction in response to NA occurring in those with the most weight loss. Thus, there is some evidence for a reduction in NA sensitivity with underfeeding in obese patients, and Jung et al. (17) had shown previously that such underfeeding reduced SNS activity, as judged by the biochemical markers measured. The apparent contradictions between the studies of Finer et al. (34) and Jung et al. (17,33) on the normality or otherwise of NA-induced thermogenesis in weight stable obese subjects is probably a reflection of the marked heterogeneity in the responsiveness to NA in untreated obese patients

←——

FIG. 2. Influence of starvation (**left panel**) or underfeeding (**right panel**) on the metabolic rate and heart rate responses to the infusion of adrenaline (25 ng/kg/min) for 30 min. Values are means. ■, starvation; ●, underfeeding; □ and ○, controls. (Adapted from Mansell et al., ref. 25 and Mansell and Macdonald, ref. 26, with permission of the American Physiological Society.)

(35). In the latter study, a group of 40 patients were studied, with nine of them having subnormal responses to NA. Further evidence of heterogeneity between groups of obese patients is provided from the studies of Katzeff and colleagues. They found no differences in NA-induced thermogenesis between lean and obese Caucasian subjects (36) or Pima Indians (37). However, underfeeding the obese Caucasian subjects appeared to increase their response to NA while in the obese Pima Indians the response was slightly reduced. The interpretation of the results in the obese Caucasians is somewhat difficult as the enhanced response is on the basis of percentage stimulation of metabolic rate; underfeeding having reduced the fasting value. Thus, the absolute increases of metabolic rate were unaltered by underfeeding those subjects.

Thus, underfeeding is accompanied by biochemical changes (plasma NA concentration and turnover, and urinary excretion of catecholamine metabolites) consistent with reduced SNS activity. In some cases there is evidence of functional impairments consistent with such reduced SNS activity. The failure of most studies to demonstrate reduced thermogenic responses to either NA or adrenaline in humans during underfeeding does not contradict these other observations. In other circumstances, when the controlling stimulus is decreased in magnitude there is normally maintenance, or even enhancement (upregulation) of tissue responsiveness. Such a change in responsiveness was demonstrated in a study of the effect of 15 days underfeeding (at 2.5 MJ/day) in 8 obese women. β-adrenoceptor sensitivity was assessed by determining the dose of isoprenaline (a synthetic catecholamine, β-agonist) needed to increase heart rate by 25 beats/min. In the underfed state the required dose was significantly lower than in the normally fed state, indicating enhanced β-adrenoceptor sensitivity after such underfeeding (38). Similar observations of enhanced β-adrenoceptor sensitivity have been made during acute starvation in non-obese subjects (39,40) and in chronically undernourished Indian laborers (41).

It is highly unlikely that underfeeding would be accompanied by decreases in both SNS activity and responsiveness to catecholamines. The latter needs to be preserved to enable an adequate response to be produced in an emergency situation. However, if underfeeding is accompanied by reduced NA responsiveness in some obese patients, this would be evidence of an adaptive reduction in thermogenesis which may be initiated to preserve the obese state. This possibility will be considered further by Professor Astrup (this volume).

The early animal (4) and human studies (11) showed enhanced SNS activity (tissue or plasma NA turnover) during overfeeding. However, subsequent studies of overfeeding (extra 5 MJ of mixed nutrients daily) non-obese subjects for 20 days failed to show any change in plasma NA concentration or urinary excretion of the catecholamines or a metabolite (VMA). There was also no effect on the thermogenic response to infused NA (42). By contrast, Katzeff et al. (37) showed that overfeeding a mixed diet for 18 days (extra 4.2 MJ per day) to lean and obese subjects increased plasma NA concentration without affecting the clearance of NA from the plasma, or the thermogenic response to infused NA. A similar study in Pima indians showed a slight increase in plasma NA during overfeeding of the obese (but not lean) subjects and also a small reduction in the thermogenic response to infused NA (36). Such a reciprocity of SNS activity and responsiveness is entirely consistent with the operation of a normal homeostatic mechanism.

CLINICAL ASPECTS OF ALTERED SNS ACTIVITY IN MALNUTRITION

A common problem in interpreting functional changes in disease states is whether any observed changes have contributed to the disease or are simply a result of it. This is certainly true so far as changes in SNS activity, and in functions such as thermogenesis, in relation to malnutrition. The clinical states of obesity and of chronic weight loss represent the extremes of "energy malnutrition." A low SNS activity, low resting metabolic rate, and reduced thermogenic responsiveness could contribute to the development of obesity in humans in a similar way as has been observed in several experimental models of obesity (43,44). Similarly, enhanced SNS activity, resting metabolic rate, and thermogenic responsiveness would lead to negative energy balance which if not compensated by increased energy intake would result in weight loss. This section will consider the extent to which such alterations in SNS activity may contribute to the development of such clinical problems, and will also outline possible reversible changes in the SNS which arise as a result of obesity or chronic weight loss.

Obesity

As mentioned above, reduced SNS activity and impaired thermogenesis are likely contributors to the development of obesity in some experimental models. The possibility that this may contribute to human obesity would appear to be supported by observations from Schwartz et al. (45). They measured the increase in thermogenesis, plasma NA, and NA appearance rate (using radiolabeled NA) in a group of 20 subjects receiving a 3.35 MJ mixed nutrient meal. They demonstrated an impressive positive correlation between the thermogenic response to the meal and the increase in the rate of NA appearance. This demonstrates a functional link between SNS activation and the stimulation of thermogenesis. Thus, individuals with a low level of SNS activation would have reduced food-induced thermogenesis and may be predisposed to the development of obesity. The necessary longitudinal studies of a large number of initially non-obese subjects with a range of SNS activity have not been performed to test this hypothesis, although non-obese Pima Indians are being studied intensively at the moment.

There is one caveat which needs to be placed on the interpretation of these results. Schwartz et al. studied subjects whose body weight ranged from 101% to 181% of ideal body weight. No information is presented as to whether there is any relation between percent overweight and either the thermogenic response or the increase in the rate of NA appearance. This is of importance because Peterson et al. (46) showed significant (although weak) correlations between body fat content and a variety of indices of SNS and parasympathetic nervous system activity. There were significantly lower plasma NA and adrenaline levels and evidence of reduced parasympathetic control of heart rate and pupil diameter with increasing fatness. The weakness of the correlations may reflect the heterogeneity of human obesity, as indicated by the marked variability in thermogenic responsiveness to NA observed by Connacher et al. (35). Thus, it is possible that the obese subjects studied by Schwartz et al. (45) had the smaller responses to the meal. A much more convincing demonstration would be provided by a study of a large group of normal weight subjects, and a separate group of obese subjects.

Further evidence of autonomic dysfunction in obesity is provided in a study by Rossi et al. (47) of 23 obese subjects and 78 non-obese controls. All subjects were evaluated with the standard cardiovascular tests of autonomic function used to screen for autonomic neuropathy. In this group of obese patients there was no evidence of SNS dysfunction, but there did appear to be impaired parasympathetic control of the heart. Thus, it would appear that obesity is associated with mild degrees of autonomic dysfunction, but that this affects the parasympathetic nervous system more than the SNS. Further studies are needed to establish whether such impairments can be reversed by weight loss. In addition, it would be useful to know if such impairments become progressively worse as obesity continues, or whether they are relatively unaffected by disease duration.

A recent study of cardiac β-adrenoceptor sensitivity and platelet α_2-adrenoceptor density in weight stable obese and non-obese women revealed interesting differences between the groups (38). In the resting state, there was no difference in β-adrenoceptor sensitivity. However, the obese women had lower resting plasma NA levels and a reduced platelet α_2-adrenoceptor density compared to the non-obese. Furthermore, 9 min of standardized exercise produced a larger rise in plasma NA in the non-obese than the obese. In the non-obese women, exercise (and the rise in plasma NA) was accompanied by a fall in platelet α_2-adrenoceptor density whereas in the obese there was no change. Thus, the different responses of plasma NA and α_2-adrenoceptor densities in the obese and non-obese are consistent with a lower stimulation of SNS activity in the obese patients.

It has recently been proposed that the obese state may be associated with enhanced SNS activity, at least in some patients, which may contribute to the development of hypertension in obesity. Patients with most of the excess adipose tissue in their abdominal region (upper body obesity) are more likely to develop hypertension than those with lower body obesity (excess gluteal and thigh adipose tissue). Landsberg (48) has argued that this development of hypertension is due to enhanced SNS activity, which itself is a result of insulin resistance and hyperinsulinemia. There is a variety of experimental evidence that increased plasma insulin concentration can stimulate SNS activity (sympathetic nerve firing rate, plasma NA levels). In upper body obesity, the adipocytes (and muscle tissue) become insulin resistant (which results in hyperinsulinemia) as part of a homeostatic response to limit the amount of fat deposited in the adipose tissue. Landsberg argues that the resultant hyperinsulinemia increases SNS activity, via effects within hypothalamus, which results in increased thermogenesis (reducing the degree of positive energy balance) and in hypertension (due to α-adrenoceptor mediated vasoconstriction). There is substantial evidence supporting this suggestion, but as yet no direct demonstration of its importance. Studies are needed comparing SNS activity in the two types of obesity, with direct assessment of the SNS, measurements of thermogenic responsiveness and determination of the cardiovascular and metabolic affects of adrenoceptor blockade.

Chronic Weight Loss

One of the most comprehensive accounts of the physiological and clinical effects of prolonged undernutrition has been provided in a book edited by Winick (49). The book, *Hunger Disease* describes the studies undertaken by the Jewish physicians in the Warsaw ghetto in 1940. Of relevance to the present topic, there are extensive chapters on the metabolic changes and the circulatory alterations in severe, prolonged undernutrition. In assessing the metabolic changes, the physicians described a markedly reduced basal metabolic rate. With glucose ingestion there was marked glucose intolerance, but an enhanced thermogenic response. They could not measure insulin levels, but one would expect them to be elevated with such glucose intolerance. If so, the enhanced glucose-induced thermogenesis could have been due to an insulin-mediated stimulation of the SNS. However, this seems unlikely as the clinical observations made by the physicians indicate markedly reduced SNS activity. It is particularly interesting that the subjects had no piloerection or "goose pimples" after cooling the skin. It is particularly intriguing that the subjects had no respiratory, cardiovascular, or blood glucose response to the subcutaneous injection of adrenaline. This would indicate markedly diminished adrenoceptor sensitivity (especially β-adrenoceptors) in chronic undernutrition, which was not observed in some more recent studies.

In a subsequent experimental investigation of the effects of semi-starvation, Keys et al. (50) underfed subjects for approximately 6 months and found impairments in the control of body temperature during cold exposure, and of blood pressure during orthostasis. As described at the start of the present review, these two processes are fundamental components of homeostasis and are regulated in part by the SNS. Thus, the observations in the Warsaw ghetto and by Keys and colleagues are consistent with reduced SNS activity or diminished effectiveness of the SNS in physiological regulation after prolonged underfeeding.

Thermoregulation in the human neonate and infant is critically dependent upon the ability to activate brown adipose tissue thermogenesis during exposure to cold. Brooke et al. (51) reported impaired thermoregulation in undernourished babies. Exposing the babies to an environment temperature of 25°C for approximately 45 min led to a fall in core temperature of 1.1°C and no thermogenic response. Some of the undernourished babies studied by Brooke et al. died, and at autopsy were found to have little discernible brown adipose tissue. However, in most of the undernourished babies, a refeeding program was successful and recovery achieved.

When such babies were exposed to the same cold stimulus after recovery, they showed a smaller fall in core temperature (−0.85°C) and marked thermogenic response (+20%). It is well established that brown adipose tissue is regulated by the SNS. However, as the undernourished babies are likely to have had a markedly reduced brown adipose tissue mass, one cannot tell whether the lack of a thermogenic response to cold exposure was due to failure to activate the SNS or the inability of the tissue to respond.

Impaired thermoregulation with chronic weight loss has also been observed in middle-aged (52) and elderly adult humans (53). In the latter study, normal weight and severely underweight women recovering from femoral fracture were exposed to cooling of the trunk and legs achieved with a suit perfused with water at 23°C. The underweight women had no thermogenic response to cooling, despite showing a fall in core temperature. By contrast the normal weight women maintained core temperature and increased their metabolic rate by 10%. It is interesting to note that forearm venous NA concentration increased during cooling in the normal weight women but did not change in the underweight women (Fig. 3). Thus, it would appear that such a degree of underweight was accompanied by impaired thermoregulation, possibly contributed to by an inadequate SNS response to cooling. It seems likely that this impaired thermoregulation is of clinical significance, as Bastow et al. (54) had previously observed that in the winter time on arrival at the hospital emergency department immediately after incurring their fracture, a substantial proportion of the underweight patients were hypothermic, whereas none of the normal weight women were.

One of the most obvious clinical conditions of chronic weight loss and undernutrition is anorexia nervosa. However, one needs to be rather cautious in assessing physiological reflex function in such patients, as this disorder may be associated with extensive hypothalamic dysfunction (which may be pathological rather than secondary to weight loss). Nevertheless, patients with anorexia nervosa do have impaired thermoregulation, showing impaired reflex vasoconstrictor responses to cold exposure (55). Such responses are almost entirely mediated by the SNS, and as the response was greater in control subjects, it seems highly likely that SNS activation is impaired in anorexia. Furthermore, patients with anorexia nervosa are reported to have lower resting plasma NA concentrations than controls (56).

Mansell et al. (52) confirmed in a younger group of patients that chronic weight loss (to 78% of ideal body weight) was accompanied by impaired thermoregulation— a fall in core temperature during cooling with no thermogenic response. The absence of a thermogenic response was not due to a generalized inability to increase thermogenesis, as on a separate occasion they demonstrated the presence of a thermogenic response to infused adrenaline (at the lower end of the normal range) in these underweight patients (52). The energy intake of these patients was increased to a sufficient extent that their weight increased to 93% of ideal. In this state they had normal thermoregulatory responses to cooling (Fig. 4) (52).

Thus, in human babies and adults, undernutrition with weight loss is accompanied by impaired thermoregulation. Refeeding and weight gain reverses their impairment.

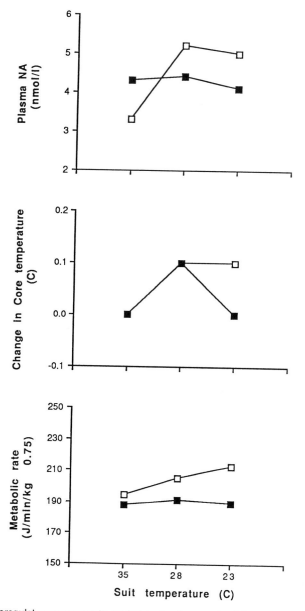

FIG. 3. Thermoregulatory responses to graded cooling in normal weight and underweight elderly women with fractured femurs. Mean values of metabolic rate per unit metabolic body size (□, normal; ■, underweight), plasma noradrenaline (□, normal; ■, underweight), and change in core temperature (□, normal; ■, underweight) are shown in relation to the external stimulus (suit temperature). Adapted from Fellows et al., ref. 53.)

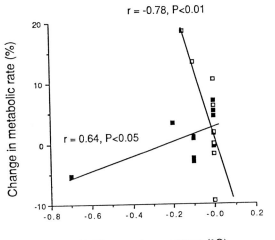

Fall in core temperature (°C)

FIG. 4. Reversible impairment of thermoregulatory response to cooling in underweight adults. Data are changes in core temperature and metabolic rate (thermogenesis) during the cooling procedure in the underweight state (■) and after weight gain (□). The two correlation coefficients are significantly different from each other. From Mansell et al. ref. 52, with permission of Oxford University Press.

It seems probable, although not proven, that reduced SNS activity contributes to the impaired thermoregulation.

We have recently observed the absence of facultative thermogenesis during insulin-glucose infusion (a glucose clamp) in a similar group of severely underweight patients (57). As pointed out earlier it seems likely that such insulin-glucose induced facultative thermogenesis is mediated by the SNS, so it seems most probable that chronic weight loss does affect the SNS. We managed to refeed three of these patients sufficiently to return their weight to normal, at which time the patients then displayed normal thermogenic responses to the glucose clamp (58).

In the section on "Experimental Studies" it was shown that the thermogenic responses to adrenaline were unaffected by 7 days underfeeding (26) and actually enhanced by 48 hours starvation (25). Furthermore, patients with chronic weight loss (but of normal height) did not have defective responses to infused adrenaline (52). By contrast, studies on chronically undernourished Indian laborers have revealed reduced thermogenic responses to infused NA, compared to normal weight controls (59). However, the undernutrition in these subjects is likely to have existed during critical periods of growth, as they were also significantly shorter than the control subjects. Furthermore, a recent preliminary report by the same group on similar subjects showed that 12 weeks of dietary supplementation did not affect the response to NA infusion (60). The latter observation implies a severe and possibly irreversible defect in NA sensitivity with long-term chronic undernutrition.

The studies discussed so far have indicated that individuals with chronic weight loss, who are severely undernourished have decreased SNS activity or impaired SNS mediated reflexes. None of these studies addressed the question of a possible role of the SNS in the development of negative energy balance. On theoretical grounds, prolonged increased SNS activity with stimulation of thermogenesis, would produce negative energy balance unless opposed by increased energy intake. Such a possibility is raised by the studies of Hofford et al. (61) in patients with chronic respiratory disease. These patients were underweight compared to matched controls, despite similar energy intakes, and had increased plasma NA levels. Thus, the negative energy balance in these patients seems likely to be due to an elevated energy expenditure which may have been due, in part, to increased SNS activity.

We have recently completed a similar study in patients with cystic fibrosis and observed resting metabolic rate approximately 40% higher in the patients than in their matched controls (Elborn et al. *unpublished data*); although we do not yet have the plasma NA results.

Thus, it seems likely that in some circumstances, enhanced SNS activity may lead to negative energy balance and weight loss, whereas the normal situation is that severe undernutrition and weight loss reduces SNS activity. This is of importance for the provision of nutritional support to patients in the post-operative or post-traumatic state. From the available evidence it seems that carbohydrate intake (enterally or parenterally) is a potent stimulus of the SNS. Nordenstrom et al. (62) compared the effects of glucose alone, or a mixture (50/50) of glucose and lipid as the sources of non-protein energy provided to post-operative patients receiving total parenteral nutrition. The patients receiving glucose alone (plus amino acids) had markedly increased urinary excretion of NA and a modest elevation in resting MR compared to the group receiving glucose and lipid. Thus, it does appear that a high carbohydrate intake stimulates the SNS and increases thermogenesis in post-operative, traumatized patients. Such effects may produce undesirable physiological demands on the cardiorespiratory system.

SUMMARY

From the evidence considered in this review, there are substantial associations between altered nutritional status and SNS activity. In some situations there are physiological changes consistent with alterations in the SNS, but these are not always accompanied by changes in the biochemical markers of the SNS. This apparent inconsistency probably reflects the fact that plasma NA concentrations are a rather insensitive index of the SNS. In addition, the SNS is a discrete regulatory system via which functions can be stimulated separately or collectively. Thus, alterations in the SNS control of thermogenesis, or of the cardiovascular system, may occur without a generalized change in SNS activity and so produce little effect on plasma NA concentration. Of greater importance is the possibility that sensitivity to catecholamines may be altered in malnutrition and so the most useful information is obtained by studying the physiological processes regulated by the SNS, rather than any of the biochemical markers in isolation.

The likelihood that altered nutritional state affects the SNS has important clinical implications, both in the acute care of patients and in more longer term situations.

REFERENCES

1. Cori CF, Buchwald KW. Effect of continuous injection of epinephrine on the carbohydrate metabolism, basal metabolism and vascular system of normal man. *Am J Physiol* 1930;95:71–78.
2. Steinberg D, Nestel PJ, Buskirk ER, Thompson RH. Calorigenic effect of norepinephrine correlated with plasma free fatty acid turnover and oxidation. *J Clin Invest* 1964;43:167–176.
3. Young JB, Landsberg L. Suppression of sympathetic nervous system during fasting. *Science* 1977;196:1473–1475.
4. Young JB, Landsberg L. Stimulation of the sympathetic nervous system during sucrose feeding. *Nature* 1977;269:615–617.
5. Wallin BG, Fagius J. The sympathetic nervous system in man—aspects derived from microelectrode recordings. *T.I.N.S.* 1986;9:63–67.
6. Fagius J, Niklasson F, Berne C. Sympathetic outflow in human muscle nerves increases during hypoglycemia. *Diabetes* 1986;35:1124–1129.
7. Berne C, Fagius J, Niklasson F. Sympathetic response to oral carbohydrate administration. Evidence from microelectrode recordings. *J Clin Invest* 1989;84:1403–1409.
8. Wallin BG, Sundlof G, Eriksson B-M, Dominiak P, Grobecker H, Lindblad LE. Plasma noradrenaline correlates to sympathetic muscle nerve activity in normotensive men. *Acta Physiol Scand* 1981;111:69–73.
9. Esler M. Assessment of sympathetic nervous function in humans from noradrenaline plasma kinetics. *Clin Sci* 1982;62:247–254.
10. Kopp U, Bradley T, Hjemdahl P. Renal venous outflow and urinary excretion of norepinephrine, epinephrine and dopamine during graded renal nerve stimulation. *Am J Physiol* 1983;244:E52–E60.
11. O'Dea K, Esler M, Leonard P, Stockigt JR, Nestel P. Noradrenaline turnover during under- and over-eating in normal weight subjects. *Metabolism* 1982;31:896–899.
12. Young JB, Mullen D, Landsberg L. Calorie restriction lowers blood pressure in the spontaneously hypertensive rat. *Metabolism* 1978;27:1771–1774.
13. Einhorn D, Young JB, Landsberg L. Hypotensive effect of fasting; possible involvement of the sympathetic nervous system and endogenous opiates. *Science* 1982;217:727–729.
14. Schwartz RS, Jaeger LF, Veith RC, Lakshminarayan S. The effect of diet or exercise on plasma norepinephrine kinetics in moderately obese young men. *Int J Obes* 1990;14:1–11.
15. Del Rio G, Marrama P, Fiorani P, Della Casa L. Very low calorie diet induces opposite effects on sympathetic nervous system and adrenomedullary responses. *Int J Obes* 1989;13(Suppl 2):173–175.
16. Bennett T, Macdonald IA, Sainsbury R. The influence of acute starvation on the cardiovascular responses to lower body subatmospheric pressure or to standing in man. *Clin Sci* 1984;66:141–146.
17. Jung RT, Shetty PS, Barrand M, Callingham BA, James WPT. Role of catecholamines in hypotensive response to dieting. *BMJ* 1979;1:12–13.
18. Welle SL, Campbell RG. Stimulation of thermogenesis by carbohydrate overfeeding. Evidence against sympathetic nervous system mediation. *J Clin Invest* 1983;71:916–925.
19. Scott AR, Macdonald IA, Bennett T, Tattersall RB. Abnormal thermoregulation in diabetics with autonomic neuropathy. *Diabetes* 1988;37:961–968.
20. Astrup A, Bulow J, Madsen J, Christensen NJ. Contribution of BAT and skeletal muscle to thermogenesis induced by ephedrine in man. *Am J Physiol* 1985;248:E507–E515.
21. Bearn AG, Billing B, Sherlock S. The effects of adrenaline and noradrenaline on hepatic blood flow and splanchnic carbohydrate metabolism in man. *J Physiol (Lond)* 1951;115:430–441.
22. Jessen K, Rabol A, Winkles K. Total body and splanchnic thermogenesis in curarized man during a short exposure to cold. *Acta Anaesth Scand* 1980;24:339–344.
23. Macdonald IA, Bennett T, Sainsbury R. The effect of a 48 hour fast on the thermoregulatory responses to graded cooling in man. *Clin Sci* 1984;67:445–452.
24. Mansell PI, Macdonald IA. Effect of 7d underfeeding on thermoregulation in healthy women. *Clin Sci* 1989;77:245–252.

25. Mansell PI, Macdonald IA, Fellows IW. 48 hour starvation enhances the thermogenic response to infused epinephrine. *Am J Physiol* 1990;258:R87–R93.
26. Mansell PI, Macdonald IA. Underfeeding and the physiological responses to epinephrine in lean women. *Am J Physiol* 1989;256:R583–R589.
27. DeFronzo RA, Jordan D, Tobin JD, Andres R. Glucose clamp technique: a method for quantifying insulin secretion and resistance. *Am J Physiol* 1979;237:E214–E223.
28. Flatt JP. The biochemistry of energy expenditure. In: Bray GA, ed. *Recent advances in obesity*, vol II. London: Newman 1978;211–218.
29. Acheson K, Ravussin E, Wahren J, Jéquier E. Thermic effect of glucose in man. Obligatory and facultative thermogenesis. *J Clin Invest* 1984;74:1572–1580.
30. Acheson K, Jéquier E, Wahren J. Influence of beta blockade on glucose induced thermogenesis in man. *J Clin Invest* 1983;72:981–986.
31. Mansell PI, Macdonald IA. Effect of starvation on insulin-induced glucose disposal and thermogenesis in man. *Metabolism* 1990;39:502–510.
32. Gallen IW, Macdonald IA. The effects of underfeeding for 7d on the thermogenic and physiological response to glucose and insulin infusion (hyperinsulinaemic euglycaemic clamp). *Br J Nutr* 1990;64:427–437.
33. Jung RT, Shetty PS, James WPT, Barrand MA, Callingham BA. Reduced thermogenesis in obesity. *Nature* 1979;279:322–323.
34. Finer N, Swan PC, Mitchell FT. Suppression of norepinephrine-induced thermogenesis in human obesity by diet and weight loss. *Int J Obes* 1985;9:121–126.
35. Connacher AA, Jung RT, Mitchell PEG, Ford RP, Leslie P, Illingworth P. Heterogeneity of noradrenergic thermic responses in obese and lean humans. *Int J Obes* 1988;12:267–276.
36. Kush RD, Young JB, Katzeff HL, et al. Effect of diet on energy expenditure and plasma norepinephrine in lean and obese Pima Indians. *Metabolism* 1986;35:1110–1120.
37. Katzeff HL, O'Connell M, Horton ES, Danforth E Jr., Young JB, Landsberg L. Metabolic studies in human obesity during overnutrition and undernutrition: thermogenic and hormonal responses to norepinephrine. *Metabolism* 1986;35:166–175.
38. Berlin I, Berlan M, Crespo-Laumonnier B, et al. Alterations in β-adrenergic sensitivity and platelet α₂-adrenoceptors in obese women: effect of exercise and caloric restriction. *Clin Sci* 1990;78:81–87.
39. Jenson MD, Haymond MW, Gerich JE, Cryer PE, Miles JM. Lipolysis during fasting. Decreased suppression by insulin and increased stimulation by epinephrine. *J Clin Invest* 1987;79:207–213.
40. Wolfe RR, Peters EJ, Klein S, Holland OB, Rosenblatt J, Gary H. Effects of short-term fasting on lipolytic responsiveness in normal and obese human subjects. *Am J Physiol* 1987;252:E189–E196.
41. Jayarajam MP, Shetty PS. Cardiovascular β-adrenoceptor sensitivity of undernourished subjects. *Br J Nutr* 1987;58:5–11.
42. Welle S. Evidence that the sympathetic nervous system does not regulate dietary thermogenesis in humans. *Int J Obes* 1985;9(Suppl 2):115–121.
43. Knehans AW, Romsos DR. Reduced norepinephrine turnover in brown adipose tissue of ob/ob mice. *Am J Physiol* 1982;242:E253–E261.
44. Himms-Hagen J. Thermogenesis in brown adipose tissue as an energy buffer: implications for obesity. *N Engl J Med* 1984;311:1549–1558.
45. Schwartz RS, Jaeger LF, Silberstein S, Veith RC. Sympathetic nervous system activity and the thermic effect of feeding in man. *Int J Obes* 1987;11:141–149.
46. Peterson HR, Rothschild M, Weinberg CR, Fell RD, McLeish KR, Pfeiffer MA. Body fat and the activity of the autonomic nervous system. *N Engl J Med* 1988;318:1077–1083.
47. Rossi M, Marti G, Ricordi L, et al. Cardiac autonomic dysfunction in obese subjects. *Clin Sci* 1989;76:567–572.
48. Landsberg L. The sympathoadrenal system, obesity and hypertension: an overview. *J Neurosci Methods* 1990;34:179–186.
49. Winick M, ed. *Hunger disease. Studies by the jewish physicians in the Warsaw ghetto*. New York: John Wiley, 1979.
50. Keys A, Brozek J, Henschel A, Mickelsen O, Taylor HO. *The biology of human starvation*. Minneapolis: University of Minnesota Press, 1950.
51. Brooke OG, Harris M, Salvosa CB. The response of malnourished babies to cold. *J Physiol [Lond]* 1973;233:75–91.
52. Mansell PI, Fellows IW, Macdonald IA, Allison SP. Defect in thermoregulation in malnutrition reversed by weight gain. Physiological mechanisms and clinical importance. *QJ of Med* 1990;76:817–829.

53. Fellows IW, Macdonald IA, Bennett T, Allison SP. The effect of undernutrition on thermoregulation in the elderly. *Clin Sci* 1985;69:525–532.
54. Bastow MD, Rawlings J, Allison SP. Undernutrition, hypothermia and injury in elderly women with fractured femur: an injury response to altered metabolism? *Lancet* 1983;1:143–145.
55. Luck P, Wakeling A. Increased cutaneous vasoreactivity to cold in anorexia nervosa. *Clin Sci* 1981;61:559–567.
56. Gross HA, Lake CR, Ebert MH, Zeigler MG, Kopin IJ. Catecholamine metabolism in primary anorexia nervosa. *J Clin Endocrinol Metab* 1979;49:805–809.
57. Gallen IW, Macdonald IA, Allison SP. Thermogenesis and glucose storage are diminished, but glucose oxidation is increased during glucose infusion in severely underweight patients. *Clin Nutr* 1989;8(Suppl):96.
58. Allison SP, Gallen IW, Macdonald IA. Impaired glucose induced thermogenesis in severely underweight patients is improved after weight gain. *Clin Nutr* 1989;8(Suppl):109.
59. Kurpad AV, Kulkarni RN, Shetty PS. Reduced thermoregulatory thermogenesis in undernutrition. *Eur J Clin Nutr* 1989;43:27–33.
60. Vaz M, Kulkarni RN, Piers LS, Soares MJ, Kurpad AV, Shetty PS. The effect of energy supplementation on noradrenaline-induced thermogenesis, thermic effect of a meal and basal metabolic rate in chronically energy deficient human subjects. *Proc Nutr Soc* 1991 *[in press]*.
61. Hofford JM, Milakofsky L, Vogel WH, Sacher RS, Savage GJ, Pell S. The nutritional status in advanced emphysema associated with chronic bronchitis. A study of amino acid and catecholamine levels. *Am Rev Respir Dis* 1990;141:902–908.
62. Nordenstrom J, Jeevandam M, Elwyn DH, et al. Increasing glucose intake during total parenteral nutrition increases norepinephrine excretion in trauma and sepsis. *Clin Physiol* 1981;1:525–534.

DISCUSSION

Dr. Rothwell: This chapter describes experimental evidence to suggest that sympathetic nervous system (SNS) activity may be altered by nutritional status and/or may contribute directly to energy balance in humans.

A major problem in this area of research is in obtaining reliable assessment of SNS activity, particularly in man. One of the most important aspects of this topic highlighted by the author is the probability that selective and discrete activation of the SNS may occur. Thus, measurement of circulating catecholamine concentration can be misleading, and alterations in cardiovascular function may be of little reliance to sympathetically mediated changes in thermoregulation, thermogenesis, and energy balance.

Acute starvation and chronic underfeeding appear to reduce SNS activity and may impair thermoregulation. It is interesting to speculate that the reduced thermoregulatory capacity which has been reported during underfeeding or in states of negative energy balance in normal subjects, may reflect an adaptive process for energy conservation. This response appears to relate to an alteration in stimulus and not in the capacity of thermogenic effector mechanisms, however increased β-adrenoceptor sensitivity during underfeeding may, in part compensate for reduced SNS activity. Facultative thermogenesis, assessed under glucose clamp conditions, appears to be decreased.

Inconsistent changes (usually increases) in SNS activity have been reported during overfeeding. One of the most potent stimuli for SNS activation and thermogenesis in experimental animals, that of protein deficiency (but adequate energy supply), has not been tested in human subjects.

Understanding of the relationship of SNS activity to clinical changes in energy balance is confounded by the difficulty in distinguishing causal and resultant factors. There is evidence to suggest that SNS activity is decreased in human obesity, and this could contribute to reduced thermogenesis and increased fat deposition. Studies on post-obese patients support this proposal. However, in order to verify the suggestion, it will be necessary to study large numbers of patients and if possible to assess SNS activity in normal weight children or young adults with genetic predispositions to obesity (i.e., strong history of familial obesity) to fully unravel the mechanisms. Some studies have reported diminished responses to infused noradrenaline in obese states. However, this has not been confirmed in all studies, and is inconsistent with data on experimental animals. It is now recognized that most, if not all, forms of spontaneous obesity in laboratory rodents result from defects in activation of the SNS rather than impaired peripheral effector mechanisms. An interesting suggestion from animal research, that reduced SNS activity together with increased parasympathetic NS activity contributes to obesity, has received little attention in humans.

The suggestion that SNS activity may actually be increased in obesity serves as a poignant illustration of the need to distinguish cause and effect, and may prove a likely explanation for some of the conflicting data obtained in obese subjects.

Observations on chronically underfed humans are consistent with reduced SNS activity or effectiveness. In neonates, underfeeding may lead to severe thermoregulatory impairment, and decreased food intake and/or body weight may contribute to alterations in thermoregulation in aging subjects or those with anorexia nervosa. However, in aging, alterations in SNS activity, thermoregulatory capacity and body weight may reflect different aspects of hypothalamic dysfunction rather than causally related changes. Altered glucocorticoid status, which often accompanies aging, could provide a common mechanism for each of these alterations. However, restoration of normal body weight often reverses reduced thermoregulatory capacity in humans, although this is rarely the case in experimental animals.

Weight loss during illness may be associated with increased SNS activity. In addition to results quoted from humans studies, there are now ample data from research in laboratory animals to show that injury, infection, and malignant disease can all stimulate SNS activity resulting in increased metabolic rate and subsequent weight loss.

Implications for Future Research

The major avenues for future research into the relationship between SNS activity and dietary status in humans can be summarized as follows:

(i) Improved methods for assessing SNS activity. Selective inhibition of SNS actions can provide a useful tool for research, and the possible availability of selective β-adrenoceptor antagonists (particularly β₃ antagonists which may selectively inhibit thermogenesis) in the future will considerably facilitate such studies.

(ii) Investigation into selective activation of sympathetically mediated processes, e.g., cardiovascular vs thermogenic.

(iii) Determination of whether alterations in thermogenesis/energy balance and SNS activity are causally related. This problem could be addressed in studies of weight loss due to illness where acute and often severe alterations in energy balance may exist. In contrast, the development of obesity usually occurs over a very long period (years). The task of investigating the underlying causes of obesity in humans is therefore a daunting one.

(iv) Effect of alterations in feeding regimes, dietary composition, and specific supplements (particularly those used clinically) on SNS activity and energy balance.

(v) Current research indicates close interactions between dietary intake, SNS activity, and thermoregulation/thermogenesis. A critical question is whether dietary or pharmacological intervention to modify SNS activity will prove beneficial for the acute and chronic outcome of the patient.

Energy Metabolism: Tissue Determinants and
Cellular Corollaries, edited by J. M. Kinney
and H. N. Tucker. Raven Press, Ltd.,
New York © 1992.

Studies of Human Adipose Tissue In Vivo

Keith N. Frayn

Sheikh Rashid Diabetes Unit, Radcliffe Infirmary, Oxford, OX2 6HE, United Kingdom

The work described in this chapter had its roots in the early 1980s, when a number of groups were studying the metabolic responses of septic, injured, or otherwise nutritionally depleted patients to intravenous nutrition. Dr. Kinney's group at Columbia University had pioneered the application of indirect calorimetry in studying such patients and had shown differing responses in those acutely ill and those suffering primarily from nutritional depletion. In the former group, infusion of large amounts of glucose (greater than the resting metabolic rate) failed to suppress fat oxidation completely so that the nonprotein respiratory quotient remained below 1.0, whereas in the latter group glucose infusion produced a progressive rise in the respiratory quotient, implying refilling of glycogen stores followed by net lipogenesis from the glucose (1).

The author, as a member of the Medical Research Council's Trauma Unit in Manchester, England, was engaged in studies that essentially confirmed the work being done at Columbia (2,3). It was easy, for a worker fairly new to human studies, to get the impression from these results that the "normal" response to carbohydrate intake was to convert it to fat for storage. A belief in net lipogenesis as a major route for laying down fat in adipose tissue was ingrained in many people from the low-carbohydrate diets popular in the 1960s and 1970s; bread and potatoes were regarded as particularly fattening, and to anyone versed in metabolism, it was obvious that carbohydrate intake stimulated insulin secretion, which then stimulated the pathway of lipogenesis. This pathway, the subject of detailed study, was—and still is—used as a model for elucidating some of the mechanisms of insulin's intracellular effects (albeit in isolated rat adipocytes).

These beliefs began to disappear at the beginning of the last decade. For the author, the first indication that human metabolism did not obey these simple rules came when Dr. David Elwyn pointed out that net lipogenesis is not something that usually occurs in normal people. It was necessary to realize that nutritionally depleted, inactive patients receiving large amounts of glucose intravenously, whom we studied, were not the same as normal, active people consuming a mixed diet via the mouth. This remark was followed by a series of elegant papers from Acheson and colleagues in Jéquier's group in Lausanne, which showed that in normal subjects the ingestion even of a large carbohydrate load produced no net fat deposition (4). Only after

267

several days on a high-carbohydrate diet did net lipogenesis become a route for depositing the excess calories (5,6).

These observations were very thought provoking. The implication was that, in humans, energy deposition in adipose tissue stores must occur primarily through uptake of dietary fat. This tallied with long-standing observations that the fatty acid composition of human adipose tissue is strongly influenced by the dietary fatty acid composition (7–9). If excess carbohydrates were not converted rapidly into lipid, then someone following a low-fat diet should find it difficult to put on weight. On the other hand, this simple strategy for weight control would have its limitations. There seemed to be some trigger that signaled, from the fullness of the glycogen stores, when lipogenesis should switch on. The process of fat uptake into human adipose tissue and its regulation had never been studied directly, and all these aspects seemed to require investigation from the point of view of the intermediary metabolic processes involved.

Alongside these aspects of the regulation of body fat stores were other reasons for wanting to study more directly the regulation of fat storage and mobilization. The lipid store in a typical human of normal body weight is between 10 kg and 20 kg, or around 400 MJ to 700 MJ. With a daily energy turnover of around 12 MJ/day, of which typically 40% (say 5 MJ) comes from fat, the turnover of total body fat is around 1% per day. A small difference in this figure would thus have major consequences for energy balance. Indeed, the hypermetabolism typical of septic and injured patients can be viewed as resulting primarily from an increased rate of fat mobilization and oxidation (10,11). Conversely, the excess fat deposition of obesity could also be viewed as a derangement of the normal regulation of adipose tissue lipid storage. The metabolic regulation of fat mobilization and fat storage must be extremely precise and is at the heart of any metabolic description of the control of body weight and composition. A more detailed understanding of how this regulation is brought about, and how it is disturbed in pathologic states, might open new possibilities for manipulation of energy balance.

It is probably fair to say that of the total world literature on fat metabolism, 85% is based on the rat, 80% is work done in vitro (of which perhaps 90% employs the rat epididymal fat pad or its isolated cells), and only a very small proportion refers to human fat metabolism in vivo (Table 1). The regulation of fat mobilization is readily studied in vitro, but the only route of fat deposition easily amenable to study in vitro is that of de novo lipogenesis from carbohydrates. This may account for the undue emphasis placed on the role of carbohydrates in the diet, as discussed earlier. Even in vivo, with turnover studies, the rate of fat mobilization is more easily studied than is the rate of fat deposition. Although it is possible to administer isotopically labeled fatty acids and to measure their incorporation into adipose tissue lipids (31), such studies are technically very difficult because of the extremely large lipid pool. Indirect calorimetry again will give evidence only on de novo lipogenesis; the processes of ingestion of dietary fat and its incorporation into chylomicrons and uptake by adipose tissue are invisible to this technique.

These considerations all seem to lead to the conclusion that a method is needed

TABLE 1. *Techniques for studying fat metabolism*

Preparation	Era	Seminal reference
In vitro		
Isolated adipose tissue		
Rat epididymal fat pad	1960s	12, 13
Human tissue	1960s, 1970s	14
Rat fat cells	1970s	15
Human fat cells	1980s	16
In vivo		
Whole-body turnover		
Fatty acids	1960s to date	17, 18
Glycerol	1980s	19, 20
Gas exchange (indirect calorimetry)[a]	1970s increasing to date	1, 4
Perfused fat pad (animals)	1960s	21, 22
Arteriovenous differences		
Human superficial veins	1950s to date	23, 24
Fat-tailed sheep	1980s	25
Canine subcutaneous fat	1970s	26, 27
Human subcutaneous fat depot	1988 to date	28,29
Microdialysis (human subcutaneous adipose tissue)	1988 to date	30

[a] This refers to the use of indirect calorimetry specifically for investigation of substrate oxidation rates in vivo.

for studying the metabolism of adipose tissue in vivo, where it will be exposed to its normal physiologic range of substrates and hormones and subject to its normal nervous control. The idea of measuring arteriovenous differences across adipose tissue, the obvious solution to this problem, is not new. In one of the studies that elucidated the important role of non-esterified fatty acids (NEFA) in energy supply, Gordon in 1957 (23) collected blood from a variety of sites including the saphenous vein draining largely the superficial tissues of the leg. The demonstration of a high-plasma NEFA level in this vein was used as evidence for adipose tissue as the source of plasma NEFA. When Andres, Zierler, and colleagues pioneered the study of the human forearm by measurement of arteriovenous differences, they studied in some cases the superficial as well as the deep (muscle-draining) veins (24). Superficial forearm veins have since been studied by several authors (e.g., refs. 32, 33), but although they are sometimes described as representing adipose tissue metabolism, they actually drain a number of tissues, including communications from muscle. Most importantly, it seems that skin metabolism plays a major role among superficial forearm tissues. In animals, clear studies have been made in the fat-tailed sheep (25). This animal's large tail, weighing up to 2 kg, is composed largely of adipose tissue, the venous drainage of which is accessible for sampling. This is useful for studies of fat mobilization, but the relevance of routes of fat deposition in the sheep to those in the human must be questionable. Similar studies have been pursued in the dog. In 1966 Rosell (26) introduced a technique for isolation of the blood supply to the

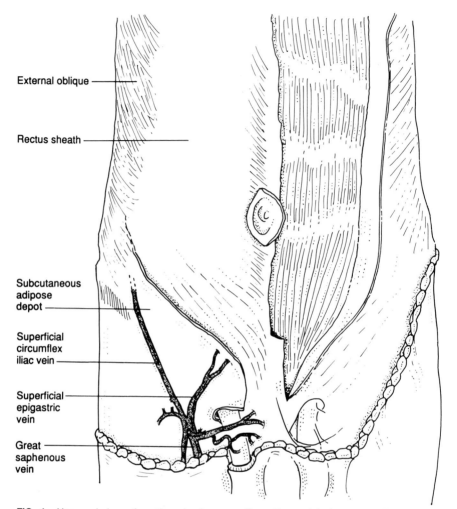

External oblique

Rectus sheath

Subcutaneous adipose depot

Superficial circumflex iliac vein

Superficial epigastric vein

Great saphenous vein

FIG. 1. Venous drainage from the subcutaneous adipose tissue of the human anterior abdominal wall. This fat depot (partially removed in the diagram) is drained by two major systems: the superficial circumflex iliac and the more medial superficial epigastric, which merge before entering the femoral triangle. The avascular fibrous aponeurosis of the *external oblique* muscle, which separates this fat depot from the underlying muscle, is shown. In the technique we have developed, (28,29) a catheter is introduced percutaneously into a tributary, usually of the superficial epigastric vein, and threaded downstream until its tip lies just superior to the inguinal ligament. Based on plate 2-6 in reference 35.

inguinal subcutaneous fat pad in the dog, so that the tissue could be perfused with blood and the venous effluent collected. This technique has been used by many workers. Bülow (27) cannulated the canine pudendal vein, which drains mainly subcutaneous adipose tissue, to measure arteriovenous differences across this tissue in vivo during exercise, and Holloway et al. (34) collected blood draining the bladder fat depot in anesthetized dogs for studies of thermogenesis.

The need for a method for pursuing such studies in the human led me and my colleagues to a serious consideration of the venous anatomy of human adipose depots a few years ago. The measurement of arteriovenous difference across a tissue requires a site that has a well-defined and accessible venous system that is not contaminated by drainage from other tissues. One site that appears to satisfy these criteria is the subcutaneous adipose tissue of the anterior abdominal wall (Fig. 1). This adipose depot is drained by two main venous systems: the superficial circumflex iliac, and the more medial superficial inferior epigastric. These veins run toward the groin, meeting inferior to the inguinal ligament before joining with the saphenous vein and returning to the inferior vena cava via the femoral triangle. We have confirmed by dissection (29) that they arise from within the adipose tissue (Color plate)

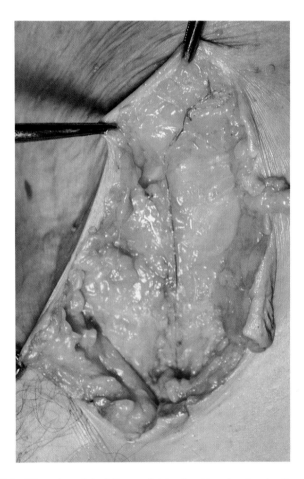

COLOR PLATE 1. Dissection of the left superficial epigastric vein, showing its origin in subcutaneous adipose tissue. To the anatomic left of the vein, the fat has been dissected away to show a small area of the aponeurosis of *external oblique*. Courtesy of Dr. S. W. Coppack.

with no noticeable communication with the underlying muscle bed, which is completely separated by an avascular, fibrous sheath, the aponeurosis of the *external oblique* muscle. Drainage from the overlying skin must be included, but in most people it seems likely that on a simple weight basis, the ratio of adipose tissue to skin would be fairly high. The more superficial veins that make up the tributaries of the veins previously named can usually be seen (albeit diffusely) percutaneously. The development of a method for cannulation of these veins (28,29) has led to a series of studies on human fat metabolism in vivo, which will be reviewed in the remainder of this chapter along with the results of other studies in the literature.

OVERVIEW OF THE METABOLISM OF WHITE ADIPOSE TISSUE

History of the Elucidation of White Adipose Tissue Metabolism

Wertheimer and Shapiro (36) were among the first to draw attention to the metabolic importance of white adipose tissue, which had until then been regarded simply as a mechanical cushion or as insulation. At that time it was clear that lipid was stored in adipose tissue in the form of "neutral fat" or triglyceride (referred to henceforth as triacylglycerol, or TAG), that fat deposition occurred in times of overfeeding (their studies on rats were largely concerned with carbohydrate feeding), and that fat was mobilized in times of shortage. Among other farsighted conclusions, they noticed the presence of glycogen in adipose tissue, the amount increasing in times of overfeeding. They believed this glycogen was an intermediate in the pathway of lipogenesis. The next important step came in the 1950s when Gordon, Dole, and others elucidated the role of the NEFA in plasma as the carriers of lipid energy from adipose tissue to the tissues where it would be oxidized (reviewed in ref. 37). Their studies included, as mentioned earlier, some of the earliest measurements of arteriovenous differences for NEFA, showing their production in superficial tissues. By the early 1960s, the rat epididymal fat pad had been introduced as a useful model for adipose tissue metabolism in vitro. This discrete fat pad possesses the advantage to experimenters of coming in pairs, so one of a pair can be incubated with a substance under test while the other serves as control. Basic features of adipose tissue metabolism and its regulation were rapidly elucidated, and the picture that emerged in the *Handbook of Physiology*'s section on adipose tissue in 1965 (13) has remained substantially unchanged since then.

Basic Features of White Adipose Tissue Metabolism

The typical white adipocyte contains a large lipid droplet, the stored TAG, surrounded by a thin layer of cytoplasm containing the nucleus and mitochondria. The metabolic activity of the cell occurs in this cytoplasm, at the surface of the lipid droplet and in the cell membrane. White adipose tissue is not, in most respects, a particularly active tissue on a per-weight basis or even on a per-volume-of-cell-water

TABLE 2. *Metabolic activities of various tissues and organs in a typical 70 kg human (resting)*[a]

Tissue/organ	Wet wt kg	Oxygen consumption ml/min		
		per kg wet wt.	per liter tissue water	whole body
Liver	1.7	44	60	75
Skeletal muscle (resting)	20–30	2.8	4	70
Gastrointestinal tract	2.6	22	30	58
Brain	1.5	31	40	46
Heart	0.3	90	120	27
Adipose tissue	10–20	0.25	2.5	4

[a] Values for tissues other than adipose are based on Table 2.2 in ref. 38. Values for adipose tissue based on Table 2 in ref. 39. Values per liter water calculated assuming water contents of 10% and 75% for adipose and all other tissues, respectively.

basis (Table 2). However, as will be pointed out, in particular respects its metabolic activity dominates those of all other tissues (especially release of NEFA and clearance of TAG postprandially).

The white adipocyte requires energy, as does any other cell, for its various metabolic activities. It has long been thought to obtain this energy primarily by oxidation of glucose. Wertheimer and Shapiro (36) and Ball and Jungas (40) reviewed studies on the respiratory quotient (RQ) of isolated adipose tissue. In tissue from fed animals and in studies in which exogenous substrate was supplied, the RQ was usually around 1.0. This has been confirmed (41) for human white adipose tissue in vitro. In human tissue the RQ is not affected by addition of insulin (41), whereas in rat tissue the RQ may rise markedly (40). Rat white adipose tissue (unlike brown adipose tissue) appears almost unable to oxidize fatty acids; the proportion of labeled fatty acid oxidized as opposed to esterified is around 1% (42,43). Our studies of human subcutaneous adipose tissue in vivo challenge these views. In normal subjects fasted overnight, adipose tissue extracts both glucose and oxygen from the blood and releases lactate (29,44). Lactate release accounts for about one-third of the glucose extracted. If the remaining glucose were all oxidized, only about one-fourth of the observed oxygen extraction would be accounted for. We have measured the contribution of other potential substrates for oxidation. Acetate, acetoacetate, and 3-hydroxybutyrate are all extracted from the blood and if also oxidized could, together with glucose, account for around 50% of the oxygen consumed (44). (Again, there is an apparent difference from rat adipose tissue, which almost entirely lacks the enzymes for ketone body utilization; ref. 45). The remaining substrate remains unidentified. Only a very small portion of the NEFA released in the fasting state would need to be oxidized in order to account for this "substrate deficit"; it may be that human adipose tissue is not so clearly white or brown as is that of the rat. Alternatively, the breakdown of stored glycogen could provide the missing substrate. We have measured glycogen concentrations in needle-biopsies of human adipose tissue after overnight fast and during the day (46), and the levels found, although, as in other species, low in comparison with muscle, are nevertheless sufficient to account for the substrate deficit.

Lipolysis in Adipose Tissue

In the fasting state, the role of adipose tissue is to release lipid-derived energy (in the form of NEFA) as a substrate for use by other tissues. The detailed properties and regulation of the intracellular enzyme responsible for hydrolysis of the stored TAG, the so-called hormone-sensitive lipase (HSL), have been thoroughly reviewed elsewhere. In brief, this enzyme hydrolyzes the TAG stored in the lipid droplet of the white adipocyte (Fig. 2). Hydrolysis of the first ester link appears to be the rate-limiting step. Hydrolysis of a second (by the same enzyme) proceeds more rapidly. The third fatty acid is removed by a monoacylglycerol lipase (49). HSL is regulated on a short-term basis by phosphorylation/dephosphorylation; the former is catalyzed by a cyclic AMP-dependent protein kinase, activated in turn by a variety of agonists including β-adrenergic agonists, glucagon, and ACTH. Adrenergic influences appear to be predominant in vivo (50–52). These actions may be opposed by a number of endogenous or exogenous factors acting to decrease the cyclic AMP concentration (adenosine, prostaglandin E2, nicotinic acid); of these, adenosine almost certainly plays a physiologic role (53). Insulin also acts to oppose lipolysis by an uncertain mechanism leading to dephosphorylation of the enzyme, whereas cortisol and growth hormone both have more long-term stimulatory actions resulting in increases in the amount of enzyme protein.

The NEFA resulting from hydrolysis of the stored TAG are thought to be bound to an intracellular fatty-acid binding protein (54) rather than being free in solution. They may either be exported, probably via a fatty acid transporter protein (54–56), or used for re-esterification within the cell. Since adipose tissue possesses little glycerol kinase activity (12,57,58), the glycerol cannot be used for re-esterification and is exported. The proportion of fatty acids re-esterified intracellularly can thus be assessed from the ratio of glycerol to NEFA release, either from isolated adipocytes or from adipose tissue in vivo. Estimates of re-esterification made in vitro depend on the incubation conditions, but in human tissue around 30% to 40% of the fatty acids released by lipolysis are re-esterified (59,60). Edens, Leibel, and Hirsch (61) have recently raised the interesting possibility that, because of compartmentalization of lipolysis and esterification within the adipocyte, re-esterification may involve an extracellular movement of the fatty acids. This may account for some of the variability of the figures measured in vitro. Estimates of re-esterification have been made in vivo both by isotopic means (62,63) and by measurement of arteriovenous differences (44,64), and all agree on a figure of around 20% re-esterification in the overnight-fasted state. Because intracellular lipolysis/re-esterification is an energy-consuming substrate cycle (discussed further by Wolfe in this volume), this result is of some interest.

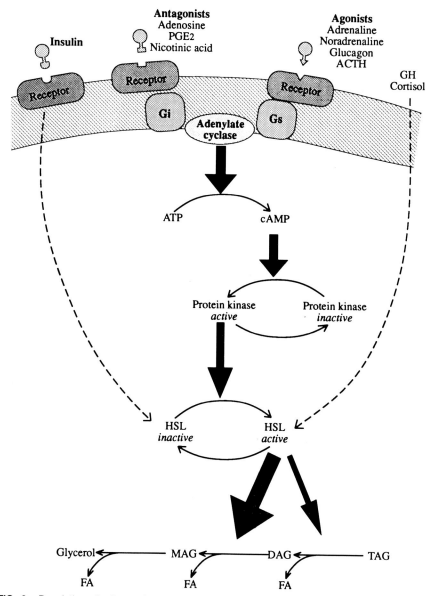

FIG. 2. Regulation of adipose tissue lipolysis. Rapidly acting stimulators of lipolysis (including circulating adrenaline, noradrenaline released at sympathetic nerve terminals, and some peptide hormones) act via membrane receptors to stimulate adenylate cyclase, which produces cyclic AMP (cAMP). Some antagonists (including nicotinic acid and related pharmacologic agents) act to inactivate adenylate cyclase, thus reducing cAMP levels. Both types of receptor are coupled to adenylate cyclase via G-proteins, either Gs (stimulatory) or Gi (inhibitory); these involve GTP binding. Elevation of cAMP leads to activation of the protein kinase which phosphorylates, and thus activates, the HSL. HSL catalyzes the first, and rate-limiting, step in lipolysis, the hydrolysis of stored TAG to a diacylglycerol and a fatty acid; it also catalyzes the next step leading to a monoacylglycerol and liberation of another fatty acid. The final fatty acid is removed by a separate enzyme. Insulin inactivates the HSL via an uncertain mechanism leading to dephosphorylation. Longer-acting stimulatory hormones, cortisol and growth hormone (GH), act via uncertain mechanisms to increase the amount of active enzyme protein. Based on Fig. 7.1 in ref. 47; reproduced from ref. 48, with permission.

Substrate Deposition in Adipose Tissue

There are two major routes by which white adipose tissue may accumulate tria-cylglycerol in times of energy surplus: by lipogenesis de novo from carbohydrate precursors and by uptake of fatty acids from circulating TAG. The latter might represent uptake of chylomicron-TAG (derived directly from ingested fat) or uptake of very-low-density-lipoprotein (VLDL)-TAG (secreted from the liver). Hepatic VLDL-TAG may in turn arise either from de novo lipogenesis or from esterification and export of preformed fatty acids; the possibility thus exists for another extracellular substrate cycle in which fatty acids are liberated from adipose tissue, taken up by the liver, and returned as VLDL-TAG.

Lipogenesis De Novo

Although the process of lipogenesis has been much studied in isolated adipose tissue, there are doubts, discussed earlier, about the physiologic importance of this process in humans. Even in situations in which whole-body net lipogenesis occurs, the liver is thought to play a larger role than adipose tissue; based on observations on adipose tissue isolated from patients receiving glucose infusions, adipose tissue lipogenesis might contribute up to 40% of that in the whole body (65). One reason for this may be the apparent lack of activity of lipogenic enzymes, particularly citrate lyase, in normal human adipose tissue (66), although others have suggested that some alternative pathway may exist for lipogenesis (67). It should, incidentally, be noted that the term "lipogenesis" is frequently used in studies of human adipose tissue in vitro but may simply refer to incorporation of carbon from glucose into TAG (16). Under normal conditions, the majority of this carbon will be present in the glycerol rather than the fatty acid moieties (65,67) so this is not de novo lipogenesis in the sense of energy storage.

Despite these reservations, we have observed glucose uptake into human adipose tissue in vivo at rates that exceed the rates of oxygen consumption, after oral glucose ingestion, during insulin infusion, or after a meal. Our observation of glycogen storage on high-carbohydrate diets (46) suggests this as a route for the disposal of excess glucose. Whether glycogen storage might be an intermediate process in lipogenesis, as suggested by Wertheimer and Shapiro 40 years ago (36), is unknown. It is interesting that some observations show an elevation of whole-body respiratory exchange ratio in the early hours of the morning (68), perhaps suggesting that carbohydrate stores laid down during the day are later converted into storage fat.

Uptake of Triacylglycerol Fatty Acids by Adipose Tissue

Uptake of fatty acids from circulating lipoprotein-TAG occurs via the action of the enzyme lipoprotein lipase (LPL) bound to the luminal surface of the capillaries of adipose tissue, heart, skeletal muscle, and other tissues (probably in that order of activity in the nonlactating animal) (69). At least a proportion of the non-esterified fatty acids produced by the action of LPL on lipoprotein particles is in some way transferred to the adipocytes. A number of models have been proposed for this process. It is clearly unlikely to involve simple diffusion of the fatty acids through the aqueous phase of the plasma and interstitial fluid. Some models envisage a highly structured system in which there is a continuous lipid layer extending out to and including the surface film of the lipoprotein particle (70,71); fatty acids diffuse through this lipid layer. Alternatively, the fatty acids may be carried on albumin molecules in the interstitial fluid; evidence for this comes from the binding of albumin to adipocytes in an apparently specific manner (reviewed in refs. 54,72). Another model (61) envisages a relatively mobile pool of NEFA within the interstitial space; fatty acids released by LPL may cross the endothelium to enter this pool, where they mix with fatty acids released in lipolysis.

Adipose tissue LPL is synthesized within the adipocytes, and its synthesis (via regulation of transcription), activation of post-translational modification, and export to the capillary all appear to be stimulated by insulin (reviewed in Williamson, ref. 73). Many measurements have been made of the activity of this enzyme in adipose and other tissues. There are, however, difficulties in the interpretation of such studies. Not all the enzyme measured in a tissue homogenate will be active at the capillary surface. Some of the problems in measurement of LPL activity in vitro have been reviewed (74). It may be assayed either in an extract of the whole tissue or after release from the tissue in vitro by heparin. In principle, the former should be a measure of total activity in the tissue, the latter, a measure of active enzyme. The two measures usually give broad agreement (74) but fundamental interpretation is difficult because LPL exists in a number of states within the tissue, presumably reflecting its progressive activation by post-translational modification. A considerable portion of total activity may be "cryptic" (75) and expressed only on dilution or treatment with heparin. In its physiologically active site LPL is bound to the endothelial cells by a heparan sulphate glycoprotein matrix and can be released into the plasma by exogenous heparin. Lipase activity in plasma after injection of heparin, therefore, gives another possible measure of its tissue activity. The most direct measure of its physiologic activity, however, would come from measurement of the hydrolysis of circulating TAG during its passage through the tissue. This necessitates either measurement of arteriovenous differences in vivo (76) or the use of a perfused preparation such as the perfused rat endometrial fat pad (22). Some of the measurements made in human adipose tissue in this way will be reviewed in the following section.

NORMAL PHYSIOLOGY OF HUMAN WHITE ADIPOSE TISSUE

In this section the results of our own studies on human adipose tissue in vivo in various physiologic situations will be discussed. In early studies we did not have a technique available to measure adipose tissue blood flow; results must be interpreted with this in mind. Lack of blood flow measurement does not, of course, alter relative rates of exchange of different substrates across adipose tissue (e.g., lactate release as a proportion of glucose uptake).

One point that should be made at this stage is that it is well established that adipose tissue from different parts of the body does not behave uniformly. In general, subcutaneous fat from the abdominal region is more actively lipolytic than that from the femoral or gluteal regions, studied both in vitro (77,78) and in vivo by the microdialysis technique (52). Intra-abdominal fat is even more metabolically active (79,80), and its special properties may have important implications in terms of risk factors for coronary heart disease. A review of this area is, however, outside the scope of this chapter; recent reviews may be found in refs. 81 through 83.

In our own studies of adipose tissue metabolism in vivo, we have used exclusively (for the anatomic reasons discussed earlier) the subcutaneous tissue of the anterior abdominal wall. In generalizing from these results, the site-specific properties of adipose tissue must be borne in mind. We have reason to believe, however, that the site we study is not atypical. For instance, local arteriovenous differences for NEFA and glycerol release across this site in a variety of conditions correlate well with systemic plasma concentrations of NEFA (Fig. 3 and ref. 44).

Another qualification to keep in mind is that the venous blood sampled in our studies inevitably includes a contribution from the overlying skin. We believe this contribution to be small for a number of reasons. On anatomical grounds, it might be expected that, except in the leanest of subjects, adipose tissue would be more

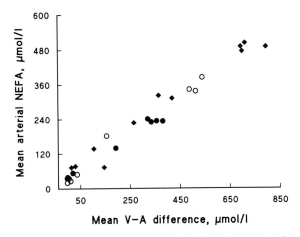

FIG. 3. Relationship between the plasma non-esterified fatty acid concentration (Y-axis) and the local arteriovenous difference for non-esterified fatty acid (NEFA) release, across the subcutaneous adipose tissue of the anterior abdominal wall in normal subjects. The results are group means at various times, taken from earlier papers: solid circles, ref. 29; open circles, ref. 64; diamonds, ref. 39. The close relationship observed implies that release of NEFA from this particular depot (as measured by the arteriovenous difference) reflects that from adipose tissue as a whole. The data are summarized in ref. 84.

important in mass terms. Metabolically, one feature of skin is that it is a highly glycolytic tissue, releasing around 80% of its glucose uptake as lactate (85). In contrast, we find (as outlined earlier) that only around one-third of the glucose taken up by the tissue we study is released as lactate. This contrasts, again, with studies of superficial forearm veins, in which much higher proportions of glucose are released as lactate (24,32,33). Using this criterion, it might be argued that with increasing adiposity of subject, a smaller proportion of the venous drainage should come from skin, and a lesser proportion of the glucose uptake should be released as lactate. In fact, we find that in the morbidly obese (body mass index $> 40 \ kg/m^2$) an equal or larger proportion of glucose is released as lactate (S.W. Coppack and K.N. Frayn, unpublished work). This suggests that the lactate release we see is a genuine feature of human adipose tissue in vivo as in vitro (86).

Human Adipose Tissue and Muscle After Overnight Fast

The relatively steady metabolic state obtaining after overnight fasting in normal subjects has enabled us to make a detailed assessment of the metabolic pattern of human adipose tissue in vivo in that state. In this section, the results for human adipose tissue will be contrasted with those for skeletal (forearm) muscle in the same experiments. The raw data are taken from Frayn et al. (29,87) and Coppack et al. (64), as summarized by Coppack et al. (44). After overnight fast, the metabolic pattern of human adipose tissue is dominated by the export of NEFA. This is accompanied by glycerol in a molar ratio of around 2.4 NEFA : 1 glycerol, indicating around 20% re-esterification of fatty acids within the tissue. The tissue is taking up glucose (with a fractional extraction from plasma of only 1–2%), ketone bodies, and acetate (fractional extractions 7–24%), and, perhaps surprisingly, there is a measurable extraction (around 4% in these experiments) of plasma triacylglycerol. In the postabsorptive state, this plasma TAG will be present mainly as VLDL-TAG. There is a technical difficulty in the measurement of TAG extraction, in that most methods for measurement of TAG concentration involve the hydrolysis of TAG with a lipase, and measurement of total glycerol. Since the concentration of free (non-esterified) glycerol is appreciably greater in the adipose tissue venous effluent than in arterial blood, a correction must be made for this. We now believe that our early studies, in which the correction of plasma TAG was based on the whole-blood glycerol concentration (88), underestimated TAG extraction by the adipose tissue; measurements made using a more direct assay (89) show fractional extraction of TAG in adipose tissue to be around 10% after overnight fast (39).

In order to assess overall substrate balance, we have calculated arteriovenous differences in terms of numbers of carbon atoms leaving or entering the tissue. The numbers shown in Fig. 4 represent exchange in μg-atoms of carbon (per liter of whole blood flow). Viewed in this way, the release of NEFA becomes even more dominant; on the uptake side, the extraction of carbon atoms from TAG considerably exceeds that from glucose. The lipid side of adipose tissue's metabolic activity clearly

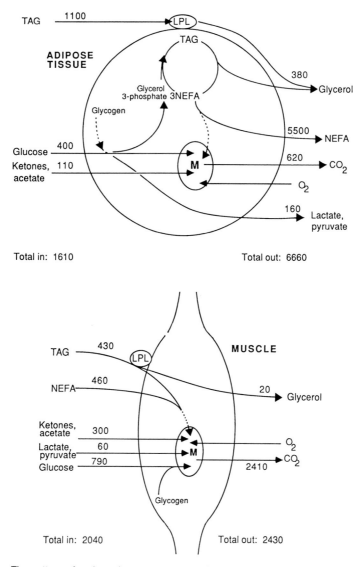

FIG. 4. The pattern of major substrate movements into and out of human forearm and subcutaneous adipose tissue after overnight fast in normal subjects. TAG, triacylglycerol (triglyceride); NEFA, non-esterified fatty acids; LPL, lipoprotein lipase; M, mitochondrion. The numbers refer to mean arteriovenous differences for each substrate expressed in μg-atoms of carbon per liter of whole blood. Based on 25 studies on normal subjects. Reproduced from ref. 44, with permission.

outweighs the carbohydrate side. Because the NEFA released may be re-esterified within the liver and returned as VLDL-TAG, the results show a potential "extra-tissue" substrate cycle equivalent to around 20% to 30% of the rate of NEFA release (44,88).

This picture may be contrasted with that for skeletal (forearm) muscle in the same state. In some respects the pictures are similar: forearm is also clearing small molecules such as ketone bodies and acetate with high fractional extractions (30–40%), and there are measurable arteriovenous differences for glucose (3% extraction) and TAG (2% extraction). In terms of inward carbon flux, that from glucose is greater than that from TAG in muscle. However, unlike adipose tissue, forearm muscle's carbon uptake in the postabsorptive state includes a substantial contribution from extraction of NEFA. In terms of overall balance, the extraction of carbon-containing substrates by muscle is just about balanced by its release of CO_2; it is in approximate carbon balance after overnight fast. Release of amino acids, not included here, would, from published data (90), make this negative to the extent of about 500 μg-atoms/l. Adipose tissue, in contrast, is a considerable net exporter of carbon. This picture of NEFA release from adipose tissue in the postabsorptive state, the NEFA being oxidized by other peripheral tissues such as skeletal muscle, tallies well with the conventional view of adipose tissue's role in whole-body metabolism.

Amino Acid Exchanges Across Human Adipose Tissue After Overnight Fast

Adipose tissue is often not considered to be important in amino acid metabolism; it is notably absent from two major reviews on amino acid metabolism (90,91). It has, however, been known for nearly three decades to have an active pattern of amino acid metabolism. Amino acids are, as in all tissues, substrates for and products of protein synthesis and breakdown respectively. These processes appear to be regulated, as in muscle, by insulin (92). Amino acids may also serve as precursors for lipogenesis. In principle, any amino acid whose metabolism can lead to acetyl-CoA formation can be converted into fat. Feller (93) reviewed a number of studies in which ^{14}C-labeled amino acids were added to adipose tissue in vitro and the appearance of ^{14}C in fatty acids was determined. Although all amino acids were able to contribute label to fatty acids, only leucine and alanine appeared to make a potentially significant contribution; all others contributed less than 5% of their label. The facet of amino acid metabolism that has attracted most attention is that of the release of the potential gluconeogenic precursors (and fuels for other tissues), alanine and glutamine. Alanine and glutamine are released from rat epididymal fat pads in vitro at rates that suggest a significant contribution to whole-body alanine production (94,95). As in muscle, a proportion of the alanine appears to arise from transamination of pyruvate, the source of the amino groups being branched-chain amino acids oxidized within the tissue (94). Studies of rat adipocytes in vitro, however, suggest utilization of glutamine (96), again at rates that if extrapolated to the whole-body, appear physiologically significant.

TABLE 3. *Amino acid concentrations and fluxes in seven normal subjects*[a]

	Alanine	Glutamine	Glutamate
Blood concentration, μmol/l			
Arterial	248 ± 16	509 ± 21	167 ± 11
Forearm venous	290 ± 17	551 ± 18	158 ± 11
Adipose venous	271 ± 18	538 ± 20	152 ± 11
Tissue flux, nmol.100 ml tissue^{-1}.min^{-1}			
Forearm	97 ± 18	157 ± 24	38 ± 8
Adipose tissue	70 ± 15	90 ± 22	42 ± 7
Estimated whole-body tissue flux, μmol/min			
Muscle	23 ± 4	39 ± 8	9 ± 2
Adipose tissue	9 ± 2	12 ± 3	6 ± 1

[a] "Adipose venous" refers to the venous drainage from abdominal subcutaneous adipose tissue. Values are means ± SEM. Tissue flux is calculated as product of arteriovenous difference and blood flow rate. Estimated whole-body tissue flux is calculated on the assumption that all skeletal muscle in the body (taken as 40% body weight) behaves like forearm tissues and that all adipose tissue (calculated from skinfold thicknesses) behaves like the subcutaneous abdominal depot studied here. These extrapolations must be interpreted cautiously. Based on ref. 97.

In collaboration with Drs. Elia and Khan (Cambridge, England), we have examined the exchange of alanine, glutamine, and glutamate across human subcutaneous adipose tissue (97). Only results in the overnight-fasted state will be discussed here. In each of 13 subjects studied (this total includes two diabetic subjects), there was net release of both alanine and glutamine across the tissue and net uptake of glutamate. In seven subjects, blood flow rates were also measured, and exchange across the forearm was examined for comparison. The results (Table 3) show that adipose tissue may well make a significant contribution to whole-body fluxes of these amino acids, at least as compared with the contribution of skeletal muscle. In considering why these results appear to disagree with the studies of rat adipocytes (as regards glutamine exchange), two important points should be kept in mind. First, measurement of arteriovenous differences gives information only on net exchanges and does not exclude the possibility of uptake by some cells and release by others. Second, it may be relevant that studies of rat fat pads in vitro appear to contradict the studies of rat adipocytes. Adipose tissue is not a pure preparation of adipocytes, and the contribution of adipocytes may be outweighed in the whole tissue by that of other cell types. Against this idea, most of the other cell types likely to be involved, including skin, have also been shown to be glutamine users, at least in vitro (references in Frayn et al., ref. 97).

Effects of Nutrient Ingestion and Insulin Infusion

We have studied the perturbation of the steady metabolic pattern after overnight fast produced by the ingestion of glucose (75 g glucose monohydrate or 1,160 kJ; eight subjects), by infusion of insulin (eight subjects), or by ingestion of ethanol (47.5

g or 1,400 kJ; seven subjects). In each case, the normal healthy subjects were studied initially after overnight fast. The data on individual substrates are presented in our papers (29,64,87); in reviewing them, the emphasis will be placed on overall substrate balance in adipose tissue. Again, the results will be contrasted with those for the forearm.

After oral glucose there was increased glucose extraction by adipose tissue, accompanied by marked suppression of NEFA and glycerol release. The increase in glucose extraction was much less, and less prolonged, than that seen in the forearm. We found a small, transient rise in plasma TAG at around 60 minutes after glucose ingestion, and this TAG appeared to be in a form that was avidly cleared by the adipose tissue. This finding is unexplained; one suggestion (T. D. R. Hockaday, Oxford, personal communication) is that it represents release of chylomicrons remaining in the intestinal wall since the previous day's fat ingestion.

In terms of overall balance of carbon-containing substrates (Fig. 5), the net export of carbon-containing material (mainly NEFA) in the postabsorptive state was converted at 60 minutes to an uptake; this returned to a state of "balance" at 2 hours after the glucose load. In the forearm, the postabsorptive state of carbon balance changed to one of marked carbon input and remained such at 120 minutes after the glucose load. This change in muscle metabolism reflected almost entirely an increase in glucose uptake and presumably represents the deposition of muscle glycogen; glucose uptake exceeded that of oxygen (in equivalent terms) about threefold at 60 and 120 minutes postglucose. In contrast, the major single change in adipose tissue metabolism, converting net export to net import, was not an increase in carbon uptake but the almost complete suppression of NEFA release. This was complemented by increases in the extraction of both glucose and TAG.

The enormous literature on the stimulation of glucose uptake by insulin in isolated adipose tissue would give the impression that the changes occurring after glucose ingestion are likely to be mediated primarily by the increase in plasma insulin. We therefore investigated the role of insulin by infusing it at 35 mU/m^2.min for 2 hours, using a euglycemic insulin clamp procedure (64). The plasma glucose concentration was clamped at the fasting level. Plasma insulin concentrations during infusion were around 50 mU/l, comparable to the peak reached in the oral glucose experiments. There was rapid and very complete suppression of NEFA release (Fig. 6), but surprisingly little stimulation of glucose extraction by the adipose tissue. In terms of overall carbon balance, the forearm behaved similarly in these experiments to those involving glucose ingestion (Fig. 5), rapidly changing to a net importer and remaining so at 2 hours. The major change in the forearm was a stimulation of glucose uptake, and again this presumably reflected glycogen storage as glucose uptake exceeded oxygen uptake (in equivalent terms) two to three times. In adipose tissue, however, the switch from export to import was much less pronounced than after oral glucose, the tissue barely reaching a state of 'carbon balance' after 2 h of insulin infusion. These results suggest that the role of insulin in stimulation of short-term nutrient uptake by adipose tissue is less clear-cut than often supposed, although insulin's

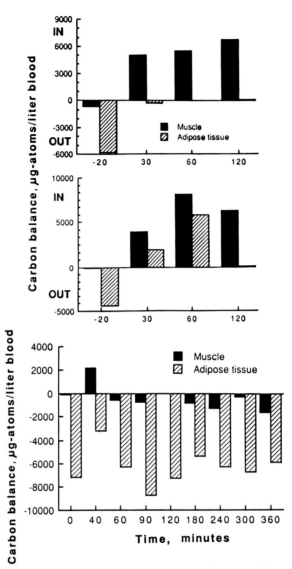

FIG. 5. Net balances of carbon-containing substrates across forearm (solid bars) and subcutaneous adipose tissue (hatched bars). The carbon balance is the algebraic sum of the uptake or release of non-esterified fatty acids, triacylglycerol, glycerol, glucose, lactate, 3-hydroxybutyrate and CO_2, expressed at μg-atoms of carbon per liter of whole blood. For the ethanol studies (lower panel), acetate, acetoacetate, ethanol, and pyruvate are also included. Bars going downward indicate net carbon efflux from the tissue; those going upwards indicate net carbon influx. Results are for seven or eight normal subjects, fasted overnight. The values shown at 0 or -20 are the mean of three baseline measurements. At time 0, one of three treatments was started. **Top:** An infusion of insulin was commenced using a euglycemic-insulin clamp procedure as described in the legend to Fig. 6. **Middle:** The subjects ingested 75 g glucose monohydrate orally. **Bottom:** The subjects ingested 47.5 g ethanol in the form of gin and low-calorie tonic water. After glucose ingestion (middle), both adipose tissue and forearm changed to net carbon uptake (i.e., substrate storage); during insulin infusion (top), although the efflux of fatty acids from adipose tissue was suppressed, net substrate storage was not seen. After ethanol ingestion, although the caloric content was rather greater than that provided by the glucose, again there was no tendency for substrate storage in adipose tissue. Based on figs. in refs. 64 and 87, with permission.

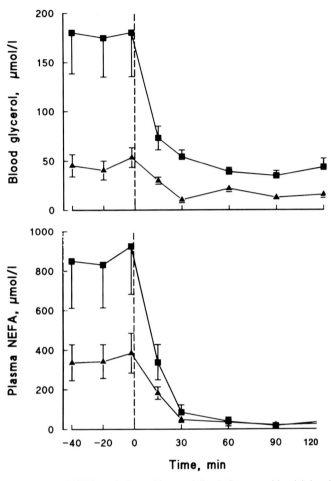

FIG. 6. Concentrations of NEFA and glycerol in arterialized plasma or blood (triangles) and in adipose tissue venous drainage (squares) in eight normal subjects. The subjects had fasted overnight. At time 0, an infusion of insulin (35 mU.m^{-2}.min^{-1}) was commenced, with the plasma glucose "clamped" at the fasting level. Release of NEFA from adipose tissue was completely suppressed from 60 minutes to 120 minutes, whereas release of glycerol was reduced but not completely suppressed, showing the role of increased fatty acid re-esterification in the suppression of fatty acid release by insulin. Based on data in ref. 64.

suppression of fatty acid release is still a major influence on overall carbon balance across the tissue.

The studies of ethanol ingestion were undertaken in part to address the question of whether net substrate deposition in adipose tissue after ingestion of nutrients is stimulated in a similar manner whatever form the nutrient takes. The load of ethanol used (in the form of gin and low-calorie tonic water) actually provided a slightly greater caloric load than did the oral glucose given in the earlier studies. Despite continuing observations for 6 hours after ethanol ingestion, we at no time recorded a positive flux of carbon-containing substrates into adipose tissue (Fig. 5C). We were not able from these studies to say whether there might have been prolonged slight sparing of fat mobilization, but even if this were the case, the mechanism for net energy storage after ethanol is clearly quite different from that observed after oral glucose. Our observations point again to the fact that, in terms of biochemical mechanisms, equal caloric loads of different nutrients may behave in entirely different ways. An "ethanol" calorie is clearly not, in metabolic terms, the same as a "glucose" calorie, and it may be oversimplistic to equate fuels on the basis of their "delta H."

Substrate Deposition in Adipose Tissue After a Mixed Meal

In our recent experiments (37) we have been unraveling the more realistic but more complicated situation of substrate movements in and out of tissues after ingestion of a typical mixed meal. The meal we have used in based on that of Elia et al. (98) but with a smaller proportion of simple sugars; it provides 3.1 MJ with 47% of energy from carbohydrates, 41% from fat. The results are taken from seven normal subjects, fasted overnight. In these experiments we have measured adipose tissue blood flow using ^{133}Xe clearance (99).

After this meal there was a relatively rapid rise in plasma glucose (peak at 60 minutes) with a much later rise in plasma TAG (peak at 240 minutes). About one-half the rise in plasma TAG concentration was accounted for by the appearance of chylomicron-TAG.

Overall carbon balance across the adipose tissue (Fig. 7) changed rapidly from a state of export after overnight fast to a state of net import; this was maintained at a surprisingly constant level until 5 hours after the meal, before returning at 6 hours to a negative value similar to the starting point. This smooth pattern was made up of two distinct phases: an early and rather transient period of stimulated glucose uptake, merging into a later and slower increase in TAG extraction. The removal of TAG made a far bigger contribution to net carbon storage overall than did the glucose uptake. Uptake of these substrates was opposed by release of NEFA and, to a lesser extent, glycerol. NEFA release from adipose tissue was suppressed after the meal, becoming undetectable at 90 minutes, but thereafter it steadily returned, again at 6 hours after the meal, reaching a value similar to that after overnight fast.

In forearm muscle, in contrast, positive carbon balance was produced mainly by increased uptake of glucose with only a small rise in TAG uptake later. In terms of the overall disposal of nutrients entering the plasma after the meal, adipose tissue played a major role in uptake of dietary-derived fat and a small one in glucose uptake; muscle played a major role in the disposal of glucose and a minor one in the disposal of fat.

One interesting outcome of these studies, still awaiting further exploration, was the surprisingly rapid return of NEFA release from adipose tissue, at a time when

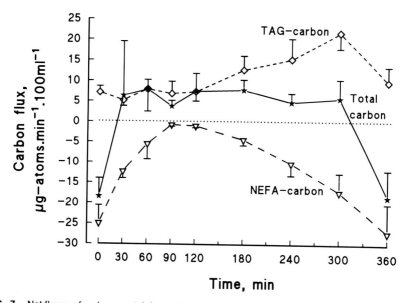

FIG. 7. Net fluxes of carbon-containing substrates across subcutaneous adipose tissue after over-night fast (0 minutes; this point represents the mean of three baseline measurements) and for 6 h after eating a mixed meal in seven normal subjects. Carbon flux is expressed as the algebraic sum of release or uptake of the eight major substrates in terms of their carbon content; these are absolute values, calculated as the product of arteriovenous difference and blood flow. The total carbon balance (stars and solid line) was negative after overnight fast (i.e., the tissue was exporting material) but became positive (i.e., the tissue stored substrates) between 30 minutes and 5 hours after the meal (eaten between 0 and 20 minutes). The total carbon balance was largely determined by the counterplay between triacylglycerol uptake (diamonds) and NEFA release (inverted triangles). Reproduced from ref. 39, with permission.

the plasma TAG concentration was still increasing postprandially and adipose tissue might have been expected *a priori* to be at its most active in net fat uptake (Fig. 7). By measurement of total glycerol release in relation to total TAG extraction, we can estimate the activity of the intracellular hormone-sensitive lipase (HSL). The assumption involved is that both LPL and HSL release one mole of glycerol into the venous effluent per mole of TAG hydrolyzed; the contribution of LPL can thus be assessed directly from TAG extraction, that of HSL by subtraction. It turns out that at 4–5 hours after the meal, the appearance of NEFA in the adipose venous plasma was greater than could be accounted for by HSL activity. We are therefore forced to conclude that the action of adipose tissue LPL is not fully efficient in terms of uptake of TAG–fatty acids into the tissue; a proportion must "leak" into the venous plasma. This phenomenon has been observed previously in perfused rat adipose tissue (100) and in dog and sheep in vivo (76). These leaked fatty acids will, of course, be available for uptake by other tissues and potential recycling as VLDL-TAG; their energy is not lost to the body. It appears, however, that adipose tissue LPL must be looked on not solely as a means for directing dietary-derived fat into that tissue for storage but also as a distribution point for making some of that fat available to the rest of the body.

PROSPECTS FOR THE FUTURE

The ability to study human white adipose tissue metabolism in vivo opens up many possibilities for studying the regulation of fat deposition and mobilization, and thus the metabolic basis of body weight regulation, in health and disease. Our studies are taking us in two main directions: the metabolism of lipoproteins and the pathophysiology of adipose tissue.

Lipoprotein Metabolism in Adipose Tissue

The activity of adipose tissue lipoprotein lipase in hydrolysis of circulating TAG has been previously discussed in terms of its role in fat deposition. The significance of this enzyme's action is, however, much wider than this role might suggest. It forms the hub of a complex series of interactions between lipoprotein particles (Fig. 8) not directly concerned with energy metabolism and thus not directly relevant to the subject of this review. In brief, hydrolysis of core TAG in the TAG-rich lipoproteins (chylomicrons and VLDL) is thought to lead to a surplus of surface components, mainly cholesterol, phospholipids, and apoproteins, and thus a "metastable" particle (101). These excess surface components may be shed by transfer to other particles, ultimately producing a new selection of stable particles (101). This is thought to be an important route of transfer of cholesterol into the high-density lipoprotein fraction (102). Our knowledge of these processes is at present indirect and based either on studies *in vitro* or on whole-body tracer studies. The ability to investigate lipoprotein lipase in vivo is enabling us to observe these processes more directly; marked changes in different lipoprotein particles are observed during their passage through adipose tissue (103).

Pathophysiology of Adipose Tissue

The very precise regulation of the vast quantity of energy flowing in and out of adipose tissue in normal daily life has previously been alluded to. It is likely that control of this process will be disturbed in some situations and that such disturbances will have major effects on whole-body energy metabolism.

The increased fat oxidation characteristic of wasting conditions such as sepsis, trauma, and cancer cachexia may be seen as an insensitivity of fat mobilization to suppression by insulin or glucose (11). Fat oxidation is also increased in relation to the rate of plasma-NEFA turnover, a change unlikely to reside in adipose tissue (10). Whether accelerated fat mobilization represents some primary change in adipose tissue such as a loss of insulin receptors or whether it represents the effects of a

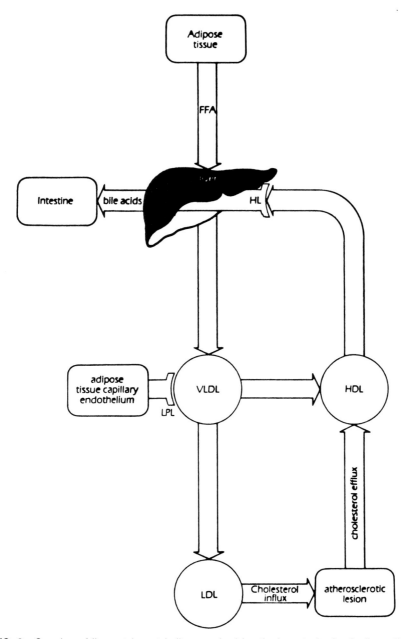

FIG. 8. Overview of lipoprotein metabolism, emphasizing the important role of adipose tissue, which both regulates the supply of free fatty acids (FFA) and plays a major role, via LPL activity, in the removal of circulating lipoprotein-TAG (shown here in the form of VLDL). The unlabeled arrow joining VLDL and HDL represents the transfer of excess surface components during the hydrolysis of TAG. These components include unesterified cholesterol, and this may be one reason for the commonly observed inverse relationship between plasma TAG and HDL-cholesterol levels. Based on literature provided by Farmitalia Carlo Erba, with permission.

sustained counter-regulatory hormone response is uncertain. Studies involving the infusion of combinations of counter-regulatory hormones into normal subjects suggest that this is one possible mechanism (104,105), but observations of many catabolic patients show that levels of counter-regulatory hormones are often not raised to the extent required to produce these changes (11,106,107). We lack direct information on adipose tissue or adipocyte metabolism, either in vitro or in vivo, in cachectic conditions. Another possible effector mechanism is the inhibition of lipoprotein lipase demonstrated in adipocytes and related cells in response to tumor necrosis factor (cachectin) and interleukin-1 (reviewed in ref. 108). Again, information on either plasma levels of tumor necrosis factor or interleukin-1 or on adipose tissue lipoprotein lipase activity in cachectic conditions is scarce. There have been reports of impaired LPL activity in biopsies of adipose tissue and muscle in septic patients (109), but the usual observation is that septic and injured patients clear triacylglycerol loads more quickly than normal (110,111).

The suggestion that a primary increase in adipose tissue LPL activity might be the cause of the increased fat deposition that leads to obesity has been thoroughly investigated but not satisfactorily answered (112). Many studies show LPL activity to be increased in adipose tissue biopsies from obese subjects, although even this demonstration depends on the mode of expression (per cell or per unit weight of tissue) (112,113). The question of cause and effect is far from resolved. If the increased LPL activity is a cause of the obesity, then it would be expected to be manifest after weight reduction. As Eckel (112) points out, studies of adipose tissue LPL activity in weight-reduced obese subjects have given extremely variable answers. What is clear, however, is that in insulin-resistant obese subjects the responsiveness of adipose tissue LPL to stimulation by insulin is blunted (112,113). This impaired insulin-activation of LPL may be important in the aetiology of the hypertriglyceridemia often associated with obesity, insulin-resistance, and glucose intolerance (114).

A further change in adipose tissue related to the pathogenesis of hypertriglyceridemia in the insulin resistance of obesity may be a decrease in the sensitivity of fat mobilization to suppression by insulin. This is an observation now made in a number of insulin-resistant conditions (115–117). The increased levels and turnover rate of NEFA in obesity have been recognized for many years (17,118). Hepatic VLDL secretion may be driven by an accelerated supply of NEFA from adipose tissue (119). With accelerated VLDL-TAG secretion and impaired TAG clearance, both arising as consequences of insulin insensitivity in adipose tissue, the link between insulin resistance and hypertriglyceridemia may be explained. These aspects of adipose tissue metabolism are now open to exploration in vivo, and such studies will, we hope, help in the coming years to elucidate some of the links among insulin resistance, adipose tissue, and coronary heart disease (114).

ACKNOWLEDGMENTS

The studies reviewed in the preceding sections have been the result of a team effort in the Sheikh Rashid Diabetes Unit and the Metabolic Research Laboratory,

Radcliffe Infirmary, Oxford. The contributions of Simon Coppak and of Sandy Humphreys have been particularly valuable: without Simon, we would never have developed the technique; without Sandy, we would not have been able to measure what we wanted in the small blood samples we obtained in our early experiments. I thank Dr. Derek Hockaday (director, Sheikh Rashid Diabetes Unit) for his encouragement and for his stimulating discussions, and Elizabeth Mansour for her secretarial assistance.

Financial assistance for these studies has been provided by the British Heart Foundation, the Juvenile Diabetes Foundation International, the Medical Research Council, the Humane Research Trust, the Oxford Regional Health Authority, and Glaxo Group Research. The Sheikh Rashid Diabetes Unit is supported by the Oxford Diabetes Trust.

REFERENCES

1. Askanazi J, Carpentier YA, Elwyn DH, et al. Influence of total parenteral nutrition on fuel utilization in injury and sepsis. *Ann Surg* 1980;191:40–6.
2. Stoner HB, Little RA, Frayn KN, Elebute AE, Tresadern J, Gross E. The effect of sepsis on the oxidation of carbohydrate and fat. *Br J Surg* 1983;70:32–5.
3. Frayn KN, Little RA, Stoner HB, Galasko CSB. Metabolic control in non-septic patients with musculoskeletal injuries. *Injury* 1984;16:73–9.
4. Acheson KJ, Flatt JP, Jéquier E. Glycogen synthesis versus lipogenesis after a 500 gram carbohydrate meal in man. *Metabolism* 1982;31:1234–40.
5. Acheson KJ, Schutz Y, Bessard T, Anantharaman K, Flatt JP, Jéquier E. Glycogen storage capacity and de novo lipogenesis during massive carbohydrate overfeeding in man. *Am J Clin Nutr* 1988; 48:240–7.
6. Acheson KJ, Schutz Y, Bessard T, Ravussin E, Jéquier E, Flatt JP. Nutritional influences on lipogenesis and thermogenesis after a carbohydrate meal. *Am J Physiol* 1984;246:E62–70.
7. Hirsch J. Fatty acid patterns in human adipose tissue. In: Renold AE, Cahill GF, eds. *Handbook of Physiology. 5. Adipose tissue.* Washington, D.C.: American Physiological Society, 1965;181–9.
8. Jacobsen BK, Trygg K, Hjermann I, Thomassen MS, Real C, Norum KR. Acyl patterns of adipose tissue triglycerides, plasma fatty acids, and diet of a group of men participating in a primary coronary prevention program (The Oslo Study). *Amer J Clin Nutr* 1983;38:906–13.
9. van Staveren WA, Deurenberg P, Katan MB, Burema J, de Groot LCPGM, Hoffmans MDAF. Validity of the fatty acid composition of subcutaneous fat tissue microbiopsies as an estimate of the long-term average fatty acid composition of the diet of separate individuals. *Am J Epidemiology* 1986;123:455–63.
10. Nordenström J, Carpentier YA, Askanazi J, et al. Free fatty acid mobilization and oxidation during total parenteral nutrition in trauma and infection. *Anns Surg* 1983;198:725–35.
11. Frayn KN. Hormonal control of metabolism in trauma and sepsis. *Clin Endocrinol* 1986;24:577–99.
12. Vaughan M. The metabolism of adipose tissue *in vitro*. *J. Lipid Res* 1961;2:293–316.
13. Renold AE, Cahill GF, eds. *Handbook of physiology. 5. Adipose tissue.* Washington, D.C.: American Physiological Society, 1965.
14. Hirsch J, Goldrick RB. Serial studies on the metabolism of human adipose tissue. I. Lipogenesis and free fatty acid uptake and release in small aspirated samples of subcutaneous fat. *J Clin Invest* 1964;43:1776–92.
15. Rodbell M. Metabolism of isolated fat cells. 1. Effects of hormones on glucose metabolism and lipolysis. *J Biol Chem* 1964;239:375–80.
16. Taylor R, Husband DJ, Marshall SM, Tunbridge WMG, Alberti KGMM. Adipocyte insulin binding and insulin sensitivity in 'brittle' diabetes. *Diabetologia* 1984;27:441–6.
17. Issekutz B Jr, Bortz WM, Miller HI, Paul P. Turnover rate of plasma FFA in humans and in dogs. *Metabolism* 1967;16:1001–9.

18. Wolfe RR, Evans JE, Mullany J, Burke JF. Measurement of plasma free fatty acid turnover and oxidation using [1-13C]palmitic acid. *Biomed Mass Spectrometry* 1980;7:168–71.
19. Carpentier YA, Askanazi J, Elwyn DH, Gump FE, Nordenström J, Kinney JM. The effect of carbohydrate intake on the lipolytic rate in depleted patients. *Metabolism* 1980;29:974–9.
20. Elia M, Zed C, Neale G, Livesey G. The energy cost of triglyceride-fatty acid recycling in nonobese subjects after an overnight fast and four days of starvation. *Metabolism* 1987;36:251–5.
21. Ho RJ, Meng, HC. A technique for the cannulation and perfusion of isolated rat epididymal fat pad. *J Lipid Res* 1964;5:203–9.
22. Rodbell M, Scow RO. Chylomicron metabolism: uptake and metabolism by perfused adipose tissue. In: Renold AE, Cahill GF, eds. *Handbook of physiology. 5. Adipose tissue.* Washington, D.C.: American Physiological Society, 1965;491–8.
23. Gordon RS. Unesterified fatty acid in human blood plasma. II. The transport function of unesterified fatty acid. *J Clin Invest* 1957;36:810–5.
24. Baltzan MA, Andres R, Cader G, Zierler KL. Heterogeneity of forearm metabolism with special reference to free fatty acids. *J Clin Invest* 1962;41:116–25.
25. Gooden JM, Campbell SL, van der Walt JG. Measurement of blood flow and lipolysis in the hind-quarter tissues of the fat-tailed sheep *in vivo*. *Quart J Exp Physiol* 1986;71:537–47.
26. Rosell S. Release of free fatty acids from subcutaneous adipose tissue in dogs following sympathetic nerve stimulation. *Acta Physiol Scand* 1966;67:343–51.
27. Bülow J. Subcutaneous adipose tissue blood flow and triacylglycerol-mobilization during prolonged exercise in dogs. *Pflügers Arch* 1982;392:230–4.
28. Frayn KN, Coppack SW, Whyte PL, Humphreys SM, Ng LL. Measurement of arteriovenous differences across an adipose depot in man. *Proc Nut Soc* 1988;47:173A (abstract).
29. Frayn KN, Coppack SW, Humphreys SM, Whyte PL. Metabolic characteristics of human adipose tissue *in vivo*. *Clin Sci* 1989;76:509–16.
30. Arner P, Bolinder J, Eliasson A, Lundin A, Ungerstedt U. Microdialysis of adipose tissue and blood for in vivo lipolysis studies. *Am J Physiol* 1988;255:E737–42.
31. Mårin P, Rebuffé-Scrive M, Björntorp P. Uptake of triglyceride fatty acids in adipose tissue in vivo in man. *Eur J Clin Invest* 1990;20:158–65.
32. Heaf DJ, Kaijser L, Eklund B, Carlson LA. Differences in heparin-released lipolytic activity in the superficial and deep veins of the human forearm. *Eur J Clin Invest* 1977;7:195–9.
33. Jackson RA, Hamling JB, Sim BM, et al. Peripheral lactate and oxygen metabolism in man: the influence of oral glucose loading. *Metabolism* 1987;36:144–50.
34. Holloway BR, Stribling D, Freeman S, Jamieson L. The thermogenic role of adipose tissue in the dog. *Int J Obes* 1985;9:423–32.
35. Anderson JE. *Grant's Atlas of Anatomy*, 8th Edition. Baltimore: Williams & Wilkins, 1983.
36. Wertheimer E, Shapiro B. The physiology of adipose tissue. *Physiol Rev* 1948;28:451–64.
37. Fredrickson DS, Gordon RS. Transport of fatty acids. *Physiol Rev* 1958;38:585–630.
38. White DA, Middleton B, Baxter M. *Hormones and metabolic control*. London: Edward Arnold, 1984.
39. Coppack SW, Fisher RM, Gibbons GF, et al. Postprandial substrate deposition in human forearm and adipose tissues *in vivo*. *Clin Sci* 1990;79:339–48.
40. Ball EG, Jungas RL. Net gas exchange and oxygen consumption. In: Renold AE, Cahill GF, eds. *Handbook of Physiology. 5. Adipose tissue.* Washington, D.C.: American Physiological Society, 1965;355–62.
41. Pozza G, Ghidoni A, Basilico C. Glucose uptake and gas exchange in human adipose tissue incubated in vitro. *Lancet* 1963;1:836.
42. Harper RD, Saggerson ED. Factors affecting fatty acid oxidation in fat cells isolated from rat white adipose tissue. *J Lipid Res* 1976;17:516–26.
43. Baht HS, Saggerson ED. Comparison of triacylglycerol synthesis in rat brown and white adipocytes. Effects of hypothyroidism and streptozotocin-diabetes on enzyme activities and metabolic fluxes. *Biochem J* 1988;250:325–33.
44. Coppack SW, Frayn KN, Humphreys SM, Whyte PL, Hockaday TDR. Arteriovenous differences across human adipose and forearm tissues after overnight fast. *Metabolism* 1990;39:384–90.
45. Williamson DH, Bates MW, Page MA, Krebs HA. Activities of enzymes involved in acetoacetate utilization in adult mammalian tissues. *Biochem J* 1971;121:41–7.
46. Rigden DJ, Jellyman AE, Frayn KN, Coppack SW. Human adipose tissue glycogen levels and responses to carbohydrate feeding. *Eur J Clin Nutr* 1990;44:689–92.

47. Lafontan M, Berlan M. Plasma membrane properties and receptors in white adipose tissue. In: Cryer A, Van RLR, eds. *New perspectives in adipose tissue*. London: Butterworths, 1985;145–82.
48. Frayn KN. Adipose tissue metabolism. *Clinics in dermatology: cutaneous adipose tissue* 1989;7:48–61.
49. Belfrage P. Hormonal control of lipid degradation. In: Cryer A, Van RLR, eds. *New perspectives in adipose tissue*. London: Butterworths, 1985;121–44.
50. Havel RJ, Goldfien A. The role of the sympathetic nervous system in the metabolism of free fatty acids. *J Lipid Res* 1959;1:102–8.
51. Smith U. Adrenergic control of human adipose tissue lipolysis. *Eur J Clin Invest* 1980;10:343–4.
52. Arner P, Kriegholm E, Engfeldt P, Bolinder J. Adrenergic regulation of lipolysis in situ at rest and during exercise. *J Clin Invest* 1990;85:893–8.
53. Lönnroth P, Jansson P-A, Fredholm BB, Smith U. Microdialysis of intercellular adenosine concentration in subcutaneous tissue in humans. *Am J Physiol* 1989;256:E250–5.
54. Potter BJ, Sorrentino D, Berk PD. Mechanisms of cellular uptake of free fatty acids. *Annu Rev Nutr* 1989;9:253–70.
55. Abumrad NA, Perkins RC, Park JH, Park CR. Mechanism of long chain fatty acid permeation in the isolated adipocyte. *J Biol Chem* 1981;256:9183–91.
56. Abumrad NA, Park JH, Park CR. Permeation of long-chain fatty acid into adipocytes. Kinetics, specificity, and evidence for involvement of a membrane protein. *J Biol Chem* 1984;259:8945–53.
57. Margolis S, Vaughan M. α-Glycerophosphate synthesis and breakdown in homogenates of adipose tissue. *J Biol Chem* 1962;237:44–8.
58. Steinberg D, Vaughan M. Release of fatty acids from adipose tissue in vitro in relation to rates of triglyceride synthesis and degradation. In: Renold AE, Cahill GF, eds. *Handbook of physiology. 5. Adipose tissue*. Washington, D.C.: American Physiological Society, 1965;335–47.
59. Leibel RL, Hirsch J. A radioisotopic technique for analysis of free fatty acid reesterification in human adipose tissue. *Am J Physiol* 1985;248:E140–7.
60. Hammond VA, Johnston DG. Substrate cycling between triglyceride and fatty acid in human adipocytes. *Metabolism* 1987;36:308–13.
61. Edens NK, Leibel RL, Hirsch J. Mechanism of free fatty acid re-esterification in human adipocytes in vitro. *J Lipid Res* 1990;31:1423–31.
62. Wolfe RR, Peters EJ. Lipolytic response to glucose infusion in human subjects. *Am J Physiol* 1987;252:E218–23.
63. Wolfe RR, Klein S, Carraro F, Weber J-M. Role of triglyceride-fatty acid cycle in controlling fat metabolism in humans during and after exercise. *Am J Physiol* 1990;258:E382–9.
64. Coppack SW, Frayn KN, Humphreys SM, Dhar H, Hockaday TDR. Effects of insulin on human adipose tissue metabolism *in vivo*. *Clin Sci* 1989;77:663–70.
65. Chascione C, Elwyn DH, Davila M, Gil KM, Askanazi J, Kinney JM. Effect of carbohydrate intake on de novo lipogenesis in human adipose tissue. *Am J Physiol* 1987;253:E664–9.
66. Shrago E, Spennetta T, Gordon E. Fatty acid synthesis in human adipose tissue. *J Biol Chem* 1969;244:2761–6.
67. Bray GA. Lipogenesis in human adipose tissue: some effects of nibbling and gorging. *J Clin Invest* 1972;51:537–48.
68. Lean MEJ, James WPT. Metabolic effects of isoenergetic nutrient exchange over 24 hours in relation to obesity in women. *Int J Obes* 1988;12:15–27.
69. Robinson DS. Lipoprotein lipase—past, present and future. In: Borensztajn J, ed. *Lipoprotein lipase*. Chicago: Evener, 1987;1–14.
70. Scow RO, Blanchette-Mackie EJ, Smith LC. Role of capillary endothelium in the clearance of chylomicrons. A model for lipid transport from blood by lateral diffusion in cell membranes. *Circ Res* 1976;39:149–62.
71. Scow RO, Chernick SS. Role of lipoprotein lipase during lactation. In: Borensztajn J, ed. *Lipoprotein lipase*. Chicago: Evener, 1987;149–85.
72. Saggerson ED. Hormonal regulation of biosynthetic activities in white adipose tissue. In: Cryer A, Van RLR, eds. *New perspectives in adipose tissue*. London: Butterworths, 1985;87–120.
73. Williamson DH. The endocrine control of adipose tissue metabolism and the changes associated with lactation and cancer. In: Forbes JM, Hervey GR, eds. *The control of body fat content*. London: Smith-Gordon, 1990;43–61.
74. Nilsson-Ehle P. Measurements of lipoprotein lipase activity. In: Borensztajn J, ed. *Lipoprotein lipase*. Chicago: Evener, 1987;59–77.

75. Pradines-Figuères A, Vannier C, Ailhaud G. Lipoprotein lipase stored in adipocytes and muscle cells is a cryptic enzyme. *J Lipid Res* 1990;31:1467–76.
76. Bergman EN, Havel RJ, Wolfe BM, Bøhmer T. Quantitative studies of the metabolism of chylomicron triglycerides and cholesterol by liver and extrahepatic tissues of sheep and dogs. *J Clin Invest* 1971;50:1831–9.
77. Rebuffé-Scrive M, Lönnroth P, Mårin P, Wesslau C, Björntorp P, Smith U. Regional adipose tissue metabolism in men and postmenopausal women. *Int J Obes* 1987;11:347–55.
78. Wahrenberg H, Lönnqvist F, Arner P. Mechanisms underlying regional differences in lipolysis in human adipose tissue. *J Clin Invest* 1989;84:458–67.
79. Smith U. Regional differences in adipocyte metabolism and possible consequences *in vivo*. *Int J Obes* 1985;9(Supplement 1):145–8.
80. Rebuffé-Scrive M, Andersson B, Olbe L, Björntorp P. Metabolism of adipose tissue in intraabdominal depots of nonobese men and women. *Metabolism* 1989;38:453–8.
81. Björntorp P. Abdominal obesity and the development of noninsulin-dependent diabetes mellitus. *Diabetes Metab Rev* 1988;4:615–22.
82. Kissebah AH, Peiris AN. Biology of regional body fat distribution: relationship to non-insulin-dependent diabetes mellitus. *Diabetes Metab Rev* 1989;5:83–109.
83. Frayn KN. Insulin resistance in obesity and in wasting disorders. In: Rothwell NJ, Stock MJ, eds. *Obesity and cachexia: physiological mechanisms and new approaches to pharmacological control.* London: John Wiley, 1991;119–48.
84. Coppack SW, Evans RD, Fisher RM, et al. Adipose tissue metabolism in obesity: lipase activity *in vivo* before and after a mixed meal. *Metabolism* (in press).
85. Johnson JA, Fusaro RM. The role of the skin in carbohydrate metabolism. In: Levine R, Luft R, eds. *Advances in metabolic disorders*, vol. 6. New York: Academic Press, 1972;1–55.
86. Mårin P, Rebuffé-Scrive M, Smith U, Björntorp P. Glucose uptake in human adipose tissue. *Metabolism* 1987;36:1154–60.
87. Frayn KN, Coppack SW, Walsh PE, Butterworth HC, Humphreys SM, Pedrosa, HC. Metabolic responses of forearm and adipose tissues to acute ethanol ingestion. *Metabolism* 1990;39:958–66.
88. Coppack SW, Frayn KN, Humphreys SM. Plasma triacylglycerol extraction in human adipose tissue *in vivo*: effects of glucose ingestion and insulin infusion. *Eur J Clin Nutr* 1989;43:493–6.
89. Humphreys SM, Fisher RM, Frayn KN. Micro-method for measurement of sub-nanomole amounts of triacylglycerol. *Anns Clin Biochem* 1990;27:597–8.
90. Felig P. Amino acid metabolism in man. *Ann Rev Biochem* 1975;44:933–55.
91. Christensen HN. Interorgan amino acid nutrition. *Physiol Rev* 1982;62:1193–233.
92. Herrera MG, Renold AE. Amino acid and protein metabolism. In: Renold AE, Cahill GF, eds. *Handbook of physiology. 5. Adipose tissue.* Washington, D.C.: American Physiological Society, 1965;375–83.
93. Feller DD. Conversion of amino acids to fatty acids. In: Renold AE, Cahill GF, eds. *Handbook of physiology. 5. Adipose tissue.* Washington, D.C.: American Physiological Society, 1965;363–73.
94. Snell K, Duff DA. Alanine release by rat adipose tissue in vitro. *Biochem Biophys Res Commun* 1977;77:925–32.
95. Tischler ME, Goldberg AL. Leucine degradation and release of glutamine and alanine by adipose tissue. *J Biol Chem* 1980;255:8074–81.
96. Kowalchuk JM, Curi R, Newsholme EA. Glutamine metabolism in isolated incubated adipocytes of the rat. *Biochem J* 1988;249:705–8.
97. Frayn KN, Khan K, Coppack SW, Elia M. Amino acid metabolism in human adipose tissue *in vivo*. *Clin Sci* 1991;80:471–4.
98. Elia M, Folmer P, Schlatmann A, Goren A. Austin S. Carbohydrate, fat, and protein metabolism in muscle and in the whole body after mixed meal ingestion. *Metablism* 1988;37:542–51.
99. Larsen OA, Lassen NA, Quaade F. Blood flow through human adipose tissue determined with radioactive xenon. *Acta Physiol Scand* 1966;66:337–45.
100. Scow RO. Metabolism of chylomicrons in perfused adipose and mammary tissue of the rat. *Fed Proc* 1977;36:182–5.
101. Havel RJ. Lipoprotein biosynthesis and metabolism. *Ann N Y Acad Sci* 1980;348:16–29.
102. Eisenberg S. Plasma lipoprotein conversions: the origin of low-density and high-density lipoproteins. *Ann N Y Acad Sci* 1980;348:30–47.
103. Potts JL, Fisher RM, Coppack SW, Gibbons GF, Frayn KN. Lipoprotein interconversions during passage through subcutaneous adipose tissue in humans *in vivo*. *Biochem Soc Trans* 1990;18:1196–7.

104. Bessey PQ, Watters JM, Aoki TT, Wilmore DW. Combined hormonal infusion simulates the metabolic response to injury. Ann Surg 1984;200:264–81.
105. Gelfand RA, Matthews DE, Bier DM, Sherwin RS. Role of counterregulatory hormones in the catabolic response to stress. *J Clin Invest* 1984;74:2238–48.
106. White RH, Frayn KN, Little RA, Threlfall CJ, Stoner HB, Irving MH. Hormonal and metabolic responses to glucose infusion in sepsis studied by the hyperglycemic glucose clamp technique. *J Parenter Enter Nutr* 1987;11:345–53.
107. Henderson AA, Frayn KN, Galasko CSB, Little RA. Dose-response relationships for the effects of insulin on glucose and fat metabolism in injured patients and control subjects. *Clin Sci* 1991; 80:25–32.
108. Evans RD, Argilés JM, Williamson DH. Metabolic effects of tumour necrosis factor-α (cachectin) and interleukin-1. *Clin Sci* 1989;77:357–64.
109. Robin AP, Askanazi J, Greenwood MRC, Carpentier YA, Gump FE, Kinney JM. Lipoprotein lipase activity in surgical patients: influence of trauma and infection. *Surgery* 1981;90:401–8.
110. Nordenström J, Carpentier YA, Askanazi J, et al. Metabolic utilization of intravenous fat emulsion during total parenteral nutrition. *Ann Surg* 1982;196:221–31.
111. Wilmore DW, Moylan JA, Helmkamp GM, Pruitt BA. Clinical evaluation of a 10% intravenous fat emulsion for parenteral nutrition in thermally injured patients. *Ann Surg* 1973;178:503–13.
112. Eckel RH. Adipose tissue lipoprotein lipase. In: Borensztajn J, ed. *Lipoprotein lipase*. Chicago: Evener, 1987;79–132.
113. Eckel RH. Lipoprotein lipase A multifunctional enzyme relevant to common metabolic diseases. *N Engl J Med* 1989;320:1060–8.
114. Frayn KN, Coppack SW. Insulin resistance, adipose tissue and heart disease. *Clin Sci* 1992;82: 1–8.
115. Chen Y-DI, Golay A, Swislocki ALM, Reaven GM. Resistance to insulin suppression of plasma free fatty acid concentrations and insulin stimulation of glucose uptake in noninsulin-dependent diabetes mellitus. *J Clin Endocr Metab* 1987;64:17–21.
116. Singh BM, Palma MA, Nattrass M. Multiple aspects of insulin resistance. Comparison of glucose and intermediary metabolite responses to incremental insulin infusion in IDDM subjects of short and long duration. *Diabetes* 1987;36:740–8.
117. Yki-Järvinen H, Taskinen M-R. Interrelationships among insulin's antipolytic and glucoregulatory effects and plasma triglycerides in nondiabetic and diabetic patients with endogenous hypertriglyceridemia. *Diabetes* 1988;37:1271–8.
118. Dole VP. A relation between non-esterified fatty acids in plasma and the metabolism of glucose. *J Clin Invest* 1956;35:150–4.
119. Kissebah AH, Alfarsi S, Adams PW, Wynn V. Role of insulin reistance in adipose tissue and liver in the pathogenesis of endogenous hypertriglyceridaemia in man. *Diabetologia* 1976;12:563–71.

DISCUSSION

Dr. Astrup: The technique developed by Keith Frayn and his group for in vivo measurement of human subcutaneous adipose tissue metabolism has been a breakthrough in this field of research. There has been a long-standing need for in vivo results produced in humans, and myths about human nutrition have already fallen based on data generated by this technique.

In this review Dr. Frayn clearly presents his view of the postabsorptive and postprandial metabolism of adipose tissue (AT). By the use of the forearm technique, simultaneous information is provided about the role of skeletal muscle in the substrate handling as well. He carefully discusses the theory and substantiates the shortcomings and pitfalls of the methodology applied. Almost all the experimental work using this in vivo methodology has been contributed by his own laboratory.

General Criticism

As stated by Dr. Frayn, considerable regional variation exists in the subcutaneous AT metabolism. Actually, different depots serve different metabolic purposes. The abdominal subcutaneous AT depot has been well characterized to be highly metabolically active, with pronounced lipolytic responsiveness to catecholamines, etc. The abdominal subcutaneous AT, together with the mesenterial depot, seems to play a central role in the pathogenesis of type-2 diabetes, hypertension, ischemic heart disease, and stroke in the presence of a local accumulation of TAG. In light of this knowledge, the localization of the studied AT depot may seem an advantage.

Methodologic Criticism

The in vivo technique for the study of human AT metabolism is based on the application of the Fick principle, which says that net substrate balance in a tissue can be assessed by measurements of arteriovenous concentration differences $(C_a - C_v)$ and blood flow (BF):

$$\text{Net balance} = BF\,(C_a - C_v)$$

The determination of each of these three variables is subject to methodologic problems, which should be taken into consideration when applying the method at any given tissue. The general drawback of the present in vivo method is the fact that each of the three variables is not directly measured but is estimated based on certain assumptions. I am not convinced that these have been dealt with sufficiently by Frayn and his co-workers.

Blood Flow Determination by Xenon Clearance

The determination of the AT blood flow (ATBF) or perfusion coefficient (ml per min per 100 g tissue) is based on the xenon clearance method, in which the fractional washout (k) is multiplied by the AT/blood partition coefficient for xenon (λ):

$$\text{ATBF} = \text{Perfusion coefficient (ml/min/100 g)} = \lambda \cdot k \cdot 100$$

The xenon method has certain advantages for use in AT, the most important being its high lipid solubility. It allows that the washout from a depot can be followed for extended periods without injection of a new isotope during the experiment. It is a major disadvantage that the tissue/blood partition coefficient is unknown and that it is highly dependent on the lipid content of each individual AT depot. The AT lipid content is subject to a considerable regional and interindividual variation as well. The partition coefficient can probably not be determined in vivo (1), so its calculation must rely on chemical analyses of biopsies or autopsies of AT and subsequent calculation of λ. Traditionally, a fixed value of 10 ml/g has been employed (2), but this value has been shown to be too high for most depots (3). In rat brown AT, the value was found to be as low as 3.6 ml/g (4), and in human perirenal AT, the lipid content varied from 29% to 90%, giving λ values from 3.7 to 10.5 ml/g (5). Most of the interindividual variation in the perirenal λ could probably be explained by differences in body fatness. The λ of the interscapular subcutaneous AT was found to be 7.6 ml/g (6), and in abdominal and thigh subcutaneous AT, the λ-value was found to be 8.2 ± 1.2 (3). However, good correlations have been found between the individual skinfold thickness and the subcutaneous blood partition coefficient, suggesting that a partition coefficient should be given on an individual basis to reduce the error on the calculated ATBF. Actually, more than 50% of the variation in λ can be accounted for by differences in skinfold thickness (3), and it is possible that this figure can be further increased by introducing the waist-hip circumference ratio in the prediction equation.

When addressing questions about relative changes in blood flow and substrate balances, information about the partition coefficient is not necessary. By contrast, the λ value used is critical when assessing the contribution of AT to the whole-body disposal of, for instance, TAG (7). Frayn has generally taken λ as 10 ml/g, which I think is at least 15% to 20% too high. This may cause an overestimation of ATBF of similar magnitude and hence of substrate uptakes and releases, as well as the AT contribution to whole-body metabolism.

Imperfect Arterialization of Venous Blood

To avoid arterial cannulation it has been increasingly common to use arterialization of venous blood by inserting the cannula retrogradingly into a hand vein and then to heat the hand either by hot air or by a heating blanket. It is well established that arterial concentrations of blood gases (8) and glucose (9) cannot be entirely achieved by these methods, but the errors associated with this approximation are generally considered small. However, when the arteriovenous concentration differences are assessed, the degree of arterialization may become crucial.

Frayn and coworkers have used hot air to obtain arterialized venous blood, and this method has been shown to cause less reflectory cardiovascular disturbance than the warming blanket (10). However, the oxygen saturations obtain by Frayn et al. have been of the order of 95% after exclusion of subjects with values of 93% and below (7). The directly measured arterial oxygen saturation in respiratory healthy subjects is very stable and lies within a narrow range of 96% to 99% (11). In the superficial abdominal veins draining the AT, the median oxygen saturation was 90.8% (7), so the oxygen uptake of the AT may be underestimated by 30%. More reasonable estimates of AT and forearm oxygen uptakes would be obtained by assuming a fixed arterial oxygen saturation value of 97% to 98% for the calculations. Clearly, a similar assumption cannot be granted for metabolites and hormones. The arterialized blood concentrations have been shown to be lower than arterial levels for glucose and insulin, and the extraction increases during hyperinsulinemia (12), a condition also present in a number of the studies by Frayn et al. in which both AT and forearm balances were assessed. It seems impossible to make corrections for the error of imperfect arterialization of venous blood, but it may result in a trend to underestimate the net balance across both the AT and the forearm.

Assessment of Local Venous Blood Concentrations

Heating the hand for arterialization of venous blood may be associated with other drawbacks. It is well known that heating the hand induces vasodilation and increased blood flow in other regions far removed from the stimulus. We found that heating the contralateral hand increased forearm AT blood flow and decreased skeletal muscle blood flow, thereby facilitating mixing of superficial blood with deep venous blood (11). Contralateral heating increased oxygen saturation in the deep vein draining forearm muscles and abolished the decrease found after an oral glucose load (11). Although Gallen and Macdonald recently showed that using hot air for hand heating had less effect on core and skin temperatures and on skin blood flow, their results suggested that both methods had pronounced effects on contralateral forearm blood flow and on forearm deep venous oxygen saturation (10). The calculated forearm oxygen consumption is highly dependent on the deep oxygen saturation, and these studies showed that contamination with superficial blood with a high oxygen saturation occurs during hand heating.

The implications for the techniques employed by Frayn et al. are obvious for the forearm studies, but it cannot be excluded that blood draining skin or muscle may be mixed with the venous blood draining the AT during heating.

It may also be difficult to draw significant amounts of blood from the small abdominal veins without causing a retrograde mixing of blood from the larger veins draining sites other than the AT. Simonsen et al. have recently shown that repeated withdrawal of 10 ml of blood from the deep forearm vein caused the oxygen concentration to increase by 16% and the carbon dioxide concentration to decrease by 3% (13).

Conclusion

A number of methodologic difficulties may cause incorrect determinations of each of the variables in the Fick equation, which is used for the calculation of net tissue uptake and release of substrates and metabolites. The use of a too high λ value may give rise to an overestimation of the balance, whereas the imperfect arterialization of venous blood combined with the mixing of venous blood from other sources to the local venous drainage may result in an underestimation of the arteriovenous extraction. Consequently, it is difficult to predict to what extent the errors may cause incorrect quantitative estimates. However, in future research more effort should be put into studies clarifying the importance of these methodologic problems.

REFERENCES

1. Jelnes R, Astrup A, Bülow J. The double isotope technique for in vivo determination of the tissue-to-blood partition coefficient for xenon in human subcutaneous adipose tissue—an evaluation. *Scand J Clin Lab Invest* 1985;45:565–8.
2. Larsen OA, Lassen NA, Quaade F. Blood flow through human adipose tissue determined with radioactive xenon. *Acta Physiol Scand* 1966;66:337–45.
3. Bülow J, Jelnes R, Astrup A, Madsen J, Vilman P. Tissue/blood partition coefficients for xenon in various adipose tissue depots in man. *Scand J Clin Lab Invest* 1987;47:1–3.
4. Astrup A, Bülow J, Madsen J. Interscapular brown adipose tissue blood flow in the rat. Determination with 133-Xenon clearance compared to the microsphere method. *Pflügers Arch* 1984;401:414–17.
5. Astrup A, Bülow J, Masen J, Christensen NJ. Contribution of brown adipose tissue and skeletal muscle to thermogenesis induced by ephedrine in man. *Am J Physiol* 1985;248:E507–15.
6. Astrup A, Bülow J, Christensen NJ, Madsen J. Ephedrine-induced thermogenesis in man: no role for interscapular brown adipose tissue. *Clin Sci* 1984;64:179–86.
7. Coppack SW, Fisher RM, Gibbons GF, et al. Postprandial substrate deposition in human forearm and adipose tissues in vivo. *Clin Sci* 1990;79:339–48.
8. Forster HV, Dempsey JA, Thomsen J, Vidruk E, doPico GA. Estimation of arterial P_{O_2}, P_{CO_2}, pH, and lactate from arterialized venous blood. *J Appl Physiol* 1972;32:134–7.
9. McGuire EAH, Helderman JH, Tobin JD, Andres R, Berman M. Effects of arterial versus venous sampling on analysis of glucose kinetics in man. *J Appl Physiol* 1976;41:565–73.
10. Gallen IW, Macdonald IA. Effect of two methods of hand heating on body temperature, forearm blood flow, and deep venous oxygen saturation. *Am J Physiol* 1990;259:E639–43.
11. Astrup A, Simonsen L, Bülow J, Christensen NJ. Measurement of forearm oxygen consumption. Role of heating the contralateral hand. *Am J Physiol* 1988;255:E572–78.
12. Krarup T, Nurnberg B, Mikkelsen K, et al. How arterialized is the blood sampled from a superficial hand vein? *Diabetes* 1990;39(suppl. 1):88A (abstract).
13. Simonsen L, Bülow J, Madsen J, Hermansen F, Astrup A. Whole body respiratory quotient in humans. The effect of an oral glucose load. *Metabolism.* [In press].

Energy Metabolism: Tissue Determinants and Cellular Corollaries, edited by J. M. Kinney and H. N. Tucker. Raven Press, Ltd., New York © 1992.

Role of the Sympathetic Nervous System in Obese and Postobese Subjects

*Arne Astrup and †Niels Juel Christensen

Research Department of Human Nutrition, The Royal Veterinary and Agricultural University, 1958 Frederiksberg, Denmark; and †Department of Internal Medicine and Endocrinology, Herlev Hospital, University of Copenhagen, Denmark

The high, and increasing, prevalence of obesity in affluent societies has become a major health problem because obesity is commonly accompanied by complications such as type-2 diabetes, hypertension, and artherosclerosis causing ischemic heart disease and stroke. In spite of a wide variety of treatment programs, the results are modest and unsatisfactory, mainly because of the high relapse rate. It seems reasonable to gain increased insight into the pathophysiology of the disorder in order to improve treatment efficiency.

GENETIC INFLUENCE ON BODY SIZE AND OBESITY

Within the last decade a number of studies have shown that the adult body weight has a strong genetic component. In the earlier Danish adoption study, the weight class of the adult adoptees was strongly related to the body mass index (BMI) of their biologic parents but was unrelated to the BMI of their adoptive parents (1). If one assumes that similarity between monozygotic twins reared apart is due to genetic effects alone, the correlation between members of such pairs may be considered a direct estimate of heritability. By studying the relation between BMI and monozygotic and dizygotic twins reared together or apart, Stunkard et al. have further shown that genetic factors may be the major determinants of BMI. According to their research, genetic factors may account for as much as 70% of the variance in BMI (2,3). By contrast, differences in BMI later in life and childhood environment had little or no influence (2). Although these studies provide evidence for an important genetic effect, they rely on BMI and provide more support for the inheritance of frame size or LBM than for the inheritance of obesity.

In obesity there is evidence for both polygenic and major gene inheritance in the mode of transmission (4). It should be stressed that the results of genetic studies do not mean that differences in dietary and other environmental factors have no effect. It does not mean that obesity is determined at conception, but rather that subjects with the genetically determined predisposition become obese when they are exposed to a particular range of environmental conditions. This implies that the heritable tendencies may be prevented and that they are potentially reversible. The mechanisms by which these genetic factors cause excess weight, however, remain unresolved. The question of which component of energy balance is responsible needs to be answered. Energy balance can be altered toward a positive energy balance by increasing energy intake (e.g., genetic factors determining appetite control); by decreasing EE, or energy expenditure (e.g., a genetically determined lower EE or an increased energy efficiency related to meals and physical activity); or by both.

DETERMINANTS OF HUMAN ENERGY EXPENDITURE

Between 60% and 80% of the total 24-hour EE is represented by basal EE (BEE), which is slightly higher than sleeping EE (SEE). It is well known that within individuals, BEE and SEE are remarkably constant over time: the variations have been reported to be as low as 1% to 2% after correction for variability attributable to the method (5,6). By contrast, even between normal weight subjects, BEE and SEE exhibited interindividual variation of the order of 16% to 20% (6). However, the interindividual variance was reduced to 5% to 6% when EE was adjusted for differences in the most important covariable, LBM, using the method described by Ravussin and Bogardus (7). A substantial proportion of the unexplained variation in BEE is due to inherited differences. After control for differences in LBM, much larger intrapair variance in BEE was found in dizygotic twins than in monozygotic twins (8,9). Further, Bogardus et al. found in Pima Indians that BEE adjusted for differences in LBM varied by 500 kcal/d between families but only by 60 kcal/d within families (10). Differences in LBM accounted for 83% of the variance in BEE, whereas family membership accounted for an additional 11%.

In a follow-up study Ravussin et al. found a markedly higher risk of subsequent weight gain in the subjects with the low adjusted BEE (11). Caucasian babies born of obese mothers were found to have a lower adjusted EE than babies born of normal weight mothers, and this was found to be associated with an increased risk for subsequent development of obesity (12).

Since these studies were reported, much effort has been put into studies to elucidate the genetic components responsible for the variation in BEE. In multiple linear regression analyses, a number of factors have been identified, which can account for some of the variation unexplained by LBM (Fig. 1). A number of studies have shown that body fat mass may explain some of the variance in BEE, even after accounting for differences in LBM (13–15). Although it is not immediately clear how fat mass increases EE, an increase in body fat mass seems to increase protein turnover and, hence, EE (16). Neither can the decline in LBM with increasing age fully account for the lower BEE in the old (10,14,17); endurance training increases BEE independently of differences in body composition (14). We have recently found that in premenopausal women with a wide range of body weights, most of the variance

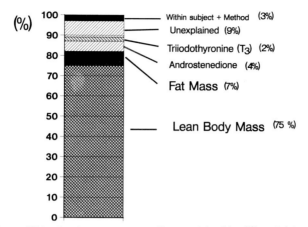

FIG. 1. Variance (%) in sleeping energy expenditure explained by different determinants in pre-menopausal women (15). Triiodothyronine and androstenedione refer to fasting venous plasma concentrations of the two hormones.

in SEE was accounted for by LBM (75%) and fat mass (7%). A further 6% of the variance in SEE was accounted for by differences in plasma concentrations of androstenedione and free T_3 (15). Thus, a total of 88% of the variation in SEE was accounted for by these four covariates (Fig. 1). It is possible that the higher levels of androstenedione in males than in females and the decline in androstenedione and T_3 concentrations with increasing age may be responsible for the sex and age effects found by others. The finding that plasma androstenedione concentration is mainly genetically determined may help explain some of the genetic effect on EE (18).

Consistent with the fact that about 25% of the excess body weight in obese subjects is LBM is the fact that the obese have higher levels of BEE and 24-hour EE. However, when adjusted for differences in body composition (LBM and fat mass), the SEE and BEE of obese subjects have generally been reported to be no different from those of normal weight subjects (13,15,19). Although we found that plasma androstenedione concentration was lower in the obese women then in the normal-weight control group, it did not result in a lower adjusted SEE or BEE in the obese group (15).

SYMPATHETIC ACTIVITY AND BASAL EE

The major physiologic role of the sympathetic nervous system (SNS) is to exert the efferent control of cardiovascular homeostasis via the arterial blood pressure. Posture and physical activity are important stimuli to increase SNS activity, but a basal tone is maintained in the resting, supine condition. It is well known that catecholamines stimulate EE through β-adrenoceptors (20), so baseline SNS activity may contribute with a component of BEE (e.g., arousal, the increment above SEE).

Indeed, a number of studies have reported that acute administration of β-antagonists reduces BEE (21,22), but others have failed (23). The diverging results have been attributed to the heterogeneity of the studied subjects. Alger et al. have reported that β-blockade reduced BEE in Caucasians but not in Pima Indians (24). However, caution should be exercised in drawing extensive conclusions from the positive observations. The study conditions in themselves may be stressful to the experimental subjects (venous cannulation, drug administration, indirect calorimetry, etc.), stressful enough to increase the SNS activity and EE, which does not necessarily result in a concomitant increase in plasma noradrenaline concentration (25). Less stressful experimental conditions using 24-hour measurements in respiration chambers have failed to detect effects of either acute or chronic β-blockade on BEE in nonobese subjects (26,27), whereas a small but significant effect has been found in reduced obese women (26). The apparent reduction in BEE by β-blockade reported by some may be partly artifactual or, at best, the contribution of SNS to BEE must be small.

SYMPATHOADRENAL ACTIVITY, THERMIC EFFECT OF FOOD (TEF), AND 24-HOUR EE

Chronic pharmacologic blockade with β-receptor antagonists has been shown to cause weight gain. Rössner reported a mean weight gain of 2.3 kg after 1 year of propranolol treatment, compared to 1.2 kg in the placebo-treated group (28). This was slightly less than found in previous studies (for review, see ref. 29). However, the entire weight gain has been found to be due to increased fat deposition (29). The β-blockers have not been suspected of stimulating appetite; the change in energy intake required to explain the surplus on daily energy balance is too small to be detectable.

In contrast, there is suggestive evidence for a role of the sympathoadrenal activity in the daily energy expenditure. Thermogenic responses owing to increased sympathoadrenal activity are evoked after stimuli such as cold exposure, stress, and food. Under normal circumstances the thermic effect of food (TEF) seems to be the quantitatively most important phenomenon. TEF can be divided into two components, the specific dynamic action of food, now named obligatory thermogenesis, and a facultative component, which seems to be mediated mainly by the sympathoadrenal system. In particular, carbohydrate intake is accompanied by indications of increased activity of SNS, such as increased heart rate and cardiac output. This can be assessed directly by measurement of sympathetic outflow in human muscle nerves by microneurography (25), by plasma noradrenaline appearance rate, and by plasma noradrenaline concentration (30). The increased SNS activity caused by carbohydrates stimulates thermogenesis via β_1-adrenoceptors (31). After oral carbohydrates the adrenal medulla also contributes with a relatively late enhanced-adrenaline secretion, which is elicited by the postprandial decrease in plasma glucose concentration (32). The major proportion of the facultative thermogenesis mediated by adrenaline was found to take place in skeletal muscle via β_2-receptors (23). TEF has been found to be influenced by several factors, such as the preceding energy balance, age, aerobic capacity, degree of insulin resistance, fat mass, and fat topography. A significant genetic effect in TEF has also been reported (33).

Twenty-four-hour measurement of EE in a respiratory chamber has been a tool for assessment of the quantitative importance of the sympathoadrenal system. Acheson et al. found an insignificant reduction in 24-hour EE by 64 kcal/day after 2 weeks of propranolol treatment (27), and Buemann et al. (26) failed to see any significant effect of propranolol on 24-hour EE in normal subjects (-17 kcal/d, $p > 0.50$). It is likely that in these studies, lack of statistic power owing to the limited number of subjects explains the negative outcome. Alger et al., however, in a study of a rather large number of subjects, found that 24-hour EE correlated with 24-hour urinary noradrenaline in Caucasians independently of LBM, fat mass, age, and sex but that it did not correlate in Pimas (24).

There seems to be good evidence for a facultative component of TEF, however, although there is no agreement in the literature on its contribution to TEF as estimated by pharmacologic inhibition of the sympathoadrenal system (29). One reason may be the many factors influencing TEF, but it also may be significant that in some of the studies that failed to detect an effect of β-blockade, measurement of EE had a too-short duration (29). More systematic studies recognizing all factors affecting TEF are required.

SYMPATHETIC ACTIVITY IN OBESITY

A large number of conflicting studies have been reported on baseline SNS activity and noradrenaline levels in obese subjects compared with normal weight controls. It is possible that increased SNS activity may play a role in hypertension in a subgroup of obese subjects with a family history of hypertension (34,35), but obesity hypertension may be more directly linked to the renal effects of hyperinsulinemia (36,37). Clearly, the inconsistent results may be due to heterogeneity of the subjects (i.e., age and body fat topography) and to poor control of the experimental conditions for factors that influence SNS activity, such as dietary carbohydrate content, sodium intake, smoking, and seasonal variation. Peterson et al. carried out a more extensive study with measurement of several indices of SNS activity (38). They found that SNS activity was inversely correlated with body fat mass (38). We found that plasma noradrenaline concentration was similarly reduced in both simple nondiabetic obese subjects and diabetic obese subjects (39). However, the glucose-induced increase in plasma noradrenaline concentration was normal in the simple obese group but was abolished in the diabetic obese group (39). Fasting noradrenaline concentration correlated inversely with degree of obesity ($r = -0.25$, $p < 0.05$), but multiple linear regression analysis showed that part of the effect of obesity was accounted for by insulin resistance (39). It is possible that enhanced sodium and water retention caused by hyperinsulinemia via a negative feedback mechanism may suppress SNS activity, indicating that the maintenance of cardiovascular homeostasis is altered in obesity.

Obesity has also been reported to be accompanied by a reduced SNS response to carbohydrate (40), cold exposure (41), and exercise (42).

However, as the reduced SNS activity and responsiveness in obese subjects are closely linked to insulin resistance and hyperinsulinemia, it is likely that we are looking at a secondary phenomenon, which may subside after normalization of body composition.

SNS AND TEF IN REDUCED OBESE

Studies in reduced obese and postobese subjects probably give more insight into the mechanisms responsible for the weight gain. The Lausanne group has conducted a number of studies, all indicating that the defective TEF persists in the reduced obese subjects (for review, see ref. 43). We have also found that severely obese patients showed an impaired TEF and a blunted increase in plasma noradrenaline concentration in response to oral glucose (40). After a 30 kg weight loss, their plasma glucose and lipid profile was almost normalized, but the increase in plasma nora-drenaline and the thermogenic response to glucose were still lower than that of the normal weight control group (44). However, both in this and in the study by Golay et al. (45), the reduced obese were still overweight and had insulin resistance com-pared to the control group. In a calorimeter study, Buemann et al. found that reduced obese women fed a high-carbohydrate low-fat diet had 24-hour EE very similar to that of the control group when EE was adjusted for differences in body composition (26). The postprandial EE, however, was found to be significantly lower in the re-duced obese women. It was also found that acute β-blockade reduced 24-hour EE (both BEE and TEF) in the reduced obese but had no effect on the controls (26). These findings indicate that the suppressed SNS activity in obese individuals is of secondary nature, but they also suggest that an abnormality in SNS may contribute to the disease. Despite the evidence of enhanced SNS action, TEF remained lower in the reduced obese subjects, which points to the involvement of factors other than SNS activity as responsible for the impaired TEF. Because TEF has been found to be inversely correlated with both percent body fat ($r = -0.80$) and plasma insulin levels ($r = -0.86$) (19), TEF may thus become normal along with an entire nor-malization of body composition.

24-HOUR EE IN POSTOBESE SUBJECTS

In their classic study in entirely normal weight, postobese women, Geissler et al. found that at three different levels of physical activity, the postobese had a 15% lower 24-hour EE than matched controls (46). This study has been criticized for having a poorly controlled activity program, but a later-reported reanalysis found that BEE was 10% lower and thermogenesis 50% lower in the postobese subjects than in the matched controls (47). McNeill et al. also reported slightly lower 24-hour EE and SEE in postobese women than in matched controls (48). Goldberg et al. measured total free-living EE by doubly labeled water and 24-hour EE in respiratory

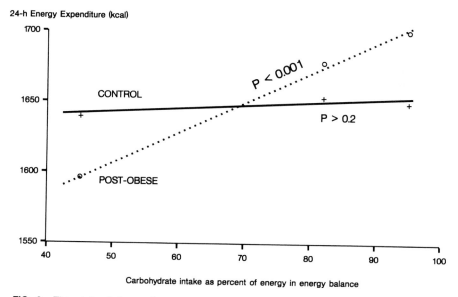

FIG. 2. The relation between dietary carbohydrate intake and 24-hour energy expenditure in post-obese women and matched normal weight controls. Data recalculated from Lean and James (50).

chamber in postobese and matched control (49). They found no difference in EE, independently of method and expression of the data.

The inconsistency of these studies may be explained by going into details in the study by Lean and James, who compared 24-hour EE and substrate utilization in obese, postobese, and normal-weight women (50). These women were studied while being in precise energy balance and consuming two isoenergetic diets, a low-fat diet (3% energy as fat, 82% carbohydrates) and a high-fat diet (40% fat and 45% carbohydrates) (50). In addition, they were studied with the same high-fat diet supplemented with carbohydrates to 150% of energy balance (51). Multiple regression analysis showed a linear relation between carbohydrate intake and 24-hour EE (Fig. 2). There was a significant positive slope in the postobese group, whereas the 24-hour EE was constant and unrelated to dietary carbohydrate intake in the control group (Fig. 2). On the high-carbohydrate diet, 24-hour EE was significantly higher in the postobese group than in the control group, but on the high-fat diet, 24-hour EE was lower in the postobese group. These results demonstrate that postobese and normal controls responded differently to changes in dietary carbohydrate content. Unfortunately, no information about diet composition has been given in most of the studies on postobese subjects (46–49).

SUBSTRATE UTILIZATION IN POSTOBESE SUBJECTS

In the study by Lean and James, striking differences were found in substrate handling by the obese, postobese, and normal weight controls (50). Whereas mean

24-hour RQ was similar in the obese and the control group, it was significantly higher in the postobese group, both during fasting and the high-fat diet. This indicates that the postobese group utilized relatively less fat and more carbohydrate than the control group during fasting and on the high-fat days. How can this finding and the dependency of EE on carbohydrate content in the postobese be explained by a common mechanism? One hypothesis holds that an inappropriate insulin action/sensitivity in response to dietary carbohydrate in the postobese would favor carbohydrate oxidation and suppress lipid oxidation. Further, SNS reactivity may be subject to a similar high sensitivity to dietary carbohydrate, resulting in hyperactivity during high-carbohydrate feeding and hypoactivity during low-carbohydrate feeding. We have recently studied postobese women after being weight stable for 7 to 25 weeks and compared them with controls matched with respect to age, height, weight, and body composition (52). On a standardized diet providing energy from 30% fat, 55% carbohydrates, and 15% protein, 24-hour EE was 11% higher in the postobese than in the controls. The difference was present both during sleep and in the daytime. The higher EE in the postobese was entirely covered by carbohydrate oxidation, which was 25% higher than in the control group. Lipid and protein oxidation were similar in the two groups. Plasma noradrenaline concentration was increased by 50% in the postobese as compared to the control group, and in a multiple regression analysis, noradrenaline levels accounted for 65% of the variance in 24-hour EE and explained the entire difference between the two groups. These results are in accordance with those reported by Lean and James (51), except that our postobese were responsive to a diet containing less carbohydrate than reported in their study. This difference may be explained by our postobese women being leaner and thus more insulin sensitive. Jung et al. reported an altered seasonal variation in SNS activity of obese and postobese women compared to normal weight controls (53). The obese and postobese women had lower plasma noradrenaline concentrations in the summer, but in the winter they had significantly higher levels than the control subjects (53). During the winter months the postobese subjects were noted to increase their body weight by 2.7 kg (53), which may be due to the well-described fall-winter changes in eating behavior with carbohydrate craving (54). Consequently, the seasonal fluctuations in plasma noradrenaline concentration may reflect variations in SNS activity imposed by dietary carbohydrate content.

The Phoenix group recently reported that in Pima Indians fed a standard diet, family membership was the principal determinant of the ratio of fat to carbohydrate oxidation (55). Furthermore, a low ratio of fat-to-carbohydrate oxidation predicted subsequent weight gain independent of low EE (55). The background for the altered substrate utilization in postobese may also be a lower proportion of slow type-1 muscle fibers utilizing fatty acids for oxidation and a higher proportion of the glycolytic fast (type-2) fibers (56).

CONCLUSION

The available knowledge may suggest that obesity is an inherited disorder associated with an altered proportion of carbohydrate/lipid oxidation rates and an abnormal SNS reactivity to dietary carbohydrate. There is evidence suggesting that the body is not "energy blind." Thus, when challenged with a typical Western high-fat diet unmatched to their metabolic requirements, EE may be suppressed, an increased proportion of the dietary fat may be stored, and the faster depletion of carbohydrate stores may stimulate appetite. According to Flatt, the development of obesity induces insulin resistance, which reduces the rate of carbohydrate oxidation and increases lipid oxidation (57). The enlargement of the adipose tissue stores raises the circulating levels of non-esterified fatty acids, which in turn enhance lipid oxidation until it is commensurate with the fat content of the diet. This concept explains the obese state as being a compensatory mechanism by which we adjust our metabolism to the high-fat content of the diet.

ACKNOWLEDGMENTS

We thank John Lind, Inge Timmermann, Lene Kristiansen, Tina Cuthbertson, Inger-Lise Grønfeldt, Kaare Jacobsen, Ole Victor, Benjamin Buemann, and Grete Thorbek for their contribution to our studies. The constructive criticism provided by Flemming Quaade was much appreciated. Our studies were supported by the Danish Veterinary and Agricultural Research Council (13-4268), the Danish Medical Research Council (12-9537), and P. Carl Petersens Foundation.

REFERENCES

1. Stunkard AJ, Sørensen TIA, Hanis C, et al. An adoption study of human obesity. *N Engl J Med* 1986;314:193–8.
2. Stunkard AJ, Harris JR, Pedersen NL, McClearn GE. The body-mass index of twins who have been reared apart. *N Engl J Med* 1990;322:1483–7.
3. Macdonald A, Stunkard AJ. Body-mass indexes of British separated twins. *N Engl J Med* 1990; 322:1530.
4. Price RA, Ness R, Laskarzewski P. Common major gene inheritance of extreme overweight. *Hum Biol* 1990;62:747–65.
5. Garby L, Lammert O. Within subjects between days and weeks variation in energy expenditure at rest. *Hum Nutr Clin Nutr* 1984;38C:395–7.
6. Astrup A, Thorbek G, Lind J, Isaksson B. Prediction of 24-h energy expenditure and its components from physical characteristics and body composition in normal-weight humans. *Am J Clin Nutr* 1990; 52:777–83.
7. Ravussin E, Bogardus C. Relationship of genetics, age, and physical fitness to daily energy expenditure and fuel utilization. *Am J Clin Nutr* 1989;49:968–75.
8. Henry CJK, Piggott SM, Rees DG, Priestley L, Sykes B. Basal metabolic rate in monozygotic and dizygotic twins. *Eur J Clin Nutr* 1990;44:717–23.
9. Bouchard C, Tremblay A, Nadeau A, Després JP. Genetic effect in resting and exercise metabolic rates. *Metabolism* 1989;38:364–70.
10. Bogardus C, Lillioja S, Ravussin E, et al. Familial dependence of the resting metabolic rate. *N Engl J Med* 1986;315:96–100.
11. Ravussin E, Lillioja S, Knowler WC, et al. Reduced rate of energy expenditure as a risk factor for body-weight gain. *N Engl J Med* 1988;318:467–72.
12. Roberts SB, Savage S, Coward WA, Chew B, Lucas A. Energy expenditure and intake in infants born to lean and overweight mothers. *N Engl J Med* 1988;318:461–6.
13. Freymond D, Larson K, Bogardus C, Ravussin E. Energy expenditure during normo- and overfeeding in peripubertal children of lean and obese Pima Indians. *Am J Physiol* 1989;257:E647–53.

14. Poelhman ET, McAuliffe TL, Van Houten DR, Danforth E. Influence of age and endurance training on metabolic rate and hormones in healthy men. *Am J Physiol* 1990;259:E66–72.
15. Astrup A, Buemann B, Christensen NJ, et al. The contribution of body composition and thermogenic hormones to the variability in energy expenditure and substrate utilization in premenopausal women. *J Clin Endocrinol Metab* (in press).
16. Welle S, Nair KS. Relationship of resting metabolic rate to body composition and protein turnover. *Am J Physiol* 1990;258:E990–8.
17. Fukagawa NK, Bandini LG, Young JB. Effect of age on body composition and resting metabolic rate. *Am J Physiol* 1990;259:E233–8.
18. Parker L, Lifrak E, Shively J, Soon-Shiong P. Control of adrenal androgen secretion. In: Lardy H, Stratman F, eds. *Hormones, thermogenesis, and obesity*. New York: Elsevier, 1989;355–63.
19. Segal KR, Lacayanga I, Dunaif A, et al. Impact of body fat mass and percent fat on metabolic rate and thermogenesis in men. *Am J Physiol* 1989;256:E573–9.
20. Macdonald IA, Bennet T, Fellows IW. Catecholamines and control of metabolism in man. *Clin Sci* 1985;68:613–9.
21. Christin L, Ravussin E, Bogardus C, Howard BV. The effect of propranolol on free fatty acid mobilization and resting metabolic rate. *Metabolism* 1989;38:439–44.
22. Vernet O, Nacht CA, Christin L. β-Adrenergic blockade and intravenous nutrient-induced thermogenesis in lean and obese women. *Am J Physiol* 1987;253:E65–71.
23. Astrup A, Simonsen L, Bülow J, Madsen J, Christensen NJ. Epinephrine mediates facultative carbohydrate-induced thermogenesis in human skeletal muscle. *Am J Physiol* 1989;257:E340–5.
24. Alger S, Saad MF, Zurlo F, et al. Symapthetic nervous system (SNS) contribution to energy expenditure. *Int J Obesity* 1990;14(2):38 (abst).
25. Hjemdahl P, Fagius J, Freyschuss U, et al. Muscle sympathetic activity and norepinephrine release during mental challenge in humans. *Am J Physiol* 1989;257:E654–64.
26. Buemann B, Astrup A, Christensen NJ. A 24-hour energy expenditure study on reduced-obese and non-obese women. The effect of beta-blockade. *Am J Clin Nutr* (in press).
27. Acheson KJ, Ravussin E, Schoeler DA, et al. Two-week stimulation or blockade of the sympathetic nervous system in man: influence on body weight, body composition, and twenty four-hour energy expenditure. *Metabolism* 1988;37:91–8.
28. Rössner S, Taylor CL, Byington RP, et al. Long term propranolol treatment and changes in body weight after myocardial infarction. *Br Med J* 1990;300:902–3.
29. Astrup A, Christensen NJ, Simonsen L, Bülow J. Effects of nutrient intake on sympathoadrenal activity and thermogenic mechanisms. *J Neurosci Methods* 1990;34:187–92.
30. Christensen NJ. Methods of studying sympathoadrenal activity in man. *Acta Med Scand* 1988; 223:481–3.
31. Thorin D, Golay A, Simonsen DC, et al. The effect of selective beta-adrenergic blockade on glucose-induced thermogenesis in man. *Metabolism* 1986;35:524–8.
32. Astrup A, Bülow J, Christensen NJ, Madsen J, Quaade F. Facultative thermogenesis induced by carbohydrate. A skeletal muscle component mediated by epinephrine. *Am J Physiol* 1986;250: E226–9.
33. Bouchard C, Tremblay A. Genetic effects in human energy expenditure components. *Int J Obesity* 1990;14:49–55.
34. Rocchini AP, Key J, Bondie D, et al. The effect of weight loss on the sensitivity of blood pressure to sodium in obese adolescents. *N Engl J Med* 1989;321:580–5.
35. Egan BM, Schork NJ, Weder AB. Regional hemodynamic abnormalities in overweight men. Focus on α-adrenergic vascular responses. *Am J Hypertens* 1989;2:428–34.
36. Reduction of blood pressure in obese hyperinsulinaemic hypertensive patients during somatostatin infusion. *J Hypertens* 1989;7:S196–7.
37. Pollare T, Lithell H, Berne C. Insulin resistance is a characteristic feature of primary hypertension independent of obesity. *Metabolism* 1990;39:167–74.
38. Peterson H, Rothschild M, Weinberg CR. Body fat and the activity of the autonomic nervous system. *N Engl J Med* 1988;318:1077–83.
39. Astrup A, Christensen NJ, Breum L. Reduced plasma noradrenaline concentrations in simple-obese and diabetic obese patients. *Clin Sci* 1991;80:53–8.
40. Astrup A, Andersen T, Henriksen O. Impaired glucose-induced thermogenesis in skeletal muscle in obesity. The role of the sympathoadrenal system. *Int J Obesity* 1987;11:51–67.
41. Astrup A, Simonsen L, Bülow J, Christensen NJ. The contribution of skeletal muscle to carbohydrate-induced thermogenesis in man: the role of the sympathoadrenal system. In: Lardy H, Stratman F, eds. *Hormones, thermogenesis and obesity*. New York: Elsevier, 1989;187–96.

42. Gustafson AB, Farrell PA, Kalkhoff RK. Impaired plasma catecholamine response to submaximal treadmill exercise in obese women. *Metabolism* 1990;39:410–7.
43. Jequier E. Energy metabolism in obese patients before and after weight loss, and in patients who have relapsed. *Int J Obesity* 1990;14:59–64.
44. Astrup A, Andersen T, Christensen NJ, Henriksen J, Quaade F. Impaired glucose-induced thermogenesis and arterial norepinephrine response persist after weight reduction in human obesity. *Am J Clin Nutr* 1990;51:331–7.
45. Golay A, Schutz Y, Felber JP, Jallut D, Jéquier E. Blunted glucose-induced thermogenesis in "overweight" patients: a factor contributing to relapse of obesity. *Int J Obesity* 1989;13:767–75.
46. Geissler CA, Miller DS, Shah M. The daily metabolic rate of the post-obese and the lean. *Am J Clin Nutr* 1987;45:14–20.
47. Shah M, Miller DS, Geissler CA. Lower metabolic rates of post-obese versus lean women: thermogenesis, basal metabolic rate and genetics. *Eur J Clin Nutr* 1988;42:741–52.
48. McNeill G, Bukkens SGF, Morrison DC, Smith JS. Energy intake and energy expenditure in post-obese women and weight-matched controls. *Proc Nutr Soc* 1990;49:14A.
49. Goldberg GR, Black AE, Prentice AM, Coward WA. No evidence of lower energy expenditure in post-obese women. *Proc Nutr Soc* 1990. [In press].
50. Lean MEJ, James WPT. Metabolic effects of isoenergetic nutrient exchange over 24 hours in relation to obesity in women. *Int J Obesity* 1988;12:15–27.
51. Lean MEJ. Current status of research: why do people get fat? In: James WPT, Parker SW, eds. *Obesity—current approaches*. Southampton: Duphar Medical Relations, 1988;1–12.
52. Astrup A, Buemann B, Christensen NJ, et al. 24-hour energy expenditure and sympathetic activity in post-obese women consuming a high carbohydrate diet. *Am J Physiol* (in press).
53. Jung RT, Shetty PS, James WPT, et al. Plasma catecholamines and autonomic responsiveness in obesity. *Int J Obesity* 1982;6:131–41.
54. Rosenthal NE, Genhart M, Jacobsen FM, et al. Disturbances of appetite and weight regulation in seasonal affective disorder. In: Wurtman RJ, Wurtman JJ, eds. *Human obesity. Ann N Y Acad Sci* 1987;499:216–30.
55. Zurlo F, Lillioja S, Puente AE-D, et al. Low ratio of fat to carbohydrate oxidation as predictor of weight gain: study of 24-h RQ. *Am J Physiol* 1990;259:E650–7.
56. Wade AJ, Marbut MM, Round JM. Muscle fiber type and aetiology of obesity. *Lancet* 1990;335: 805–8.
57. Flatt JP. Differences in the regulation of carbohydrate and fat metabolism and their implications for body weight maintenance. In: Lardy H, Stratman F, eds. *Hormones, thermogenesis and obesity*. New York: Elsevier, 1989;3–18.

DISCUSSION

Dr. Macdonald: It has been proposed many times in recent years that reduced thermogenesis may contribute to the development and maintenance of obesity. Studies in experimental animals have revealed a variety of nutritional and metabolic factors that can alter the activity of the sympathetic nervous system and affect energy expenditure. This has led to the proposition that sympathetic nervous control of thermogenesis may be an important means of regulating energy balance. Such a hypothesis gains support from studies of genetically obese rodents, which appear to have impaired thermogenesis and reduced sympathetic control of their major thermogenic organs. There is extensive evidence in support of a sympathetic nervous control of thermogenesis in the regulation of body temperature in rodents.

These demonstrations of an important role for the sympathetic nervous system in the control of thermogenesis in experimental animals has led to great interest in the possibility that similar effects may occur in humans. It was suggested from the early studies of Neumann (1) that energy expenditure in humans may alter as an adaptation to changes in energy intake to minimize the disturbance of energy balance. The term "luxuskonsumption" was used to describe this phenomenon. This idea was largely ignored until the 1960s, when studies by

Miller and Munford (2) and Sims et al. (3) showed that experimental overfeeding of healthy nonobese subjects was accompanied by far less weight gain than had been predicted. This was explained by the occurrence of luxuskonsumption during overfeeding. These experiments stimulated vigorous debate at the time and led to many attempts to repeat and extend the studies in order either to refute or to further explain the phenomenon. Further review of this topic is beyond the scope of this commentary, but it was this proposed control of energy expenditure to regulate energy balance that stimulated interest in the possible involvement of the sympathetic nervous system. Together with the reduced energy expenditure and sympathetic activity in genetically obese rodents, this led to the hypothesis that impaired sympathetic control of thermogenesis may contribute to obesity in humans. However, studying the development of obesity in humans is restricted to investigations of the Pima Indians, who are not representative of the majority of obese patients. Thus, the rationale behind the approach of Drs. Astrup and Christensen is to study patients when obese, and then after they have lost weight, to establish whether they display features of altered sympathetic nervous activity or reduced thermogenic responsiveness in either state.

Astrup and Christensen make the important point that the studies of body weight and obesity in monozygotic and dizygotic twins show a more impressive inheritance of frame size or lean body mass (LBM), than of obesity itself. Furthermore, in most cases of human obesity, any genetic component is likely to be a predisposition to developing obesity in the appropriate environmental circumstances and should not be equated with the genetic obesity in rats and mice.

In considering the determinants of resting energy expenditure, it is apparent that the lean body mass of an individual is the most important factor. Correcting for lean body mass reduces substantially the variability between individuals. The magnitude of this effect depends on the group of subjects studied and is a potential source of confusion when comparing studies. For example, a study of nonobese subjects in a respiration chamber on a fixed activity pattern showed LBM accounting for 91% of the variance in basal energy expenditure (4). In contrast, studies in nonobese and obese Pima Indians revealed LBM accounting for only 83% of the variance in basal energy expenditure. The summary diagram from one of their recent studies, the first figure presented by Astrup and Christensen, shows only 75% of the variance in sleeping energy expenditure accounted for by LBM. It is likely that some of the confusion in the literature arises from the fact that some investigators use estimated LBM, whereas other use fat-free mass. The two are of course not identical, because the latter includes the cytoplasm from adipocytes and the nonadipocyte material in adipose tissue. Astrup and Christensen also draw attention to recent suggestions that basal energy expenditure may be influenced by an individual's fat mass (possibly through an increase in protein turnover) and that aging is accompanied by parallel reductions in LBM and basal energy expenditure. These factors may fully account for the variations in prediction of resting energy expenditure from the various elements of body composition. However, one point that is also worthy of consideration is the extent to which body composition is a continuum from very low to very high percentage body fat content. The underlying assumption in all of the attempts to account for interindividual variations in energy expenditure on the basis of LBM, body fat, age, gender, etc., holds that leanness and obesity are part of the same continuum. However, any fundamental differences between the extremes, or interaction between contributing factors in one extreme but not the other, would produce weaker predictive relationships when studying groups with markedly differing body composition. Until such possibilities are refuted, one should be cautious in attempting to account for differences in energy expenditure between obese and nonobese subjects on the basis of differences in body composition.

There have been numerous attempts to demonstrate effects of the sympathetic nervous system on basal energy expenditure by administering β-adrenoceptor antagonists in order to block any catecholamine-induced thermogenesis. Astrup and Christensen point out that the studies that have administered such drugs acutely and seen a fall in energy expenditure have often involved very invasive procedures, which may have increased the level of sympathetic activity. In contrast, the studies involving chronic oral dosing with these drugs and minimal invasive procedures have generally failed to see any alteration in energy expenditure. However, some caution is needed in interpreting these studies because the β-adrenoceptor antagonists are competitive drugs, with different acute and chronic effects, and it is well established that higher doses have to be used to reduce the metabolic effects of catecholamines compared to the cardiovascular effects. Furthermore, the studies with obese patients who have lost weight have shown that in most cases the patients were still overweight and had insulin resistance. Thus, the absence of normal thermogenic and sympathetic nervous responses is not convincing evidence that defective sympathetic stimulation of thermogenesis is an underlying contributor to the development of obesity. Astrup and Christensen suggest that complete normalization of body weight and composition may lead to normal thermogenic responses to food. However, the study they cite as evidence for this proposal compared overweight and normal subjects in showing that the thermogenic response to food was negatively correlated with body fat and plasma insulin levels. One would need to show such a relationship in the same individuals before and after normalization of body weight in order to have convincing evidence for this hypothesis.

The most intriguing aspect of Astrup and Christensen's work is the differences in substrate oxidation observed between postobese and control subjects. The indication is that the postobese had lower rates of fat oxidation than control subjects during fasting or a high-fat diet. By contrast, the postobese were more responsive to an increased carbohydrate intake, showing a rise in plasma noradrenaline concentration and in 24-hour energy expenditure. Although it is possible that such differences in substrate utilization may be related to alterations in muscle fiber type in obesity (and thus in the postobese), it would be most dangerous to use the study of Wade et al. (5) as supporting evidence. That study purported to show a reduction in type-1 muscle fibers (which are slow and oxidative and predominantly utilize fatty acids) with increasing fatness. However, the highest percent body fat in their subjects was 20%, and the study failed to control for the age of the subjects or the relative work intensity. The latter is particularly important, because using the same absolute work load (as the authors did) would be more demanding for those with a lower maximum aerobic capacity and would require a higher rate of carbohydrate oxidation.

On the basis of the evidence currently available, the postobese do seem to have altered patterns of substrate utilization and of sympathetic nervous system response to nutrient intake. This may have important implications not only for helping such patients maintain their reduced weight, but also for understanding the development of obesity.

REFERENCES

1. Neumann RO. Experimentelle Beitrage zur lehre von den taglichen nahrungsbedarf des menschen unter besonderer. Berusksich tigung der notwendigen einweissmenge. *Arch Hyg* 1902;45:1–87.
2. Miller DS, Munford P, Gluttony I. An experimental study of overeating low or high protein diets. *Am J Clin Nutr* 1967;20:1212–22.

3. Sims EAA, Danforth E, Horton ES, et al. Endocrine and metabolic effects in experimental obesity in man. *Recent Prog Horm Res* 1979;29:457–96.
4. Astrup A, Thorbek G, Lind J, Isaksson B. Prediction of 24 h energy expenditure and its components from physical characteristics and body composition in normal weight humans. *Am J Clin Nutr* 1990; 52:777–83.
5. Wade AJ, Marbut MM, Round JM. Muscle fibre type and aetiology of obesity. *Lancet* 1990;335: 805–8.

Energy Metabolism: Tissue Determinants and Cellular Corollaries, edited by J. M. Kinney and H. N. Tucker. Raven Press, Ltd., New York © 1992.

Overview: Neurohormonal Influences on Thermogenesis

W. P. T. James

Rowett Research Institute, Aberdeen, United Kingdom

The magnitude of thermogenesis and its control have been of interest since studies by the Japanese of the seasonal cycling of the basal metabolic rate (BMR) demonstrated the potential for environmental stimuli enhancing the metabolic rate (1). Thereafter, Cuthbertson (2) studied the magnitude and nature of the metabolic response to trauma and other stresses, but it was some time before the distinction between physiologic responses to cold, diet, and hormonal changes and the pathologic responses to infection and trauma was accepted as appropriate. Even now, however, it remains unclear to what extent the response to pathologic change reflects the induction of new regulatory and effector mechanisms in addition to a stimulation of the normal physiologic processes.

The maximum physiologic range in thermogenesis rarely achieves more than an increase of 30% above the BMR. This increase was occasionally seen in the early cyclical studies on seasonal changes in BMR, but Jessen's studies on cooling curarized men showed increases of only about 10% (3). This implies that greater adaptive seasonal changes in thermogenic capacity could be involved if there were long-term entraining of some thermogenic organ or a rebalancing of the neural control of thermogenesis. Adaptive inductions of thermogenesis were demonstrated in Canadian cooling studies (4) and Korean divers habituating to the cold (5). A rise of 20% is also evident when subjects are tested by infusions of catecholamines (6,7) at levels that may not necessarily reflect the true concentration of neurotransmitters at the effector sites under normal circumstances. Nevertheless, these studies, the recent demonstration that dietary spices can also lead to a 25% increase in BMR (8), and the 40% increase in BMR on sustained forced overfeeding with sucrose and other carbohydrates (33% of excess intake) (9) suggest that these are the usual limits of thermogenesis even if the mechanisms involved differ.

These physiologic responses seem very different from the enhancement of metabolic rate in severely traumatized, burned, or infected humans, in whom the release of metabolites, cytokines, and the other mediators in inflammatory responses seem dominant. With the rise of core temperature, one can then expect a general enhancement of the metabolic rate of all those organs which achieve similar increases in cellular temperature. These changes probably occur in addition to the stress responses, which involve the induction of specific (e.g., sympathomimetic) responses. However, the distinction between physiologic and pathologic thermogenesis cannot be based on the failure to induce a rise in core temperature in the former with this as the hallmark of pathology because the menstrual cycle rhythmicity of metabolic rate is closely linked to the resetting of core temperature (10). Ravussin has also recently linked the interindividual differences in metabolic rate to the different settings of core temperature in different subjects (11).

Rothwell has documented many of the peripheral and central signals for the induction of thermogenesis via neurohumoral mechanisms. These signals do not reflect the only mechanisms for inducing the thermogenesis in response to diet, because nutrients can have direct peripheral substrate-inducing effects on organ metabolism. These peripheral responses may account for a substantial part of the effects of overfeeding in humans. Ravussin noted that only 25% of the 24-hour energy expenditure remained unaccounted for once he had assigned costs to the need to move in the chamber and to the synthetic process for storing the ingested nutrients (12) during a 9-day overfeeding period. This carefully controlled study may be taken to suggest that diet has little effect on special induced mechanisms of thermogenesis, but such a conclusion is readily discarded once the analyses presented by Macdonald and Astrup in this book are considered.

Macdonald summarizes our current understanding of sympathetic activity in humans and how it is affected by diet. Attempts to analyze sympathetic activity by studying peripherally monitored noradrenaline turnover is attractive, but the clear demonstration that noradrenaline turnover alters proportionately to neuronal firing would be surprising with the multiplicity of sympathetic effector pathways and their differential modulation of blood flow and cellular activity. Thus, Macdonald emphasizes that tissue turnover is an index only of the level of sympathetic nervous system activity to that tissue and that the organs' differential responses will all be collated in any circulatory monitoring of noradrenaline turnover by isotopic techniques. Wallin's studies of sympathetic nerve firing rates and their increase in response to glucose feeding provide one of the first attempts to link dietary responses in humans with direct sympathetic monitoring (13). Macdonald notes the changes in circulating noradrenaline turnover on overfeeding and underfeeding (14), findings that we have confirmed. But the links between the responses to cooling and to diet, so readily demonstrable in animal studies, have had limited attention in humans. Macdonald shows that short-term starvation alters the ability of the body to resist central cooling; the intake of some food seems to enhance the thermogenic responsiveness, which is seemingly dependent on the maintenance of afferent sensitivity rather than the effectiveness of the thermogenic mechanisms. This work may concur with the surprising findings of Brundin and Wahren (15), who note that dietary thermogenesis seems to depend on the splanchnic heat exchange induced by feeding. Thus, abdominal insulation enhances hepatic vein temperatures after a meal and reduces overall body metabolism, particularly in the periphery. We may therefore be returning to consider the detail of heat exchange within the body and how this affects the central control of body temperature through vasoconstrictor and thermogenic mechanisms. If there are hepatic temperature sensors as well as metabolic sensors potentially relating to appetite control (16), then the continued ingestion of food seems to maintain the afferent sensing system. Upregulation of this sensing system may occur on semistarvation because Shetty and Kurpad have shown that undernourished Indians have an enhanced thermogenic response to a standard meal (17). The tissue responsiveness to standard infusions of noradrenaline can also be upregulated or downregulated within 15 to 30 minutes of changing the stimulus. The reduced basal metabolism of energy-restricted subjects is also partly attributable to reductions in sympathetic nervous activity, which Shetty has monitored by pupillometric responsiveness and by blood pressure responses to sustained isometric exercise rather than by direct neural recording. Thus, we need to develop further the studies that have allowed subjects to be monitored under precisely controlled conditions of nutritional state, environmental temperature, and diet. Meticulous attention to detail is important if we are to obtain clear evidence of the small changes in metabolic rate linked to alterations in autonomic control and organ metabolism. Only then can short-term effects be discriminated from more long-term adaptive changes.

Astrup describes carefully conducted studies that begin to reveal differences between individual patient responses to specific nutrient groups such as carbohydrates. His concern about the different results of selective β-adrenergic blockade is important. The use of glucose clamp techniques and propranolol infusions to assess the dietary-induced thermogenic response attributable to sympathetic activation may, I believe, be a mistake because not only is the substrate infused rather than given orally but the infusion rate to the periphery may be very different from normal. Nevertheless, the fall in metabolic rate after propranolol is likely to reflect β-adrenergic activity per se, whereas our use of chronic propranolol feeding to reduce the metabolic rate includes the effect of propranolol in reducing thyroxine to triiodothyronine conversion (18). Astrup makes much of the differences in respiratory quotient (RQ) in postobese subjects and links this with Flatt's hypothesis (19) that a diet rich in fat with a lower food quotient (FQ) will enhance energy storage because there is a discrepancy between the low food quotient and the higher (RQ) of the subjects. The concept holds that the higher RQ of postobese subjects signifies a greater rate of carbohydrate oxidation, so the drive to eat may be greater on a low-FQ, high-fat diet as people seek to satisfy their carbohydrate needs. Our own paper (20) did indeed highlight the importance of the differential response of postobese individuals to carbohydrate feeding, but we were more cautious in interpreting the data because we already had subsequently published evidence (21) that RQ does vary between individuals on a standard diet and that the fasting RQ takes several days to respond to an altered nutrient balance in the diet. The higher RQ of postobese subjects may then reflect their having responded to advice to consume a low-fat, high-carbohydrate diet. Nevertheless, Flatt's hypothesis is attractive, and if true, then interindividual differences in fasting RQ may predict behavior, notwithstanding the truism that FQ and 24-hour RQ must be the same if the subjects are in energy balance.

Finally, we are reminded by Frayn's new approach to adipose tissue metabolism that the in vivo regulation of organ metabolism in humans is far from being resolved. Whereas we were originally keen on the potential for brown adipose tissue activity in humans (22), Astrup favors a muscular site. Clark supports the possibility that the smooth muscle contractibility of arterioles induced by sympathetic activity could be involved (23), and Frayn reminds us that sympathetic control of adipose tissue metabolism must also be considered. The technical details of the methods of studying the abdominal pad of adipose tissue are still evolving, but we are beginning to move toward the time when the effects of hepatic, skeletal, and adipose tissue metabolism can be distinguished and given their due role in thermogenesis in short-term and long-term feeding studies. Frayn notes that adipose tissue depots vary in their responsiveness to adrenergic stimuli, as documented by Ottosson et al. (24), so the quantitative role of adipose tissue in the neural control of thermogenesis may take some time to emerge. Nevertheless, these cannulation studies present a new avenue for analyzing the complex interactions between diet and thermogenesis in physiologic and pathologic conditions.

REFERENCES

1. Kashiwazaki H. Seasonal fluctuation of BMR in populations not exposed to limitations in food availability—reality or illusion? *Eur J Clin Nutr* 1990;44(suppl 1):85–93.
2. Cuthbertson DP. Physical injury and its effects on metabolism. In: Munro HN, Allison JB, eds. *Mammalian protein metabolism*, vol 2. New York: Academic Press, 1964;373–414.
3. Jessen K, Rabol A, Winkler K. Total body and splanchnic thermogenesis in curarised man during a short exposure to cold. *Acta Anaesth Scand* 1980;24:339–44.
4. Joy RJT. Responses of cold-acclimatized men to infused norepinephrine. *J Appl Physiol* 1963;18:1209–12.
5. Kang BS, Han DS, Paik KS, et al. Calorigenic action of norepinephrine in the Korean women divers. *J Appl Physiol* 1970;29:6–9.
6. Steinberg D, Nestel PJ, Buskirk ER, Thompson RH. Calorific effect of norepinephrine correlated with plasma free fatty acid turnover and oxidation. *J Clin Invest* 1964;43:167–76.
7. Jung RT, Shetty PS, James WPT, Barrand MA, Callingham BA. Reduced thermogenesis in obesity. *Nature* 1979;279:332.
8. Henry CJK, Emery B. Effect of spiced food on metabolic rate. *Hum Nutr Clin Nutr* 1986;40C:165–8.
9. Schutz Y, Acheson KJ, Jéquier E. Twenty-four-hour energy expenditure and thermogenesis: response to progressive carbohydrate overfeeding in man. *Int J Obes* 1985;9(suppl 2):111–4.
10. Bisdee JT, James WPT, Shaw MA. Changes in energy expenditure during the menstrual cycle. *Br J Nutr* 1989;61:187–99.
11. Rising R, Keys A, Ravussin E, Bogardus C. The human thermostat: individual variability and relationship to metabolic rate. [In press].
12. Ravussin E, Schutz Y, Acheson KJ, Dusmet M, Bourquin L, Jéquier E. Short-time mixed-diet overfeeding in man: no evidence for "luxuskonsumption." *Am J Physiol* 1985;249:E470–4.
13. Wallin BG, Fagius J. The sympathetic nervous system in man—aspects derived from microelectric recordings. *TINS* 1986;9:63–7.
14. O'Dea K, Esler M, Leonard P, Stockigt JR, Nestel P. Noradrenaline turnover during under- and over-eating in normal weight subjects. *Metabolism* 1982;31:896–9.
15. Brundin T, Wahren J. Thermal insulation of the abdominal wall reduces meal-induced thermogenesis. *Int J Obes* 1989;13(suppl 1):1.
16. Forbes JM. Metabolic aspects of the regulation of voluntary food intake and appetite. *Nutr Res Rev* 1988;1:145–68.

17. Shetty PS, Kurpad AV. Role of the sympathetic nervous system in adaptation to seasonal energy deficiency. *Eur J Clin Nutr* 1990;44(suppl 1):47–53.
18. Jung RT, Shetty PS, James WPT. The effect of beta adrenergic blockade on metabolic rate and peripheral thyroid metabolism in obesity. *Eur J Clin Invest* 1980;10:179–82.
19. Flatt JP. Differences in the regulation of carbohydrate and fat metabolism and their implications for body weight maintenance. In: Lordy H, Stratman F, eds. *Hormones, thermogenesis and obesity.* New York: Elsevier, 1989.
20. Lean MEJ, James WPT. Metabolic effects of isoenergetic nutrient exchange over 24 hours in relation to obesity in women. *Int J Obes* 1988;12:15–27.
21. McNeill G, Bruce AC, Ralph A, James WPT. Inter-individual differences in fasting nutrient oxidation and the influence of diet composition. *Int J Obes* 1988;12:455–63.
22. James WPT, Trayhurn P. Thermogenesis and obesity. *Br Med Bull* 1981;37:43–8.
23. Ye JM, Colquhoun EQ, Hettiarachchi M, Clark MG. Flow-induced oxygen uptake by the perfused rat hindlimb is inhibited by vasodilators and augmented by norepinephrine: a possible role for the microvasculature in hindlimb thermogenesis. *Am J Physiol Pharmacol* 1989;68:119–25.
24. Ottosson M, Enerback S, Olivercrona T, Bjorntorp P. The effects of cortisol on the regulation of lipoprotein lipase activity in human adipose tissue. *Int J Obes* 1991;15(suppl 1):314.

Energy Metabolism: Tissue Determinants and Cellular Corollaries, edited by J. M. Kinney and H. N. Tucker. Raven Press, Ltd., New York © 1992.

Energy Costs of ATP Synthesis

J. P. Flatt

Department of Biochemistry, University of Massachusetts Medical School, Worcester, Massachusetts 01655

As verified by the classical studies of calorimetry (1,2), the stoichiometric relationships between oxygen consumption and heat release associated with biologic substrate oxidations are the same as those observed during chemical reactions or combustions (Table 1). Rates of energy expenditure and substrate oxidation can therefore be established by measuring heat losses (i.e., by direct calorimetry) and work output and by measuring oxygen consumption, CO_2 production, and urinary nitrogen excretion. It is possible to establish the changes in the body's content of carbohydrates, fats, and proteins owing to metabolism. Because the energy liberated per gram of substrate oxidized is known, this also permits an assessment of energy expenditure, i.e., by indirect calorimetry. In this regard, it is useful to understand that calculations based on respiratory exchange and nitrogen excretion data yield estimates of *changes in content* rather than amounts of protein, carbohydrate, and fat *oxidized*, as commonly stated. Making this distinction helps to resolve possible concerns about the validity of indirect calorimetry when lipogenesis and fat oxidation or gluconeogenesis and glucose oxidation occur concomitantly. It should also be kept in mind that indirect calorimetry involves assumptions about the nature of the carbohydrates, fats, and protein metabolized, notably including assumptions that CO_2, water, and urea are the only quantitatively significant endproducts of substrate degradation (6). Measurements of energy expenditure and of the composition of the substrate mixture oxidized have contributed much important information for our current understanding of energy metabolism and the manner in which regulatory phenomena interact and coordinate metabolic fuel utilization in the whole organism.

Measurements of whole-body metabolism have also provided quantitative information about the increments in energy expenditure caused by physical and metabolic tasks, which have yielded the numeric data needed to describe in quantitative terms the relationship between ATP turnover and substrate oxidation in intact cells or *in vivo*. It is under such circumstances that the cost of replacing the ATP used for a given process and the cost of the process can be evaluated. Much less is known about the factors that determine metabolic rates and ATP turnover in the resting state. It is also not evident to which extent the energy expended to maintain the body's integrity should be counted as part of the energy costs for ATP synthesis. This issue is somewhat analogous to the problem encountered in trying to describe

TABLE 1. *Stoichiometry of substrate oxidation and high-energy bond production*

$C_6H_{12}O_6$ + 6 O_2 **Glucose**	$\xrightarrow[\text{(4.99 kcal/L }O_2)]{\text{RQ = 1.00}}$	6 CO_2 + 6 H_2O + 670 kcal[a] [+38 − 2 = +36 ~][b]
$C_6H_{10}O_5$ + 6 O_2 **Glucosyl-**	$\xrightarrow[\text{(5.05 kcal/L }O_2)]{\text{RQ = 1.00}}$	6 CO_2 + 6 H_2O + 678 kcal [+38 − 1 = +37~]
[c]4.5 $C_6H_{12}O_6$ + 4 O_2 **Glucose**	$\xrightarrow[\text{(7.06 kcal/L }O_2)]{\text{RQ = 2.75}}$	1 $C_{16}H_{32}O_2$ + 11 CO_2 + 11 H_2O + 630 kcal *Palmitate* [+40 − 34 = +6~]
$C_{16}H_{32}O_2$ + 23 O_2 **Palmitate**	$\xrightarrow[\text{(4.68 kcal/L }O_2)]{\text{RQ = .696}}$	16 CO_2 + 16 H_2O + 2,398 kcal [+131 − 2 = +129~]
$C_{57}H_{107}O_6$ + 78 O_2 **Triglyceride**[d]	$\xrightarrow[\text{[e](4.69 kcal/L }O_2)]{\text{[e]RQ = .71}}$	57 CO_2 + 52 H_2O + 8,139 kcal [+459 − 7 = +452~]
$C_{4.6}H_{8.4}O_{1.8}N_{1.25}$ + 1.5 O_2 + 0.2 H_2O **Protein**[f]	$\longrightarrow$	0.6 Urea + 0.6 CO_2 + 0.35 Gluc + 0.3 KB [+8.2 − 4.6 = +3.6~]
.35 Gluc + .3 KB + 3.3 O_2	$\longrightarrow$	3.3 CO_2 + 3.1 H_2O [+20.6 − 1 = +19.6~]
$C_{4.6}H_{8.4}O_{1.8}N_{1.25}$ + 4.8 O_2 **Protein**[f]	$\xrightarrow[\text{[e](4.66 kcal/L }O_2)]{\text{[e]RQ = .835}}$	0.6 Urea + 4.0 CO_2 + 2.9 H_2O + 520 kcal [+28.8 − 5.6 = +23.2~]

[a] From ref. 3.
[b] Brackets show the number of high-energy (~) produced, minus those utilized, as well as the overall ~ yield.
[c] Based on stoichiometry reported for lipogenesis in rat adipose tissue (4).
[d] Palmityl-stearyl-oleyl triglyceride, which is representative of the usual fatty acid pattern in human adipose fat.
[e] Coefficients given by Livesey and Elia (6), according to whom protein oxidation yields 4.70 kcal/g and occurs with an RQ of .835, which differ from the commonly used values of 4.32 and .80, respectively, based on Loewy (48).
[f] Approximate composition of a protein mixture chosen to contain 1,000 mmoles of amino-acyl residues in 110 g of protein, to have 16% of its weight as N and 50% as C, to be oxidized with an RQ of .835 (6) and to generate 3.6 g glucose per g of N. ATP stoichiometry is based on ref. 5.

the cost of patient hospitalization. The figure obtained by averaging the increments in operating costs incurred for the care of each patient provides a more specific, but also a very different, answer from that obtained by dividing total hospital expenditures by the total number of patient days.

ROLE OF ATP AND HIGH-ENERGY INTERMEDIATES

Adenosine triphosphate (ATP) serves as the major energy carrier in the intermediary metabolism of animals, plants, and micro-organisms. The essential role that ATP plays in capturing energy during the oxidation of metabolic fuels and carrying it to sites where it can be released to drive chemical reactions is due to the special properties of its phosphate-oxygen-phosphate (or *pyrophosphate*) bonds (7). As is the case with other anhydrides of acids, considerable energy is released when these bonds are split, be it by hydrolysis or by transfer of one moiety to another molecule. In contrast to other anhydrides, however, pyrophosphate bonds are relatively stable in aqueous solutions, making their breakdown contingent on the presence of particular enzymes. A few other types of molecules have evolved that contain stable high-energy bonds (e.g., other diphosphate or triphosphate nucleotides, Coenzyme A derivatives). They allow the formation of *activated* or *reactive* intermediates capable of providing the chemical energy needed to make particular reactions occur, notably those involved in biosynthesis.

At rest, about one-half of the body's ATP content (some 25–35 grams in an adult) is hydrolyzed to ATP + P_i every minute to drive the life-sustaining reactions that serve to transport molecules, maintain concentration gradients and muscle tone, accomplish the synthesis and secretion of biologic molecules, and produce the mechanical work required for respiration and blood circulation. During physical exercise, several hundred grams of ATP may be utilized per minute. It is thus essential that ATP resynthesis from ADP and P_i adjust itself very promptly to the rate of ATP utilization. This is made possible by a network of intracellular regulatory phenomena that is poised for effectively maintaining high ATP/ADP ratios (8) and by the fact that the cell's enzymatic machinery usually operates far below its maximal capacity. With the availability of various intracellular substrates, notably glycogen, as well as adequate tissue oxygenation, substrate oxidation is in effect generally limited by the rate at which ADP is formed. This explains why ATP hydrolysis and its resynthesis from ADP and P_i can remain closely matched. These intracellular features of energy metabolism are complemented by systemic and local regulation of blood flow to maintain tissue oxygenation and by a hormonal regulatory system capable of controlling the mobilization, distribution, and storage of metabolic fuels (9).

The increase in energy expenditure elicited by performing specific tasks under standardized conditions is highly reproducible and generally proportional to body weight. Thus, it is possible to predict the rate of energy expenditure of a walking individual (by taking into account body weight, speed of walking, slope of the track, weight carried, and nature of the terrain) more accurately than that individual's resting metabolic rate (10). This indicates that the efficiency of metabolism in regenerating the ATP used during muscle contractions is relatively constant. This does not imply, however, that different individuals will necessarily expend the same amount of energy to perform the same tasks, on account of differences in body weight and skill. At the end of a period of exertion, the rate of oxygen consumption decays rapidly but remains elevated above the resting rate for some time. This *excess postexercise oxygen consumption* (EPOC) serves to repay the oxygen debt—i.e., to restore myoglobin oxygenation, ATP, and creatine-P to resting levels—and to reconvert to glucose some of the lactate. Lactate may have accumulated by anaerobic energy production, although lactate oxidation by the heart is a more important process of lactate disposal (11). After vigorous exertion, a small increase in the metabolic rate can be noted even 24 hours later, possibly due in part to increased muscle protein synthesis. It has been estimated that about 15% of the increase in energy expenditure induced by physical exertion occurs after the period of exertion itself (11). Furthermore, expansion of the muscle mass induced by regular physical activities also causes a long-term increase in the resting metabolic rate (12).

ENERGY GENERATION/ATP GENERATION

A substantial fraction of the energy liberated during substrate oxidation can be captured because several reactions in the degradative pathways are linked to the transformation of ADP + P_i into ATP. These processes are often referred to as ATP generation, or even as energy generation. Energy, like matter, is conserved, and the use of the words *energy production* or *energy dissipation* merely reflects the fact that one focuses only on one part of the overall process. In the context of metabolism, *ATP synthesis* usually means ATP regeneration from ADP + P_i (and not ATP biosynthesis), whereas *energy expenditure* is used to describe the degradation of ATP to ADP + P_i, or the use of high-energy bonds. The chemical energy exchanges associated with chemical reactions are quantified in terms of free energy change, or ΔG. ΔG is related to the enthalpy change (ΔH) associated with chemical reactions by the equation $\Delta G = \Delta H - T\Delta S$. Because changes in entropy (ΔS) during oxidative degradations are comparatively small relative to ΔH, the numerical values for ΔG and ΔH are very nearly the same. The extensive data available on heats of combustion (i.e., ΔHs) are therefore useful in discussing energy exchanges in cells, even though chemical reactivity is linked to ΔG rather than to ΔH. ΔGs are influenced by temperature and by the concentration of reactants and products. In the case of ATP hydrolysis in erythrocytes (8), the reaction and its ΔG are described by the following equations;

$$ATP^- + H_2O \quad ADP^- + P_i^- + H^+ \Delta G$$

$$= \Delta G^{o\prime} + RT \text{ in } \frac{(ADP)\,(P_i)}{(ATP)}$$

$$= -7,300 + 2.303 \times 1.987 \times 298 \log \frac{(ADP)\,(P_i)}{(ATP)}$$

$$= -7,300 + 2.303 \times 1.987 \times 298 \log \frac{(25 \times 10^{-3})\,(1.65 \times 10^{-3})}{(2.25 \times 10^{-3})}$$

$$= -12,400 \text{ calories/mol}$$

Where $\Delta G^{o\prime}$ describes the free energy change when the reaction occurs under standard conditions for biologic systems (i.e., at 25°C and neutral pH) with all reactants present at a concentration of 1 $-M$. However $H^+ = 10^{-7} -M$ instead of $H^+ = 1-M$, as when ΔG° is defined for standard conditions in chemistry; the ΔG° for ATP hydrolysis is -16.8 kcal/mol at pH $= 0$. The second term in the equation takes into account the influences of temperature and of the reactant and product concentrations of the free energy change with the reaction. Chemical bonds whose hydrolysis is associated with a large free energy change in absolute terms (i.e., for which $\Delta G^{o'} = -7$ kcal/mol or less) are usually referred to as high-energy bonds (often represented by the symbol ~). One should be aware of the fact the ΔG for ATP hydrolysis is almost twice the $\Delta G^{o'}$ when the reactants are present in physiologic concentrations, as shown by the preceding example.

Some ATP is formed from ADP and P_i by substrate level phosphorylation in the glycolytic pathway, but the bulk of ATP resynthesis occurs on the inner mitochondrial membrane by oxidative phosphorylation. This process couples the reaction between oxygen and hydrogen atoms removed from organic molecules by various *dehydrogenases* to the conversion of ADP + P_i into ATP. The enzymes commonly referred to as dehydrogenases catalyze oxidoreductions involving hydrogen-carrying coenzymes, such as NAD^+ (Nicotinamide adenine dinucleotide) or FAD (Flavin adenine dinucleotide) in their oxidized forms or NADH + H^+ and $FADH_2$ in their reduced forms. These hydrogen-carrier coenzymes allow the transfer of H atoms from substrate molecules (two at a time) to the mitochondrial electron-transmitter system (ETS). This name reflects the fact that its most characteristic components, the cytochromes, manage the transfer of electrons (formed by dissociation of H into $H^+ + e^-$) rather than of H atoms. The transfer of hydrogen atoms from NADH to the mitochondrial respiratory chain is initiated by NADH reductase and completed by cytochrome oxidase, which catalyzes the ultimate reaction with the oxygen carried to the tissues by the blood. These mitochondrial processes occur at near equilibrium conditions (13), and their rates are usually limited by the availability of ADP. Respiratory control is thus exerted by the rate of ATP utilization, a situation designed to allow maintenance of a high ATP/ADP ratio as well as prompt replacement of the ATP used.

For many years the formation of ATP was believed to proceed though a sequence of coupled chemical reactions generally known as the chemical theory of oxidative phosphorylation (14). In view of the believed existence of three sequential phosphorylation sites in the mitochondrial electron transmitter chain, it became general usage to consider that 3 molecules of ATP are generated for each pair of hydrogen atoms (i.e., one *reducing-equivalent*) passing through the entire respiratory chain. This would correspond to a P:O ratio of 3 (number of high-energy bands ~ formed per g-atom of oxygen [1/2 mol O_2] consumed). This concept has now been replaced by the chemiosmotic theory of oxidative phosphorylation proposed by Mitchell (15), according to which the transfer of hydrogen atoms removed from substrates though the mitochondrial electron-transmitter chain generates a proton gradient across the inner mitochondrial membrane. Reentry of protons provides the driving force for ATP resynthesis. There has been some debate about the precise number of protons pumped out of the inner mitochondrial membranes during the passage of two hydrogen atoms through the respiratory chain and about the number of protons needed to induce the formation of a high-energy bond (16,17). Furthermore, it has become evident that energy is also needed to transfer ATP from the mitochondrial to the cytoplasmic compartment, where the ATP/ADP ratio is higher (18). According to Lehninger (8), 12 protons are moved out of the mitochondria during the reoxidation of 1 molecule of mitochondrial $NADH_2$. The reentry of 9 protons would allow the synthesis of 3 molecules of ATP from ADP + P_i, while the remaining 3 protons are used to transport the 3 ATPs from the mitochondrial to the cytoplasmic compartment. Although the concept of a precise stoichiometry between the number of pairs of hydrogen atoms oxidized and high-energy bond formation became less rigid with the advent of this theory, the use of the traditional P:O ratios in calculating the amounts of ATP yielded by the oxidation of metabolic fuels appears to have remained an essentially unquestioned practice.

EFFICIENCY OF OXIDATIVE PHOSPHORYLATION AND THE P:O RATIO

Few direct attempts to evaluate the efficiency of oxidation phosphorylations have been possible in intact cells, because the rapid turnover of ATP involved in the maintenance of the cell's metabolic activities is not readily measurable, making it impossible to relate the number of moles of high-energy bonds formed to the amount of oxygen consumed. A particularly elegant study relevant to this issue was performed by Pahud et al. (19) on young men pedaling on a bicycle ergometer at different levels of work output, with simultaneous measurements of rates of heat production by direct calorimetry and establishment of rates of substrate oxidation by indirect calorimetry. During sustained aerobic work, the mechanical work performed was equivalent to 27% of the energy contained in the increment in substrate oxidation elicited by pedaling. During the first minutes of pedaling against a suddenly increased resistance, work demanding an increase in power output from 45 W to 150 W, the mechanical work produced (measured electrically with the bicycle ergometer) plus the energy appearing in the form of heat (measured by direct calorimetry and from the increase in the subjects' body temperature) exceeded the energy liberated by substrate oxidation (determined by indirect calorimetry) (Fig. 1). This implies that performed high-energy bonds (ATP and creatine phosphate) were utilized to accomplish part of the mechanical work during this phase of the test. The characteristics of this latter process were assessed by subtracting from the overall exchanges the contribution made by aerobic metabolism during this phase. It was found that 41% of the energy liberated by breakdown of preformed high-energy bonds could be converted into mechanical energy. This yields an experimental value of the *coupling coefficient*, which describes the efficiency with which chemical energy can be converted into work in muscles (21). The difference in the two observed efficiencies (i.e., 41% for the production of mechanical energy from preformed high-energy bonds versus 27% in generating such energy by substrate oxidation) is due to the fact that a fraction of the energy liberated by the oxidation of metabolic fuels is recovered in the form of ATP. The 0.66 ratio, 27% to 41%, thus provides an estimate of the

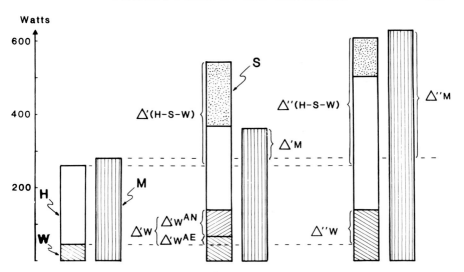

FIG. 1. Evaluation of efficiencies of aerobic and anaerobic work output and of efficiency of oxidative phosphorylation in humans (based on ref. 19). Aerobic ▨ and anaerobic ▧ work performed on a bicycle ergometer by a group of young men during the last 5 minutes of a 45-minute period of priming exercise against a low resistance (45 W), during the first minute after pedaling against a high resistance (150 W), and 20 minutes later. Heat output □ measured by direct calorimetry. Heat storage ▨ from data obtained with thermometric probes at 10 sites, calculated with a thermometric model. Metabolic energy production ▥ measured by indirect calorimetry. Efficiency of aerobic work $\eta^{AE} = \Delta''W/\Delta''M = 27\%$; anaerobic work $\Delta'W^{AN} = \Delta'W - \Delta'M \times \eta^{AE}$, efficiency of anaerobic work $\eta^{AN} = \Delta'W^{AN}/[\Delta'(H + S + W) - \Delta'M] = 41\%$; efficiency of oxidative phosphorylation $\eta P = \eta^{AE}/\eta^{AN} = 27\%/41\% = 65\%$. (From ref. 20, with permission.)

efficiency with which the energy liberated by substrate oxidation is recovered in the form of ATP in human muscles—i.e., about 65% (19).

Accordingly, one would expect that 450 kcal of free energy would be recovered in the form of high-energy bonds during the complete oxidation of 1 mole of glucose ($\Delta G = -689$ kcal/mol). Based on data on the creatine phosphate/Mg-ATP equilibrium, the ΔG for ATP hydrolysis in muscle can be evaluated at about -14.3 kcal/mol (22). Because oxidative phosphorylation appears to be operating at near equilibrium conditions (13), one would expect 450/14.3 = 31.5 mol ATP to be formed, which corresponds to a P:O ratio of 31.3/12 = 2.6 (23). The ATP/ADP ratio falls somewhat during vigorous muscular contraction, so the value of 14.3 kcal/mol for the ΔG of ATP formation is perhaps somewhat high. The value of 2.6 for the P:O ratio during carbohydrate oxidation is thus possibly underestimated.

The value yielded by this assessment in vivo is in reasonably good agreement with the limited number of situations where evaluations of the P:O ratio in intact cells has been possible (Table 2). Considering the number of assumptions and sources of possible errors inherent in these attempts, it is difficult to decide whether these values differ significantly from the traditional value of 3. As pointed out by Livesey (30), these experiments actually provide an evaluation of the $\Delta P:\Delta O$ *ratio* rather than of the P:O ratio. Higher values should be expected to be obtained for the former (such

ENERGY COSTS OF ATP SYNTHESIS

TABLE 2. P:O estimates in intact cells or tissues

Experimental situation	P:O	References
Δ O_2 consumption after glucose pulse in ascites cells	2.6	24
Δ FFA re-esterification versus O_2 consumption in adipose tissue		
of fasted/refed rats	3.0	25
of hypo-, eu-, and hyperthyroid rats	2.4	26
NMR measured ^{31}P transfer and O_2 consumption		
in isolated perfused rat heart	3.5 ± 0.8	27
in rat brain	2.0–2.4	28
in rat kidney	2.4 ± 0.2	29
$\eta^{aerobic}$work, $\eta^{anaerobic}$ work, η oxidative phosphorylation following Δ work load in humans, and ΔG for ATP hydrolysis in muscle	2.6	23
Glycogen deposition versus Δ metabolic rate		
in normal subjects	2.4 ± 0.5	30
in obese subjects	3.4 ± 1.1	Based on data from 31

as those given in Table 2) because they are less affected than the latter by proton slippage and proton leakage, which occur in mitochondria and lower the overall P:O ratio, particularly when oxygen consumption and ATP turnover are proceeding at low rates (30). Because some proton leakage always occurs, ATP turnover cannot in fact be accurately predicted from oxygen uptake or heat exchanges data when rates of ATP generation are low. ATP turnover in the resting state will thus be overestimated when it is based on estimates of the ΔP:ΔO ratio, as generally is the case. This uncertainty is probably of minor importance when increments in ATP turnover are to be considered. In order to maintain consistency with common practices, we have therefore continued to use the traditional values for the P:O ratios (i.e., 3 high-energy bonds regenerated/mitochondrial NADH reoxidized, or 2 high-energy bonds per $FADH_2$ or cytoplasmic NADH reoxidized) in computing the amounts of ATP yielded by the oxidation of metabolic fuels and in the assessment of the metabolic costs of processes based on their ATP-related stoichiometries (as done in Table 1 and in Fig. 4). If P:O ratios are in fact lower than 3, the actual metabolic costs would be somewhat greater than those presently predicted (i.e., 15–20% for a P:O ratio of 2.6 instead of 3.0).

UNCOUPLING OF OXIDATIVE PHOSPHORYLATION

Except for some reactions catalyzed by peroxidases and for diverse hydroxylations catalyzed by oxygenases (where the ultimate reaction with oxygen is often catalyzed by the cytoplasmic cytochrome P450), reaction with oxygen is mediated only by cytochrome oxidase, the ultimate enzyme in the mitochondrial respiratory chain. Oxygen consumption is thereby coupled to the flux of reducing equivalents through the electron-transmitter system, to the associated proton extrusion, as well as to their reentry, which occurs in association with ATP reformation from ADP + P_i. A number of agents are known to interfere with ATP regeneration by inhibiting specific reactions in the respiratory chain. For example, cyanide blocks cytochrome oxidase, rotenone prevents electron transfer to cytochrome b from NADH, and antimycin A prohibits the transfer from cytochrome b to cytochrome c_1. Oligomycin inhibits the coupling factor, the large multienzyme complex attached to the inner mitochondrial membrane that carries out the reconversion of ADP + P_i into ATP by coupling it to proton reentry (32), whereas, atractyloside inhibits ATP export from the mitochondria. These agents all inhibit or block oxygen consumption. On the other hand, dinitrophenol (DNP) permits protons to cross the inner mitochondrial membrane and thereby to return to the mitochondrial compartment without concomitant ATP formation, discharging the pH gradient created by the proton-pumping action of the electron-transmitter system. DNP thus permits oxygen consumption to occur without being limited by ADP availability, and this substance is accordingly considered to be an encoupling agent. Substrate oxidation in vivo is believed to be closely controlled by ADP availability under most circumstances, except in brown adipose tissue. Its mitochondria is equipped with a unique proton-conducting pathway, which is activated when fatty acids are produced by catecholamine-stimulated lipolysis (33). This allows NADH reoxidation to occur at rates much higher than necessary for oxidative phosphorylation, permitting rapid substrate oxidation and heat production. The major role of this elaborately controlled mechanism appears to be in helping to maintain body temperature in small animals during cold exposure, as well as in raising body temperature during arousal from hibernation (33). Activation of this protein conductance pathway during overfeeding can play an important role in enhancing energy dissipation, thereby limiting the development of obesity in small animals (34). This mechanism for energy dissipation does not appear to operate to a significant extent in humans, however (35).

SUBSTRATE CYCLES AND FUTILE CYCLES

Interconversion of intracellular substrates involving ATP-consuming reactions (e.g., kinases), such as fructose-1,6-diphosphate hydrolysis by fructose diphosphatase, and resynthesis by phosphofructokinase (PFK), can cause ATP dissipation. Because substrate cycles of this type cause no net change in the organism, they have sometimes also been referred to as futile cycles, which potentially might play a role in energy dissipation. Very elaborate mechanisms have evolved that regulate the activity of enzymes involved in catalyzing opposite transformation, preventing them from being both active simultaneously, so as to prevent high rates of wasteful substrate interconversions. However, complete suppression of these interconversions is not achieved because it may not be compatible with the fast response times desirable to allow for rapid changes in flux, as may be needed in the glycolytic pathway (36). Other intracellular substrate cycles include interconversions of glucose and glucose-6-P or synthesis and breakdown of phosphoenolpyruvate by enzymes involved in the gluconeogenic pathway. When fatty acids are produced by triglyceride hydrolysis in adipose tissue, some are re-esterified on the spot (37). In spite of this, free fatty acids are released from adipose tissue in amounts greater than those used for energy production; the excess if re-esterified in the liver, to be re-exported to adipose tissue in the form of lipoproteins. Lipolysis and fatty acid re-esterification thus also cause ATP dissipation without net change in the system, but higher-than-minimal rates of lipolysis help to ensure an adequate supply of circulating FFA and to promote fat oxidation, which is enhanced by high circulating FFA levels (38,39). It has been very difficult to design tracer studies that could provide accurate estimates of substrate cycling rates. Current information suggests that they account for only a small percentage of total energy expenditure (40). The increase in peripheral substrate mobilization caused by higher catecholamine levels during overfeeding and the increased release of various mobilizing hormones during periods of stress cause an increase in substrate traffic, which may account for about 25% of the rise in resting metabolic rates under these conditions (41).

The energy-dependent sodium extrusion constantly carried out by the cell membranes' sodium-potassium ATPase is quantitatively by far the most significant process causing ATP expenditure and energy dissipation at rest. Yet one would not readily consider this a "futile" cycle because it is essential in keeping intracellular [NA$^+$] low in spite of constant Na$^+$ leakage back into the cells, thereby maintaining membrane potential and cell integrity. This phenomenon may account for 30% to 40% of basal energy expenditure (42), but data to establish this with some certainty are not available. Increases in sodium-potassium ATPase activity induced by thyroxine suggest that enhanced Na$^+$ pumping may account for increases in energy expenditure caused by elevation of thyroxine levels, although a high number of ATPase molecules does not by itself prove that Na$^+$ fluxes are increased (43).

METABOLIC COSTS ASSOCIATED WITH ATP PRODUCTION

In order to evaluate the costs of metabolic processes, the stoichiometry of ATP consumption must be known as well as the amount of substrate that needs to be oxidized to regenerate a given amount of ATP, rather than the energy liberated by ATP hydrolysis. Such estimates depend therefore not only on the P:O ratio, but also on the amounts of ATP expended for the transport and handling of the metabolic fuels whose oxidation provides the energy for ATP regeneration. The numbers of mol of ATP formed per mol of glucose, fatty acid, and amino acid oxidized are summarized in Table 1; the negative numbers describe how much ATP is required to initiate their degradation, and in the case of amino acid oxidation, the amount needed to carry out gluconeogenesis and ureagenesis.

Additional ATP is expended in making these metabolic fuels available to the various tissues. For instance, 38 ATPs are produced during the oxidation of 1 glucose molecule, but 2 are used for its activation to glucose-6-P and fructose-di-P, so the

ATP yield is $36/38 = 95\%$. If one allows for the fact that some 15% to 25% of the glucose released by the liver is recycled via the *Cori cycle* and the *glucose-alanine cycle* (44) (at a net cost of 4 ATP/glucose recycled), only 90% of the ATP generated by oxidation of glucose derived from liver glycogen is available to replace ATPs used in peripheral tissues (Fig. 2). Significant portions of the carbohydrates supplied by the diet are now believed to be stored initially in the form of muscle glycogen (45,46), so that a substantial part of the glucose released by the liver is in fact regenerated from lactate released by breakdown of muscle glycogen. The cost of gluconeogenesis would then consume additional ATP. If one assumes that this applies to one-half of the glucose released by the liver, the net ATP yield during glycogen oxidation is reduced to about 82% (Fig. 2). The heats of combustion (ΔH) for glucose is 670 kcal/mol (3), and the ΔH for fructose-1,6-di P may be estimated at 685 kcal/mol. The turnover of 38 mol of ATP is thus indicated by the release of 685 kcal, or $685/38 = 18$ kcal/mol ATP when glucose is the metabolic fuel oxidized. However, because 18% of the ATP generated merely replaces the ATP spent for substrate handling, an amount of glucose containing $18/.82 = 22$ kcal must be oxidized to *replace* one mole of ATP consumed by a given metabolic process. To evaluate the energy expended in regenerating ATP by oxidation of fat, one has to consider that some of the free fatty acids produced by triglyceride hydrolysis adipose tissue are re-esterified before leaving adipose tissue at a cost of 7 ATP/triglyceride made (2 ATP for the activation of FFA to fatty-acyl CoA, multiplied by 3, plus 1 ATP for the formation of glycerol-P). Some of the FFA released into the circulation are removed and re-esterified by the liver, to be re-exported in the form of lipoproteins, which requires another cycle of hydrolysis and re-esterification for their redeposition into adipose tissue, or 2×2.33 ATP/FFA (Fig. 2). The extent to which the lipolytic rate exceeds the rate of fatty acid oxidation appears to be rather variable (34,47). If one assumes that lipolysis proceeds at twice the rate of fat oxidation and that one-half of the fatty acids that escape oxidation are re-esterified in adipose tissue while the other one-half is returned to adipose tissue via lipoproteins secreted by the liver, 3.5 ATP are expended per mol of fatty acid oxidized. Oleate is the most common fatty acid in human triglycerides. During its oxidation 146 ATP/mol are generated, and 2 ATP are expended for its activation to oleyl-CoA. The ATP yield for fat oxidation is thus approximately $140.5/146 = 96\%$. In view of the large amount of ATP generated per mol of fatty acid oxidized, some variations in the relative rate of FFA reesterification will not greatly modify this yield. The ΔH for oleate oxidation is 2,657 kcal/mol (3), and that for oleyl-CoA can be estimated at 2,670 kcal/mol, so that $2,670/146 = 18.3$ kcal are released per mole of ATP turned over. The energy expenditure per mol of ATP utilized and replaced by fatty acid oxidation thus comes to $18.3/.96 = 19$ kcal/mol ATP (as compared to 22 kcal/mol ATP during glycogen oxidation) (Fig. 2).

By taking into account the known heats of combustion and the amino acid content of various proteins, Elia and Livesey concluded that the RQ during protein oxidation is 0.835 and that 4.7 kcal are released per gram of protein metabolized to CO_2, water, and urea (6). These coefficients should replace those traditionally used (1,2) (i.e.,

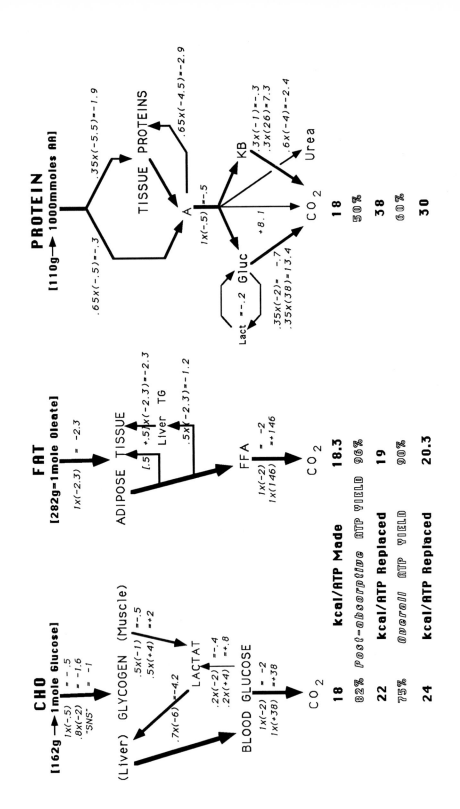

RQ = .80) and 4.32 kcal released per gram of protein oxidized, based on the original work of Loewy (48). In the course of amino acid oxidation, 5.5 moles of ATP are expended for ureagenesis and gluconeogenesis per mol (110 g) of protein oxidized. This is equivalent to about 20% of the 28.8 moles of ATP generated by their oxidation (Table 1). With the oxidative degradation of the 1,000 mmoles of amino acids derived from 110 g of protein to CO_2, water and urea being accompanied by the release of 110 g × 4.70 kcal/g = 517 kcal, 1 mole of ATP is generated by the oxidation of 517/ 28.8 = 18 kcal. (With the old coefficient the corresponding figure is 16.5 kcal released per mole of ATP generated, which seems inconsistent with the values of 18.0 to 18.3 kcal/mol ATP during carbohydrate and fat oxidation.) Because the costs of gluconeogenesis and ureagenesis consume an amount of ATP equal to 20% of the amount produced during amino acid oxidation, an expenditure of 18/.8 = 22.5 kcal of protein is required to replace 1 ATP by oxidation of amino acids. But only a fraction of the amino acids produced by protein breakdown is oxidized (possibly about one-third), (49), so oxidation of amino acids derived from endogenous protein turnover is always accompanied by protein resynthesis, a process requiring about 5 ATP/amino acid reincorporated into protein (4 for the synthesis of the peptide bond plus an estimated 1 additional mole for amino acid transport, mRNA synthesis, etc.). This would consume 10 ATP in addition to the 5.5 utilized for glucose and urea synthesis per mole of amino acid oxidized. The net ATP yield associated with the oxidation of amino acids derived from the turnover of endogenous proteins would accordingly be in the order of (28.8 − 15.5)/28.8 = 45%. Thus, in situations in which amino acids contribute 15% or 20% of the fuel mix oxidized, if this is considered to imply commensurate differences in protein turnover rates, one would expect a 3% difference in metabolic rates. As shown recently, part of the variability in basal metabolic rates is indeed explained by differences in protein turnover (50). Furthermore, it is well known that elevations in urinary nitrogen excretion and in resting metabolic rates run a parallel course following trauma or during sepsis (51).

FIG. 2. *ATP yields during oxidation of carbohydrate, fat, and protein.* The numbers printed in outlines show moles of substrate flowing through various metabolic pathways; those in parenthesis show the moles of ATP produced and expended per mole of substrate metabolized, assuming a P:O ratio of 3 for the reoxidation of mitochondrial NADH. The following assumptions were made. For glucose: postprandial stimulation of the sympathetic nervous system (SNS) causes an energy dissipation equivalent to an amount of ATP slightly less than the obligatory ATP expenditure for glucose absorption followed by storage of 80% of absorbed glucose as glycogen—one-half in liver, one-half in muscle. The latter is subsequently released as lactate and reconverted to glucose in the liver; one-sixth of the glucose released by the liver is recycled via the Cori cycle. For fat: postprandial ATP expenditure is required for fatty acid (e.g., oleic acid) esterification into triglycerides to form chylomicrons and for triglyceride deposition in adipose tissue. During fatty acid mobilization, one-half of the fatty acids produced by lipolysis are re-esterified, either before leaving adipose tissue or during VLDL formation in the liver and subsequent redeposition in adipose tissue. For protein: ATP expenditure for gluconeogenesis and ureagenesis during AA degradation is the same as for protein synthesis. After one accounts for the cost of active transport, this amounts to 5.5 moles of ATP per 1,000 mmoles of dietary amino acids; two-thirds of the AA formed by breakdown of proteins in tissues are reutilized for protein synthesis.

METABOLIC COSTS FOR NUTRIENT STORAGE AND THE THERMIC EFFECT OF FOOD

The ATP yielded by different nutrients is further decreased when one takes into account the costs incurred for their initial transport and storage after ingestion. If one assumes that in addition to the 2 ATPs used for the synthesis of glycogen, .5 ATP is expended for active transport and intestinal enzyme synthesis and motility, this would entail an energy expenditure equivalent to 2.5 × [22.5 kcal per mole ATP replaced at a postprandial RQ of .89] = 56 kcal, or 56/670 = 8%, for the storage of dietary carbohydrates as glycogen. The fact that some of the ingested glucose is used without prior conversion into glycogen (assumed to be 20% in Fig. 2) is more than offset by the stimulation of the sympathetic nervous system induced by carbohydrate intake. In studies in which the amount of glycogen synthesis could be calculated from indirect calorimetry data, the energy expended for glucose storage was evaluated at 4% to 6% of the glucose energy infused, accounting for about two-thirds of the observed increase in energy expenditure above the fasting rate. The remainder is attributable primarily to increased catecholamine secretion. When this phenomenon was curtailed by administration of adrenergic blocking agents, the thermic effect observed was consistent with the predicted metabolic expense for glucose storage (52). Thus, one can understand why the increase in resting energy expenditure elicited by carbohydrate ingestion, i.e., the thermic effect of food (TEF), is generally found to vary somewhat around 8% to 10%. If one takes into account this energy dissipation during the postprandial phase, the net ATP yield from dietary carbohydrate comes to about .91 × 82% (the net ATP yield for glycogen oxidation) = 75%. In the case of fat, the predictable cost for the initial deposition of dietary fat comes to about 3% of the energy provided by dietary fat, which is too low to be experimentally assessed (53). Various experiments indicate that the addition of fat raises the TEF of meals by 5% to 10% of the energy provided by the added fat (54,55). The net ATP yield from dietary fat would thus be reduced to .93 × 96%, (the yield from endogenous fat), or about 90%. These considerations suggest that the oxidation of 18/.75 = 24 kcal of dietary carbohydrate, or the oxidation of 18.3/.90 = 20.3 kcal of dietary fat, is needed to replace one mole of ATP. This indicates that 15% to 20% more energy may be required to sustain metabolism with dietary carbohydrate than with dietary fat, even in the absence of lipogenesis, a point that will be further considered.

The TEF elicited by protein usually falls into the 20% to 30% range (1,2,53). The ATP required to absorb and transport dietary amino acids into cells and then to convert them into protein may be estimated at about 5.5 moles of ATP per mole of amino acid mixture. If the amino acids are oxidized instead, the ATP expenditure for transport, ureagenesis, and gluconeogenesis also comes to about 5.5 moles of ATP (5). The TEF of protein is therefore essentially the same when either (or any combination) of these two processes is involved—that is, 5.5 × 22.5 kcal/ATP replaced = 125 kcal per 100 g of ingested protein, or 125/(110 g × 4.70 kcal/g) = 125/517 = 25%. However, depending on the proportion of amino acids initially converted into protein, subsequent costs for protein turnover will vary, until an amount of amino acids equivalent to that initially incorporated into protein has in turn been degraded and converted into glucose and urea. Protein intake can thus be expected to influence energy expenditure beyond the postprandial phase. For instance, in patients receiving fixed amounts of energy by intravenous infusion, but in whom .31 g of dextrose per kg body weight per day was replaced by an equicaloric amount of amino acids (to provide 364 mg instead of 180 mg amino acid nitrogen/kg body weight/day), an increase in energy expenditure of 2.2 kcal/kg/day was observed (56). This is equivalent to 40% of the energy content of the additional dose of amino acids. Considering that the amino acids were provided intravenously and that there was a concomitant decrease in metabolic costs for handling glucose, one should apparently expect dietary protein to raise the metabolic rate by an amount approaching one-half of its energy content. On this basis, a change in protein intake from 75 g per day to 100 g per day would be expected to increase energy expenditure by about 50 kcal per day.

METABOLIC COSTS OF LIPOGENESIS

Several reactions in the fatty acid synthesizing pathway require ATP, so conversion of glucose into fat requires a substantial energy investment, estimated at about 20% of the energy channeled into the lipogenic pathway (4). If the costs for prior conversion of glucose into glycogen, as well as for the transport of fatty acid synthesized in the liver to adipose tissue, are also included, the cost for conversion of dietary carbohydrate into fat may be assessed at some 25% (57). In subjects consuming 1,500 kcal/day of excess carbohydrate during 7 consecutive days, de novo fat synthesis reached 150 g per day. This was accompanied by a 35% increase in daily energy expenditure, equivalent to the dissipation of about 30% of the calories consumed in excess. About 25% of this 30% could be attributed to the obligatory costs for de novo fat synthesis (57). Such an uncommonly high rate of nutrient energy dissipation in humans becomes manifest only when lipogenesis is stimulated by deliberate and sustained overconsumption of carbohydrates in large amounts. In subjects consuming a Western diet, fatty acid synthesis from glucose appears to have minor quantitative significance, because even the ingestion of an unusually large carbohydrate load of 500 g will be accommodated by expansion of the glycogen reserves, without increases in body fat (58). It is noteworthy that this observation illustrates that glycogen reserves are spontaneously maintained in a range far below their maximal capacity even under *ad libitum* food intake conditions, which implies that satiety occurs well before glycogen stores are maximally filled and well before lipogenesis becomes an important pathway for carbohydrate disposal.

Dissipation of dietary energy by conversion of glucose into fat is often considered a factor in explaining why high-carbohydrate diets are less conducive to obesity than high-fat diets (59). With the limited quantitative significance of de novo lipogenesis when mixed diets are consumed (58), this is probably quite irrelevant. Furthermore, the possible significance of lipogenesis for energy dissipation under conditions of energy balance is actually quite small when one considers that glucose energy channeled into fat, at a cost equivalent to 25% of its caloric content, is followed by oxidation with the net ATP yield applicable to endogenous fat (96%) for an overall net ATP yield of .75 × 96% = 72%. This is not much less than the 75% net ATP yield estimated for carbohydrate oxidation in the absence of lipogenesis! As will be shown, the fact that weight gain occurs more readily on high-fat than on high-carbohydrate diets should be attributed primarily to the fact that food can more readily be consumed in great excess when its fat content is high. The excess may be due to the higher caloric density of fatty foods compared to glycogen accumulation on high-carbohydrate diets.

METABOLIC EFFICIENCY

When compared to daily energy turnover, the amount of energy retained during the development of obesity is rather small. Averaged over a long period, the imbalance amounts to a difference of only a few percent between energy intake and energy expenditure. Because a positive energy balance can, in principle, be attributed to excessive intake or to reduced expenditure of energy, there has been considerable interest in the possible significance of even small differences in *metabolic efficiency* in the development or the prevention of obesity (59,60).

Metabolic efficiency can be defined in many ways (Table 3). The most readily applied approach is to relate physical work output to energy expenditure. During low-intensity exertion, the efficiency of the process appears to be low, because most of the energy expended serves to regenerate the ATP dissipated for maintenance metabolism. The intensity of the workload, relative to resting energy expenditure, is thus the major variable determining the apparent overall metabolic efficiency. For one to obtain a better measure of metabolic efficiency, it is important to relate the amount of work produced to the change in metabolic rate that it causes. Typical net efficiency values obtained in this manner for aerobic exertion range from 25% to 27% in humans and animals (2,19). When the effect of differences in body weight is minimized, as during bicycle ergometry, net efficiencies for the production of muscular work are essentially the same in normal and obese subjects over a considerable range of work intensities (61). Costs for weight-bearing activities, being roughly proportional to body weight (10), are, however, higher in obese than in lean subjects for comparable tasks.

Relating energy deposited in the carcass to total amount of food energy consumed is an important practical consideration in judging feed efficiency in the production of meat. As in the case of increasing workloads, gross nutrient efficiencies rise markedly as the amount of excess energy consumed becomes larger relative to maintenance energy expenditure (Fig. 3). In a situation characterized by small changes in body size over time, such as in adult humans, gross metabolic efficiency is close to zero, which is essentially meaningless. In trying to assess the efficiency with which

TABLE 3. *Some possible definitions of metabolic efficiency*

1. η_{work}	$= \dfrac{\text{Work produced}}{\text{Energy intake}}$	Depends primarily on amount of physical activity performed; varies from very low to nil
2. $\eta_{\Delta\,work}$	$= \dfrac{\Delta \text{ Work produced}}{\Delta \text{ Metabolic rate}}$	Reproducible under well-defined conditions and thus meaningful where it is about 27%
3. $\eta_{coupling}$	$= \dfrac{\text{Mechanical work produced}}{\text{High-energy bond energy utilized}}$	About 40%
4. η_{gross}	$= \dfrac{\text{Energy retained}}{\text{Energy intake}}$	Depends primarily on intake/expenditure ratio; important in judging feed efficiency during meat production; negative when intake $<$ expenditure
5. η_{net}	$= \dfrac{\text{Energy retained}}{\text{Energy int. above maint. req.}}$	Similar in principle to Eq. 2 but difficult to assess with accuracy (particularly when intake is not substantially greater than expenditure) because maintenance requirements cannot be reliably established
6. $\eta_{storage}$	$= \dfrac{\text{Cost of nutrient absorption and storage}}{\Delta \text{ Energy expenditure}}$	Somewhat variable; depends primarily on importance of catecholamine (SNS)-mediated stimulation of metabolism relative to obligatory storage costs (i.e., ATP needed for synthesis of glycogen, protein, and adipose tissue triglycerides)
7. $\eta_{ox.\,phos.}$	$= \dfrac{\text{Energy recovered in} \sim \text{of ATP}}{\begin{array}{c}\text{Heat of combustion}\\\text{of substrates oxidized}\end{array}}$	Depends primarily on P:O ratio; reaches 67% for P:O ratio of 3. (Because some proton leakage across the mitochondrial membrane always occurs, the P:O ratio can be substantially less than 3 at low rates of substrate oxidation)
8. $\eta_{metabolism}$	$= \dfrac{\text{ATP replaced}}{\text{ATP generated}}$	Depends on metabolic costs incurred for substrate handling (i.e., ATP expenditure for transport, activation, substrate cycles; cf. Fig. 4)
9. $\eta_{ATP\,prod.}$	$= \eta_{ox.\,phos.} \times \eta_{metabolism}$	

food energy is processed, it is therefore important here as well to assess energy retention relative to the amount consumed in excess of maintenance requirements. The accuracy of such an approach is limited, particularly in humans, because the required correction for maintenance energy requirements involves a rather large fraction of the energy turnover and because these requirements keep changing as body weight and physical activities vary during the weeks needed to produce measurable changes in body composition. Even small errors in estimating maintenance requirements have a considerable impact on the net efficiency value obtained (Fig.

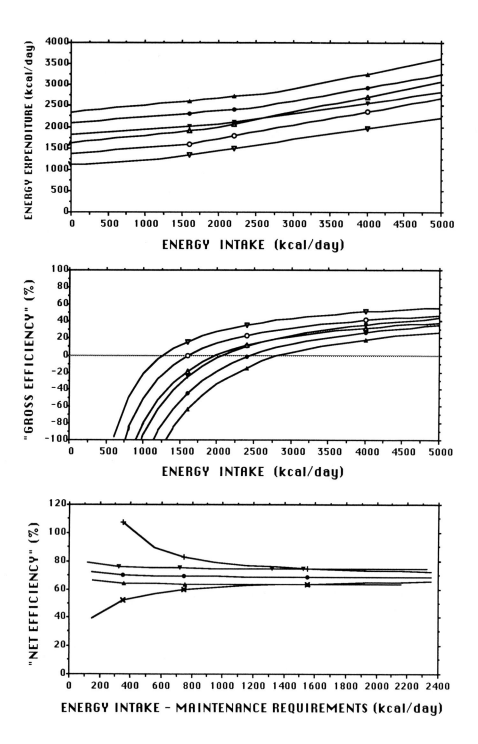

3), so the accuracy of such evaluations must be expected to be quite uncertain and ill-suited to detect minor variations in metabolic efficiencies.

Discussion of possible differences in metabolic efficiency in humans is thus generally confined to comparisons of resting metabolic rates (RMRs) and of TEFs. RMRs are quite closely correlated with fat-free mass (FFM), but the correlation line intercepts the vertical axis (63). RMR is therefore not proportional to FFM, and RMR expressed per kg FFM must be logically expected to be lower for individuals of large body size (64). Lower TEFs have been reported for some but not all obese subjects, particularly following weight reduction (60). Because the nonobligatory component of TEF dissipates at most 3% to 5% of food energy, the impact of a partial reduction in this postprandial phenomenon on overall resting energy expenditure is relatively small, compared to the effects of exercise or of changes in body size (65).

Variations in the metabolic costs incurred for processing different nutrients and substrates are relatively readily assessed. Considering the diet consumed and the time elapsed since food was last consumed, one should expect the cost for the replacement of one mole of ATP to vary between 20 and 22 kcal/mol, rather than the 13–14 kcal/mol corresponding to the ΔG of ATP hydrolysis or the 18 kcal/mol of ATP turned over. In fact, one would expect energy turnover to be slightly higher when a carbohydrate-rich fuel mix is oxidized, though a 10% shift in the energy provided by carbohydrate at the expense of fat, or vice versa, would be expected to alter overall energy expenditure by only 1.5%. Hurni et al. (66) found sleeping metabolic rates, BMRs, and 24-hour energy expenditure to be 5% to 8% higher in a group of volunteers when they were consuming a high-carbohydrate diet (80% of energy as CHO, 5% as fat) as compared to a mixed diet (55% CHO and 30% fat). On the other hand, Abbot et al. (67) could find no difference in 24-hour expenditure among obese Pima Indians adapted to diets providing 42% fat and 43% carbohydrate or diets with 20% fat and 65% carbohydrate.

FIG. 3. Conditions affecting the measurement of gross and net nutrient efficiency. **Top:** Daily energy expenditure varies as a function of energy intake, assuming a basic metabolic rate of 1,440 kcal/day (i.e., 1 kcal/min), a TEF of 10%, a decrease in metabolic rate attenuating energy deficits by 5%, and a dissipation of 20% of the energy consumed in excess (line identified by open circles; maintenance energy requirement = 1,490/0.9 = 1,600 kcal/day). The effect of a ±20% difference in resting and food-induced energy expenditure is shown by the open triangles. The filled-in circles are calculated for similar conditions except that physical activity is considered to raise energy expenditure by 720 kcal/day. The same identifying symbols are used in all three graphs. **Middle:** The apparent *gross nutrient efficiency* is determined primarily by the level of energy intake; differences in physical activity can have a greater impact on gross efficiency values than even large (i.e., ±20%) differences in metabolic efficiency. **Bottom:** The apparent *net nutrient efficiency* for the case with exercise and the normal rate of energy dissipation (maintenance requirement = 2,160 kcal/day; filled-in circles in all panels). The lines identified by filled-in triangles show net efficiencies when resting metabolic rates differ by ±20%, assuming that maintenance energy requirements are based on actual measurements. The two lines with crosses show the impact of ±5% errors in evaluating maintenance energy requirements. The figure illustrates that errors in estimating maintenance requirements have an overwhelming impact when energy intake is less than 50% higher than maintenance requirements. Even at higher intakes, 5% errors have as great an impact on the apparent net nutrient efficiency as a ±20% difference in metabolic efficiency. (From ref. 62, with permission).

TABLE 4. *Effect of CHO and FAT content of fuel mix oxidized on energy expenditure of* ad libitum *fed mice[a]*

$$1.^{b} \; \text{EnExp} = .046 + .332 \times 10^{-5} \, \text{rev/d} + \overbrace{1.10 \, \text{CHO ox} + 1.01 \, \text{fat ox}}^{1.09 \times}$$
$$\pm .005 \times 10^{-5c} \qquad \pm .01^{c} \qquad \qquad \pm .01^{c}$$

$$[R^2 = .95^c \qquad N = 1553]$$

$$2.^{d} \; \text{EnExp} = .02 + .338 \times 10^{-5} \, \text{rev/d} + \overbrace{1.22 \, \text{CHO ox} + 1.09 \, \text{fat ox}}^{1.12 \times}$$
$$\pm .005 \times 10^{-5d} \qquad \pm .01^{d} \qquad \qquad \pm .01^{d}$$

$$[R^2 = .96^d \qquad N = 3,225]$$

---

[a] From ref. 62, with permission.
[b] Daily energy expenditures, CHO, and fat oxidations (in terms of kcal/g BWt/day), and spontaneous running activity (number of revolutions/day) observed in 10 female CD1 mice during 160 consecutive days, on diets providing 18% of energy as protein, 13% or 45% as fat, and the remainder as sucrose and starch (1:1).
[c] $p \leq .0001$.
[d] Same parameters, as observed in 10 male CD1 mice studied during 345 consecutive days under similar conditions, except that the diets provided 13%, 27%, or 41% of dietary energy as fat.

In animal studies, Donato and Hegsted (68) reported that 35% of the energy consumed in excess of maintenance requirements were retained when the excess was provided in the form of fat, as compared to 28% when the excess was carbohydrate. In mice whose 24-hour energy expenditure was measured individually for many consecutive days, the use of carbohydrate as a fuel, as compared to fat, was accompanied by 9% to 12% higher rates of energy expenditure (Table 4).

COSTS FOR MAINTAINING ENERGY RESERVES

Finally, it is important to appreciate that the costs for nutrient storage include not only the ATP expenditure required for their initial incorporation into the body's stores but also the costs for maintaining and moving the tissues that contain these reserves. If the resting metabolic rate is considered to increase by about 10 kcal/day per kg of additional body weight in adults (63), each kg of additional body weight will cause an increase in energy expenditure of some 12 to 15 kcal/day in sedentary individuals. These costs will be in the range of 20 to 30 kcal/day per kg of additional body weight for individuals engaging in moderate to substantial physical activities. The degree of physical activity thus appears as yet another factor affecting the efficiency with which ingested energy appears to be retained, even though it does not imply any change in the efficiency with which metabolic processes or ATP turnover occur! Furthermore, the self-correcting effect that changes in body weight exert in compensating for deviations from the energy balance are greater in physically active and in fidgety subjects (69) than in sedentary individuals, a phenomenon that totally escapes detection when resting metabolic rates are compared.

CONCLUSIONS AND IMPLICATIONS

Approximately two-thirds of the energy liberated in the course of oxidative degradation of carbohydrates, fats, and proteins are recovered in the form of high-energy bonds. Based on a number of "best guesses," the ATP expended for substrate handling (transport, storage, recycling, and activation) dissipates about 10%, 25%, or 45% of the energy provided by dietary fat, carbohydrates, and protein, respectively. The net ATP yields are thus estimated to decline from 90% with fat to 75% with carbohydrate and 55% with protein. Depending on the composition of the diet consumed and the time elapsed after food intake, the cost for replacing one mole of ATP would thus vary between 20 and 22 kcal, or some 20% more than the 18 kcal released per mol of ATP turned over.

Differences in net ATP yields provide a logical basis from which to assess possible differences in metabolic efficiency; the approach involves specified assumptions that can be challenged or modified. By contrast, attempts to rationalize observations on nutrient energy retention in terms of metabolic efficiency and/or ATP turnover are fraught with intractable uncertainties, notably because they are greatly affected by the ratio of intake to expenditure and by the level of physical activity. In the attempt to understand the metabolic causes of obesity, the concept of metabolic efficiency has been a conceptual trap rather than a tool! Furthermore, preoccupation with the possible impact of differences in metabolic efficiencies in promoting or preventing obesity or in playing a role in body weight maintenance tends to hide the fact that energy balance and changes in energy balance under *ad libitum* feeding conditions are determined overwhelmingly by factors influencing food intake and adjustments of food intake. Changes in energy expenditure exert only minimal leverage on the energy balance and its corrective adjustments (Fig. 4). It is only when energy intake

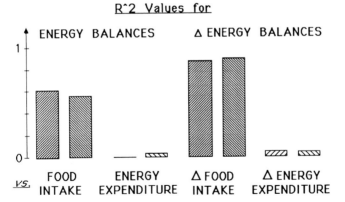

FIG. 4. Impact of energy intake and expenditure on energy balance and of changes (Δ) in energy intake and expenditure from one day to the next in altering the energy balance in ad libitum fed mice. The data were obtained in 10 female CD1 mice maintained on diets providing 18% of dietary energy as protein, 13% (left) or 45% (right side of the pair) as fat, and the balance as starch plus sucrose (1:1). The 24-hour energy expenditures and food intake were determined for each mouse during 160 consecutive days (70).

is "clamped" at some fixed amount that differences in rates of energy dissipation will influence body weights, to the extent that a 5% difference in metabolic rate would have to be offset by a 5 kg to 8 kg difference in body weight. The impact of different physical activity levels is readily far greater. The exaggerated importance often attributed to differences in metabolic efficiencies appears to be founded on the unjustified presumption that a change in energy expenditure will not be offset by a change in energy intake when food intake is self-determined.

ACKNOWLEDGMENT

This work was supported by NIH Grant DK 33214.

REFERENCES

1. Lusk G. *Science of Nutrition*. New York: Johnson Reprint, 1976.
2. Kleiber M. *The Fire of Life. An introduction to animal energetics*. New York: RE Krieger, 1975.
3. Weast RC. *Handbook of chemistry and physics*, 57th ed. Cleveland, OH: CRC Press, 1976.
4. Flatt JP. Conversion of carbohydrate to fat in adipose tissue: an energy-yielding and, therefore, self-limiting process. *J Lipid Res* 1970;11:131–43.
5. McGilvery RW, Goldstein G. *Biochemistry. A functional approach*. Philadelphia: WB Saunders, 1979.
6. Livesey G, Elia M. The estimation of energy expenditure, net carbohydrate utilization and net fat oxidation and synthesis by indirect calorimetry; evaluation of some errors with special reference to the detailed composition of fuels. *Am J Clin Nutr*, 1988;47:608–28.
7. Westheimer FH. Why nature chose phosphates. *Science* 1987;235:1173–8.
8. Lehninger AL. *Principles of biochemistry*. New York: Worth Publishers, 1982.
9. Flatt JP, Blackburn GL. The metabolic fuel regulatory system: implications for protein-sparing therapies during caloric deprivation and disease. *Am J Clin Nutr* 1974;27:175–87.
10. Pandolf KB, Givoni B, Goldman RF. Predicting energy expenditure with loads while standing or walking very slowly. *J Appl Physiol* 1977;43:577–81.
11. Bahr R, Ingnes I, Vaage O, Sejersted OM, Newsholme EA. Effect of duration of exercise on excess postexercise O_2 consumption. *J Appl Physiol* 1987;62:485–90.
12. Tremblay A, Fontaine E, Poehlman ET, Mitchell D, Perron L, Bouchard C. The effect of exercise-training on resting metabolic rate in lean and moderately obese individuals. *Int J Obes* 1986;10:511–7.
13. Lemasters JL. Near thermodynamic equilibrium of oxidative phosphorylation by inverted inner membrane vesicles of rat liver mitochondria. *FEBS* 1979;51:15–28.
14. Slater EC. Mechanisms of phosphorylation in the respiratory chain. *Nature* 1953;172:975–8.
15. Mitchell P. Keilin's respiratory chain concept and its chemiosmotic consequences. *Science* 1979;206:1148–59.
16. Murphy MP, Brand MD. Variable stoichiometry of proton pumping by the mitochondrial respiratory chain. *Nature* 1987;329:170–2.
17. Hinkle PC, Yu ML. The phosphorus/oxygen ratio of mitochondrial oxidative phosphorylation. *J Biol Chem* 1979;254:2450–5.
18. Heldt HW, Klingenberg M, Milovancev M. Differences between the ATP/ADP ratios in the mitochondrial matrix and in extramitochondrial space. *Eur J Biochem* 1972;30:434–40.
19. Pahud P, Ravussin E, Jéquier E. Energy expended during oxygen deficit period of submaximal exercise in man. *J Appl Physiol*, 1980;48:770–5.
20. Flatt JP. Energetics of intermediary metabolism. In: Garrow JS, Halliday D, eds. *Substrate and energy metabolism in man*. London: John Libbey, 1985:58–69.
21. Whipp BJ, Wasserman K. Efficiency of muscular work. *J Appl Physiol*, 1965;26:644–8.
22. Manchester KL. Muscle ATP and creatine-P. *Biochem Educ* 1980;8:70–2.
23. Flatt JP, Pahud P, Ravussin E, Jéquier E. An estimate of the P:O ratio in man. *TIBS* 1984;9:251–5.

24. Hess B, Chance B. Phosphorylation efficiency of the intact cell. I. Glucose-oxygen titrations in ascites tumor cells. *J Biol Chem* 1959;234:3031–5.
25. Jungas RL, Ball EG. Studies on the metabolism of tissue. XVII. In vitro effects of insulin upon the metabolism of the carbohydrate and triglyceride stores of adipose tissue from fasted-refed rats. *Biochemistry* 1964;3:1696–1702.
26. Fisher JN, Ball EG. Studies on the metabolism of adipose tissue. XX. The effect of thyroid status upon oxygen consumption and lipolysis. *Biochemistry* 1967;6:637–47.
27. Matthews PM, Bland JL, Gadian DG, Radda GK. The steady-state rate of ATP synthesis in the profused rat heart measured by 31 P NMR saration transfer. *Biochem Res Commun* 1981;103: 1052–9.
28. Shoubridge EA, Brige RW, Radda GK, Ross B. 31 P NMR saturation transfer measurements of the steady state rates of creatine kinase and ATP synthesis rat brain. *FEBS Lett* 1982;140:288–92.
29. Freeman D, Bartlett S, Radda G, Ross B. Energetics of sodium transport in the kidney. Saturation transfer 31P NMR. *Biochim Biophys Acta* 1983;762:325.
30. Livesey G. ATP yields from proteins, fats and carbohydrates and mitochondrial efficiency in vivo. *Recent Adv Obes Res* 1986;5:131–4.
31. Ravussin E, Acheson KJ, Vernet O, et al. Evidence that insulin resistance is responsible for the decreased thermic effect of glucose in human obesity. *J Clin Invest* 1985;76:1268–73.
32. Boyer PD. A perspective of the binding change mechanism for ATP synthesis. *FASEB J* 1989;3:2164–78.
33. Himms-Hagen J. Brown adipose tissue thermogenesis and obesity. *Prog Lipid Res* 1989;28:65–115.
34. Rothwell NJ, Stock MJ. Regulation of energy balance. *Ann Rev Nutr* 1981;1:235–56.
35. Astrup A, Christensen NJ, Simonsen L, Bülow J. Thermogenic role of brown adipose tissue and skeletal muscle in humans. In: Müller MJ, Danforth E, Burger AG, Siedentopp U, ed. *Hormones and nutrition in obese and cachexia*. Berlin: Springer-Verlag, 1990.
36. Newsholme EA, Leech AR. *Biochemistry for the medical sciences*. Chichester: John Wiley, 1983.
37. Edens NK, Leibel RL, Hirsch J. Mechanism of free fatty acid re-esterification in human adipocytes in vitro. *J Lipid Res*, 1990;31:1423–31.
38. Randle PJ, Hales CN, Garland PB, Newsholme EA. The glucose fatty-acid cycle. Its role in insulin sensitivity and metabolic disturbances of diabetes mellitus. *Lancet* 1963;1:785–9.
39. Meylan M, Henny C, Temler E, Jéquier E, Felber JP. Metabolic factors in the insulin resistance in human obesity. *Metabolism* 1987;36:256–61.
40. Wolfe RR. The role of triglyceride-fatty acid cycling and glucose cycling in thermogenesis and amplification of net substrate flux in human subjects. In: Müller MJ, Danforth E, Burger AG, Siedentopp U, eds. *Hormones and nutrition in obesity and cachexia*. Berlin: Springer-Verlag, 1990.
41. Wolfe RR, Herndon DN, Jahoor F, Miyoshi H, Wolfe M. Effect of severe burn injury on substrate cycling by glucose and fatty acids. *N Engl J Med* 1987;317:403–8.
42. Grande F, Keys A. Body weight, body composition and calorie status. In: Goodhart RS, Shils ME, eds. *Modern nutrition in health and disease*. Philadelphia: Lea, Febiger, 1980:3–34.
43. Smith TJ, Edelman IS. The role of sodium transport in thyroid thermogenesis. *Fed Proc* 1979;38: 2150–3.
44. Wolfe RR. Isotopic measurement of glucose and lactate kinetics. *Ann Med* 1990;22:163–70.
45. McGarry JD, Kuwajima M, Newgard CB, Foster DW. From dietary glucose to liver glycogen: the full circle round. *Ann Rev Nutr* 1987;7:51–73.
46. DeFronzo RA, Ferrannini E. Regulation of hepatic glucose metabolism in humans. *Diabetes Metab Rev* 1987;3:415–59.
47. Elia M, Zed C, Neale G, Livesey G. The energy cost of triglyceride-fatty acid recycling in non-obese subjects after an overnight fast and four days of starvation. *Metabolism* 1987;36:251–5.
48. Loewy A. *Handbuch der biochemie*. Oppenheimer ed. Jena 1911;1:279.
49. Garlick PJ, Glugston GA, Swick RW, Waterlow JC. Diurnal pattern of protein and energy metabolism in man. *Am J Clin Nutr* 1980;33:1983–6.
50. Welle S, Nair KS. Relationship of resting metabolic rate to body composition and protein turnover. *Am J Physiol* 1990;258:E990–8.
51. Kinney JM, Elwyn DH. Protein metabolism and injury. *Ann Rev Nutr* 1983;3:433–66.
52. Acheson KJ, Ravussin E, Wahren J, Jéquier E. Thermic effect of glucose in man, obligatory and facultative thermogenesis. *J Clin Invest* 1984;74:1572–80.
53. Karst H, Steiniger J, Noack R, Steglich HD. Diet-induced thermogenesis in man: thermic effects of single protein, carbohydrate and fats depending on their energy amounts. *Ann Nutr Metab* 1987;31:117–25.

54. Flatt JP, Ravussin E, Acheson KJ, Jéquier E. Effects of dietary fat on postprandial substrate oxidation and on carbohydrate and fat balances. *J Clin Invest* 1985;76:1019–24.
55. Shaw SN, Elwyn DH, Askanazi J, Iles M, Schwarz Y, Kinney JM. Effects of increasing nitrogen intake on nitrogen balance and energy expenditure in nutritionally depleted adult patients receiving parenteral nutrition. *Am J Clin Nutr* 1983;37:930–40.
56. Dallosso HM, James WPT. Whole-body calorimetry studies in adult men. 1. The effect of fat overfeeding on 24 h energy expenditure. *Br J Nutr* 1984;52:49–64.
57. Acheson KJ, Schutz Y, Bessard T, Anantharaman K, Flatt JP, Jéquier E. Glycogen storage capacity and *de novo* lipogenesis during massive carbohydrate overfeeding in man. *Am J Clin Nutr* 1988;48:240–7.
58. Acheson KJ, Flatt JP, Jéquier E. Glycogen synthesis versus lipogenesis after a 500-g carbohydrate meal. *Metabolism* 1982;31:1234–40.
59. Sims EAH. Energy balance in human beings: the problems of plenitude. *Vit and Horm* 1986;43:1–101.
60. Schutz Y, Bessard T, Jéquier E. Diet-induced thermogenesis measured over a whole day in obese and nonobese women. *Am J Clin Nutr* 1984;40:542–52.
61. Segal K, Presta E, Gutin B. Thermic effect of food during graded exercise in normal weight and obese men. *Am J Clin Nutr* 1984;40:995–1000.
62. Flatt JP. The biochemistry of energy expenditure. In: Brodoff BN, Björntorp P, eds. *Obesity.* New York: JB Lippincott [In press].
63. Owen OE. Regulation of energy and metabolism. In: Kinney JM, Jeejeebhoy KN, Hill GL, Owen OE, eds. *Nutrition and metabolism in patient care.* New York: WB Saunders, 1988.
64. Forbes GB. *Human body composition: growth, aging, nutrition, and activity.* New York: Springer-Verlag, 1987.
65. Waterlow JC. Metabolic adaptation to low intakes of energy and protein. *Ann Rev Nutr* 1986;6:495–526.
66. Hurni M, Burnand B, Pittet P, Jéquier E. Metabolic effects of a mixed and a high-carbohydrate low-fat diet in man, measured over 24 h in a respiration chamber. *Br. J Nutr* 1982;47:33–43.
67. Abbott WGH, Howard BV, Ruotolo G, Ravussin E. Energy expenditure in humans: effects of dietary fat and carbohydrate. *Am J Physiol* 1990;258:E347–51.
68. Donato KA, Hegsted DM. Efficiency of utilization of various energy sources for growth. *Proc Natl Acad Sci USA* 1985;82:4866–70.
69. Ravussin E, Lillioja S, Andersen TE, Christin L, Bogardus C. Determinants of 24-h energy expenditure in man. *J Clin Invest* 1986;78:1568–78.
70. Flatt JP. Assessment of daily and cumulative carbohydrate and fat balances in mice. *J Nutr Biochem* 1991;2.

DISCUSSION

Dr. Edwards: As a physiologist I would like to pick up this concept of efficiency and take it a little further, because clearly from the point of view of work efficiency there has been a very interesting and varied history. The problem is that if one considers what was the mechanical efficiency of exercise as defined by Hill, Long, and Lufton and A. V. Hill's earliest collaborators, based on the mechanical power output of muscle in relation to its actual heat measurements, figures were quoted in the region of 20%. From then on it became a matter of defining it according to the relationship between the energy cost in terms of oxygen intake and the energy cost of some reference state, whether that was basal metabolic rate—resting on the bicycle or some form of other equivalent resting state such as loadless pedaling—or, as one group has studied, unloaded exercise on a horizontal treadmill. The problem then goes further, because it depends on how the measurements are made, whether they are steady-state gas collections (of course any assumptions about efficiency depend on the assumption of steady-state). Are these steady-state oxygen intake measurements made and referred to the steady-state of the control state, or are they made from, for example, more modern techniques allowed by breath analysis and computer integration? Well, that may be absolutely marvelous for looking at transients, but the problem is that we are aware that the time required to obtain the satisfactory consistent reading for these is long and that it offers the opportunity of integration of errors. Then the other method of doing it is to make a total gas collection over a very considerable length of time and to compare and contrast those total costs in terms of oxygen intake of the exercise period against an equivalent control period. The trouble is that the answers obtained are different. This has raised the question of whether the energy cost of resynthesis is the same as the energy cost of maintenance. I would like to ask Jean-Pierre Flatt whether he sees any possibility of a difference in the efficiency of recovery processes compared to maintenance processes in relation to exercise. We heard yesterday from Professor Pi-Sunyer that the excess oxygen of exercise was not likely to be of very great importance because of the recovery processes being complete in 40 minutes to 1 hour after the exercise. The reality of exercise in life is that it is not a single period of exercise followed by a single recovery but multiple small episodes of exercise with multiple small recovery periods. This modeling of real life by an intermittent exercise study was one which Eric Hultman, Roger Harris, and colleagues at the Swedish Aviation Institute carried out in a detailed metabolic and gas exchange study when I worked there in 1970. There we found the difference between the carefully analyzed work efficiency of intermittent exercise compared with continuous exercise for the same average power output. It was interesting to us that the difference was small, which seemed to agree with what had been published from measurements of the oxygen consumption of the isolated canine muscle studied in situ and the restoration of high-energy phosphate in that muscle. They found the P:O ratio of the recovery process to be less than that of the maintenance process. Since this seems to have some relevance to the role of exercise and energetics in real life and a possible role in relation to energy balance, I wonder whether Jean-Pierre Flatt could comment on whether his work now supports or does not support the idea of a difference in the energy efficiency of recovery processes compared with maintenance processes.

Jean-Pierre Flatt: You could imagine that if substrate handling is greater there could be a small difference. For example, glycogen converted to lactate and remade to glucose would have additional energy costs than substrate burned by direct oxidation. However, I think it would be relatively minor. The total postexercise energy expenditure has been estimated to be about 15% of the energy expenditure induced while the exercise is performed. It is going to involve a relatively minor fraction of the total energy dissipation. The answer to your question is, there could be some differences explained by differences in the cost for substrate handling. There could be other causes of differences that I have not considered and which I am not able to consider from the data that I have, but my interpretation is that it will not be a very significant factor compared to the total energy expenditure induced by exercise.

*Energy Metabolism: Tissue Determinants and
Cellular Corollaries*, edited by J. M. Kinney
and H. N. Tucker. Raven Press, Ltd.,
New York © 1992.

Energy Metabolism in Muscle: Its Possible Role in the Adaptation to Energy Deficiency

Jan Henriksson

Department of Physiology III, Karolinska Institute, S-114 33 Stockholm, Sweden

The body's strategy for coping with a low energy intake involves several distinct adaptive changes, the most important of which is a reduction in body weight and a reduction of physical activity. Other sources of economy, such as a reduction in the basal metabolic rate (BMR) and metabolic changes leading to the sparing of glucose, are also of considerable importance in maintaining body functions during periods of energy shortage.

Skeletal muscle accounts for a large portion of the body's energy expenditure both at rest and during exercise. Compared to other tissues, such as the viscera or the brain, the resting skeletal muscle has a low metabolic rate per unit mass. Owing to its large mass, however, it accounts for as much as 25% of the body's oxidative metabolism at rest. The muscle cell is unique in the sense that its metabolic rate can vary over a very wide range, increasing more than 200 times from rest to maximal exercise. Previous investigations involving chronic muscle stimulation have revealed that skeletal muscle cells possess a quite remarkable capacity for adapting to extreme metabolic demands, so it is conceivable that adaptations in skeletal muscle may contribute to the saving of energy during periods of energy deficiency.

This chapter focuses on some possible mechanisms for economizing energy in resting and contracting skeletal muscles and on the information available about the importance of these mechanisms in the energy-deficient body.

MAJOR METABOLIC PATHWAYS OF THE MUSCLE CELL: AN OVERVIEW

The energy metabolism of skeletal muscle can be simplified as consisting of a rather small number of biochemical pathways that have a significant impact on the cellular metabolic equilibrium. These include (A) the complete oxidation of carbohydrates, fats, and proteins; (B) the net formation of lactic acid from carbohydrates (glycogen), i.e., the pathway known as anaerobic glycolysis; and (C) the net transformation of carbohydrates into fats and of proteins into carbohydrates (gluconeogenesis) and fats (see ref. 1 for further reading). The oxidative capacity is limited by the cellular mitochondrial content (i.e., the enzymatic capacities of the citric acid cycle, the

345

respiratory chain, and the fatty acid degradation systems) as well as by the capacity of the muscle microcirculatory system. The anaerobic capacity of skeletal muscles is mainly limited by the enzymatic capacity of the glycogenolytic system. These biochemical pathways, as well as the energy exchange involving adenosine triphosphate and phosphocreatine, are considered in the following discussion. Protein is not normally a major fuel for skeletal muscles (2,3). This makes sense physiologically, because proteins constitute the building blocks of the cells of the body. This is especially true of skeletal muscle cells because of their high content of the contractile proteins (myosin and actin). When the body's energy supply is compromised, however, such as in long-term starvation, proteins (including those derived from muscle tissue itself) will also be used as a fuel in the energy metabolism of muscle.

MUSCLE FIBER TYPES

On the basis of the myofibrillar ATPase technique, muscle fibers can be classified as type I (slow-twitch) or type II (fast-twitch). The latter are generally divided into IIA and IIB subgroups (Fig. 1) (for further reading see ref. 4). An alternative terminology has been proposed, based on data on laboratory animals pertaining to the metabolic characteristics of these fibers: slow-twitch-oxidative (type I), fast-twitch-oxidative-glycolytic (type IIA), and fast-twitch-glycolytic (type IIB). Fiber type classifications are useful in describing muscle characteristics, but it should be kept in mind that they represent a simplification. Thus, for many variables, there is an almost continuous variation also within each fiber type or subtype.

In a large proportion of human muscles the ratio between the numbers of fast- and slow-twitch fibers ranges from 40/60 to 60/40, but with a large interindividual variation. In the most studied human muscles, the IIA fibers make up approximately two-thirds of the fast-twitch fraction (see ref. 4). In humans, the difference in contractile speed between the fast- and the slow-twitch fibers has not been clearly established; in the rat and in the cat the difference in the time to peak isometric tension has been reported to be twofold to threefold between the different fiber types (see 4). In these species, however, fiber-type differences tend to be greater than in human skeletal muscle. A probable reason is that in most experimental animals, the different fiber types are largely located in different muscles or in different parts of one muscle, whereas most human muscles are mixed muscles, with all fiber types intermingled in a mosaic pattern. There has been considerable discussion as to whether the maximum isometric force developed per unit of cross-sectional area differs in fast- and slow-twitch fiber types of skeletal muscle, but the available evidence does not support the existence of a clear difference between the muscle fiber types in this respect (for a discussion see refs. 4 and 5). In the thigh muscle of a sedentary person, slow-twitch fibers have an oxidative capacity approximately 50% higher than that of fast-twitch fibers, whereas the glycolytic capacity may be half of that in fast-twitch fibers (see ref. 4). Human muscle fiber types differ less in metabolic characteristics than fiber types in the rat, and the terms *fast-twitch-oxidative-glycolytic* and *fast-twitch-*

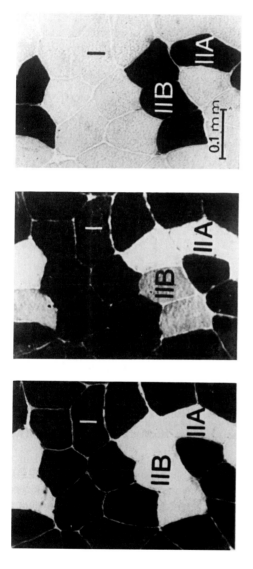

FIG. 1. Photomicrographs of transverse sections of a biopsy of the human thigh muscle. Sections stained for myofibrillar ATPase after preincubation at pH 4.3 (slow-twitch type I fibers darkly stained) (left), pH 4.6 (type I fibers and fibers of the IIB fast-twitch subgroup darkly stained) (middle), and pH 10.3 (all fast-twitch fibers –type IIA and IIB– darkly stained) (right). The same three fibers are identified in the three sections. Courtesy of P. Schantz.

the total number of muscle capillaries by 50% (9). The difference between endurance athletes and untrained individuals with respect to the capillary count per muscle fiber (leg muscles) has been found to be twofold to threefold (4). When stains for myofibrillar ATPase have been used as the basis for fiber type classification, most longitudinal studies in humans have failed to demonstrate an interconversion of fiber types (i.e., fast-twitch to slow-twitch) in response to endurance training (10). Endurance training is known, however, to lead to a complete type transformation within the fast-twitch (type II) fiber subgroup from type IIB to type IIA (11,12). The concept that endurance training does not change the relative occurrence of fast-twitch and slow-twitch fibers has been challenged in recent years, and it seems reasonable to conclude from the available data that extensive endurance training will result in an enhanced percentage of slow-twitch fibers. The probable reasons that fiber type transformation was not seen in the early studies are that these studies were of too short duration, and the fact that the muscles investigated were postural muscles, and therefore relatively trained even in the pretraining state (for a detailed discussion, see ref. 10). The training-induced adaptation of skeletal muscle has been shown to be metabolically significant in leading to a greater reliance on fat as an energy substrate (see references in refs. 4 and 13). This is the case despite the fact that, at a given rate of work, the plasma levels of free fatty acids are often lower in the trained state. The mechanism by which this occurs has not been conclusively shown; one conceivable mechanism has been put forward by Holloszy (13) (Fig. 4).

FIBER TYPE RECRUITMENT

During muscle contraction, muscle fibers are recruited in an orderly manner with the slow-twitch fibers having the lowest activation threshold (4). In humans, there is quite detailed information available on cycle ergometer exercise at different workloads (see 4). It has been shown that the slow-twitch (type 1) muscle fibers are the first to be activated and remain activated even at higher exercise intensities. Only thereafter is there a recruitment of the fast-twitch motor units, type IIA followed by type IIB. It is believed that fibers (motor units) of all types are recruited at exercise intensities demanding more than 80% to 85% of the VO_2max. However, very strenuous exercise is probably required for maximal activation of all the type IIB motor units in a given muscle.

In all probability, this fiber type recruitment pattern also applies to other activities, such as running. It may be, however, that the recruitment of high-threshold IIB units is less pronounced in running than it is in cycling, especially at high exercise intensities, at which cycling may involve quite forceful pedaling.

DIFFERENCES IN ENERGY EFFICIENCY BETWEEN THE FIBER TYPES

There is evidence that slow-twitch muscles use less ATP per unit of isometric tension developed than fast-twitch muscles (14,15). Similarly, Crow and Kushmerick

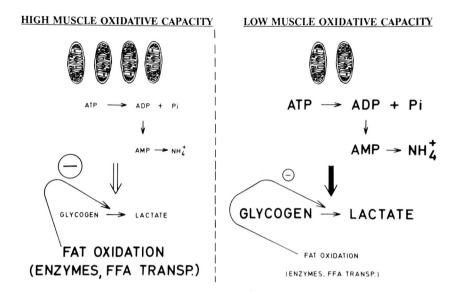

FIG. 4. A hypothetical biochemical mechanism whereby a large concentration of oxidative enzymes (i.e., citric acid cycle and fat oxidation enzymes and respiratory chain components), such as those in a slow-twitch muscle fiber, would lead to a greater reliance on fat metabolism, a lower rate of lactate formation, and sparing of muscle glycogen during exercise. An increased content of oxidative enzymes in a muscle cell is explained to a large extent by a larger mitochondrial volume (volume fraction). In the figure this is indicated schematically with mitochondrial symbols. Suppose that in one muscle (right), there are only one-half as many enzyme molecules of the citric acid cycle and one-half as many components of the respiratory chain as in another muscle (left). At a given rate of work (i.e., at a given rate of oxygen uptake), each mitochondrial unit therefore must be activated twice as much in this muscle than in the muscle with an oxidative capacity twice as high. An important component of this activation is the increased levels of the degradation products of ATP (e.g., ADP), which are the result of muscle contractions. These compounds must therefore be stabilized at a higher level in the right than in the left muscle. However, in addition to stimulating mitochondrial respiration, these ATP degradation products are also powerful stimulators of the glycolytic pathway. This leads to a higher glycolytic rate in the low oxidative muscle, resulting in a greater lactate formation and carbohydrate oxidation. The fat oxidation rate is higher in the muscle with the higher oxidative capacity, and the higher content of the enzymes of fatty acid transport and oxidation contribute to this. The increased rate of fat oxidation leads to a more pronounced inhibition of glycolysis in the high than in the low oxidative muscle, where the rate of fat oxidation is lower. In concert, these factors lead to a sparing of glycogen during exercise in muscles with a high oxidative capacity. Based on ref. 13.

(16) found that in the mouse the energy cost (per unit tension) for a brief maintained tetanus was much less for the slow-twitch soleus than for the fast-twitch extensor digitorum longus (EDL) muscle. This difference persisted when the contraction was maintained for 5 to 10 seconds, although it was reduced to approximately 10% owing to a pronounced decrease in the energy cost for the EDL muscle. It has been shown that during isometric contraction, the rise of maximal temperature in human skeletal

muscle is significantly higher in a muscle composed of mainly fast-twitch fibers than in a predominantly slow-twitch muscle (17).

During dynamic (concentric) contractions, the situation is more complicated because the energy cost will then also depend on the speed of contraction; the higher the speed of shortening, the lower the biochemical efficiency (18), and, furthermore, at high contraction speeds, fast-twitch fibers may well be the most energy efficient (19). Although corresponding data for human muscle fiber types are limited, the available data suggest that, if rapid movements are avoided, a loss through atrophy of fast-twitch fiber mass would be more advantageous in terms of fuel economy during intermediate or prolonged starvation than when the same amount of atrophy occurs in slow-twitch fibers. In addition to a proposed difference in the energy cost of contraction between the muscle fiber types, the higher oxidative capacity of slow-twitch fibers tends to make them rely more on fat as an energy substrate (Fig. 4) (4,13) (in analogy with the effects of training; see the preceding discussion). They are therefore better adapted than fast-twitch fibers to a situation in which the body's carbohydrate stores are depleted and, owing to the high cost of gluconeogenesis (1), the use of glucose by the muscles must be limited.

ENERGY EXPENDITURE IN RESTING MUSCLE

The reported rates of oxygen uptake of the resting human leg or forearm range from 1.1 ml $\times$ 1^{-1} to 3.6 ml $\times$ 1^{-1} tissue $\times$ min^{-1} (20,21,22). Interestingly, interindividual variations in the forearm resting oxygen uptake has been reported to correlate significantly with deviations from predicted values of the basal or sleeping metabolic rate. This suggests that differences in resting muscle metabolism account for part of the variance in metabolic rate among individuals (23). Studies in the rat also lend some support to this idea (24).

It may be speculated that part of the variation in resting muscle energy expenditure could be attributed to fiber-type differences, but it is not known how much the different fiber types vary in this respect. There is a known fiber-type difference in protein turnover, with higher values in the slow-twitch fibers. There is evidence that the basal metabolic rate increases with exercise training, independently of body composition and of the last bout of exercise (25), so it may be that energy expenditure in resting muscle is increased at high levels of physical training. In accord with the evidence that the resting muscle energy expenditure is increased in the trained state, Molé et al. (26) observed that daily exercise can reverse the drop in resting metabolic rate associated with the consumption of a very low-calorie diet. The effect of exercise training on the basal metabolic rate is controversial, however, and several studies have yielded conflicting results (27,28; see Ravussin and Rising). This may indicate that a possible effect of exercise training is small relative to a normal variation of the order of 10% in the population.

There is evidence that the basal metabolic rate decreases with caloric restriction (for references see 26). This decrease and the increased reliance on metabolism of the calorically dense fat stores minimizes the negative energy balance and the weight loss in connection with dieting. Furthermore, there is evidence that starvation may lead to some reduction in the basal metabolic rate (BMR) per unit of active tissue mass (29). One possible mechanism behind this change is a decrease in the plasma triiodothyronine (T_3) concentration following insufficient nutrition (30,31). Another likely contributing factor is the decreased sympathetic activity that accompanies energy deficiency. Interestingly, there is evidence that the hypothyroid state and the diminished sympathetic drive in malnutrition may be balanced by an increased sensitivity to physiologic concentrations of catecholamines (32,33,34).

In a microcalorimetric study of human thigh muscle biopsies, Fagher et al. (35) observed a markedly lower production of heat (per unit of tissue mass) in muscle samples from patients with anorexia nervosa than in samples from controls. Likewise, Nichols et al. (36) demonstrated diminished in vitro muscle respiratory rates in malnourished infants. Although these effects remain to be demonstrated in vivo, it is conceivable that a reduction in the basal metabolic rate of muscle during starvation could result from several different adaptive changes, including reductions in protein turnover, ion pumping, or a decreased rate of substrate cycling. All of these processes are known to be stimulated by thyroid hormones and would therefore be expected to respond to the hypothyroid state accompanying starvation.

MUSCLE PROTEIN DEGRADATION

One obvious change during the first 24 to 48 hours of starvation is an increased protein degradation in muscle, partly mediated by a decreased concentration of insulin and increases in glucocorticoid hormones (1). A substantial portion of the degraded muscle protein is ultimately made available to the liver as amino acids (predominantly alanine), which are precursors for the necessary increased rate of gluconeogenesis. It has been estimated that the central nervous system oxidizes about 100 g of glucose per day; and during the first 2 to 4 days of starvation, amino acids released from muscle can be expected to provide the carbon source for roughly one-half of this amount (40–50 g of glucose, corresponding to the degradation of approximately 75–90 g of muscle protein). This high rate of muscle protein loss (in the order of 2–3% per day) is not sustained, however, and a subsequent decline in muscle protein degradation has been observed when starvation is prolonged for more than a few days (1). The main cause of this is believed to be a switch from glucose to ketone bodies as a fuel for the brain, which leads to a diminished demand for gluconeogenic glucose production. The normal ketone body concentration in overnight-fasted subjects is 0.1 mM to 0.4 mM. If fasting proceeds, the plasma ketone body concentration rapidly increases to a new steady-state concentration of 7 mM to 10 mM (37). Nair et al. (38) have presented evidence that the fasting-induced increases in blood ketone bodies serve to spare muscle protein by reducing amino acid oxidation and influencing the balance between protein breakdown and synthesis. Thus, with prolonged starvation, the rate of whole-body protein turnover is subsequently reduced, and balance is achieved at a lower turnover rate. Another mediator of this adaptation could be the lower triiodothyronine levels, which accompany undernutrition. When obese subjects are treated with T_3 there is an increase in whole-body protein turnover (39,40). Muscle protein turnover in the rat has also been reported to be influenced by the thyroid status (41). A lowered protein turnover in skeletal muscle would contribute to the body's overall fuel economy, but, theoretically, it might impair the potential for amino acid mobilization during trauma or severe infections (42), conditions in which these processes may be of vital importance (43).

Normally, the protein turnover for the body as a whole is believed to account for 15% to 20% of the basal metabolic rate (42), although the figure may be higher. This indicates that a reduction may involve a significant saving of energy. A potential for adaptation is supported by the observation of an up to twofold variation in the rates of protein turnover of different individuals (44). For muscle there have been reports of both decreased (45) and increased (46,47) rates of protein turnover as a result of food deprivation. A consistent finding, however, is that the ratio of myofibrillar/nonmyofibrillar protein degradation markedly increases in the starved state (46,47,48). Changes in muscle protein turnover probably differ between the fiber types. The rates of protein synthesis and breakdown in skeletal muscle are known to be higher in slow-twitch fibers than in fast-twitch ones; in addition, there is a decline in protein synthesis and degradation in both fiber types with increasing age (49; 50, study on the rat).

In the postabsorptive state, muscle is considered to be a major source of circulating glutamine, an amino acid known to be indispensable for normal function of the immune system as well as other rapidly dividing cells (1). With prolonged fasting, the release of glutamine from muscle has been reported to be significantly increased. Interestingly, this occurs although starvation results in a pronounced decrease in muscle intracellular glutamine concentration (51). The latter finding is of interest also in the light of the reported (positive) relationship between muscle intracellular glutamine concentration and protein synthetic rate (41).

ION PUMPING

The maintenance of the membrane potential demands that sodium be extruded from the cell in exchange for potassium. This occurs through the action of the sodium-potassium pump, which consumes ATP. The energy cost of this process remains uncertain, and, for resting muscle, values ranging from 5% to 59% of the total energy turnover have been reported (52). Other investigators claim that the energy cost is comparatively small, corresponding to only a few percent of the total energy turnover both at rest and during maximal exercise (53,54). In the hypothyroid state accompanying energy deficiency, there is decreased activity of the Na-K pump (55). In this respect, however, the low T_3-induced reduction in calcium pumping is potentially more important, because the concentration of calcium ATPase in skeletal muscle is one to two orders of magnitude higher than that of the Na-K ATPase (56). The importance of the calcium pumping stems from the facts that the intracellular calcium concentration is much lower than that in the extracellular space and that Ca^{2+} must be pumped back into the sarcomplasmic reticulum during relaxation.

SUBSTRATE CYCLING

A decreased rate of substrate cycling may be one means by which skeletal muscle could contribute to the energy-saving process. This term, also called futile cycling, denotes a situation in which a key enzyme in a metabolic pathway is opposed by another enzyme that catalyzes the reverse reaction. One such enzyme couple is the fructose-6-phosphate/fructose bisphosphate cycle. It is believed that such substrate cycles are important in enhancing the sensitivity of metabolic regulation. Because the two complementary enzymes can maintain a high cycling flux (e.g., in anticipation of exercise), it is evident that a change in the concentration of an enzyme modulator (such as ADP for the F6P-FBP cycle) would affect the net flux of the main reaction much more than if no substrate cycling occurred. The role of substrate cycling in metabolic regulation has been discussed by Newsholme and Leech (1) and is also discussed in the chapters by Drs. Newsholme and Wolfe in this book. Other potentially important substrate cycles are the triglyceride/fatty acid and the protein/amino acid cycles.

The price for the improvement in metabolic sensitivity provided by the substrate cycling would be a marked increase in energy expenditure. The fructose-6-P/fructose bisphosphate cycle alone has been estimated to demand up to 50% of the daily caloric intake if it were constantly activated maximally (57). This is evidently not the case; it seems more likely that these cycles are activated only when a high sensitivity in the respective pathways is needed. In starvation the extra energy expenditure accompanying substrate cycling would seem less beneficial. There are indications that the efficiency of carbohydrate use is higher when the food intake is low: a change compatible with a lower degree of substrate cycling (58). If it is hypothesized that starvation decreases substrate cycling (e.g., in the fructose-6-phosphate/fructose bisphosphate cycle), this could result both from hormonal changes accompanying the state of starvation (such as the low insulin concentration) and from enzyme changes in the muscle per se. According to Russel et al. (59), starvation reduces muscle 6-phosphofructokinase (PFK) and therefore, in all probability, also fructose bisphosphatase (FBPase), since these two enzymes are highly correlated with each other in muscle (60). If, in fact, starvation leads to a reduction in substrate cycling, it appears likely that in these cases the sensitivity of metabolic control may be sacrificed in order to conserve energy.

Clearly, more research is needed to evaluate the importance of these and other potential means of reducing the energy expenditure in resting muscle.

CHANGES IN MUSCLE METABOLISM RESULTING FROM UNDERNUTRITION

During intermediate and prolonged starvation, ketone bodies, as previously stated, substantially replace glucose as a fuel for the brain, which leads to a markedly diminished demand for gluconeogenesis. Because gluconeogenesis can be said to represent a waste of energy—approximately 1.7 g of protein must be broken down to synthesize 1 g of glucose (1)—it is essential that other organs such as skeletal muscle should diminish their use of glucose as a fuel. There is evidence that glucose oxidation at rest and during exercise is markedly depressed during starvation (61). The mechanism underlying this inhibition of muscle glucose metabolism has not been clearly established, but there is considerable evidence that fatty acid and ketone body oxidation, through inhibition of glucose transport and of 6-phosphofructokinase and pyruvate dehydrogenase, decreases glucose utilization (1). There is also evidence that, during starvation, an insulin-resistant state develops in skeletal muscle with respect to carbohydrate metabolism (62,63). The metabolic response is influenced by the lower insulin concentration in fasted subjects (which is most pronounced at rest, but which prevails also during exercise) (64) and the higher plasma catecholamine concentrations during exercise (65,66). These hormonal changes serve to increase lipolysis and hence muscle fat oxidation during exercise in the fasted state (64,66–68). A low pyruvate dehydrogenase activation may explain the higher plasma lactate values noted in connection with exercise in the fasted state, but the higher concentration of plasma catecholamines is likely to have contributed. Interestingly, there have also been several reports that starvation increases the ratio of lactate to pyruvate in resting muscle (59,69,70).

Ketone bodies do not significantly contribute as a fuel for the exercising muscle even at high ketone body concentrations (37). It is known that ketogenesis in prolonged starvation is not additionally stimulated by exercise and, furthermore, that the ketone bodies may limit their own utilization in muscle by inhibiting the first enzyme in their degradation, 3-ketoacidCoA transferase (37). This could direct the ketone bodies to the central nervous system.

The described glucose-sparing process is mainly governed by changes outside the muscle itself, chiefly by the increased plasma fatty acid concentration that regularly accompanies starvation. There is, however, evidence that the metabolic characteristics of the muscle cell itself are important in this respect. As previously stated and illustrated in Fig. 4, a high muscle oxidative capacity, as normally occurs in slow-twitch fibers or in physically trained muscle, is believed to be metabolically significant in leading to a greater reliance on fat as an energy substrate. For a more detailed discussion, see Holloszy (13). Slow-twitch fibers (or well-trained muscle) can thus be said to be better adapted than fast-twitch fibers (or untrained muscle) to a situation in which the use of glucose by the muscles must be limited. In accord with this, Wade et al. (71) recently reported a significant (positive) correlation between the percentage of slow-twitch fibers in the quadriceps femoris muscle of healthy men and the rate of fat combustion during standardized exercise. In addition, there was a negative correlation between the percentage of slow-twitch fibers and the percentage of body fat content. The authors hypothesize that muscle fiber type is an etiologic factor for obesity; another possible explanation seems to be that more active individuals develop a higher percentage of slow-twitch fibers via fiber-type transformation (see the preceding section on the effects of training). In the following section on muscle enzyme adaptation, some evidence is given that indicates that starvation may also induce enzymatic adaptations within the muscle that assist in the glucose-saving process.

Anaerobic Glycolysis

Although the amount of ATP produced per kJ of substrate used is of a comparable magnitude—though not identical—for fat and carbohydrate oxidation, the corresponding value for anaerobic glycolysis is less than one-tenth of this amount (1). Some of the lactic acid produced during anaerobic glycolysis will be oxidized subsequently so that the actual difference in ATP yield/kJ of substrate used will be less than tenfold. It should be emphasized that the energy yield for the resynthesis of ATP is the same whether the degradation of glycogen goes directly via pyruvate into the mitochondrion or detours to lactate first. Normally, however, not all the lactate formed during intense contractions is subsequently oxidized, so anaerobic glycolysis is a less economical pathway than glucose oxidation (1). This is one important factor, in addition to the force-velocity relationship per se, that explains why high rates of intensities of muscle contraction are not compatible with high energy efficiency. This fact probably automatically leads to a lifestyle in which activities demanding a high power output and an accompanying high activation of anaerobic glycolysis are avoided and in which movements are performed slowly rather than quickly. If heavy tasks must be performed, intermittent work patterns are likely to be chosen, because anaerobic glycolytic activation will then be minimal, and the relative contribution of fat oxidation will be higher (see 72).

MUSCLE ATROPHY: EVIDENCE OF FIBER TYPE DIFFERENCES

There is evidence from the rat that the level of activity influences the responsiveness of a muscle to starvation. Tonically active muscles (e.g., the slow-twitch soleus) therefore show less atrophy than phasic muscles (such as the fast-twitch EDL muscle) (73). This may also hold true for human muscles. In a study on six healthy men (74), we investigated the response of the triceps brachii and the quadriceps femoris muscles to endurance training of low intensity and long duration. During the second and third weeks of the training, the diet consisted of standard

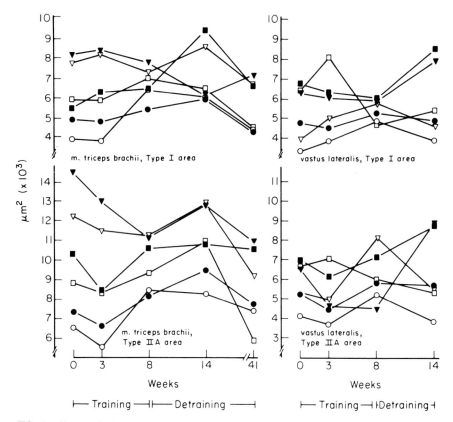

FIG. 5. Changes in the area of fiber type I and IIA in m. triceps brachii, and m. quadriceps femoris, vastus lateralis during training and detraining. The training consisted of dynamic exercise of long duration and low intensity (skiing with a backpack, 30 km/day). During the second and third weeks of training, the subjects were energy deficient (see text). Each subject is designated by a specific symbol. Owing to their small percentage, IIB fibers were not analyzed. From ref. 74.

Swedish army rations of 18 MJ/day, resulting in a calculated energy deficit of 4 MJ to 5 MJ per day. As can be seen from Fig. 5, this was accompanied by a reduction in the size of the fast-twitch fibers, but the size of the slow-twitch fibers was not affected. In line with these results are the findings of Russel et al. (59) in malnourished patients and of Essén et al. (75) in patients with anorexia nervosa. These groups found that the size of the slow-twitch fibers in the human calf and thigh muscles, respectively, was better preserved than that of the fast-twitch fibers. Considering the fiber type recruitment pattern, this change, per se, would not lead to a better economy during low-intensity exercise, but, as previously discussed, it would in all probability be more advantageous than if the same atrophy occurred in the slow-twitch fibers.

Fiber Type Proportions

Theoretically, the hypothyroid state induced by food shortage could lead to some degree of fast-to-slow muscle-fiber transformation, because the thyroid state has been shown to markedly affect muscle fiber type proportions in this direction (76). The proportions of myofibrillar ATPase fiber types in muscle have been shown to be quite stable, although chronic stimulation (for references, see ref. 77) and, to some extent, endurance training can result in a fast-to-slow fiber type transformation.

There is one report (59) of a fast-to-slow transformation in malnourished patients, but there is not enough evidence at present to establish that this occurs regularly as a consequence of long-term energy deficiency. In anorexia nervosa patients, whose body weights were 2 to 3.5 standard deviations less than expected from the normal weight/height relationship, the ratio of slow-twitch to fast-twitch fibers was clearly higher (66/34) than in a control group (53/47) (75). However, these severely malnourished patients were considerably more physically active than the controls, and it is not known how this might have influenced the results. In connection with intermittent feeding in rats (3 days of fasting followed by 3 days of refeeding for 10 weeks), Favier and Koubi (70) observed another pattern of fiber type change, namely a decrease in percentages of types I and IIA. The IIB fiber fraction increased.

It cannot be ruled out that the economy of muscle contraction might be influenced even though fiber types, based on the myofibrillar ATPase stain, are not affected. There have been reports of a changed force-frequency response to stimulation and a pronounced slowing of the rate of muscle relaxation in malnourished rat and human muscle (59,78; see also references in 79). Russel et al. (59) attributed this not to a changed fiber type profile, but to an increased intracellular Ca^{2+} content. In line with these results, Bruce et al. (79) recently concluded that the slow muscle relaxation rate is the most consistently abnormal muscle variable in subnourished patients but that the maximal force generated is not decreased relative to the remaining muscle bulk. Although the reports of a slowing of muscle relaxation are interesting, it is not known whether this change might result in an augmented muscle economy.

Muscle Enzyme Adaptation

Russel et al. (59), studying the effect of 2 weeks of 1.7 MJ/day carbohydrate dieting in humans, observed significant decreases in muscle glycolytic capacity (6-phosphofructokinase, -48%) and citrate cycle capacity (succinate dehydrogenase, -33%). The indicator of the capacity of the fat oxidation system, 3-hydroxyacylCoA dehydrogenase (HAD), remained unchanged. Similar data were found in 5-day-fasted and 21-day-starved rats, although HAD increased after starvation and showed some decrease after hypocaloric dieting (80). These findings were not verified in the study by Ardawi et al. (81). In anorexia nervosa patients, Essén et al. (75) found that the activities of glycolytic enzymes were 50% lower than those in sedentary controls, whereas the activities of enzymes of the mitochondrial oxidative pathways were decreased only by 10% to 20%. To some extent, these data support the hypothesis that an enzymatic adaptation (or at least a selective enzyme loss) may occur in muscle, which tends to favor fat at the expense of carbohydrate oxidation. It is quite possible, however, that this adaptation is simply a consequence of an increase in fatty acid availability and that the adaptation will subside within a few weeks following normalization of the plasma free fatty acid concentration upon refeeding.

Interestingly, Favier and Koubi (70), in their study of 10 weeks of intermittent fasting in the rat, observed a significant decrease in hexokinase activity. This change had also been reported earlier in intermittently fasting obese women (82) and also in rats after hypocaloric dieting (81). This decrease is in accord with the insulin-resistant state earlier noted in response to starvation and would assist in limiting the utilization of blood glucose by the muscles. Another interesting observation in this study (70) was that the muscle triglyceride concentration in the intermittently starved rats was significantly increased; only in this group of rats did exercise lead to a significant depletion of muscle triglycerides.

CONCLUSION

Although it is likely that some of the discussed adaptive changes are important in saving energy in the resting muscle and probably to an even greater extent in the contracting muscle, it is clear that much more research is needed into the significance as well as costs of these and other potential adaptive changes in malnourished muscle. This knowledge will constitute an important step in the further understanding of the pathophysiology of starvation.

REFERENCES

1. Newsholme EA, Leech AR. *Biochemistry for the medical sciences.* Chichester: John Wiley & Sons, 1983.
2. Wolfe RR, Wolfe MH, Nadel ER, Shaw JHF. Isotopic determination of amino acid urea interaction in exercise in humans. *J Appl Physiol* 1984;56:221–9.
3. Pettenkofer M, Voit C. Untersuchungen über den Stoffverbrauch des normalken Menschen. *Z Biol* 1866;2:537.
4. Saltin B, Gollnick PD. Skeletal muscle adaptability: significance for metabolism and performance. In: *Handbook of physiology. 10. Skeletal muscle.* Bethesda, MD: American Physiology Society, 1983; 555–631.
5. Brown JMC, Henriksson J, Salmons S. Restoration of fast muscle characteristics following cessation of chronic stimulation: physiological, histochemical and metabolic changes during slow-to-fast transformation. *Proc R Soc Lond* 1989;B235:321–46.
6. Essén-Gustavsson B, Henriksson J. Enzyme levels in pools of microdissected human muscle fibres of identified type. Adaptive response to exercise. *Acta Physiol Scand* 1984;120:505–15.
7. Chi MM-Y, Hintz CS, Coyle EF, et al. Effects of detraining on enzymes of energy metabolism in individual human muscle fibers. *Am J Physiol* 1983;C276–87.
8. Henriksson J, Reitman J. Time course of changes in human skeletal muscle succinate dehydrogenase and cytochrome oxidase activities and maximal oxygen uptake with physical activity and inactivity. *Acta Physiol Scand* 1977;99:91–7.

9. Andersen P, Henriksson J. Capillary supply of the quadriceps femoris muscle of man. Adaptive response to exercise. *J Physiol* 1977;270:677–90.
10. Schantz PG. Plasticity of human skeletal muscle. *Acta Physiol Scand* 1986;128(Suppl 558):22–3.
11. Andersen P, Henriksson J. Training induced changes in the subgroups of human type II skeletal muscle fibers. *Acta Physiol Scand* 1977;99:123–5.
12. Jansson E, Kaijser L. Muscle adaptation to extreme endurance training in man. *Acta Physiol Scand* 1977;100:315–24.
13. Holloszy JO. Metabolic consequences of endurance exercise training. In: Horton ES, Terjung RL, eds. *Exercise, nutrition and energy metabolism.* New York: Macmillan, 1988;116–31.
14. Wendt IR, Gibbs CL. Energy production of rat extensor digitorum longus muscle. *Am J Physiol* 1973; 224:1081–6.
15. Goldspink G. Biochemical energetics for fast and slow muscles. In: Bolis S, Maddrell HP, Schmidt-Nielsen K, eds. *Comparative physiology—functional aspects of structural materials,* Amsterdam: North Holland Publishing, 1975;173–85.
16. Crow M, Kushmerick MJ. Chemical energetics of slow- and fast-twitch muscles of the mouse. *J Gen Physiol* 1982;79:147–66.
17. Bolstad G, Ersland A. Energy metabolism in different human skeletal muscles during voluntary isometric contractions. *Eur J Appl Physiol* 1978;38:171–9.
18. Nwoye LO, Goldspink G. Biochemical efficiency and intrinsic shortening speed in selected vertebrate fast and slow muscles. *Experientia* 1981;37:856–7.
19. Suzuki Y. Mechanical efficiency of fast- and slow-twitch muscle fibers in man during cycling. *J Appl Physiol* 1979;47:263–7.
20. Jorfeldt L, Wahren J. Leg blood flow during exercise in man. *Clin Sci* 1971;41:459–73.
21. Baker PGB, Mottram RF. Metabolism of exercising and resting human skeletal muscle, in the post-prandial and fasting states. *Clin Sci* 1973;44:479–91.
22. Astrup A, Bülow J, Madsen J, Christensen NJ. Contribution of BAT and skeletal muscle to thermogenesis induced by ephedrine in man. *Am J Physiol* 1985;248:E507–15.
23. Zurlo F, Larson K, Bogardus C, Ravussin E. Skeletal muscle metabolism is a major determinant of resting energy expenditure. *J Clin Invest* 1990;86(5):1423–7.
24. De Luise M, Harker M. Skeletal muscle metabolism: effect of age, obesity, thyroid and nutritional status. *Horm Metab Res* 1989;21(8):410–5.
25. Poehlman ET, Horton ES. The impact of food intake and exercise on energy expenditure. *Nutr Rev* 1989;47(5):129–37.
26. Molé PA, Stern JS, Schultz CL, Bernauer EM, Holcomb BJ. Exercise reverses depressed metabolic rate produced by severe caloric restriction. *Med Sci Sports Exerc* 1989;21(1):29–33.
27. Freedman-Akabas S, Colt E, Kissileff HR, Pi-Sunyer FX. Lack of a sustained increase of VO₂ following exercise in fit and unfit subjects. *Am J Clin Nutr* 1985;41:545–9.
28. Warwick M, Garrow JS. The effect of addition of exercise to a regime of dietary restriction on weight loss, nitrogen balance, resting metabolic rate, and spontaneous physical activity in three obese women in metabolic ward. *Int J Obes* 1981;2:25–32.
29. James WPT, Shetty PS. Metabolic adaptations and energy requirements in developing countries. *Hum Nutr Clin Nutr* 1982;36C:331–6.
30. Cox MD, Dalal SS, Heard CRC, Millward DJ. Metabolic rate and thyroid status in rats fed diets of different protein-energy values: the importance of free T3. *J Nutr* 1984;114:1609–16.
31. Payne Robinson HM, Betton H, Jackson AA. Free and total triiodothyronine and thyroxine in malnourished Jamaican infants. *Hum Nutr Clin Nutr* 1985;39C:245–57.
32. Drott C, Persson H, Lundholm K. Cardiovascular and metabolic response to adrenaline infusion in weight-losing patients with and without cancer. *Clin Physiol* 1989;9:427–39.
33. Wolfe RR, Peters EJ, Klein S, Holland OB, Rosenblatt J, Gary H Jr. Effect of short term fasting on lipolytic responsiveness in normal and obese human subjects. *Am J Physiol* 1987;252:E189–96.
34. Jayarajan MP, Shetty PS. Cardiovascular β-adrenoceptor sensitivity of undernourished subjects. *Br J Nutr* 1987;58:5–11.
35. Fagher B, Monti M, Theander S. Microcalorimetric study of muscle and platelet thermogenesis in anorexia nervosa and bulimia. *Am J Clin Nutr* 1989;49:476–81.
36. Nichols BL, Barnes DJ, Ashworth A, Alleyne GAO, Hazlewood CF, Waterlow JC. Relationship between total body and muscle respiratory rates in infants with malnutrition. *Nature* 1968; 217(5127):475–6.
37. Balasse EO, Féry F. Ketone body production and disposal: effects of fasting, diabetes, and exercise. *Diabetes Metab Rev* 1989;5(3):247–70.

38. Nair KS, Welle SL, Halliday D, Campbell RG. Effect of β-hydroxybutyrate on whole-body leucine kinetics and fractional mixed skeletal muscle protein synthesis in humans. *J Clin Invest* 1988;82:198–205.

39. Nair KS, Halliday D, Lalloz M, Garrow JS. Rate of protein turnover in obese women on energy restriction and its relationship to extra-thyroidal T4 metabolism. *Proc Nutr Soc* 1981;40:94A.

40. Wolman S, Sheppard H, Fern M, Waterlow JC. The effect of triiodothyronine (T3) on protein turnover and metabolic rate. *Int J Obesity* 1985;9:459–63.

41. Jepson MM, Bates PC, Broadbent P, Pell JM, Millward DJ. Relationship between glutamine concentration and protein synthesis in rat skeletal muscle. *Am J Physiol* 1988;255:E166–72.

42. Waterlow JC. Metabolic adaptation to low intakes of energy and protein. *Annu Rev Nutr* 1986;6:495–526.

43. Pearl RH, Clowes GHA Jr, Hirsch EF, Loda M, Grindlinger GA, Wolfort S. Prognosis and survival as determined by visceral amino acid clearance in severe trauma. *J Trauma* 1985;25:777–81.

44. Waterlow JC. Observations on the variability of man. In: Blaxter KL, Macdonald IA, eds. *Comparative nutrition*, London: John Libbey, 1988.

45. Garlick PJ, Millward DJ, James WPT, Waterlow JC. The effect of protein deprivation and starvation on the rate of protein synthesis in tissues of the rat. *Biochim Biophys Acta* 1975;414:71–84.

46. Li JB, Wassner S. Effects of food deprivation and refeeding on total protein and actomyosin degradation. *Am J Physiol* 1984;246:E32–7.

47. Lowell BB, Ruderman NB, Goodman MN. Regulation of myofibrillar protein degradation in rat skeletal muscle during brief and prolonged starvation. *Metabolism* 1986;35:1121–7.

48. Goodman MN, Del Pilar Gomez M. Decreased myofibrillar proteolysis after refeeding requires dietary protein or amino acids. *Am J Physiol* 1987;253:E52–8.

49. Waterlow JC, Garlick PJ, Millward DJ. *Protein turnover in mammalian tissues and in the whole body*. Amsterdam: Elsevier North-Holland, 1978.

50. Garlick PJ, Maltin CA, Baillie AGS, Delday MI, Grubb DA. Fiber-type composition of nine rat muscles. II. Relationship to protein turnover. *Am J Physiol* 1989;257:E828–32.

51. Abumrad NN, Williams P, Frexes-Steed M, et al. Inter-organ metabolism of amino acids in vivo. *Diabetes Metab Rev* 1989;5(3):213–26.

52. Guernsey DL, Edelman IS. Regulation of thermogenesis by thyroid hormones. In: Oppenheimer J, Samuels H, eds. *Molecular basis of thyroid hormone action*. New York: Academic Press, 1983;293–324.

53. Chinet A, Clausen T, Girardier L. Microcalirometric determination of energy expenditure due to active sodium-potassium transport in the soleus muscle and brown adipose tissue of the rat. *J Physiol* 1977;265:43–61.

54. Medbø JI, Sejersted OM. Plasma potassium changes with high intensity exercise. *J Physiol* 1990; 421:105–22.

55. Kjeldsen K, Nørgaard A, Gøtzsche CO, Thomassen A, Clausen T. Effect of thyroid function on number of Na-K-pumps in human skeletal muscle. *Lancet* 1984;2:8–10.

56. Everts ME, Andersen JP, Clausen T, Hansen O. Quantitative determination of Ca^{2+}-dependent Mg^{2+}-ATPase from sarcoplasmic reticulum in muscle biopsies. *Biochem J* 1989;260:443–8.

57. Newsholme EA. A possible metabolic basis for the control of body weight. *N Engl J Med* 1980; 302:400–5.

58. Blaxter KL. Methods of measuring the energy metabolism of animals and interpretation of results obtained. *Fed Proc* 1970;30:1436–43.

59. Russel DMcR, Walker PM, Leiter LA, et al. Metabolic and structural changes in skeletal muscle during hypocaloric dieting. *Am J Clin Nutr* 1984;39:503–13.

60. Henriksson J, Chi M-MY, Hintz CS, et al. Chronic stimulation of mammalian muscle: changes in enzymes of six metabolic pathways. *Am J Physiol* 1986;251:C614–32.

61. Ruderman NB, Goodman MN, Berger M, Hagg S. Effect of starvation on muscle glucose metabolism: studies with the isolated perfused rat hindquarter. *Fed Proc* 1977;36:171–6.

62. Gallen IW, Macdonald IA. The effects of underfeeding for 7 d on the thermogenic and physiological response to glucose and insulin infusion (hyper-insulinaemic euglycaemic clamp). *Brit J Nutr* 1990; 64:427–37.

63. Mansell PI, Macdonald IA. The effect of starvation on insulin-induced glucose disposal and thermogenesis in humans. *Metabolism* 1990;39(5):502–10.

64. Dohm GL, Beeker RT, Israel RG, Tapscott EB. Metabolic responses to exercise after fasting. *J Appl Physiol* 1986;61(4):1363–8.

65. Pequignot JM, Peyrin L, Pérès G. Catecholamine-fuel interrelationships during exercise in fasting men. *J Appl Physiol* 1980;48:109–13.
66. Koubi HE, Desplanches D, Gabrielle C, Cottet-Emard JM, Sempore B, Favier RJ. Exercise endurance and fuel utilization: a reevaluation of the effects of fasting. *J Appl Physiol* 1991;70(3):1337–43.
67. Björkman O, Eriksson LS. Splanchnic glucose metabolism during leg exercise in 60-h-fasted human subjects. *Am J Physiol* 1983;245:E443–8.
68. Galbo H, Christensen NJ, Mikines KJ, et al. The effect of fasting on the hormonal response to graded exercise. *J Clin Endocrinol Metab* 1981;52:1106–12.
69. Goodman MN, Larsen PR, Kaplan MM, Aoki TT, Young VR, Ruderman NB. Starvation in the rat. II. Effect of age and obesity on protein sparing and fuel metabolism. *Am J Physiol* 1980;239:E277–86.
70. Favier RJ, Koubi HE. Metabolic and structural adaptations to exercise in chronic intermittent fasted rats. *Am J Physiol* 1988;254:R877–84.
71. Wade AJ, Marbut MM, Round JM. Muscle fibre type and aetiology of obesity. *Lancet* 1990;335:805–8.
72. Åstrand P-O, Rodahl K. *Textbook of work physiology*, 3rd ed. New York: McGraw-Hill, 1986;304–8.
73. Goldspink DF. The influence of contractile activity and the nerve supply on muscle size and protein turnover. In: Pette D, ed. *Plasticity of muscle*. Berlin: Walter de Gruyter, 1980;525–39.
74. Schantz P, Henriksson J, Jansson E. Adaptation of human skeletal muscle to endurance training of long duration. *Clin Physiol* 1983;3:141–51.
75. Essén B, Fohlin L, Thorén C, Saltin B. Skeletal muscle fibre types and sizes in anorexia nervosa patients. *Clin Physiol* 1981;1:395–403.
76. Ianuzzo D, Patel P, Chen V, O'Brien P, Williams C. Thyroidal trophic influence on skeletal muscle myosin. *Nature* 1977;270:74–6.
77. Salmons S, Henriksson J. The adaptive response of skeletal muscle to increased use. *Muscle Nerve* 1981;4:94–105.
78. Lopes J, Russel DM, Whitwell J, Jeejeebhoy KN. Skeletal muscle function in malnutrition. *Am J Clin Nutr* 1982;36:602–10.
79. Bruce SA, Newton D, Woledge RC. Effect of subnutrition on normalized muscle force and relaxation rate in human subjects using voluntary contractions. *Clin Sci* 1989;76:637–41.
80. Russel DMcR, Atwood HL, Whittaker JS, et al. The effect of fasting and hypocaloric diets on the functional and metabolic characteristics of rat gastrocnemius muscle. *Clin Sci* 1984;67:185–94.
81. Ardawi MSM, Majzoub MF, Masoud IM, Newsholme EA. Enzymic and metabolic adaptations in the gastrocnemius, plantaris and soleus muscles of hypocaloric rats. *Biochem J* 1989;261:219–25.
82. Vondra K, Rath R, Bass A, Kutela L, Slabochova Z. Effect of protracted intermittent fasting on the activities of enzymes involved in energy metabolism, and on the concentrations of glycogen, protein and DNA in skeletal muscle of obese women. *Nutr Metab* 1976;20:329–37.

DISCUSSION

Dr. Flatt: Dr. Henriksson has reviewed evidence suggesting that the fast-twitch muscle fibers (type II fibers) that depend primarily on glucose as a fuel may tend to waste away somewhat more rapidly during energy deprivation than the slow-twitch type I fibers using primarily fat as a fuel. This would seem to be an advantage, not only because of the need to use glucose sparingly during periods of caloric deprivation, but also because ATP expenditure for a given effort may be less when slow-twitch rather than fast-twitch fibers are recruited. The biologic strategy for minimizing energy expenditure during food deprivation would thus appear to be to reduce "jerky" muscle movements while relying as much as possible on work produced by the more slowly contracting type I fibers.

Because of the fact that the relative proportions of type I and type II fibers in human muscles vary among different muscle beds and among individuals, it is rather difficult to evaluate the quantitative significance of changes in the relative proportions of type I and type II fibers for energy conservation during undernutrition. It would seem to have to be considered as a minor factor compared to the substantial other adaptive changes that occur during periods of restricted food intake. However, differences in the proportion of fiber types may play a more significant role on weight maintenance under conditions of unrestricted caloric intake. I will return to this point later. As far as adaptation to food deprivation is concerned, considerable economies in energy expenditure are achieved as a result of weight loss and decreased physical activity. In the Minnesota experiment on human starvation, Keys et al. (1) studied the energy balance in volunteers whose energy intake was restricted to 45% of their normal consumption. After 24 weeks, their basal energy expenditure had declined by 40% (from 1,600 to 960 kcal/day). Of this change, 75% was due to the loss of lean body mass, and 25% to a 15% decrease in the rate of energy expenditure per kg of cell mass. The amount of energy spent daily for physical activities decreased from 1,610 to 490 kcal per day. This reduction was brought about by a 60% decline in the amount of physical activities performed, although it led to a 70% reduction in energy spent for physical activities on account of the reduction in body size (e.g., a loss in body weight from 70 kg to 53 kg). The biggest factor in the subjects' adaptation to a 1,900 kcal reduction in daily energy intake was thus a decrease in the energy spent for physical activities.

Economy of movement, whose impact is further enhanced by the decrease in cost of motions owing to the reduction in body size, thus assumed much greater significance in reducing energy expenditure (i.e., $-1,120$ kcal/day) during starvation than the decline in basal energy expenditure (-630 kcal/day) and the decrease in specific dynamic action (-140 kcal/day). This seems to be the prevalent form of adaptation, documented for example by the reduced capacity to perform physical work when food allowances are insufficient (2). Such reduction in work output can be delayed as long as the laborers still have sufficient endogenous fat stored in their adipose tissue, providing that they have sufficient incentives to maintain a high work output (3). In view of these numbers, the reduction in physical activity brought about by undernutrition should be expected to have a far greater impact on limiting energy expenditure than the fuel economy that can be achieved by changing the proportions of type I or type II recruited to accomplish various physical activities.

Differences in the relative rates of carbohydrate and fat utilization by different types of muscle fibers seem to take on perhaps greater interest in view of their potential leverage on body weight regulation during periods of unrestricted access to food. As pointed out elsewhere (4) and in the chapter by Flatt, maintenance of body weight requires not only equality between energy intake and energy expenditure but also a proper adjustment of the composition of the fuel mix oxidized to the nutrient distribution in the diet. The latter condition is satisfied when the average RQ is equal to the FQ of the average diet. Weight maintenance under ad libitum food intake conditions is dominated by regulation of food intake rather than by changes in energy expenditure, and the modulation of food intake from one day to the next occurs in a manner serving primarily the goal of maintaining carbohydrate balance (5). This will lead to maintenance of the overall energy balance as well, if glucose, fat, and amino acids are oxidized in proportions equivalent to the carbohydrate, fat, and protein contents of the diet. If the fuel mix oxidized does not contain as much fat as provided by the diet, for example, fat will accumulate until expansion of the adipose tissue mass ultimately raises FFA levels and promotes fat oxidation to the point where the average RQ matches the diet's FQ. Muscle is the major compartment in the body capable of burning fat as well as carbohydrates. Yet not all forms of physical activity appear to be equally effective in limiting the accumulation of excessive adipose tissue. Thus, sustained efforts of moderate intensity, often referred to as "aerobic exercise," tend to restrain (or reverse) the development of adiposity much better than short bouts of intense exertion. The difference in their effect on body weight can be attributed to the fact that sustained efforts promote the use of fat to a greater extent than they do the use of carbohydrate (4), whereas violent muscle contractions enhance primarily glucose consumption. The impact of habitual physical activities on body weight could be further influenced by a subject's relative proportions of type I (primarily fat-oxidizing) and type II (primarily glucose-utilizing) fibers. Wade et al. (6) have reported that subjects with high proportions of type I muscle fibers tended to have lower respiratory quotients during standardized work on a bicycle ergometer and that these subjects also had significantly less body fat than individuals having primarily type II fibers in their vastus lateralis muscle. These very interesting findings led these authors to conclude that "the metabolic profiles of the skeletal muscle fibre types may be the cause of the relation that we have observed between fibre type proportion and fatness" (6). This conclusion is consistent with the view that the carbohydrate-to-fat ratio in the fuel mix oxidized assumes greater importance on body weight regulation, under conditions of unrestricted food intake, than overall energy turnover.

In conclusion, it would appear that studies on the differences in fuel utilization by type I and type II muscle fibers are of considerable interest, but more because of their potential significance on body weight regulation under conditions of unrestricted food intake than because of their impact on fuel economy and survival under conditions of food deprivation.

REFERENCES

1. Keys A, Brozek J, Henschel A, Mickelson O, Taylor H. *The biology of human starvation.* Minneapolis: University of Minnesota Press, 1950.
2. Kraut HA, Müller EA. Calorie intake and industrial output. *Science* 1986;104:495–7.
3. Diaz E, Goldberg GR, Taylor M, Savage JM, Sellen S, Corvard WA. Effects of dietary supplementation on work performance in Gambian laborers. *Am J Clin Nutr* 1991;53:803–11.
4. Flatt JP. Importance of nutrient balance in body weight regulation. *Diabetes Metab Rev* 1988;4:571–81.
5. Flatt JP. Differences in the regulation of carbohydrate and fat metabolism and their implications for body weight maintenance. In: Lardy H, Stratman SF, eds. *Hormones, thermogenesis and obesity.* New York: Elsevier, 1989;3–17.
6. Wade AJ, Marbut MM, Round JM. Muscle fiber type and aetiology of obesity. *Lancet* 1990;335: 805–8.

Energy Metabolism: Tissue Determinants and
Cellular Corollaries, edited by J. M. Kinney
and H. N. Tucker. Raven Press, Ltd.,
New York © 1992.

Muscle Phosphagen Status Studied by Needle Biopsy

*Roger C. Harris and †Eric Hultman

*Department of Comparative Physiology, Animal Health Trust,
Newmarket, Suffolk, CBB 7DW, United Kingdom; †Institute of Clinical Chemistry II,
Huddinge University Hospital, Huddinge, Sweden

MUSCLE PHOSPHAGEN CONTENT AT REST

The Biopsy Technique

The publication in 1962 by Dr. Jonas Bergström of St. Erik's Hospital, Stockholm, of a paper describing the electrolyte status in human skeletal muscle (1) marked the introduction of the percutaneous needle biopsy technique as a tool for muscle research. A similar biopsy needle had been described some 90 years before by Duchenne (2) for pathologic diagnosis of muscle but had not gained common usage. Dr. Bergström needed a simple, rapid, relatively atraumatic sampling technique enabling serial biopsies to be taken of the body's largest soft tissue reserve of electrolytes. In this first investigation, as in most others that followed, the organ sampled was the lateral portion of the quadriceps femoris muscle (the vastus lateralis), chosen because of the relative lack of major blood vessels and nerves. The application of the biopsy technique to the study of the changes in muscle glycogen by Dr. Eric Hultman (3–5), also of St. Erik's Hospital, marked the first use of the technique in exercise physiology. In 1967 the first description of the phosphagen contents in resting and exercised human muscle were published by Hultman, Bergström, and McLennan-Anderson (5,6). At the time this offered the only means to view the phosphagen status in human muscle, and this remained so for a further 15 years until the advent of topical NMR.

The taking of a muscle biopsy has changed little since first described by Bergström (1), although in an attempt to increase sample size, biopsy needles today are usually 5 mm to 6 mm in diameter, and suction is frequently applied. Despite their appearance, the wider needles are as equally well tolerated as the earlier 3 mm to 4 mm needles and, when used, even with suction, are not associated with any increase in discomfort or muscle damage other than that resulting in occasional mild local stiffness on the following day. In over 1,000 muscle biopsies taken by E. Hultman, only one instance of a painful hematoma has been recorded.

367

Estimates of the time taken in removing a biopsy (timed from insertion of the needle to its removal) vary from 2.5 seconds to 5 seconds, depending on the skill of the operator and whether a one-handed (fastest) or two-handed technique was used. Biopsies are normally taken from the relaxed, unstretched muscle, though some volunteer studies have been undertaken with no greater discomfort or obvious sign of damage while subjects undergo contraction induced through percutaneous electrical stimulation (7).

Analysis of Biopsies

In an attempt to minimize any postexcision chemical changes, biopsy samples are usually plunged directly into liquid nitrogen or some other freezing media such as isopentane maintained at its freezing point. The use of liquid freon at $-150°C$ no longer seems necessary. Freezing carries the risk of ice-crystal formation within the tissue, possibly causing disruption of the membranes with transient Ca^{2+} activation of actomyosin ATPase. In a study by Gilbert et al. (8), highest PCr values were obtained in frog muscle when freezing was completed within 100 ms using a hammer apparatus precooled in liquid nitrogen. Clearly this is not possible in studies of human muscle. However, no difference was found in the phosphagen contents of biopsy samples homogenized without freezing in perchloric acid or extracted following freezing *and* freeze-drying (9) (Table 1). The inclusion of freeze-drying offers numerous advantages to the management of samples. Samples are easily divided into portions for differing analysis. Non–muscle cell elements such as connective and fat tissues can largely be removed, as well as a major portion of any contaminating blood, a particular problem in postexercise samples. A simple method of removing contaminating blood—which we have not previously published—is to roll fragments of the biopsy across a paper tissue. This causes the dried blood to fracture and fall away as a fine dust from the muscle fibers. Changes in the water content of muscle cells, again a problem in exercise studies, are automatically compensated for by drying. More recent studies aimed at the analysis of phosphagen contents in different muscle fiber types (10,11) must by necessity use freezing and freeze-drying as first steps.

TABLE 1. *Effect on muscle phosphagen contents of direct homogenization in perchloric acid of unfrozen samples compared to extraction of sub-samples following freezing and freeze-drying[a]*

	Direct homogenization of biopsy ($n = 9$)	Frozen/freeze-dried biopsy ($n = 8$)
ATP	24.8 (2.5)	24.8 (2.3)
PCr	86.7 (4.0)	87.7 (4.3)
PCr/TCr	0.63 (0.09)	0.65 (0.03)
Lactate	8.8 (5.2)	9.8 (5.9)

[a] Data from ref. 9. Values are means (Sd), mmol/kg d.m.

The final procedures adopted by this group in the early 1970s for the analysis of phosphagen contents of muscle biopsies are described in reference 12 and have been adopted by numerous other groups with minimal change.

Phosphagen Status in Normals

Phosphagen contents in the resting quadriceps femoris muscle of 50 to 81 healthy subjects aged 18 to 30 years, determined using the preceding procedures, are presented in Table 2. Values of ATP, PCr, Cr, and PCr + Cr (TCr) all showed a normal distribution. Although they represent a limited age range, subsequent data from active volunteer subjects up to 62 years have not indicated any age-related trends. No difference has been noted between male and female subjects.

There is, however, a clear discrepancy between values of PCr determined in biopsy samples and those measured in situ using NMR. NMR studies have consistently recorded higher resting muscle PCr contents. A sample of studies show a range of 24.1 to 28.5 mmol/kg w.m. (13–15), which compares with a biopsy content of 17.6 mmol/kg w.m. (Table 2). Assuming a normal TCr content of around 29 mmol/kg w.m., the NMR studies indicate approximately 90% in the form of PCr in resting muscle.

This discrepancy in values has been attributed to the effects of muscle damage during biopsy (though probably not during tissue-freezing). The effect of such damage is again Ca^{2+} activation of actomyosin ATPase, leading to formation of ADP, from ATP hydrolysis, and immediate restitution of ADP back to ATP at the expense of PCr. In an investigation of the effects of delayed freezing of muscle biopsies, Söderlund and Hultman (9) observed that holding a biopsy in air for 1 minute resulted in a 13% increase in the PCr content but no change in that of ATP (Table 3). As a percentage of TCr, PCr increased from 57% to 64%. No further change was observed when biopsies were incubated for an additional 5 minutes in air. The synthesis of

TABLE 2. *Phosphagen contents determined in biopsy samples of the quadriceps femoris muscle at rest*[a]

Phosphagen	n	mmol/kg d.m.		mmol/kg w.m.
ATP	81	24.0	(2.64)	5.58
ADP	66	3.2	(0.45)	0.74
AMP	50	0.1	(0.05)	0.02
TA	50	27.4	(2.52)	6.37
PCr	81	75.5	(7.63)	17.56
Cr	81	49.0	(7.62)	11.40
TCr	81	124.4	(11.21)	28.93
PCr/TCr	81	0.61	(0.001)	
Lactate	81	5.10	(2.43)	1.19

[a] Data from ref. 12. Values are means (sd).

TABLE 3. *Effects of delayed freezing on muscle phosphagen contents in biopsy samples incubated in normal air at room temperature[a]*

	Incubation period			
	Control	1 min	2 min	6 min
ATP	23.7 (1.9)	25.4 (1.5)	24.0 (3.1)	25.2 (2.5)
PCr	72.9 (4.4)	84.9 (2.8)[b]	81.7 (9.5)	85.0 (6.7)[c]
Cr	55.8 (5.7)	47.3 (3.7)	47.2 (6.5)	48.5 (5.4)
PCr/TCr	0.57 (0.02)	0.64 (0.01)[b]	0.63 (0.03)[b]	0.64 (0.04)[c]
Lactate	2.8 (1.0)	5.2 (1.4)[c]	7.8 (3.3)[b]	9.4 (3.5)[b]

[a] Data from ref. 9. Values are means (sd) mmol/kg d.m.
[b] $p < 0.001$
[c] $p < 0.01$

PCr did not appear to be secondary to any readjustment of creatine kinase equilibrium due to increase in pH as a result of CO_2 or bicarbonate loss but was blocked by the prior depletion of myoglobin-bound O_2 (9). These results were interpreted as showing (partial) restoration of PCr lost as a result of damage incurred during muscle sampling, through the pumping back of Ca^{2+} liberated during sampling into the sarcoplasmic reticulum.

The initial loss of 10–12 mmol PCr/kg d.m. within the 3s of actual sampling is well within the capacity of the muscle. Although Söderlund and Hultman considered the PCr contents of 1-minute air-equilibrated biopsy samples to be a more accurate reflection of the true content in resting muscle, values were still considerably lower than those reported in NMR studies.

One other possibility not adequately explored is the chance that the error lies in the NMR values. The ^{31}P-NMR spectra are calibrated against assumed absolute values (frequently derived from biopsy studies) for the ATP or P_i peaks (e.g., 13–17). This assumes that all of the ATP or P_i measured chemically in acid-extracted muscle is equally visible to NMR, which will not be the case if partially bound to proteins or located within the mitochondria (18). The result in this case would be an overestimation of the PCr content. This problem would be easily resolved if Cr could be simultaneously determined with PCr. In view of the stability of the PCr content of muscle biopsies incubated in air between 2 minutes and 6 minutes, it would be interesting to compare values determined on the same sample by NMR and by chemical analysis.

REFERENCE BASES

In both clinical and nonclinical studies, a variety of reference bases and corrective procedures have been used with the result that it is often difficult to compare absolute measurements reported by different groups. Where serial biopsies are involved (e.g., before and after muscle contraction), total creatine (TCr = PCr + Cr) has proved useful as a reference standard. However, an absolute TCr standard should not be used when comparing values between different subjects because of variability between individuals.

In studies of prolonged exercise, loss of glycogen, which accounts for 4% to 5% of the sample dry weight and, in exceptional circumstances, 13% (3,4), may cause an apparent rise in metabolite concentrations. In this case values may be expressed per kg glycogen-free muscle or corrected to a constant TCr.

Muscle biopsies of patients, particularly if malnourished, frequently show increased contamination with fat and connective tissue, which can never be fully removed. This has led to the use of a number of alternative reference bases in addition to the usual expression of values per kg wet or dry muscle. These include kg fat-free solids (e.g., 19,20) obtained by prior extraction of the freeze-dried samples with light petroleum, DNA (21), protein, and NAD (22). In the study of Tresadern et al. (21), fat extraction was followed by determination of hydroxyproline to enable further correction of the reference base for connective tissue content.

Phosphagen Status in Patients

Studies of the effects of severe injury, surgical trauma, sepsis, and acute and chronic illness have showed a marked resilience in the TCr content of muscle but less so in the case of the adenine nucleotides, principally ATP. In patients with circulatory or respiratory insufficiency, the pattern observed shows a 15% to 25% decrease in PCr, which is partly compensated for by an increase in Cr (19,23,24) (Table 4). As a result, TCr shows a decrease of about 5%. The ratio of PCr/TCr is significantly lower than that in normal subjects at rest. ATP content is decreased by around 20% but this is not compensated for by any equivalent increase in ADP or

TABLE 4. *Phosphagen status of the quadriceps femoris muscle at rest in patients with circulatory or respiratory insufficiency*[a]

	Normals (12)		Möller et al. (19)	Bergström et al. (23)		Gertz et al. (24)
n	50–81		8	8		12
ATP	24.0	(2.64)	19.89 (1.89)	19.4	(2.66)	80%
ADP	3.2	(0.45)	2.73 (0.11)	2.92	(0.36)	—
AMP	0.1	(0.05)	0.1 (0.01)	0.16	(0.11)	—
TA	27.4	(2.52)	22.72 (2.98)	22.48	(2.92)	—
PCr	75.5	(7.63)	62.27 (2.98)	60.88	(6.93)	74.8%
Cr	49.0	(7.62)	57.83 (4.12)	59.10	(9.90)	—
TCr	124.4	(11.21)	120.10 (5.00)	119.88	(4.53)	—
PCr/TCr	0.61	(0.001)	0.52 (0.02)	0.51	(0.07)	—
Lactate	5.10	(2.43)	4.53 (0.97)	17.9	(13.24)	287.5%

[a] With the exception of data of Gertz et al., values are means (sd), mmol/kg d.m. Values of Gertz et al. are expressed as % of control.

TABLE 5. *Changes in phosphagen concentrations on the quadriceps femoris muscle following occlusion of the circulation for up to 2 hours and during 5 min recovery following release of occlusion[a]*

	0	Min of occlusion		120.3 (26.9)	Min of release of 2 hr occlusion		
		10	20		1	2	5
ATP	23.28 (0.27)	−0.13 (0.24)	−0.29[b] (0.13)	−1.42[b]	−0.61[b]	−0.19	−0.21
ADP	3.28 (0.27)	+0.11 (0.24)	+0.24[b] (0.13)	+1.23[b]	+0.51[b]	+0.21	+0.16
AMP	0.13 (0.02)	+0.03 (0.01)	+0.05[b] (0.01)	+0.19[b]	+0.11[b]	+0.02	+0.05
TA	26.7 (0.6)	—	—	+0.06	−1.00	+0.05	+2.00
PCr	72.3 (3.7)	−8.8[b] (4.9)	−22.9[b] (4.6)	≈−62[b]	≈−42[b]	≈−22[b]	≈0
TCr	122	—	—	≈−2	≈−2	≈−4	≈+1
Lactate	2.5 (0.9)	≈+1.0	≈+4.0[b]	≈+48[b]	≈+42[b]	≈+40[b]	≈+30[b]
Estimated Values							
pHi	7.10	7.10	7.10	6.85	6.87	6.88	6.95
ADPf (umol/ kg d.m.)	40.5	53.6	85.4	343.2	102.1	50.1	28.4

[a] Also shown are the estimated changes in intracellular pH (pH_i) and ADP_f calculated from an assumed creatine kinase equilibrium of 1.66×10^9 l/mol and intracellular water content of 3 l/kg d.m. With the exception of pH_i and ADP_f, all values are mmol/kg d.m. Where possible, the means (sd) are given. Data from refs. 25 and 26.
[b] $p < 0.05$.

AMP. This pattern is somewhat similar to that observed in anoxic muscle resulting from short-term occlusion of the blood supply (25) and has been interpreted as evidence of increased anaerobic metabolism. Raised concentrations of lactate found in the studies of Bergström et al. (23) and Gertz et al. (24) further support this.

The initial fall in PCr following occlusion of muscle at rest (24,25) (Table 5) is almost certainly a response to disturbance in the creatine kinase equilibrium as a result of an increase in the concentration of free ADP (ADP_f) in the sarcoplasm. ADP concentrations measured in muscle biopsies following acid extraction reflect both the free and bound forms. ADP_f concentrations calculated from ATP, PCr, and Cr and assuming a resting pH of 7.1 and equilibrium constant for the creatine kinase reaction of 1.66×10^9 l/mol (from ref. 27) are probably no greater than 40 μmol/kg d.m. (circa 13 μM) at rest, rising to 85 μmol/kg d.m. (28 μM) after 20 minutes of occlusion. Longer periods of occlusion (Table 5) resulted in further increases in ADP_f to 300–400 μmol/kg d.m. and marked accumulation of lactate. A pH decrease will further augment the effect of rising ADP_f in lowering the PCr concentration.

As might be expected, release of occlusion results in a rapid fall in ADP_f, possibly to values less than those prior to occlusion as temporary hyperoxia following hyperemia sets in.

Although no net loss of adenine nucleotide was observed during 2 hours of circulatory occlusion in normal subjects, this might be anticipated in persistent low-grade hypoxia, where increase in ADP_f, acting through AMP_f, would lead to increased deamination of adenine nucleotide to IMP. Thus, the 20% reduction in ATP seen in patients with circulatory or respiratory insufficiency most probably reflects an alteration in the balance between the synthesis and breakdown of adenine nucleotide secondary to the effects of mild local hypoxia.

TABLE 6. *Phosphagen status of the quadriceps femoris at rest (or RA, rectus abdominis) of chronically ill patients and those with extensive trauma following multiple injury*[a]

	Harris et al. (12) normals	Tresadern et al. (21) septic	RA	Bergström et al. (23) prolonged disease	patient 14	patient 16	Liaw et al. (28) severe injury	critical illness
n	50–81	12	14	8			12	5
ATP	24.0 (2.64)	89.0%	64.1%	12.8 (3.37)	9.7	7.8	17.8 (6.5)	10.6 (3.2)
ADP	3.2 (0.45)	—	—	2.14 (0.44)	1.55	2.90	1.8 (1.0)	0.9 (0.6)
AMP	0.1 (0.05)	—	—	0.18 (0.09)	0.05	0.20	0.28 (0.15)	0.7 (0.3)
TA	27.4 (2.52)	95.0%	67.7%	15.13 (3.23)	11.26	10.90	19.88	—
PCr	75.5 (7.63)	99.2%	70.7%	56.14 (10.52)	40.7	59.4	—	—
Cr	49.0 (7.62)	—	—	54.54 (11.87)	39.3	73.8	—	—
TCr	124.4 (11.21)	107.5%	84.2%	110.63 (16.65)	80.0	133.2	—	—
PCr/TCr	0.61 (0.001)	94.6%	85.7%	0.51 (0.07)	0.51	0.45	—	—
Lactate	5.1 (2.43)	290.0%	109.3%	4.39 (1.75)	4.2	5.2	21.0 (9.0)	25.3 (12.7)

[a] With the exception of values of Tresadern et al., values are means (sd) mmol/kg d.m. Values of Tresadern et al. are expressed as % of control.

In chronically ill patients and those with extensive trauma following multiple injury, phosphagen status shows a different pattern of change to the previous. In a high proportion of patients there is evidence of extensive loss of adenine nucleotide with ATP contents only 50% of those found in normal subjects (Table 6). In the original report of Tresadern et al. (21), data are expressed both per g fat-free dry muscle and per mg DNA; in both cases a marked reduction in ATP content was apparent. If anything, expression of the data per mg DNA accentuated the apparent reduction in ATP in comparison to the content in normal subjects. In the three studies reviewed in Table 6, patients with severe or chronic illness showed the greatest losses in ATP. This is illustrated in patients 14 and 16 from the study of Bergström et al. (23), where ATP contents of the quadriceps femoris were 30% to 40% of normal. Patient 14 died 2 weeks after biopsy, and patient 16, 2 days after biopsy.

Despite the marked changes in ATP, loss of PCr, and TCr as a whole, was much less. The near normality of TCr values further indicates that the much-reduced ATP contents in these patients was not an artifact of increased contamination by fat or connective tissues in the biopsies. PCr/TCr ratios were generally lower than normal, and lactate was moderately raised in some but not all patient groups.

In the study of Tresadern et al. (21), malnourished nonseptic patients showing an involuntary loss of 10% of usual body weight showed no change (quadriceps femoris) or modest loss (rectus abdominis) in ATP, and essentially normal TCr contents. Four days bed-rest of normal subjects had no effect on phosphagen status in the quadriceps femoris (20).

It is unlikely that the dramatic reduction in ATP content in these patients is secondary to any low-grade muscle hypoxia, but it may be indicative of impaired de novo synthesis of purine nucleotide. This may reflect an inadequate supply of the amino acid glutamine in these patients necessary to meet the cells' needs for purine synthesis. Starvation and trauma are known to result in disturbances in glutamine metabolism (29,30), and preliminary studies indicate a rapid decline in plasma levels in racehorses exposed to viral infection (Harris and Sweatman, unpublished data).

The advantages of the needle biopsy technique are its simplicity of use, low cost, and flexibility in the range of measurements that can be made. However, in the case of the phosphagens, there remains some doubt over the reliability of values of PCr measured at rest, although values of PCr + Cr are considered correct. Although the trauma associated with the taking of a muscle biopsy is considered slight by well-motivated volunteers, many of whom have returned repeatedly to the laboratory for further studies, it is doubtful that the technique will ever be accepted for routine use in the clinic. However, it has and will continue to find application in clinical investigation.

Few clinical studies of phosphagen status in resting muscle have been undertaken to date, but in general these point to a massive loss of adenine nucleotide, principally ATP, during chronic illness or following severe injury. This may be due to impairment of de novo purine synthesis and may be linked to altered glutamine status. In patients with circulatory or respiratory insufficiency, changes in muscle phosphagens are consistent with prolonged low-grade hypoxia in the skeletal muscles.

Useful clinical applications of the biopsy technique in the future are likely to be in the continuing development of specific nutrition for maintenance of energy homeostasis in disease and trauma, and the extension of current findings to the level of single muscle fibers. Is alteration in muscle phosphagen status in disease and trauma homogeneous throughout the muscle, or is it confined to one or other muscle fiber type?

PHOSPHAGEN UTILIZATION DURING EXERCISE IN DIFFERENT MUSCLE FIBER TYPES

It has been known for more than 140 years that the red and white colors of muscle fibers are associated with slow and fast contractions (31). Later studies have related different biochemical profiles of whole muscle and single motor units to physiologic properties like speed of contraction and resistance to fatigue. For references see Close (32) and Burke and Edgerton (33).

A detailed study of muscles from animal species by Beis and Newsholme (34) showed a positive correlation between ATP content and ATP/AMP ratio and the capacity to accelerate energy utilization and thus energy production. Similarly, Goldspink et al. (35), studying hamster muscles, found that muscles that fatigue quickly have higher contents of ATP at rest than fatigue-resistant muscles.

In a study of human and animal muscle, Edström et al. (36) made a comparison between fiber type composition in different muscles and their contents of high-energy phosphates. The muscles were characterized histochemically, including staining for succinate dehydrogenase (SDH), which is an accepted enzyme marker for oxidative capacity.

The results showed a higher ATP/ADP ratio in fast-twitch than in slow-twitch muscles, with the exception of the tongue muscle, in the rat. There was also a higher content of ATP and PCr in type II fibers and an inverse relation between PCr and the stainability for succinate dehydrogenase. The content of PCr was related to the glycolytic capacity of the fibers but not to the contraction time. It was also pointed out that PCr, in addition to being an immediate energy source, also functions as a buffer against lactic acidosis.

In a recent study of human fibers separated from biopsy material obtained from the quadriceps femoris muscle, it was shown that the ATP content did not differ significantly but that PCr content was as a mean 15% higher in type II fibers. Also, the glycogen content at rest was higher in fast-twitch fibers ($\approx$20%).

The anaerobic energy production in the two fiber types was studied by measuring substrate utilization during electrical stimulation of the quadriceps muscle in situ (37). Muscle samples were obtained by percutaneous biopsy at rest and after 10-second and 20-second intermittent stimulation at 50 Hz. Individual fibers were separated, characterized, and analyzed for content of ATP, PCr, and glycogen. It was shown that the PCr degradation rate during the first 10 seconds of contraction was 40% higher in type II fibers than in type I and that the rate of glycogen degradation during the whole 20-second contraction was about 10 times higher in type II than in type I. This study was done with intact blood flow to the leg. When the study was repeated with the circulation occluded, the glycogenolytic rate in type I fibers increased to about 50% of the rate in type II fibers, in which the glycogenolytic rate was practically unchanged.

The regulation of glycogenolysis is known to be determined by the transformation of the phosphorylase enzyme to an active form, but it also depends on the availability of inorganic phosphate in the muscle and on the concentration of AMP in the sarcoplasm. AMP is an allosteric activator of the enzyme (38). It was previously shown that the intensity of the muscle contraction regulated the glycogenolytic rate when the enzyme was in its active form. This finding suggested that there was a direct relation between ATP turnover rate and AMP accumulation in the sarcoplasm of contracting muscle (39).

The high ATP turnover rate in type II fibers during stimulation will result in an ADP increase in the sarcoplasm and eventually AMP formation via the adenylate kinase reaction. Owing to a lower ATP turnover rate in type I fibers combined with a higher capacity for oxidative phosphorylation of ADP, AMP formation will lower in this fiber type. Consequently, stimulation of glycogen phosphorylase will be less. In the experiment with occluded circulation, the lack of oxidative ADP resynthesis increased ADP accumulation and in turn, AMP formation in type I fibers, resulted in stimulation of glycogenolysis. The lack of further increase of glycogenolysis in type II fibers suggests that AMP stimulation was already maximal during stimulation with intact blood flow.

During the intense stimulation there was a decrease in force generation by the muscle. The decrease amounted to 40% of the initial force after 30 seconds of stimulation. Parallel with the decrease in force was a fall in the rate of anaerobic ATP production, both from PCr degradation and glycolysis. The fastest drop in energy provision came from the PCr store. This was particularly so in the case of type II fibers, in which 70% of the PCr was utilized within 10 seconds of contraction and the store approached depletion after 20 seconds. At this point it would appear that glycogenolysis-glycolysis has already reached its maximal rate in type II fibers and cannot be increased further to compensate for the decrease in ATP production from PCr degradation. Had force generation remained constant, an imbalance between ATP utilization and ATP resynthesis would have ensued. The metabolic check that prevents this is the reason for the observed decrease in force production and may explain the greater fatiguability of type II fibers.

These studies show a possible mechanism explaining the differences in substrate utilization and fatiguability in muscle fiber types I and II in situations with increased ATP demand. Detailed studies of the physiologic and biochemical response of muscle to contraction require separate analyses of the different fiber types.

REFERENCES

1. Bergström J. Muscle electrolytes in man. Determination by neutron activation analysis on needle biopsy specimens. A study on normal subjects, kidney patients and patients with chronic diarrhea. *Scand J Clin Lab Invest* 1962;14:(Suppl 68).
2. Edwards RHT, Jones DA, Harris RC. The biochemistry of muscle biopsy in man: clinical applications. In: Alberti KGMM, Price CP, eds. *Recent advances in clinical chemistry.* New York: Churchill Livingstone, 1981;243–69.
3. Bergström J, Hultman E. Muscle glycogen synthesis after exercise. An enhancing factor localized to the muscle cells in man. *Nature* 1966;210:309–10.
4. Hultman E. Muscle glycogen in man determined in needle biopsy specimens. *Scand J Clin Lab Invest* 1967;19:209–17.
5. Hultman E. Studies on muscle metabolism of glycogen and active phosphate in man with special reference to exercise and diet. *Scand J Clin Lab Invest* 1967;19:(Suppl 94).
6. Hultman E, Bergström J, and McLennan-Anderson N. Breakdown and resynthesis of phosphorylcreatine and adenosine triphosphate in connection with muscular work in man. *Scand J Clin Lab Invest* 1967;19:56–66.
7. Chasiotis D, Bergström M, Hultman E. ATP utilization and force during intermittent and continuous muscle contractions. *J Appl Physiol* 1987;63:167–71.
8. Gilbert C, Kretzschmar KH, Wilkie DR, Woledge RC. Chemical change and energy output during muscular contraction. *J Physiol* 1971;218:163–93.
9. Söderlund K, Hultman E. Effects of delayed freezing on content of phosphagens in human skeletal muscle biopsy samples. *J Appl Physiol* 1986;61:832–5.
10. Foster CVL, Harman J, Harris RC, Snow DH. ATP distribution in single muscle fibres before and after maximal exercise in the thoroughbred horse. *J Physiol* 1986;378:63P.
11. Söderlund K, Hultman E. ATP content in single fibres from human skeletal muscle after electrical stimulation and during recovery. *Acta Physiol Scand* 1990;131:459–66.
12. Harris RC, Hultman E, Nordesjöm L-O. Glycogen, glycolytic intermediates and high-energy phosphates determined in biopsy samples of musculus quadriceps femoris of man at rest. Methods and variance of values. *Scand J Clin Lab Invest* 1974;33:109–20.
13. Bertocci LA, Haller RG, Lewis SF, Fleckenstein JL, Nunnally RL. Abnormal high-energy phosphate metabolism in human muscle phosphofructokinase deficiency. *J Appl Physiol* 1991;70:1201–7.
14. Edwards RHT, Dawson MJ, Wilkie DR, Gordon RE, Shaw D. Clinical use of nuclear magnetic resonance in the investigation of myopathy. *Lancet* 1982;1:725–31.
15. Taylor DJ, Bore PJ, Styles P, Gadian DG, Radda GK. Bioenergetics of intact human muscle. A ^{31}P nuclear magnetic resonance study. *Mol Biol Med* 1983;1:77–94.
16. Wilkie DR, Dawson MJ, Edwards RHT, Gordon RE, Shaw D. ^{31}P-NMR studies of resting muscle in normal human subjects. In: Pollack GH, Sugi H, eds. *Contractile mechanisms in muscle.* New York: Plenum, 1984;333–47.

17. Meyer RA, Brown TR, Kushmerick MJ. Phosphorous nuclear magnetic resonance in fast- and slow-twitch muscle. *Am J Physiol* 1985;248:C279–87.
18. Takumi H, Faruga E, Tagawa K, et al. NMR—invisible ATP in rat heart and its change in ischaemia. *J Biochem* 1988;104:35–9.
19. Möller P, Bergström J, Furst P, Hellström K, Uggla E. Energy-rich phosphagens, electrolytes and free amino acids in leg skeletal muscle of patients with chronic obstructive lung disease. *Acta Med Scand* 1982;211:187–93.
20. Liaw K-Y, Askanazi J, Mitchelsen CB, Furst P, Elwyn DH, Kinney JM. Effect of postoperative nutrition on muscle high energy phosphates. *Ann Surg* 1982;195:12–8.
21. Tresadern JC, Threlfall CJ, Wilford K, Irving MH. Muscle adenosine 5¹-triphosphate and creatine phosphate concentrations in relation to nutritional status and sepsis in man. *Clin Sci* 1988;75:233–42.
22. Sabina RL, Swain JL, Bradley WG, Holmes EW. Quantitation of metabolites in human skeletal muscle during rest and exercise: a comparison of methods. *Muscle Nerve* 1984;7:77–82.
23. Bergström J, Boström H, Furst P, Hultman E, Vinnars E. Preliminary studies of energy-rich phosphagens in muscle from severely ill patients. *Crit Care Med* 1976;4:197–204.
24. Gertz I, Hedenstierna G, Hellers G, Wahren J. Muscle metabolism in patients with chronic obstructive lung disease and acute respiratory failure. *Clin Sci Mol Med* 1977;52:395–403.
25. Harris RC, Hultman E, Kayser L, Nordesjö L-O. The effect of circulatory occlusion on isometric exercise capacity and energy metabolism of the quadriceps muscle in man. *Scand J Clin Lab Invest* 1975;35:87–95.
26. Larsson J, Hultman E. The effect of long-term arterial occlusion on energy metabolism of the human quadriceps muscle. *Scand J Clin Lab Invest* 1979;39:257–64.
27. Lawson JWR, Veech RL. Effects of pH and free Mg²⁺ on the Keq of the creatine kinase reaction and other phosphate hydrolyses and phosphate transfer reactions. *J Biol Chem* 1979;154:6528–37.
28. Liaw K-Y. Effect of injury, sepsis, and parenteral nutrition on high-energy phosphates in human liver and muscle. *J Parenter Enter Nutr* 1985;9:28–33.
29. Wernerman J, von der Decken A, Vinnars E. Size distribution of ribosomes in biopsy specimens of human skeletal muscle during starvation. *Metabolism* 1985;34:665–9.
30. Essen P, Wernermar J, Ali MR, Vinnars E. Changes in the concentrations of free amino acids in skeletal muscle during 24h immediately following elective surgery. *Clin Nutr* 1988;7(special suppl.):67.
31. Ranvier L. De quelques faite relatifs à l'histologie et à la: à la physiologie des muscles striés. *Arch Physiol Norm Pathol* 1874;6:1–13.
32. Close RJ. Dynamic properties of mammalian skeletal muscles. *Physiol Rev* 1972;52:129–97.
33. Burke RE, Edgerton VR. Motor unit properties and selective involvement in movement. *Exerc Sport Sci Rev* 1975;3:31–81.
34. Beis J, Newsholme E. The contents of adenine nucleotides, phosphagens and some glycolytic intermediates in resting muscles from vertebrates and invertebrates. *Biochem J* 1975;152:23–32.
35. Goldspink G, Larson RE, Davies RE. The intermediate energy supply and the cost of maintenance of isometric tension for different muscles in the hamster. *Z Vergl Physiol* 1970;66:389–97.
36. Edström L, Hultman E, Sahlin K, Sjöholm H. The contents of high-energy phosphates in different fibre types in skeletal muscles from rat, guinea-pig and man. *J Physiol* 1982;332:47–58.
37. Hultman E, Greenhaft PL, Ren J-M, Söderlund K. Energy metabolism and fatigue during intense muscle contraction. *Biochem Soc Trans* 1991;19:347–53.
38. Lowry OH, Schulz TW, Passoneau JV. Effects of adenylic acid in the kinetics of muscle phosphorylase *a*. *J Biol Chem* 1964;239:1947–53.
39. Ren J-M, Hultman E. Regulation of phosphorylase *a* activity in human skeletal muscle. *J Appl Physiol* 1990;69:919–23.

DISCUSSION

Dr. Elia: I was interested too, in your data about the discrepancy between phosphate as measured by NMR spectroscopy and biochemical measurements, which might possibly be related to the mobility of the phosphate molecule. But I have heard the theoretical possibility, at least, that glycogen might exist as far as NMR is concerned in mobile and nonmobile forms. The question really is, Does the C-13 NMR measure total glycogen, or only a component of the total glycogen? In other words, how do the biochemical measurements there compare with the NMR measurements?

Dr. Gadian: The statements I've read in the literature say that, for reasons that aren't totally clear, the glycogen is 100% NMR-visible. This presumably implies that the glycogen has a lot of internal mobility, such that the signal is narrow enough to see. However, I was at a meeting in Zurich just a few weeks ago. Somebody was suggesting that in the fasted state, in the liver the glycogen was 100% visible but in the fed state it was possibly less visible. It would have been nice had Bob Schulman been there to comment on this. There weren't enough people there really to comment on this in detail, but obviously it's an important question.

Dr. Elia: Does that actually imply that the structure of the newly synthesized glycogen differs in some way from the previously stored glycogen?

Dr. Gadian: It may just be that there's more motion on the outside of the glycogen structure than the inside, so it may not be the chemistry but the random molecular motion.

Dr. Wolfe: In Dr. Harris's presentation, the reduction in ATP in the patients that had the chronic disease seemed to be quite dramatic and, in fact, was actually almost the same magnitude as the reduction in the ATP in the horses immediately following exhaustive exercise. There are two aspects to the question. I wasn't clear as to the type of patients and if the ATP reduction was a common finding. I wasn't aware that patients had such a dramatic reduction in ATP while at rest. What is the basis for such a large reduction in ATP? In a more general sense, what is the physiologic significance of that level of reduction of ATP? In other words, at what point does ATP availability become rate-limiting in the ability for the muscles to contract?

Dr. Harris: First of all, there are values showing equal decreases in the adenine nucleotide pool in humans also during intense exercise. Eric has observed similar decreases during electrical stimulation. So it is possible to find in voluntary exercise a 50% reduction in the ATP content. The patients were from a study by Bergström et al. published in 1976. Those eight patients were described as "critically ill." In fact, I had a description at the bottom of that overhead giving the details of their particular condition. That obviously is a chronic condition. The factors bringing about that reduction in total adenine nucleotide pool are obviously quite different from those that bring about the reduction in ATP in exercise. . . . It was a dramatic drop. I have no idea what the physiologic consequence of it would be, but two patients died very shortly after those biopsies had been taken. It was an extremely bad situation and clearly shows a stressful energy situation inside the cells. Eric was actually part of that study. Do you want to make any comments on it?

Dr. Holtzmann: We have published other papers (and John Kinney has a paper on this also) that show, in severely ill, prolonged care patients, that these are decreases in ATP. If I could do the study again I would look at the inosine monophosphate and hypoxanthine released over a long period, because apparently there is loss of all of the adenine nucleotides. It's not the same as a fast decrease in ATP. It's a special situation. But I know that you have also patients that die.

Dr. Harris: In the acute situation it is a dynamic loss of ATP adenine nucleotide downward toward inosine monophosphate. In the chronic situation almost certainly that loss of adenine nucleotide is not the mechanism, there must be some interruption with purine salvage and purine synthesis coming up from the bottom and therefore probably quite different.

Dr. Edwards: Work in my department among acutely ill patients is showing that you get necrosis of cells in patients who are in an intensive care unit—necrosis of muscle cells. It's quite striking how much is in fact taking place, which would be the structural correlate of what you're describing.

Dr. Milligan: Professor Hultman, I was very interested in your results, particularly the work you showed of correlation, very strong correlation, between glycogen use and ATP turnover in your preparation. It appeared to me by the slope of your graph that you had approximately 3 millimoles of ATP turnover per millimole of glycogen use. Do you have an explanation for that relationship?

Dr. Hultman: No, I haven't thought about that relationship, but what we were interested in was just to see if we could relate it to IMP formation. I think that is the most interesting thing, but the relation between ATP and glycogen integration I don't have.

Dr. Milligan: In terms of total ATP turnover, synthesis and expenditure, I would expect 5.

Dr. Hultman: Of the total ATP turnover, the highest is about 11 millimole per kilo dry muscle per second, and then it goes down on the line. Do you have any suggestions for me?

Dr. Milligan: No, I was just wondering. It's such a good relation.

Dr. Holtzmann: Yes, it is a very nice relation, that's true.

Dr. Newsholme: First of all I was concerned—perhaps *concerned* is the wrong word, but a little worried—about the fact that we're beginning to accept without question that the ATP-ADP ratio in muscle may be of the order of a thousand, ATP concentration being about 10 millimolar. If we calculate the ADP, because we can't measure it, there's 10 micromolar. Those concentrations give you a ratio, if my arithmetic is right, of approximately 1,000/1, which positions muscle quite uniquely in my experience as a tissue. Red cells, white cells, liver cells, adipose tissue cells do not, as far as I know, have a similar ratio. We have a fundamentally important question here: Is muscle that different? That's not a trivial question I would like to put forward. It does raise questions of available concentration of ADP. Can enzymes that use ADP like pyruvate kinase, mitochondrial adenine nucleotide transporter, and glycerol 3-phosphate dehydrogenase actually function with 10 micromolar or 20 micromolar ADP? I've no doubt that ADP is bound. I worry that we tend now to accept glibly that 99% is bound or approaching that level, because it does raise fundamental questions about our understanding of energy. However, having said that, I'd like to come back to Bob Wolfe's point, and perhaps suggest provocatively that I would worry that ATP is limiting, because as long as the ATP-ADP ratio, whatever that is in muscle, is maintained, I don't think muscle would suffer a major problem. I would worry more that the low ADP level, if it does occur, in patients is a reflection of something else going on in muscle, perhaps as Roger Harris was suggesting, an inability of the resynthesis of purine nucleotides over a long period of time, possibly because of a demand for amino acids for other areas of metabolism. But I wouldn't like to allow us to feel that the concentration of ATP per se is so important for muscle, which was the impression that was coming away. I might provocatively suggest it's probably reflecting something else.

Energy Metabolism: Tissue Determinants and Cellular Corollaries, edited by J. M. Kinney and H. N. Tucker. Raven Press, Ltd., New York © 1992.

NMR and Tissue Energetics

David G. Gadian

Hunterian Institute, The Royal College of Surgeons of England, London, WC2A 3PN, United Kingdom

Nuclear magnetic resonance (NMR) is increasingly used in diagnostic radiology and in biomedical research as a noninvasive method of obtaining human images and of studying tissue metabolism. NMR imaging, based primarily on the detection of signals from water and fats, has become an established radiologic technique, with over 3,000 systems currently installed worldwide. NMR spectroscopy provides a method of studying metabolism, with an emphasis on research applications rather than diagnosis. This chapter is concerned with the role of NMR as a noninvasive probe of tissue energetics.

The physical basis of NMR was described in 1946 (1,2), and from the early 1950s NMR became commonly used for the analysis of chemical structure. The use of NMR to generate cross-sectional images and to study tissue metabolism followed much later, in the 1970s (3–5). The non-invasive study of muscle and brain metabolism in small animals became feasible with the development of the surface coil (6), which is a type of detecting coil that can be placed adjacent to a superficial region of interest. Extension to human studies (first of limbs and then of the neonatal brain) followed soon afterward with the construction of larger magnets (7,8). With the development of whole-body spectroscopy systems and additional or alternative methods of spatial localization, more extensive clinical studies followed. In this chapter, illustrative examples describe the use of NMR for the investigations of tissue energetics, primarily in skeletal muscle but also in other tissues.

THE BASIC PRINCIPLES OF NMR

This chapter begins with a brief outline of the basic principles of NMR; there are several texts covering the theory and in vivo applications of NMR spectroscopy in far greater detail (9–11). In common with other spectroscopic techniques, NMR detects the interaction of radiation with matter. The technique relies on the fact that certain atomic nuclei such as hydrogen (the proton, ^1H), phosphorus (^{31}P), and fluorine (^{19}F) have intrinsic magnetic properties. When a sample containing such nuclei is placed in a magnetic field, the nuclear magnets tend to align along the direction of the field. This magnetic interaction between the nuclei and the applied field can be detected by applying pulses of radiofrequency radiation to the sample and observing the frequencies at which radiation is absorbed and subsequently re-emitted.

The resonance frequency of a nucleus is directly proportional to the *local* magnetic field experienced by the nucleus. If this field were equal to the applied field, and if it were perfectly uniform over the entire sample, then all protons, for example, would absorb energy at the same frequency. Under such circumstances, NMR would be a relatively uninformative technique incapable of resolving between protons in different chemical or spatial environments. In practice, however, there are frequency shifts associated with field variations; these are exploited in spectroscopy to provide chemical information and in imaging to provide spatial information.

NMR spectroscopy makes use of the observation that nuclei in different chemical environments give rise to signals of slightly different frequencies. This reflects the fact that the local field experienced by any nucleus differs slightly from the applied field because of the secondary fields generated by the local electrons. This frequency separation is commonly expressed (in dimensionless units of parts per million) in terms of the parameter known as the chemical shift. It should be emphasized that this is just one of the several parameters that characterize NMR signals. Among the others are the spin-spin coupling constant and the relaxation times T_1 and T_2. T_1 and T_2 are particularly important as contrast parameters in magnetic resonance imaging.

Whereas NMR spectroscopy detects signals of differing frequencies from a range of metabolites, NMR imaging is based primarily on the detection of ^1H signals from the water protons, with additional contributions from fats. Imaging makes use of magnetic field gradients to provide spatial information.

If the body were in a totally uniform magnetic field, then on application of the pulses of radiofrequency radiation that are used to generate the NMR signals, all of the water protons would give a signal of the same frequency, and no spatial information would be available. In imaging studies, well-defined magnetic field gradients are superimposed on the applied magnetic field. As a result, different points in space can be identified with specific field values and hence with specific signal frequencies. The frequency distribution therefore reflects the spatial distribution of the molecules rather than their chemical features. By far the easiest molecule to image is water because of the abundance of water molecules and because protons give stronger signals than other nuclei. The generation of a cross-sectional image is achieved by computer analysis of data obtained with a range of different gradient conditions, in analogy with image reconstruction in x-ray scanning. One of the advantages of NMR is the fact that the gradients can be applied equally easily along each axis, so that transverse, coronal, or sagittal images can all be obtained directly. The signal intensities in magnetic resonance images depend on many properties of the tissue water, including its concentration and its relaxation times T_1 and T_2. In general, images that are weighted according to one or other of the relaxation times offer far more contrast than images that simply reflect proton density.

For many studies, particularly in humans, it is important to obtain spectra from well-defined localized regions within the body. This can be achieved by using frequency to encode for both space and chemistry (i.e., to combine imaging techniques with spectroscopic methods). However, it has to be accepted that, whatever methods are used for localized spectroscopy, the spatial resolution that can be achieved is necessarily very much poorer than that for imaging of the water signal. This is primarily due to the concentration difference between water and the metabolites of interest. The average water concentration in tissues is about 40 M (i.e., 80 M in protons), whereas the metabolites detected by spectroscopy are in the millimolar range (i.e., a factor of 10,000 to 100,000 lower). In practice, this means that in order to obtain sufficient signal from metabolites, the localized volume needs to be about 10,000 to 100,000 times larger, which in turn means that the linear resolution is of the order of centimeters rather than 1 mm.

It should be noted that the nuclei previously mentioned (^{1}H, ^{19}F, and ^{31}P) are the naturally occurring stable isotopes, so signals are detected directly without any need for isotopic enrichment. In the case of carbon, the commonly occurring isotope ^{12}C has no magnetic properties, so it is necessary to use ^{13}C, which is stable and occurs naturally but which represents only 1.1% of the total carbon. As a result, the use of ^{13}C NMR often requires the introduction of ^{13}C-labeled compounds. In general, however, NMR has the advantage over many other analytic techniques that signals are observed noninvasively from species that occur naturally within the body.

WHAT CAN WE MEASURE BY NMR SPECTROSCOPY?

^{31}P NMR

The nucleus that has been used most extensively for metabolic studies is ^{31}P, which is the naturally occurring phosphorus nucleus. The reasons for this are apparent from the ^{1}H and ^{31}P spectra of rat leg muscle, shown in Fig. 1. Although the basic ^{1}H spectrum is somewhat uninformative, showing signals just from water and fats, the main signals detected by ^{31}P spectroscopy happen to be from metabolites that play central roles in muscle energetics.

The signal at about -16 ppm in the ^{31}P spectrum has a chemical shift that is characteristic of the β-phosphate group of nucleoside triphosphates and, on the basis of the known biochemistry of muscle, can be assigned to ATP. Similarly, the signals at 0 ppm and 5 ppm can be attributed to phosphocreatine (PCr) and inorganic phosphate (P_i), respectively. The signal at -2.5 ppm is characteristic of the γ-phosphate of ATP but could also contain a contribution from the β-phosphate of ADP. Similarly, the signal at -7.5 ppm could contain contributions from the α-phosphate groups of both ATP and ADP. (In fact, the ATP and ADP signals are shifted slightly from each other, but in many spectra of living systems not sufficiently for them to be resolved.) In addition, a shoulder to the right of the α-phosphate peak can often be seen as a chemical shift characteristic of the phosphate signals from NAD$^+$ and NADH.

The simplicity of the spectrum may appear surprising in view of the large number of phosphorus-containing compounds that are present in muscle. One reason for the

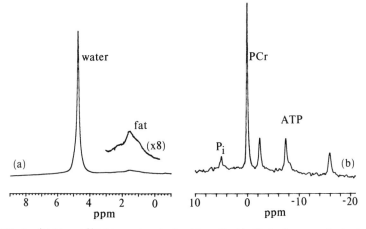

FIG. 1. ^{1}H (a) and ^{31}P (b) spectra obtained from the hindlimb of an anesthetized rat.

relatively small number of peaks is the fact that narrow signals are observed only from relatively mobile compounds; highly immobilized species such as membrane phospholipids will normally give very broad signals that show up as a baseline hump. Thus, it is commonly assumed that NMR spectroscopy monitors cytoplasmic metabolites, although there has been one report in which a second P_i contribution was attributed to mitochondrial P_i(12).

Another reason for the simplicity of the spectra is the fact that NMR is an insensitive technique and therefore detects only metabolites that are present at fairly high concentrations (typically 0.2–0.5 mM or greater). Apart from P_i, ATP, and phosphocreatine, signals are commonly observed in vivo from phosphomonoesters (around 6–8 ppm) and phosphodiesters (around 2–4 ppm). If we consider the phosphomonoester signal, the major contribution in spectra of the brain is believed to come from phosphorylethanolamine. This signal is particularly large in the neonatal brain, both in humans and in rats. However, many other metabolites (including, for example, glucose 6-phosphate in muscle) can contribute to this region of the spectrum and in particular could contribute to any changes that occur in disease or in response to physiologic stress. Further details and references relating to the phosphomonoester and phosphodiester signals can be found elsewhere (13,14).

It is a particularly useful feature of ^{31}P spectra that the chemical shift of the inorganic phosphate signal is sensitive to pH variations in the physiologic range. This signal therefore provides a monitor of intracellular pH. The sensitivity to pH arises because the state of ionization of inorganic phosphate changes in the physiologic pH range. Similarly, the chemical shifts of the ATP signals are influenced by whether or not the ATP is complexed to divalent metal ions, and in general it can be concluded from in vivo spectroscopy that ATP is predominantly complexed to Mg^{2+} ions.

If appropriate controls are performed, the concentrations of the various metabolites are proportional to the areas of their respective signals. Relative concentrations can be determined in this way, and any changes that may occur in these metabolites (e.g., loss of high-energy phosphates during exercise or ischemia) can be followed noninvasively simply by monitoring how the signal areas vary with time. The measurement of absolute concentrations is more difficult but has been achieved in studies of isolated tissues (15,16) and more recently in humans (17,18).

^{1}H Spectroscopy

Several additional nuclei are appropriate for NMR studies of tissue metabolism, and ^{1}H NMR in particular is now receiving much interest. The development of ^{1}H NMR for metabolic studies in vivo has been rather slower than that of ^{31}P NMR. This is partly due to technical reasons: although ^{1}H NMR is about 15 times more sensitive than ^{31}P NMR, it is technically more difficult because of the need to suppress the large signal from water, and in some cases, from fats and because of the large number of metabolites that produce signals in a relatively narrow chemical shift range. (The need to suppress the water and fat signals is apparent from the spectrum in Fig. 1A). However, techniques for solvent suppression and spectral "editing" are now sufficiently well developed to permit the noninvasive monitoring of several metabolites of interest, and ^{1}H spectroscopy is now being widely used for studies of the brain.

Brain metabolites that have been detected by ^{1}H spectroscopy include lactate, alanine, N-acetylaspartate, glutamine, glutamate, total creatine (i.e., creatine + PCr), and choline-containing compounds. For studies of tissue energetics, the methyl signal from lactate is particularly interesting, but unfortunately it has a similar frequency to that of the CH_2 groups of triglycerides; when the fat signal is intense (as is often the case for skeletal muscle studies), the unambiguous detection of lactate becomes difficult. The detection of lactate in the brain is much simpler, as normal brain generates no signal from fats.

Other Nuclei

For the purposes of this chapter, the only other nucleus that we shall consider is ^{13}C. ^{13}C NMR provides a method of studying metabolism that has analogies with the use of ^{14}C for radioactive tracer studies, with the advantages that well-resolved signals can be attributed to different carbons with individual molecules. In view of the poor sensitivity of ^{13}C relative to ^{1}H NMR, there are advantages in following the ^{13}C nuclei indirectly by observing protons that are coupled to the ^{13}C nuclei. However, because NMR is an intrinsically insensitive technique, the ^{13}C nucleus still needs to be present in bulk rather than trace concentrations, and this has inhibited its widespread use in vivo. Nevertheless, interesting results are emerging, particularly in relation to glucose and glycogen metabolism, as discussed in the section on skeletal muscle studies in this chapter.

Measurements of Reaction Rates in the Steady State

NMR can be used to measure the rates of certain reactions taking place under steady state or equilibrium conditions. One approach, used in ^1H and ^{13}C studies, involves isotope exchange and incorporation. A second approach uses the technique of magnetization transfer NMR, which is a type of magnetic labeling experiment. In such an experiment, the magnetization of one species is perturbed, and this perturbation can be transferred to a second species if the two are in exchange with each other. The extent to which the second species is affected (together with a measurement of the spin-lattice relaxation time T_1) can, with appropriate controls, give a measure of the rate of interconversion.

For example, Fig. 2A; shows a ^{31}P spectrum obtained from frog gastrocnemius

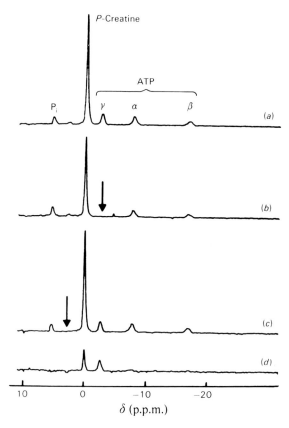

FIG. 2. ^{31}P spectra of frog gastrocnemius muscle showing the effects of magnetization transfer from the γ-phosphate of ATP to phosphocreatine. **A:** A spectrum obtained in the absence of selective irradiation. **B,C:** Spectra obtained with selective irradiation applied at the frequencies indicated by the arrows. **D:** The difference spectrum obtained by subtracting B from C. From ref. 19 (where further details can be found).

muscles at rest. Figure 2B shows spectra obtained under similar conditions, except that the signal from the γ-phosphate of ATP was caused to disappear by applying additional irradiation selectively at the frequency of this signal. Effectively, the γ-phosphate is being labeled with zero magnetization. Because the γ-phosphate of ATP is in chemical exchange with the phosphate of phosphocreatine (PCr) through the creatine kinase reaction, some of the label (i.e., loss of signal) is transferred to the PCr, which therefore has a lower intensity in Fig. 2B than in the spectrum of Fig. 2A. Figure 2C shows a control spectrum, with irradiation on the opposite side of the PCr peak, and Fig. 2D represents the difference between the spectra of Figs. 2B and 2C, illustrating the loss of intensity of the PCr signal. From a series of such spectra accumulated under specified conditions, it is possible to measure the rate of interconversion of phosphocreatine and ATP through the creatine kinase reaction. Furthermore, in some tissues it has been possible to observe magnetization transfer between the ATP and P_i signals and hence to obtain information about the rate of ATP turnover. Unfortunately, however, only a limited number of enzyme-catalyzed reactions can be studied in this way, partly because they need to be rapid and also because they must involve at least one substrate that gives rise to a detectable signal. However, it should be emphasized that this technique does provide a totally non-invasive means of measuring the steady state kinetics of certain key reactions as they take place in vivo, and some interesting conclusions have emerged, as discussed in following sections.

APPLICATIONS OF ^{31}P SPECTROSCOPY

Measurement of Metabolite Levels

Early in the development of ^{31}P spectroscopy, it was naturally important to compare the absolute or relative concentrations of energy metabolites as measured by NMR with those measured by freeze-clamping. In making these comparisons, it should be noted that freeze-clamping estimates usually rely on measurements of *total* amounts of metabolites, whereas NMR generally measures only the mobile components. The values obtained by the two techniques could therefore differ, for example, because of tight binding of metabolites to intracellular macromolecules.

For frog sartorius muscle, it was shown that freeze-clamping and NMR provide similar values for the concentrations of ATP, phosphocreatine, and P_i (15), indicating that only a small fraction of any of these compounds can be substantially immobilized. These muscles are thin and can therefore be rapidly frozen. For this reason, there are no problems associated with the possible breakdown of high-energy phosphates during the freeze-clamping procedure. In contrast, a wide range of studies on various tissues, including skeletal muscle, shows that the analytically measured ADP concentration is generally much greater than that measured by NMR. Furthermore, in skeletal muscle it is possible to determine the concentration of free ADP from the creatine kinase equilibrium, and the free ADP measured in this way is only a small percent of the total ADP. The same conclusion regarding free ADP has been reached by Veech et al. (20) on the basis of similar arguments involving enzymes such as creatine kinase that are believed to catalyze reactions that are near to equilibrium.

There are several possible reasons for the discrepancy in the ADP measurements. First, it has been believed for some time that a large percentage of the muscle ADP is tightly bound to the proteins of the myofilaments, and it is reasonable to assume that this component of the intracellular ADP is too immobilized to generate detectable NMR signals. Alternatively, in some cases there may be an unavoidable breakdown of high-energy phosphates in invasive measurements (e.g., in human biopsy analyses where there is an inevitable delay between removal and freezing of the sample). It is a further possibility that a significant fraction of the intracellular content of ADP might be sequestered (e.g., in the mitochondria), in such a way that it generates no detectable signals. This might account for the low levels of NMR-visible ADP that have been reported in the kidney (16) and liver (21).

In mammalian muscle, the concentration of free P_i as measured by NMR is often less than that determined chemically. This has analogies with the ADP measurements and could be accounted for in the same way as the ADP observations. Furthermore, the NMR-visible P_i is low in the kidney (16) and liver (21).

As discussed in more detail in later sections, these NMR measurements of free P_i and ADP have important kinetic and thermodynamic implications. In particular they strongly influence our understanding of those reactions that are subject to control by P_i and ADP, and their low values also mean that the free energy of hydrolysis of ATP in vivo is rather higher than might have been anticipated.

Applications to Human Muscle

Normal Subjects

NMR is ideally suited to investigating the metabolic changes that are associated with exercise, because the metabolic state can be monitored noninvasively and sequentially throughout a period of rest, exercise, and recovery. Although a number of animal studies have been carried out, the advantages of spectroscopy are most apparent for investigations of exercise in humans, for whom there are obvious benefits over biopsy procedures. Here a discussion is given of some of the observations that have been made in control subjects. Studies of patients are described in the following section.

Figure 3 shows four of a series of ^{31}P spectra obtained at rest, during aerobic finger-flexing exercise, and during recovery. The spectra were obtained using a surface radiofrequency coil of diameter 25 mm, positioned over the finger flexor muscle (*flexor digitorum superficialis*).

Figure 3A shows a typical resting spectrum. From such spectra, Taylor et al. (22) found that the intracellular pH of the finger flexor muscle at rest is 7.04 ± 0.03 (SD,

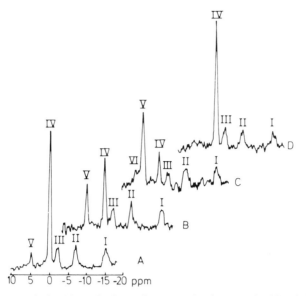

FIG. 3. ^{31}P spectra obtained from the finger flexor muscle of a normal subject before exercise **(A)**, during exercise **(B,C)**, and after exercise **(D)**. Exercise was carried out for 19 minutes by squeezing a rubber bulb to a pressure of 300 mm Hg 22 to 30 times per minute. Spectrum B was collected during the first minute of exercise, and C, during the last minute. D was obtained 5–6 minutes after exercise ceased. Spectrum A was collected over 256 seconds, and all others, over 64 seconds. Peak assignments are I, β-ATP; II, α-ATP plus pyridine nucleotides; III, γ-ATP; IV, phosphocreatine; V, P_i; VI, phosphomonoesters. From ref. 23.

$n = 20$), and that the concentration ratios PCr/ATP and P_i/ATP are 4.5 and 0.46. Absolute concentrations were evaluated from these ratios using the assumption (from biopsy studies) that the concentration of ATP seen by NMR is 5.5 mmol/kg wet wt. More recently, quantitative NMR measurements were made of the ATP concentrations in forearm muscle, confirming the validity of this assumption (18). During aerobic exercise, PCr declines and P_i increases (as seen in Figs. 3B and 3C), and there is a decline in intracellular pH. A fairly good correlation was found between intracellular pH and the ratio PCr/PCr + P_i (22). The recovery of PCr following exercise is normally half completed in about 1 minute (22), but it is slower when there is a significant depletion of ATP during exercise (23).

These observations agree well with previous biopsy studies with the exception that, as previously discussed, the PCr/P_i ratio is much higher when measured by NMR than by biopsy. Similarly, the concentration of free ADP—estimated to be about 6 μmol per liter intracellular water (22,23)—is much lower than the total values assessed from biopsy analyses. In addition, ^{31}P NMR shows that the intracellular pH can fall to as low as 6.0; one subject could exercise for more than 10 minutes with an intracellular pH of close to 6.0 (22). In contrast to this, biopsy studies have shown that after exercise to exhaustion, the intracellular pH in the quadriceps muscle falls to about 6.4–6.5. This difference may reflect the different muscles that were investigated. The NMR results suggest that glycolysis, and therefore phosphofructokinase, must be at least partially active at pH 6.0, whereas it has been thought that the enzyme might be inactivated at such a low pH.

It was also found that there was no detectable metabolic recovery during a 10-minute ischemic period following exercise (22). This is interesting because it means that glycolysis is inactivated at the end of exercise, despite elevated levels of AMP and ADP, and also because metabolic recovery must therefore be almost exclusively oxidative. This lack of glycolytic activity after exercise is consistent with the additional finding that glycolysis is very slow in human forearm muscle when exposed to a prolonged period of ischemia in the absence of exercise (24), and it suggests that Ca^{2+} ions are required for activation of the phosphorylase system. A similar conclusion was reached from NMR studies of frog gastrocnemius muscles at 4°C (25).

^{31}P spectroscopy offers an opportunity to investigate the mechanisms underlying reduced muscle performance, as in normal aging and in fatigue. In one study, young adult subjects were compared with healthy elderly subjects aged 70 to 80 years, using ^{31}P spectroscopy to monitor tissue metabolites both at rest and during aerobic dynamic exercise (26). The results suggested that the energetics of human skeletal muscle are not altered by the aging process; the decline in muscular strength and performance may simply be a reflection of reduced muscle mass.^{31}P NMR also provides a useful approach to the investigation of muscular fatigue because a number of the possible metabolic determinants can be monitored simultaneously in exercising muscle. Following earlier studies of fatiguing frog muscle (27,28), studies have been carried out in humans (29). The problem is the fact that because a large number of metabolic changes are necessarily associated with exercise, it is difficult to establish which change, if any, plays a major role in the fatiguing process. One suggestion asserts that the accumulation of P_i in its monobasic form, $H_2PO_4^-$, is the cause of the decline in force, but this is open to discussion (see ref. 29 for references). Presumably, it is possible that a range of metabolites may be associated with the fatigue process and that under various circumstances different factors may be important. For example, patients with McArdle's disease fatigue rapidly despite retaining some of their high-energy phosphate, producing very little lactate, and having a pH that is not acid (8). It can be calculated that the concentration of free ADP is unusually high under such circumstances and that this could strongly influence muscle performance (30). In normal subjects, other metabolic changes, including an increase in $H_2PO_4^-$, may play a dominant role in the fatigue process.

Skeletal Muscle Studies in Disease

The NMR studies of normal subjects discussed in the preceding sections have provided a fresh insight into several different aspects of muscle biochemistry and physiology, but they also give essential baseline information for studies of disease.

Abnormalities in tissue energetics have been observed in patients with disorders of oxidative or glycolytic metabolism. For example, in patients with McArdle's syndrome (in which there is a glycogen phosphorylase deficiency), the muscle pH becomes alkaline during exercise, rather than acid (8), which is totally consistent with the inability of these patients to generate lactic acid from glycogen. A patient with phosphofructokinase deficiency not only became alkaline on exercise but also accumulated sugar phosphate, as anticipated (24). In two sisters with a mitochondrial disorder (31), recovery of phosphocreatine following exercise was very slow, demonstrating a reduced rate of oxidative metabolism. However, pH recovery was faster than in controls. Furthermore, in view of the high blood lactate levels that had been observed in one of the patients, the changes in intracellular pH on exercise were somewhat milder than might have been expected, suggesting that such patients might have an adaptive system for eliminating excess acid. Recent reviews discuss the range of muscle disorders that have been investigated by ^{31}P spectroscopy (30,32).

It is perhaps not surprising that the most obvious abnormalities in tissue energetics are observed in patients with specific disorders of glycolytic or oxidative metabolism. As discussed in the section on metabolic control, the spectral abnormalities exhibited by these patients are of interest because they help researchers understand the disease in more detail and also because they help us to understand the relationships between metabolism and function in healthy muscle.

So far, we have restricted our discussion of muscle metabolism to ^{31}P spectroscopy. However, as previously mentioned, other nuclei have potential roles to play in the investigation of tissue energetics, and we now turn to some applications of ^{13}C NMR. Several years ago it was shown that glycogen gives a well-resolved ^{13}C NMR spectrum in which the carbons are almost completely NMR-visible (33). This was somewhat surprising in view of the fact that large molecules with relatively little mobility tend to give very broad signals. Presumably, glycogen has a high degree of internal mobility such that its carbons give fairly narrow signals. Although ^{13}C has a natural abundance of only 1.1%, the high concentration of glycogen in liver and muscle means that ^{13}C signals can be detected from glycogen in these tissues without any need for istopic enrichment (34). For example, it has been shown that ^{13}C NMR can distinguish patients suffering from McArdle's disease from normal subjects by measuring their muscle glycogen at rest (35).

^{13}C NMR has recently been used to investigate the disposal of glucose in normal and non–insulin-dependent diabetic humans (36). In this work, combined hyperglycemic-hyperinsulinemic clamp studies with ^{13}C glucose were carried out in healthy subjects and in subjects with non–insulin-dependent diabetes mellitus. The rate of incorporation of intravenously infused [1-^{13}C] glucose into muscle glycogen was measured in the gastrocnemius muscle using a [13] C-tuned surface coil, with time resolution of about 15 minutes. It was concluded that muscle glycogen synthesis provides the main pathway for disposal of glucose in both the normal and diabetic subjects and that defects in muscle glycogen synthesis play a major role in the insulin resistance that occurs in patients with non–insulin-dependent diabetes mellitus.

CONTROL OF ENERGY METABOLISM IN SKELETAL MUSCLE

The transition from rest to exercise involves a large and rapid increase in the ATP utilization of skeletal muscle. One of the questions that arises is how the ATP-producing reactions and pathways are regulated in such a way as to generate ATP strictly according to demand. NMR spectroscopy can contribute in a number of ways to our understanding of these regulatory processes.

The most immediate source of ATP occurs through the hydrolysis of phospho-creatine catalyzed by the enzyme creatine kinase. As previously described, ^{31}P NMR provides a method of measuring the activity of this enzyme within skeletal muscle noninvasively. In this way it has been confirmed that in resting muscle, the creatine kinase reaction is close to equilibrium and that the activity of this reaction is sufficiently high to ensure (provided that adequate phosphocreatine is still present) that the ATP level is maintained approximately constant during exercise (19,37,38).

With regard to glycogen metabolism, a number of NMR studies have suggested that Ca^{2+} ions are required for activation of the phosphorylase system, as previously discussed above. But perhaps the most interesting results relate to the possible role of ADP in the regulation of oxidative metabolism in muscle.

The concentration of free cytoplasmic ADP can be calculated via the creatine kinase equilibrium, because NMR allows simultaneous measurements of all the other reactants (i.e., phosphocreatine, creatine from the known concentration of PCr + creatine, ATP, and H^+). In different types of skeletal muscle at rest, typical values of about 5 μM to 20 μM are found for the free ADP concentration (19,22,23,39). On exercise, this concentration can increase to values well above 50 μM. Because it is generally accepted that the K_m for ADP control of mitochondrial ATP synthesis is of the order of 30 μM (see ref. 40 for review), ADP provides an obvious candidate for regulating oxidative metabolism in skeletal muscle. However, if the concentration of free ADP rises too much, as it can do in disease, it may then begin to inhibit muscle contraction (30).

ENERGY METABOLISM AND ITS CONTROL IN OTHER TISSUES

^{31}P NMR is ideally suited to investigating the large changes in phosphorus-containing metabolites and intracellular pH that are associated with muscular exercise. The large changes in energy demand and in the concentrations of these metabolites make it reasonable to expect that metabolites such as ADP should play a key role in the control of energy metabolism, as the preceding studies have indicated. However, it is less obvious that this should be the case for other tissues such as cardiac muscle, liver, and brain, which do not have such extensive variations in energy demand. Here we discuss some of the relevant studies that have been carried out on other tissues, which suggest that regulation of oxidative phosphorylation in these tissues cannot be explained adequately simply in terms of the actions of ADP and P_i.

As pointed out in a recent review (40), ^{31}P NMR studies of the heart, brain, and kidney have shown that there is little correlation between the rate of oxidative phosphorylation in the steady state and the cytoplasmic concentrations of ADP, P_i, and ATP. For example, studies of the normal heart suggest that the phosphorylation potential and the concentrations of ADP and P_i remain very stable despite large (approximately fourfold) increases in the rates of utilization of ATP (41,42). This does not mean that these metabolites no longer have the capacity to control oxidative phosphorylation in these tissues. However, it does suggest that, at least under the circumstances that have been investigated, there are other factors, including substrate and oxygen delivery, that presumably have a stronger influence on the regulation of oxidative phosphorylation (40).

It should be emphasized that in diseased tissue, there may be aspects of energy metabolism and its control that differ from those seen in normal tissue. For example, in patients with coronary artery disease, ^{31}P spectroscopy showed a reduced PCr/ATP ratio in the left ventricular wall during hand-grip exercise, which was not seen in normal subjects (43). This suggests that exercise testing with ^{31}P NMR may provide a useful method for assessing the effects of ischemia on cardiac energy metabolism and for monitoring the response to therapy.

^{31}P NMR can make further contributions to our understanding of the kinetics and thermodynamics of oxidative phosphorylation through its ability to monitor the unidirectional flux between ATP and P_i in intact tissues. As mentioned in the preceding section on measurements of reaction rates, this measurement can be achieved by magnetization transfer techniques in a manner analogous to the measurement of creatine kinase activity. For example, it has been shown that the unidirectional rate of ATP synthesis in the heart is similar to the net flux of ATP production calculated on the basis of the oxygen consumption of the tissue (44). This indicates that the cytochrome chain is operating under non-equilibrium conditions, which has direct relevance to mechanisms whereby ATP and in particular its products of hydrolysis might exert their control.

THE ROLE OF ^{1}H SPECTROSCOPY

The observations previously described suggest that although ^{31}P spectroscopy might provide an ideal approach to the investigation of energetics in skeletal muscle, its impact in terms of monitoring changes in the energetics of other tissues might be less obvious. An additional NMR approach, which is looking extremely interesting for investigations of brain metabolism, is to use ^{1}H spectroscopy. This section is concerned with the ways in which ^{1}H NMR is now being used to probe tissue energetics, primarily through the noninvasive detection of lactate.

As mentioned in a preceding section, the development of ^{1}H NMR for metabolic studies lagged behind ^{31}P NMR for a number of technical reasons that, particularly for the brain, have now been overcome. From a biochemical viewpoint, too, ^{1}H

NMR developed more slowly because of the perceived strength of ^{31}P NMR in monitoring energy metabolism. It has become apparent, however, that there are many disease states in which ^{1}H spectroscopy might reveal abnormalities despite a relatively normal energy status as measured by ^{31}P NMR. Therefore, at the very least, ^{1}H spectroscopy can complement the information that is available from ^{31}P studies.

A key feature of ^{1}H spectroscopy is the high sensitivity of the ^{1}H nucleus in comparison with other nuclei. In principle this means that the metabolites could be detected at relatively low concentrations. However, it is not necessarily straightforward to observe metabolites at low concentrations, because their signals may be masked by larger signals from other compounds that are present at higher concentrations. In practice, therefore, the higher sensitivity is generally exploited by trading signal-to-noise ratio with spatial resolution. The higher sensitivity of ^{1}H spectroscopy means that adequate signal-to-noise ratios can be obtained from smaller volume elements, and the consequent improvement in spatial resolution (linear resolution of 1–2 cm is being achieved for studies of the human brain) is proving to have considerable value.

Animal Studies

Following the first in vivo studies reported by Behar et al. (45), numerous research groups have used ^{1}H NMR, often together with ^{31}P NMR, to investigate metabolic abnormalities in animal models of disease. For example, in studies of a gerbil stroke model, it has been possible to correlate changes in ^{31}P and ^{1}H spectra during and following ischemia with changes in regional cerebral blood flow measured simultaneously with the hydrogen clearance technique (46–48). It was demonstrated that there is a flow threshold of about 20 ml/100g/min at which energy failure ensues, with large increases in P_i and lactate and a decrease in intracellular pH. This flow value is similar to that at which, in a variety of species, electric activity ceases, and it is also similar to the flow level at which water accumulates in the gerbil brain. These results therefore provide evidence suggesting that the thresholds for electrical function and edema are a direct consequence of energy failure. The model could be valuable in studying modifications to flow and metabolism produced by pharmaceuticals and other forms of therapy.

During recirculation following ischemia, it was found that there is a period when the lactate is still elevated, while the ^{31}P spectrum and intracellular pH are close to normal. These data suggest that ^{1}H NMR spectroscopy of lactate may be a more sensitive monitor than ^{31}P NMR of a previous ischemic episode or of repeated transient ischemia.

In parallel studies of cerebral hypoxia in the gerbil, it was found that as the P_aO_2 was reduced below 40 mm Hg, there was a significant increase in lactate in some of the animals prior to any detectable change in the phosphorus spectra (49). This suggests that glycolysis can be controlled independently of the concentrations of the phosphorus energy metabolites. Furthermore, in a rat model of hyperammonemia,

[31]P spectroscopy showed that the brain can maintain normal energy metabolite ratios despite the metabolic challenge produced by an increase in blood ammonia to about 500 μM. [1]H spectra that were edited for the detection of specific metabolites showed a significant increase in brain glutamine and lactate and a decrease in glutamate (50).

All of these studies illustrate the point that there could be many situations in which the ^{1}H spectra are more responsive than ^{31}P signals to brain disease. As a result of recent technical developments, clinical applications of ^{1}H spectroscopy for the investigation of brain metabolism are now being explored, to the extent that ^{1}H spectroscopy has probably become more popular than ^{31}P NMR for studies of brain disease.

[31]P and [1]H Spectroscopy of the Human Brain

Because of the importance of understanding the mechanisms of hypoxic-ischemic injury in newborns, ^{31}P spectroscopy of neonates was started soon after magnets of large enough dimensions became available (51,52). The PCr/P_i ratio proved to be a good prognostic indicator of the likely clinical outcome following birth asphyxia; below a certain value for the ratio, infants either die or survive with impaired neurologic function (53). With ^{31}P spectroscopy, an apparently normal spectrum (in terms of metabolite ratios) is recorded soon after the birth asphyxia episode (8–17 h), but over the next few days the energy status declines. This raises the possibility that intervention during the intermediate "normal" stage may be able to ameliorate the clinical outcome (53). However, it should be noted that in general, the normality of metabolite ratios does not always imply that the high-energy phosphate concentrations are normal throughout the brain: it is possible that severely infarcted areas may produce no signal at all. Thus, decreases of up to 40% in the total ^{31}P NMR metabolite signals have been seen in chronic adult infarctions, with no accompanying changes in metabolite ratios or intracellular pH (54). This would be consistent with a substantial loss of viable brain cells.

In studies of acute ischemic stroke, changes in the ^{31}P metabolites were observed during the acute or subacute (up to 72 hours) stages (55). No significant abnormalities in high-energy phosphates were measured in the intermediate or later stages (7–40 days), despite the persistent neurologic deficit and evidence for infarction from imaging. It was suggested that apart from partial recovery of some neurons, the return of high-energy phosphates may also originate from glial cells that are relatively resistant to ischemia or macrophages that infiltrate the infarct. These studies of ischemic disease therefore emphasize the importance of measuring absolute signal intensities in addition to signal ratios, and they demonstrate that caution is needed in relating recovery of high-energy phosphates to recovery of function.

From the preceding discussion, one could argue that ^{31}P spectroscopy provides a less complete indication of tissue energetics in the brain than it does in skeletal muscle. Complementary information is now available from ^{1}H spectroscopy. Numerous groups have reported excellent ^{1}H spectra from localized regions of the human brain, showing well-resolved signals from lactate, N-acetylaspartate (NAA), creatine + PCr, and choline-containing compounds. Much of the interest has focused on the NAA and lactate signals.

A reduced ratio of NAA to total creatine has been seen in gliomas, meningiomas, cerebrovascular disease, multiple sclerosis, and a variety of other disorders of the brain (56–61). Although the function of NAA is unclear, this compound is believed to be located primarily in neurons (62). This suggests that an abnormally low NAA signal might be attributable to neuronal loss or dysfunction. Thus, ^{1}H spectroscopy should be useful in many disorders involving neuronal degeneration and glial proliferation. As is apparent from the preceding discussion, ^{31}P spectroscopy is unlikely to be as useful in this respect because there are no equivalent phosphorus-containing markers that can be exploited. Indeed, cell culture studies suggest that neurons and glia may have similar PCr/ATP ratios (63).

For pediatric studies, interpretation of a reduced NAA signal is less straightforward because its signal intensity relative to the other major signals increases during normal development. In studies of brain disorders, comparisons with age-matched normal data are therefore essential. On the basis of recent studies of infants who had suffered birth asphyxiation, it seems likely that ^{31}P spectroscopy will be most valuable in the acute and subacute phases as a monitor of energy failure, whereas ^{1}H spectroscopy will be most informative in the chronic phase as an indicator of neuronal loss (64).

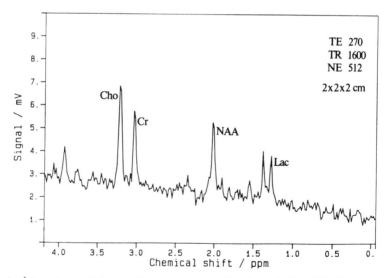

FIG. 4. ^{1}H spectrum obtained in vivo from the brain of an 8-month-old child with suspected pyruvate dehydrogenase deficiency. The spectrum was obtained from a $2 \times 2 \times 2$ cm volume using a spin echo radiofrequency pulse sequence incorporating a 90° pulse followed by two frequency-selective 180° pulses, with presaturation for solvent suppression. The study included 512 data acquisitions with an echo time of 270 ms and repetition time of 1,600 ms. (Courtesy of the Hospital for Sick Children). From ref. 65.

Another role for ^{1}H spectroscopy is apparent in the investigation of inborn errors of metabolism. For example, Fig. 4 shows a ^{1}H spectrum from an 8-month-old child with suspected pyruvate dehydrogenase deficiency, demonstrating the characteristic doublet of lactate centered at 1.32 ppm. In addition, the NAA/Cr and NAA/Cho ratios are reduced relative to age-matched normal data, presumably reflecting neuronal damage. This spectrum was obtained from a 2 × 2 × 2 cm localized volume; smaller regions (approaching 1 ml in volume) are accessible to study, and it is now possible to accumulate and process the data in such a way as to present an image (albeit of much cruder resolution than images based on the water signal) displaying the different metabolite signal intensities. Investigations of the regional variations of these metabolites should add significantly to our understanding of the mechanisms of a variety of brain disorders and could have considerable value in the evaluation and monitoring of therapy.

CONCLUDING REMARKS

The early NMR studies of tissue metabolism focused mainly on ^{31}P spectroscopy of tissue energetics in skeletal muscle, but by combining the NMR observations with data obtained from complementary analytic techniques, researchers have discovered a great deal of new information about energy metabolism and its control in vivo. As NMR techniques have evolved, greater emphasis has been placed on clinical applications of spectroscopy—not just in skeletal muscle but in, for example, cardiac muscle, liver, and brain—and we are beginning to learn more about the energetics of these tissues in both normal and diseased subjects. For example, there have been two preliminary reports of the detection by ^{1}H spectroscopy of increased lactate in the human visual cortex in response to visual stimulation (66,67). There is every reason to believe that future NMR studies will offer further insights into our understanding of energy metabolism and its control in humans.

REFERENCES

1. Bloch F, Hansen WW, Packard M. The nuclear induction experiment. *Phys Rev* 1946;70:474–85.
2. Purcell EM, Torrey HC, Pound RV. Resonance absorption by nuclear magnetic moment in a solid. *Phys Rev* 1946;69:37–8.
3. Lauterbur PC. Image formation by induced local interactions: examples employing nuclear magnetic resonance. *Nature* 1973;242:190–1.
4. Moon RB, Richards JH. Determination of intracellular pH by ^{31}P nuclear magnetic resonance. *J Biol Chem* 1973;248:7276–8.
5. Hoult DI, Busby SJW, Gadian DG, Radda GK, Richards RE, Seeley PJ. Observations of tissue metabolites using ^{31}P nuclear magnetic resonance. *Nature* 1974;252:285–7.
6. Ackerman JJH, Grove TH, Wong GG, Gadian DG, Radda GK. Mapping of metabolites in whole animals by ^{31}P NMR using surface coils *Nature* 1980;282:167–70.
7. Cady EB, Costello AMdeL, Dawson MJ, et al. Non-invasive investigation of cerebral metabolism in newborn infants by phosphorus nuclear magnetic resonance spectroscopy. *Lancet* 1983;1:1059–62.
8. Ross BD, Radda GK, Gadian DG, Rocker G, Esiri M, Falconer-Smith J. Examination of a case of

suspected McArdle's syndrome by ^{31}P nuclear magnetic resonance. *N Engl J Med* 1981;304:1338–42.

9. Gadian DG. *Nuclear magnetic resonance and its applications to living systems.* Oxford: Oxford University Press, 1982.
10. Morris PG. *Nuclear magnetic resonance imaging in medicine and biology.* Oxford: Clarendon Press, 1986.
11. Cady EB. *Clinical magnetic resonance spectroscopy.* New York: Plenum Press, 1990.
12. Garlick PB, Brown TR, Sullivan RH, Ugurbil K. Observation of a second phosphate pool in the perfused heart by ^{31}P NMR; is this the mitochondrial phosphate? *J Mol Cell Cardiol* 1983;15:855–8.
13. Williams SR, Crockard HA, Gadian DG. Cerebral ischemia studied by nuclear magnetic resonance spectroscopy. *Cerebrovasc Brain Metab Rev* 1989;1:91–114.
14. Gadian DG. Magnetic resonance spectroscopy as a probe of tumour metabolism. *Eur J Cancer.* [In press].
15. Dawson MJ, Gadian DG, Wilkie DR. Contraction and recovery of living muscles studied by ^{31}P nuclear magnetic resonance. *J Physiol* 1977;267:703–35.
16. Freeman D, Bartlett S, Radda GK, Ross BD. Energetics of sodium transport in the kidney: saturation transfer ^{31}P-NMR. *Biochim Biophys Acta* 1983;762:325–36.
17. Bottomley PA, Hardy CJ. Rapid, reliable in vivo assays of human phosphate metabolites by nuclear magnetic resonance. *Clin Chem* 1989;35:392–95.
18. Cady EB. Absolute quantitation of phosphorus metabolites in the cerebral cortex of the newborn human infant and in the forearm muscles of young adults using a double-tuned surface coil. *J Magn Reson* 1990;87:433–46.
19. Gadian DG, Radda GK, Brown TR, Chance EM, Dawson MJ, Wilkie DR. The activity of creatine kinase in frog skeletal muscle studied by saturation transfer nuclear magnetic resonance. *Biochem J* 1981;194:215–28.
20. Veech RL, Lawson JWR, Cornell NW, Krebs HA. Cytosolic phosphorylation potential. *J Biol Chem* 1979;254:6538–47.
21. Iles RA, Stevens AN, Griffiths JR, Morris PG. Phosphorylation status of liver by ^{31}P-n.m.r. spectroscopy, and its implications for metabolic control. *Biochem J* 1985;229:141–51.
22. Taylor DJ, Bore PJ, Styles P, Gadian DG, Radda GK. Bioenergetics of intact human muscle: a ^{31}P nuclear magnetic resonance study. *Mol Biol Med* 1983;1:77–94.
23. Taylor DJ, Styles P, Matthews PM, et al. Energetics of human muscle: exercise-induced ATP depletion. *Magn Reson Med* 1986;3:44–54.
24. Edwards RHT, Dawson MJ, Wilkie DR, Gordon RE, Shaw D. Clinical use of NMR in the investigation of myopathy. *Lancet* 1982;1:725–31.
25. Dawson MJ, Gadian DG, Wilkie DR. Studies of the biochemistry of contracting and relaxing muscle by the use of ^{31}P n.m.r. in conjunction with other techniques. *Philos Trans R Soc London [Biol]* 1980;289:445–55.
26. Taylor DJ, Crowe M, Bore PJ, Styles P, Arnold DL, Radda GK. Examination of the energetics of aging skeletal muscle using nuclear magnetic resonance. *Gerontology* 1984;30:2–7.
27. Dawson MJ, Gadian DG, and Wilkie DR. Muscular fatigue investigated by phosphorus nuclear magnetic resonance. *Nature* 1978;274:861–6.
28. Dawson MJ, Gadian DG, Wilkie DR. Mechanical relaxation rate and metabolism studied in fatiguing muscle by phosphorus nuclear magnetic resonance. *J Physiol* 1980;299:465–84.
29. Newham DJ, Cady EB. A ^{31}P study of fatigue and metabolism in human skeletal muscle with voluntary, intermittent contraction at different forces. *NMR Biomed* 1990;3:211–9.
30. Radda GK. Some new insights into biology and medicine through NMR spectroscopy. In: Mansfield P, Hahn EL, eds. *NMR imaging.* Royal Society Discussion meeting 5–6 June 1990;515–24.
31. Radda GK, Bore PJ, Gadian DG, et al. ^{31}P NMR examination of two patients with NADH-CoQ reductase deficiency. *Nature* 1982;295:608–9.
32. Bottomley PA. Human in vivo NMR spectroscopy in diagnostic medicine: clinical tool or research probe? *Radiology* 1989;170:1–15.
33. Sillerud LO, Shulman RG. Structure and metabolism of mammalian liver glycogen monitored by carbon-13 nuclear magnetic resonance. *Biochem J* 1983;221:1087–94.
34. Jue T, Rothman DL, Tavitian BA, Shulman RG. Natural-abundance ^{13}C NMR study of glycogen repletion in human liver and muscle. *Proc Natl Acad Sci USA* 1989;86:1439–42.
35. Jehenson P, Duboc D, Bloch G, Fardeau M, Syrota A. Diagnosis of muscular glycogenosis by in vivo natural abundance ^{13}C NMR spectroscopy. *Neuromusc Disorders* 1991;1:99–101.

36. Shulman GI, Rothman DL, Jue T, Stein P, DeFronzo RA, Shulman RG. Quantitation of muscle glycogen synthesis in normal subjects and subjects with non–insulin-dependent diabetes by ^{13}C nuclear magnetic resonance spectroscopy. *N Engl Med* 1990;322:223–8.
37. Shoubridge EA, Bland JL, Radda GK. Regulation of creatine kinase during steady-state isometric twitch contraction in rat skeletal muscle. *Biochim Biophys Acta* 1984;805:72–8.
38. Rees D, Smith MB, Harley J, Radda GK. In vivo functioning of creatine phosphokinase in human forearm muscle, studied by ^{31}P NMR saturation transfer. *Magn Reson Med* 1989;9:39–52.
39. Meyer RA, Kushmerick MJ, Brown TR. Application of ^{31}P-NMR spectroscopy to the study of striated muscle metabolism. *Am J Physiol* 1982;2423:C1–11.
40. Balaban RS. Regulation of oxidative phosphorylation in the mammalian cell. *Am J Physiol* 1990;258:C377–89.
41. Balaban RS, Kantor HL, Katz LA, Briggs RW. Relation between work and phosphate metabolites in the in vivo paced mammalian heart. *Science* 1986;232:1121–3.
42. Katz LA, Swain JA, Portman MA, Balaban RS. Relation between phosphate metabolites and oxygen consumption of heart in vivo. *Am J Physiol* 1989;256:H265–74.
43. Weiss RG, Bottomley PA, Hardy CJ, Gerstenblith G. Regional myocardial metabolism of high-energy phosphates during isometric exercise in patients with coronary artery disease. *N Engl J Med* 1990;323:1593–1600.
44. Kingsley-Hickman PB, Sako EY, Mohanakrishnan P, et al. ^{31}P NMR studies of ATP synthesis and hydrolysis kinetics in the intact heart myocardium. *Biochemistry* 1987;26:7501–10.
45. Behar KL, Den Hollander JA, Stromski ME, et al. High-resolution ^{1}H nuclear magnetic resonance study of cerebral hypoxia in vivo. *Proc Natl Acad Sci USA* 1983;80:4945–8.
46. Gadian DG, Frackowiak RSJ, Crockard HA, et al. Acute cerebral ischaemia: concurrent changes in cerebral blood flow, energy metabolites, pH and lactate measured with hydrogen clearance and ^{31}P and ^{1}H nuclear magnetic resonance spectroscopy. I. Methodology. *J Cereb Blood Flow Metab* 1987;7:199–206.
47. Crockard HA, Gadian DG, Frackowiak RSJ, et al. Acute cerebral ischemia: concurrent changes in cerebral blood flow, energy metabolism, pH and lactate measured with hydrogen clearance and ^{31}P and ^{1}H nuclear magnetic resonance spectroscopy. II. Changes during ischaemia. *J Cereb Blood Flow Metab* 1987;7:394–402.
48. Allen K, Busza AL, Crockard HA, et al. Acute cerebral ischaemia: concurrent changes in cerebral blood flow, energy metabolites, pH and lactate measured with hydrogen clearance and ^{31}P and ^{1}H nuclear magnetic resonance spectroscopy. III. Changes following ischaemia. *J Cereb Blood Flow Metab* 1988;8:816–21.
49. Allen KL, Busza AL, Proctor E, Gadian DG, Crockard HA. *Studies of brain metabolism and blood flow in acute cerebral hypoxia using simultaneous NMR spectroscopy and hydrogen clearance.* Society of Magnetic Resonance in Medicine New York meeting, 1990;1028 (abst).
50. Bates TE, Williams SR, Kauppinen RA, Gadian DG. Observation of cerebral metabolites in an animal model of acute liver failure in vivo: a ^{1}H and ^{31}P nuclear magnetic resonance study. *J Neurochem* 1989;53:102–10.
51. Cady EB, Costello AMdeL, Dawson MJ, et al. Non-invasive investigation of cerebral metabolism in newborn infants by phosphorus nuclear magnetic resonance spectroscopy. *Lancet* 1983;1:1059–62.
52. Younkin DP, Delivora-Papadopoulos M, Leonard JC, et al. Unique aspects of human newborn cerebral metabolism evaluated with phosphorus nuclear magnetic resonance spectroscopy. *Ann Neurol* 1984;6:581–6.
53. Hope PL, Reynolds EOR. Investigation of cerebral energy metabolism in newborn infants by ^{31}P NMR spectroscopy. *Clin Perinatol* 1985;12:261–75.
54. Bottomley PA, Drayer BP, Smith LS. Chronic adult cerebral infarction studied by phosphorus NMR spectroscopy. *Radiology* 1986;160:763–6.
55. Welch KMA, Gross B, Licht J, et al. Magnetic resonance spectroscopy of neurologic diseases. *Curr Neurol* 1988;8:295–331.
56. Bruhn H, Frahm J, Gyngell ML, Merboldt KD, Hanicke W, Sauter R. Cerebral metabolism in man after acute stroke: new observations using localised proton NMR spectroscopy. *Magn Reson Med* 1989;9:126–31.
57. Bruhn H, Frahm J, Gyngell ML, et al. Noninvasive differentiation of tumors with use of localized H-1 MR spectroscopy in vivo: initial experience in patients with cerebral tumours. *Radiology* 1989;172:541–8.

58. Luyten PR, Marien AJH, Heindel W, et al. Metabolic imaging of patients with intracranial tumours: H-1 MR spectroscopic imaging and PET. *Radiology* 1990;176:791–9.
59. Arnold DL, Matthews PM, Francis G, Antel J. Proton magnetic resonance spectroscopy of human brain *in vivo* in the evaluation of multiple sclerosis: assessment of the load of disease. *Magn Reson Med* 1990;14:154–9.
60. Miller DH, Austin SJ, Connelly A, Youl BD, Gadian DG, McDonald WI. Proton magnetic resonance spectroscopy of an acute and chronic lesion in multiple sclerosis. *Lancet* 1991;337:58–9.
61. Menon DK, Cassidy MJD, Baudouin CJ, Sandford RN, Bell JD, Sargentoni J. Proton magnetic resonance spectroscopy in chronic renal failure. *Lancet* 1991;337:244–5.
62. Birken DL, Oldendorf WH. N-acetyl aspartate: a literature review of a compound prominent in ¹H-NMR spectroscopic studies. *Neurosci Behav Rev* 1989;13:23–31.
63. Gill SS, Small RK, Thomas DGT, et al. Brain metabolites as ¹H NMR markers of neuronal and glial disorders. *NMR Biomed* 1989;2:196–200.
64. Peden CJ, Cowan FM, Bryant DJ, et al. Proton MR spectroscopy of the brain in infants. *J Comput Assist Tomogr* 1990;14:886–94.
65. Gadian DG. Proton NMR studies of brain metabolism. *Philos Trans R Soc Lond A* 1990;333:561–70.
66. Prichard J, Rothman D, Novotny E, et al. *Photic stimulation raises lactate in human visual cortex.* Society of Magnetic Resonance in Medicine Amsterdam meeting, 1989;1071 (abst).
67. Sappey-Marinier D, Calabrese G, Hugg J, Deicken R, Fein G, Weiner M. *Increased lactate in human visual cortex during photic stimulation.* Society of Magnetic Resonance in Medicine New York meeting, 1990;106 (abst).

DISCUSSION

Dr. Henriksson: Nuclear magnetic resonance permits the continuous monitoring of tissue metabolism in a completely noninvasive manner. It represents a new, very important metabolic technique for use in humans. This discussion focuses on the use of NMR in skeletal muscle.

Other Established Methods for the Study of Muscle Metabolism in Humans

Muscle metabolism in humans has generally been studied indirectly via analyses of blood samples or the expired air. The catheterization technique (1) has enabled researchers to study the relative importance of substrates stored in the muscle cells versus that of substrates brought to the muscle cells by the blood stream. The usefulness of this technique has been further extended by the use of labeled compounds, notably ¹⁴C or ³H compounds. The needle biopsy technique was reintroduced in 1962 (2) and has since then been extensively used in metabolic research in combination with a variety of analytic techniques. The addition of the NMR method to this arsenal of techniques represents an important step forward, and together with other recent techniques, such as positron emission tomography (3) and microdialysis (4), it is likely to give a much improved in-depth understanding of the metabolic processes occurring in resting and exercised muscle.

NMR in Muscle Metabolic Research

It is evident that, owing to its atraumatic nature, NMR may often be the only way to study muscle metabolism directly with repeated sampling. This may be the case in ¹H spectroscopy studies in small children with inborn errors of metabolism or in patients during the postoperative phase.^{31}P NMR furthermore seems to be the method of choice in studies of muscle phosphagen metabolism, because relative changes in ATP, phosphocreatine, and P_i are easily measured without the need to disturb the tissue during sampling. In addition, by the use of magnetization transfer, the rate of interconversion of phosphocreatine and ATP through the creatine kinase reaction and the ATP turnover rate may be measured. Studies of the glycogen concentration in liver or muscle based on the ^{13}C NMR spectrum are also very promising, especially because ^{13}C signals can be detected from glycogen in these tissues without the need for isotopic enrichment. For the study of fiber type differences in muscle high-energy phosphate metabolism, NMR must be combined with the biopsy technique. This is so because the linear resolution of the NMR technique is insufficient to account for the mosaic type of fiber type distribution present in human muscle. Another potential problem with some NMR applications seems to be the fact that time resolution may be hampered by the need to avoid too-low signal-to-noise ratios.

Although the general pattern of changes in high-energy phosphates is similar in biopsy and NMR studies, there are some important differences. One difference exists with respect to ADP, which, although practically invisible to the NMR, may be calculated by the application of the creatine kinase equilibrium. However, as discussed in the chapter, the muscle ADP concentration estimated in this way is much lower compared to results from biochemical ADP analyses of biopsy extracts. There may be several reasons for this discrepancy. One is likely to be that a large percentage of the cellular ADP is immobilized (e.g., bound to proteins or sequestered in mitochondria) and therefore may not yield detectable NMR signals. Some investigators (e.g., ref. 5) have used the substitution of P_i/PCr for the ADP concentration, because PCr + creatine must otherwise be estimated from biopsy data. It is a drawback with this method that changes in the cellular P_i concentration (e.g., with contractile activity) are not due solely to the degradation of PCr but are also influenced by other processes, such as the incorporation of P_i into the hexose monophosphates. NMR spectroscopy is believed to be mainly a cytoplasmic monitor, but as discussed in the chapter it seems likely that molecules in other cellular compartments, as well as partly immobilized molecules, could contribute. With the biopsy technique, there is an unavoidable time delay before freezing. In comparisons of instantly freeze-clamped and biopsied muscle, the differences are generally small (see references in the chapter), but there is known to be some PCr breakdown during the biopsy sampling procedure. Another discrepancy between NMR and muscle biopsy data concerns pH determinations during exercise, where clearly lower values are detected with NMR (pH 6.0 at exhaustion) than with the biopsy technique (pH 6.4–6.5).

The observed differences between NMR and muscle biopsy data illustrate that more research is needed to obtain a better understanding about which molecules and cellular compartments are in fact monitored with the different types of NMR spectroscopy. Comparisons between results of different techniques, especially between NMR and biochemical determinations on whole or fractionated muscle tissue, will therefore be important in the further development of the NMR spectroscopy technique in muscle.

REFERENCES

1. Seldinger SI. Catheter replacement of the needle in percutaneous arteriography. A new technique. *Acta Radiol* 1953;39:368–76.
2. Bergström J. Muscle electrolytes in man. *Scand J Clin Lab Invest* 1962;14(Suppl. 68).
3. Phelps M, Mazzeota J, Schelbert H, eds. *Positron emission tomography. Principles and application for the brain and heart.* New York: Raven Press, 1986.
4. Henriksson J, Fuchi T, Oshida Y, Ungerstedt U. Microdialysis for in vivo studies of skeletal muscle glucose metabolism. *Acta Physiol Scand* 1990;140(1), 9A.
5. Kent-Braun JA, McCully KK, Chance B. Metabolic effects of training in humans: a ^{31}P-MRS study. *J Appl Physiol* 1990;69(3):1165–70.

Energy Metabolism: Tissue Determinants and Cellular Corollaries, edited by J. M. Kinney and H. N. Tucker. Raven Press, Ltd., New York © 1992.

Overview: Thermogenesis and Muscle Tissue

Richard Edwards

Department of Medicine, Muscle Research Centre; and Magnetic Resonance Research Centre, University of Liverpool, Liverpool, L69 3BX, United Kingdom

The section of this volume "Thermogenesis and Muscle Tissue" has allowed an assembly of different muscle interests to be discussed. The subjects covered by the distinguished authors could perhaps better be fitted under the title "Thermogenesis *in* Muscle Tissue." To clarify the relevance of muscle metabolism to whole body thermogenesis it is intended to continue, after a brief review of the salient points raised by each of the authors, with considerations under two closely related sections: "The Effects of Thermogenesis *on* Muscle Tissue" and "The Effects of Muscle Tissue on Thermogenesis." It is hoped that in this way the possible relevance of recent developments in the study of energy metabolism in skeletal muscle may be seen in perspective. It will remain to be seen how relevant these considerations are to the wider interest in, and the possible clinical relevance of, thermogenesis in nutrition.

THERMOGENESIS IN MUSCLE TISSUE

The energy costs of ATP synthesis have been elegantly summarized by Professor J.P. Flatt (1) from detailed studies of indirect calorimetry in mice. His calculations based on the stoichiometry of the ATP produced or hydrolyzed in the several biochemical pathways involved in substrate metabolism have highlighted the need to recognize different concepts of "efficiency" when applied to metabolic pathways. In this connection it is a continuing conundrum as to the metabolic correlates of the excess postexercise oxygen consumption (EPOC). Is the oxygen equal to or larger than the oxygen deficit? Clearly the answer depends on the type of exercise. If, as suggested by Professor Flatt, the cost of replacing one mole of ATP can vary between 20 and 22 kcal or some 20% more than the 18 kcal released for each mole of ATP turned over it would perhaps begin to explain the different total oxygen cost of intermittent compared with continuous exercise at the same average power output (2). Intermittent exercise would appear to have more relevance to the contribution of muscular activity to overall energy balance in every day life than the single exercise and recovery model usually studied.

Energy metabolism in human muscle during exercise has been mapped out over the course of the last 25 years largely as a result of the research of our Swedish colleagues using the needle biopsy technique. Professor Jan Henriksson presented a comprehensive account (3) of the studies in normal volunteers which showed the patterns of muscle fiber type recruitment in different forms of exercise. He showed the relevance of the metabolic characteristics of the constituent fiber types and the effects of physical training and of muscle wasting associated with severe calorie restriction. The question arises as to whether long term changes in nutritional status may be associated with changes in muscle fiber composition or indeed whether inherited or otherwise determined muscle fiber composition may predispose to the development of obesity (4). Here it must be emphasized that while alterations in the average energy economy of muscle in carrying out every day activities may vary with alteration of fiber type composition it is likely that such a change in efficiency is going to be quantitatively less important than the amount of activity performed.

Doctor Roger Harris reviewed the analytical methods and sampling errors in the determination of the metabolic contents in needle biopsy samples of human muscle (5). The same techniques have been applied to studying muscle metabolism during exercise in horses. He showed that there is a very slow rate of recovery of adenine nucleotides in horse muscle after very intense exercise. Low ATP content was observed in chronically ill human patients. The clinical conditions associated with impaired oxygen transport were found to give a raised lactate in addition to low contents for the high energy phosphates in muscle. This can be contrasted with chronic conditions such as rheumatoid arthritis which had a low ATP but no increase in lactate. A poor prognosis appears to be indicated when high energy phosphate depletion is associated with increased anaerobic glycolysis as evidenced by raised lactate in muscle. The depletion of adenine nucleotides follows hydrolysis of ATP to AMP with further degradation via inosine monophosphate (IMP) to hypoxanthine and eventually uric acid. Further research with intense exercise rather than with prolonged exercise (6) is obviously required to determine the importance of this pathway. This event also appears to underlie the slow metabolic recovery from intense exercise in the horse and the clinical conditions in man which have been found to be associated with low adenine nucleotide contents in muscle. It remains to be seen whether there is a nutritional explanation [as hypothesized by Jeejeebhoy's group (7)] which might signal an opportunity for a parenteral or enteral treatment of such low metabolic states.

The detailed biochemical changes associated with fatigue of human quadriceps muscle were described by Professor Eric Hultman (5). He and his colleague Professor Jonas Bergström in the early 1960s pioneered the use of the needle biopsy technique to study human muscle metabolism during exercise. It was my privilege and pleasure to work in their laboratory in Stockholm in 1970. In particular I worked with Eric Hultman and Roger Harris to study the biochemical changes associated with muscle fatigue under conditions of different muscle temperatures (8). Subsequently it was gratifying to see that Eric Hultman's group has adopted the techniques for electrically stimulating the quadriceps muscle developed by my group (9) as a means of analyzing muscle weakness and fatigue. Eric Hultman's studies showed conclusively that anaerobic glycolysis starts within the first few seconds of contraction. The activation of phosphorylase is seen to require AMP and an increased ionic calcium concentration. Ischemia alone at rest is a much weaker stimulant of glycolysis. The rate of ATP turnover was found to correlate very highly with the rate of anaerobic glycolysis.

Analytical techniques have been greatly improved so that not only can energy metabolites, glycogen, and lactate be measured on small (10–30 mg) needle biopsy samples of muscle but they can also be determined on ATPase-typed single fiber fragments weighing as little as 1 microgram. Modifications of technique have also allowed mitochondrial enzyme activity to be measured in needle biopsies. Former techniques for studying mitochondrial function required samples too large (grams) for the percutaneous biopsy approach.

Though invasive, these techniques have mapped out in much detail the biochemical pathways involved in exchanging energy during muscular activity and allowed physiological correlates to be made. The exciting noninvasive new technique of nuclear magnetic resonance has been used in the last ten years to study essentially the same metabolic changes in human muscle during muscular activity. A pioneer in the development of the biological applications of 31-phosphorus magnetic resonance spectroscopy (31P-MRS), Professor David Gadian presented a dramatic perspective of the rapidly growing fields of magnetic resonance spectroscopy of muscle and several other human tissues (10). While energy metabolism is conveniently followed by 31P-MRS. This is an insensitive method capable of resolving only relatively large tissue volumes compared with the orders of magnitude greater sensitivity of proton spectroscopy. The latter may have greater relevance to nutrition in view of the already well developed capability of measuring lipid and tissue water composition by chemical shift imaging and by spatially located spectroscopic imaging techniques. With suppression of the dominating spectral peaks of protons in water and protons in fat it is possible to measure spectral peaks for protons in lactate, n-acetyl-aspartate, creatine, choline, and other compounds. Clearly the techniques of imaging and spectroscopy are coming closer as powerful new methods are being developed to quantitate tissue composition. Other nuclei being studied are the naturally (1%) abundant carbon isotope (13C) though again the sensitivity is low but not so low that it has not proved possible to measure changes in liver glycogen (11) in man. While skeletal muscle has continued to be a source of much interest for spectroscopic studies, it is also perhaps more relevant to the wide nutritional interests that measurements can be made of proton density in water or lipid as well as in particular chemical compounds such as n-acetyl aspartate which is a relatively abundant constituent of the brain.

The metabolite measurements by either technique are not easily correlated with oxygen uptake by muscle. Energy exchanges are determined by observing the alterations in the local energy stores in muscle during short (seconds or minutes) periods of exercise with ischemia or longer periods of ischemia at rest. A recent experimental model allows power output by the human quadriceps muscle to be related closely to the exchanges of blood borne substrates and oxygen with local energy stores during exercise (12). The calculated stoichiometry is only valid in a closed system. This is obviously a very great limitation to the applicability of these methods to the longer term (hours, days, weeks) periods of importance in whole body energy balance in everyday life in which cellular energy balance is dominated by oxidative phosphorylation of blood borne substrates.

What has not been covered despite the title of this section referring to "Thermogenesis" are measurements of metabolic heat production in muscle. Important determinants of muscle heat are the flow of heat from arterial blood at "core" temperature to muscle, or reverse flow from metabolically heated muscle to the local venous circulation in relation to the flow of heat down the gradient to the ambient temperature. Metabolic heat production during maximum isometric contractions amounts to about 1 degree centigrade per minute (Fig. 1) which amounts to a maximum of heat production of about 50 W/kg wet muscle (13). The technique of myothermography of human muscle was developed largely by our research group during the 1970s. It was found to give results which agreed well with the enthalpy changes calculated from the changes in the muscle metabolites determined in needle biopsy samples in formal thermal balance studies when the quadriceps muscle contracted isometrically during ischemia (13). It was a promising and relatively atraumatic technique (little more troublesome for the subject, patient, or investigator than needle electrode electromyography) as an indicator of cellular metabolism in muscle (14,15). It is perhaps of interest that the heat rate correlates closely with the maximum relaxation rate from tetanic isometric contractions (16). It was superceded only because

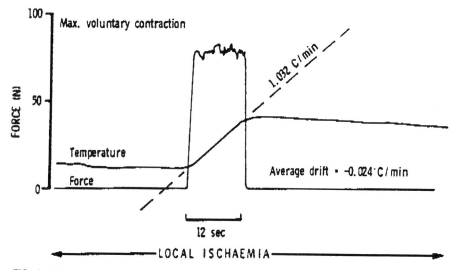

FIG. 1. Myothermogram recorded with a fine thermocouple needle, sensitive to 1/1000°C, inserted into the belly of the adductor pollicis muscle of a normal volunteer. Similar values for the maximum rate of temperature rise (dT/dt) are seen with tetanic stimulation of the muscle via its motor nerve.

of our very early interest (17) in the application of nuclear magnetic spectroscopy to the clinical study of muscle metabolism in human myopathy (18,19).

Agreement between the biopsy and magnetic resonance spectroscopic determinations may be found for the rate of recovery of phosphorylcreatine following exercise (20) and heat and maximum relaxation rates. It is a striking fact that when each has been reduced in the course of fatiguing exercise with ischemia none recover without restoration of the circulation (15,16,19,20). There is evidently no anaerobic recovery of metabolism or contractile function in human muscle despite remaining (anaerobic) energy stores (glycogen, phosphorylcreatine, and ATP). This is clearly a fruitful area for research of metabolic regulatory factors. For instance, it can be shown by 31P-MRS that the glycolysis initiated by ischemia is 200 times less than that accompanying a maximum voluntary contraction (21).

Determinations of phosphorylcreatine are found to be higher in MRS than in muscle biopsy studies, for reasons which are attributed to delays in obtaining the biopsy sample (18). A rigorous thermodynamic balance based on the stoichiometry of the biochemical reactions can only be done in a closed system (13). Such stoichiometry is more difficult if not impossible in the case of 31P-MRS because lactate, the end product of anaerobic glycolysis, is not directly measured as it is in the biopsy studies. Time resolution and volume localization are in conflict in MRS because 31P-MRS is intrinsically insensitive (10). These considerations also apply but in a different way to diseased tissue in which there is inhomogeneity of cellular or other structures causing dilution of signal intensity due to what are known as "partial volume effects" as exemplified in the difficulty in determining to what extent there may or may not be abnormalities of energy metabolism in muscles of patients with Duchenne's muscular dystrophy (22). While it may be tempting to make a direct comparison between needle biopsy and 31P-MRS determinations this has not been done and probably will not be attempted because of the statistical problems of representative sampling by needle biopsy (yielding samples of up to 300 mg) and of partial volume effects of the much larger MRS sensitive volumes (30–50 gm).

EFFECTS OF (WHOLE BODY) THERMOGENESIS ON MUSCLE

Muscle temperature, as determined directly by whole body thermogenesis or indirectly by concomitant circulatory readjustments, is a major determinant of the metabolic rate of muscle (8), and contractile function (14–16). The temperature coefficient for ATP production from glycolysis was about 3 (7) and for relaxation rate was 1.8 which closely correlated with heat rate (15,16).

Still dependent on, and influencing local temperature in muscle are the effects of thyroid hormones on thermogenesis and function in muscle. Relaxation rate and ATP turnover rate are well known to be raised in hyperthyroidism and reduced in hypothyroidism (23) with interesting consequences for fatigability in that hypothyroid muscle is less liable to fatigue due to greater efficiency of ATP utilization on holding a given force (14). While this is true for isometric contractions it seems that it may not be so for dynamic exercise in which no loss of work efficiency (defined as increment in oxygen intake $\times$ 100/increment in power output) is found in hyperthyroidism (24) though there was the expected increase in the resting oxygen intake.

Attempts to relate contractile function to metabolism of human muscle have shown significant changes in relaxation rate and fatigability in malnutrition (7,25) but these are small (26,27) and always subject to possible confusion due to alterations (including inhomogeneity) of muscle temperature secondary to disturbances in body fluid volumes or peripheral circulation.

EFFECTS OF MUSCLE ON WHOLE BODY THERMOGENESIS

We shall not dwell on the well known increase in whole body oxygen intake due to muscular exercise. It is important however to note that any alterations in muscle fiber composition in obesity (4) which might be interpreted as reducing the ATP turnover requirements of muscular activity are likely to play a small part in resting whole body thermogenesis (given the low-metabolic rate of resting muscle). Whether it may still be only a relatively small part of the activity-related thermogenesis compared to the variations in total activity (intensity or duration) between obese and normal weight persons remains to be seen.

Practical implications of reduced effects of muscle on whole body thermogenesis are readily seen in patients with Duchenne's muscular dystrophy in whom the average loss of muscle (estimated from 24 hour urinary excretion of creatinine and total body potassium determinations) is about 4% per year. This has allowed weight charts to be constructed (28) which are now in practical clinical use in muscle clinics in Britain and elsewhere to determine target weights given the gross changes in body composition as the disease progresses. The previous anxieties about accelerating muscle protein catabolism with restriction of energy intake seem to be unfounded if the findings in detailed metabolic balance studies (29) can be applied more generally. These studies showed continuing positive nitrogen balance in the presence of negative energy balance. Clearly there is in all patients with neuromuscular diseases the risk of a "vicious circle" of reduced activity—weight gain, further immobilization with loss of spontaneous associated movements, e.g., fidgeting, further weight gain with risk of embarrassing respiratory function (30).

REFERENCES

1. Flatt JP. Energy costs of ATP synthesis. In: Kinney JM, ed. *Energy metabolism: tissue determinants and cellular corollaries,* First Clintec International Horizons Conference. New York: Raven Press, 1992.
2. Edwards RHT, Ekelund LG, Harris CM, et al. Cardiorespiratory and metabolic costs of continuous and intermittent exercise in man. *J Physiol [Lond]* 1973;234:481–497.
3. Henriksson J. Energy metabolism in muscle: its possible role in the adaptation to the energy deficiency. In: Kinney JM, ed. *Energy metabolism: tissue determinants and cellular corollaries,* First Clintec International Horizons Conference. New York: Raven Press, 1992.

4. Wade AJ, Marbut MM, Round JM. Muscle fibre type and aetiology of obesity. *Lancet* 1990;1:805–808.
5. Harris CH, Hultman E. Muscle phosphagen status studied by needle biopsy. In: Kinney JM, ed. *Energy metabolism: tissue determinants and cellular corollaries*, First Clintec International Horizons Conference. New York: Raven Press, 1992.
6. Hellsten-Westing Y, Sollevi A, Sjodin B. Plasma accumulation of hypoxanthine, uric acid and creatine kinase following exhausting runs of differing durations in man. *Eur J Appl Physiology* 1991;62:380–384.
7. Pichard C, Jeejeebhoy KN. Muscle dysfunction in malnourished patients. *Q J Med* 1988;69:1021–1045.
8. Edwards RHT, Harris RC, Hultman E, Kaijser L, Koh D, Nordesjo LO. Effect of temperature on muscle energy metabolism and endurance during successive isometric contractions, sustained to fatigue of the quadriceps muscle in man *J Physiol [Lond]* 1972;335–352.
9. Edwards RHT, Young A, Hosking GP, Jones DA. Human skeletal muscle function: description of tests and normal values. *Clin Sci Mol Med* 1977;52:283–290.
10. Gadian DG. NMR and tissue metabolism. In: Kinney JM, ed. *Energy metabolism: tissue determinants and cellular corollaries*, First Clintec Horizons Conference. New York: Raven Press, 1992.
11. Shulman GI, Rothman DL, Jue T, Stein P, DeFronzo RA, Shulman RG. Quantitation of muscle glycogen synthesis in normal subjects and subjects with non–insulin-dependent diabetes by ^{13}C nuclear magnetic resonance spectroscopy. *N Engl J Med* 1990;322;223–228.
12. Bangsbo J, Gollnick PD, Graham TE, et al. Anaerobic energy production and O_2 deficit-debt relationship during exhaustive exercise in humans. *J Physiol [Lond]* 1990;422:539–559.
13. Edwards RHT, Hill DK, Jones DA. Heat production and chemical changes during isometric contractions of the human quadriceps muscle. *J Physiol [Lond]* 1975;251:303–315.
14. Edwards RHT, Wiles CM. Energy exchange in human skeletal muscle during isometric contraction. *Circ Res* 1981;48(suppl 1):11–17.
15. Wiles CM, Edwards RHT. The effect of temperature, ischaemia and contractile activity on the relaxation rate of human muscle. *Clin Physiol* 1982;2:485–491.
16. Wiles CM, Edwards RHT. Metabolic heat production in isometric ischaemic contractions of human adductor pollicis. *Clin Physiol* 1982;2:499–512.
17. Cresshull I, Dawson JM, Edwards RHT, et al. Human muscle analysed by ^{31}P nuclear magnetic resonance in intact subjects. *J Physiol [Lond]* 1981;317:18P.
18. Edwards RHT, Dawson MJ, Wilkie DR, Gordon RE. Clinical use of nuclear magnetic resonance in the investigation of myopathy. *Lancet* 1982;1:725–732.
19. Edwards RHT, Griffiths RD, Cady EB. Topical magnetic resonance for the study of muscle metabolism in human myopathy. *Clin Physiol* 1985;5:93–109.
20. Harris RC, Edwards RHT, Hultman RHT, Nordesjo EL-O, Nylind B, Sahlin K. The time course of phosphorylcreatine resynthesis during recovery of the quadriceps muscle in man. *Pflugers Arch* 1976;367:137–142.
21. Wilkie DR, Dawson MJ, Edwards RHT, Gordon RE, Shaw D. ^{31}P NMR studies of resting muscle in normal human subjects. In: Pollack GH, Sugi H, eds. *Contractile mechanisms in muscle*. New York: Plenum, 1984;333–347.
22. Griffiths RD, Cady EB, Edwards RHT, Wilkie RD. Muscle energy metabolism in Duchenne dystrophy studied by ^{31}P-NMR: controlled trials show no effect of allopurinol or ribose. *Muscle Nerve* 1985;8:760–767.
23. Wiles CM, Young A, Jones DA, Edwards RHT. Muscle relaxation rate, fibre-type composition and energy turnover in hyper- and hypo-thyroid patients. *Clin Sci* 1979;57:375–384.
24. Ben-Dov K, Sietsema E, Wasserman K. Uptake in hyperthyroidism during constant work rate and incremental exercise. *Eur Appl Physiol* 1991;62:261–267.
25. Lennmarken C, Sandstedt S, Schenck HV, Larssen J. The effect of starvation or skeletal muscle function in man. *Clin Nutr* 1986;5:99–103.
26. Newham DJ, Tomkins AM, Clark CG. Contractile properties of the adductor pollicis in obese patients in a hypo-caloric diet for two weeks. *Am J Clin Nutr* 1986;44:756–760.
27. Newham DJ, Harrison RA, Tomkins AM, Clark CG. The strength, contractile properties and radiological density of skeletal muscle before and 1 year after gastroplasty. *Clin Sci* 1988;74:79–83.
28. Griffiths RD, Edwards RHT. A new chart for weight control in Duchenne muscular dystrophy. *Arch Dis Child* 1988;63:1256–1258.
29. Edwards RHT, Round JM, Jackson MJ, Griffiths RD, Lilburn MF. Weight reduction in boys with muscular dystrophy. *Dev Med Child Neurol* 1984;26:384–390.
30. Edwards RHT. Management of muscular dystrophy in adults. *Br Med Bull* 1989;45:802–818.

Energy Metabolism: Tissue Determinants and Cellular Corollaries, edited by J. M. Kinney and H. N. Tucker. Raven Press, Ltd., New York © 1992.

Energetics and Cell Membranes

H. S. Park, J. M. Kelly, and L. P. Milligan

Department of Animal and Poultry Science, University of Guelph, Guelph, Ontario, N1G 2W1, Canada

THERMODYNAMICS

Living organisms can certainly be viewed as energy conversion systems (5). When energy derived from nutrients is transformed into a metabolically useful form, there is some loss as heat and entropy. As shown in Fig. 1, input energy is equal to the work achievement plus the energy dissipated as heat and entropy to the surroundings. The surrounding environment can receive energy from a biological system and vice versa, but the total amount of spatial energy, i.e., that of the system and surroundings, remains constant. Thus, the first law of thermodynamics defines that energy can neither be created or destroyed.

The above relationship may be expressed as $\Delta H = q - w$, where q is the heat absorbed into the system, and w is the work done by the system. ΔH is the change in enthalpy in the system with enthalpy being defined as the total energy content. It is the sum of the internal energy (E; chemical energy) and the product of its pressure (P) times its volume (V). In biological systems, however, pressure remains constant both within and out of the system, therefore

$$\Delta H = \Delta E + P\Delta V.$$

The second law of thermodynamics states that the amount of entropy (S) in a system and its surroundings always increases in a spontaneous reaction. Entropy is defined as isothermally unavailable energy divided by the absolute temperature (5). Living animals comprise nonequilibrium systems and spontaneous processes occur in the direction towards equilibrium by using free energy taken from its surroundings. Schrodinger (107) stated that "what an organism feeds upon is negative entropy." Organisms increase the entropy of their surroundings by discharging end products (increased entropy) of metabolism of nutrient molecules (low entropy) ingested. For a more detailed discussion, readers are referred to Morowitz (79) and Crabtree and Taylor (17).

411

Surroundings

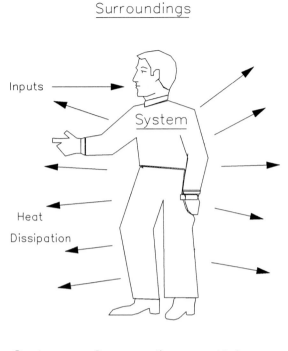

System + Surroundings = Universe

FIG. 1. Energy flow in the universe.

Application of Thermodynamic Laws to Metabolism

Numerous authors have calculated the energy requirement needed to transport a molecule across a membrane using one of two equations:

$$\Delta G = RT \ln(C_2/C_1) \qquad [1]$$

or

$$\Delta G = RT \ln(C_2/C_1) + ZF\Delta\psi \qquad [2]$$

for an ionized molecule, where ΔG is the Gibbs free energy change; R is gas constant; T is absolute temperature (°K); C_1 is concentration of substance on side 1, C_2 is concentration on side 2; Z is the valence of the ion, F is the Faraday constant, and $\Delta\psi$ is the potential difference across the membrane. However, the significance of ΔG is often misunderstood. ΔG is useful in predicting the directionality of a reaction. The use of ΔG as a quantitative or absolute measure is generally not practically possible. Additionally, ΔG has been used to calculate the efficiency of nutrient utilization. For instance, when we assume that one mole of glucose is completely combusted by oxygen in the reference state (760 torr, 298.15°K) according to the reaction:

$$C_6H_{12}O_6 + 6O_2 \longrightarrow 6CO_2 + 6H_2O + 2803.1 \text{ kJ}$$

ΔH in this exothermic reaction is -2803.1 kJ mol^{-1}. However, 36 or 38 ATP may be synthesized during direct oxidation of one mole of glucose within the cell. According to the first law of thermodynamics, the energy not conserved in the synthesis of ATP dissipates to the surrounding environment. There is frequent indication that ΔH for ATP hydrolysis is -21 kJ mol^{-1} (17). Thus, the standard efficiency of transformation is 27.0–28.5%. This calculation implies that only some 28% of the available energy during glucose oxidation is conserved in the synthesis of ATP. Using ΔG to calculate the energy transfer in metabolic reactions quantitatively is somewhat misleading because, unlike ΔH or ΔE, ΔG ($\Delta H - T\Delta S$) is not a conventional form of energy which obeys the first law of thermodynamics (83). Additionally, ΔS is affected by the substrate and product concentration therefore ΔG cannot be calculated without knowledge of these concentrations.

OXIDATIVE PHOSPHORYLATION

Any discussion of energetics and membranes in mammals must make early reference to the mechanism of energy conservation in oxidative phosphorylation (77). In summary, free energy release from the passage of a pair of electrons at a high energy level immediately after their removal from the carbon of energy substrate through the electron transfer system to a low energy level upon induction of O_2 to H_2O is utilized to form a proton (electrochemical) gradient across the inner mitochondrial membrane, with the intermembrane space being acidified. This gradient serves as a means of storage of potential energy. Subsequent passage of protons from the high concentration in the intermembrane space down their electrochemical gradient across the inner mitochondrial membrane provides free energy necessary to propel endergonic dehydration of ADP and inorganic phosphate catalyzed by F_1ATPase which yields ATP. Clearly then, the movement of ions (protons) across a biological membrane (the inner mitochondrial membrane) is at the very heart of aerobic energy transformation.

The system of oxidative phosphorylation has often been viewed as being of constant effectiveness with the entry level of electrons (NADH, FADH) determining formation of either three, or two, ATP per pair of electrons transferred to O_2. This would of course be a "currency" constancy rather than energetic constancy because the precise energy value of the ATP will depend upon the solute environment pertaining at the time of hydrolysis of its pyrophosphate bond (s). Constancy of effectiveness of oxidative phosphorylation has however been questioned. Pietrobon and colleagues (94,128) have argued that there is a variable effectiveness both of proton pumping by the electron transport chain and of utilization of the proton gradient in ATP formation. Brand (11) contends that the inner mitochondrial membrane is not impermeable to protons that have been pumped across and that protons do indeed leak down their concentration gradient yielding heat and entropy and not ATP synthesis. This leak was suggested to account for as much as 30% of the resting heat production of isolated rat hepatocytes and also a significant portion of that of whole organisms. In addition, Brand (11) concluded that proton leakage across the inner mitochondrial membrane varies with qualitative and quantitative changes in the membrane and is greater with higher proton motive force.

There can be no doubt that there is indeed heat and entropy production during mitochondrial proton pumping and use of the proton gradient. It is also presumptuous to expect that there is always a constancy of effectiveness of energy currency regeneration during oxidative phosphorylation. There must now be efforts to establish the possibility of in vivo variation in effectiveness of proton pumping and in leakage of protons across the inner mitochondrial membrane.

A dissipation of the mitochondrial proton gradient that is certainly conceptually related to proton leakage appears to take place in the mitochondria isolated from brown adipose tissue. These mitochondria contain a protein that is located in the inner mitochondrial membrane and is activated by fatty acids (60). It allows protons to move down their concentration gradient across the membrane without being coupled to ATP formation. This protein is closely related to the ATP/ADP and inorganic phosphate carriers. The result of uncoupled proton movement is, like leakage, simply production of heat and entropy from the oxidation of ingested substrates. This would appear to account for a significant portion of energy expenditure, particularly nonshivering heat production during cold stress and arousal from hibernation, in those small mammals that clearly have significant amounts of brown adipose tissue. It remains to be established that brown fat plays any significant role in energy metabolism in most active humans (44).

ENERGETICS IN CELLS

As briefly reviewed, life is a very highly organized thermodynamic energy conversion system into which energy must be constantly supplied. For example, the energy derived from ingested food is converted into various forms (chemical bonds, solute gradients, mechanical work) to support a favorable milieu to sustain life.

Milligan (74) noted that the direct pathways for incorporation of precursors into products do not differ between animals. Therefore, although it is possible that there could be differences in diversions from direct pathways, differences in efficiency of formation of products appear to depend largely upon the ancillary or supportive energy expenditures occurring at the time of the synthetic processes, which include ion transport and the turnover of cell constituents. In the ovine parotid gland, for example, the proportion of Na^+, K^+-ATPase-dependent to total energy expenditure in non-secretory state (in vitro) was significantly lower (40%) than that in active secretory state (66%, in vivo; (118)). In the following sections, energetic implications of transport of ions (one of the major energy consuming processes) and organic molecules (initial building blocks of synthesis or the release of end products of metabolism) across the biological membrane will be considered.

ION TRANSPORT

Movement of biomolecules and ions across biological membranes is a fundamental event in cellular metabolism and is very often precisely controlled by specific transport systems. In addition to supply of nutrients and excretion of wastes and toxic materials, ATPases involved in ion translocation are necessary for the regulation of cell volume and modulation of the cytosolic H^+ concentration and osmolarity within narrow limits to provide a favorable environment for enzymatic activities. For example, intracellular Na^+ is pumped against a concentration gradient across the plasma membrane by the conformational change of Na^+,K^+-ATPase caused by hydrolysis of ATP, whose energy is derived from glucose oxidation (Fig. 2).

Table 1 presents various types of ATPases found in nature. Pedersen and Carafoli (91) classified ATPases into three groups: P (those which form a covalent phosphorylated intermediate), V (those associated with membrane bound organelles other than the mitochondria and the endoplasmic or sarcoplasmic reticulums), and F (those of F_0F_1 type found in bacteria, chloroplasts, and mitochondria). Na^+,K^+-ATPase and Ca^{2+}-ATPase (both P-type ATPases) and Na^+,H^+-exchange will be reviewed in terms of their respective quantitative significance of ATP utilization in total cell energy use or qualitative importance of metabolic regulation.

Na^+,K^+-Transport

One of the predominant consumers of energy within the cell membrane is the enzyme Na^+,K^+-ATPase (EC 3.6.1.3). As a transporter of Na^+ and K^+, the major cations of extra- and intracellular fluids in animals, this enzyme aids in the maintenance of the electrochemical gradient across the plasma membrane (a low Na^+ and high K^+ intracellular concentration; 89,110). Milligan (74) considered this pro-

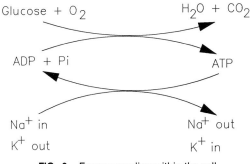

FIG. 2. Energy coupling within the cell.

TABLE 1. *ATPases found in different cell types and organelles*

ATPase	Source	Membrane	ATPase class
H^+	Yeast, Fungi	Plasma	P
H^+	Plants	Plasma	P
H^+	Animals	Plasma (bladder, tumor)	P
K^+	E. coli, S. faecalis	Inner	P
H^+/K^+	Animals	Plasma (intestine)	P
Na^+/K^+	Animals	Plasma	P
Ca^{2+}	Animals	Plasma	P
Ca^{2+}	Animals	Sarcoplasmic reticulum	P
Ca^{2+}	Animals	Lysosomes, Golgi	P
H^+	Yeast, Fungi	Vacuoles	V
H^+	Plants	Tonoplasts	V
H^+	Animals	Lysosomes	V
H^+	Animals	Endosomes	V
H^+	Animals	Secretory granules	V
H^+	Animals	Storage granules	V
H^+	Animals	Clathrin-coated vesicles	V
H^+	Most bacteria	Inner	F
H^+	Plants	Mitochondrial inner	F
H^+	Animals	Mitochondrial inner	F
H^+	Plants	Chloroplast thylakoid	F

From Pederson and Carafoli, ref. 91.

cess to account for a substantial portion of maintenance energy expenditures within the animal.

Function of Na^+,K^+-ATPase

At the cost of one high energy phosphate bond per turn of the cycle, this enzyme is responsible for the extrusion of 3 Na^+ from the cell while at the same time introducing 2 K^+ into the cell with both ions being transferred against their respective concentration gradients (6). ATP hydrolysis occurs via a sequence of intermediate steps following Na^+-dependent protein phosphorylation and K^+-dependent degradation of the phosphoenzyme (Fig. 3; 90).

Na^+,K^+-ATPase sustains ionic homeostasis within the cell, facilitates transmembrane uptake of solutes (47) such as amino acids or glucose via Na^+-symport systems and participates in cellular proliferation by functioning in provision of substrates for protein synthesis. Membrane potential is due to the intra- and extracellular ion concentration differences. Ion (Na^+,K^+) pumping enables maintenance of this differential; which is an absolute requirement for membrane signaling.

Determination of Na^+,K^+-ATPase

Efforts to quantify the existence and metabolic activity of Na^+,K^+-ATPase have, for the most part, relied on in vitro assessment of excised biopsies or cultured cells.

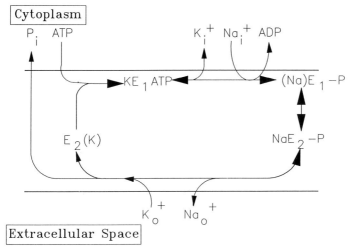

FIG. 3. Hydrolysis of ATP by Na$^+$,K$^+$-ATPase. From ref. 90.

Recently, Pedemonte and Kaplan (90) produced a thorough review of the approaches to arrive at structure/function correlates, but did not discuss the in vivo energetic significance of Na$^+$,K$^+$-ATPase. Generally, the existence of the enzyme has been quantitatively determined by the attachment of ^{3}H-ouabain via a timed incubation. For a thorough description of the methodology involved, the reader is referred to Hootman and Ernst (47).

Sodium-potassium pump activity has been assessed by measurement of ouabain-sensitive oxygen consumption (64); ouabain binding having an allosteric inhibiting effect on the Na$^+$,K$^+$-ATPase conformation (36). Other inhibitors have been used, such as vanadate and oligomycin, however the former is not specific to Na$^+$,K$^+$-ATPase and inhibits other ATPases, and the latter does not give complete inhibition only decreasing the rate of hydrolysis and transport (111). The metabolic costs of this enzyme's activity have been elicited in suspensions within a temperature-controlled chamber using a Clark-style, polarographic O$_2$ electrode (68–71,88). Cells, or biopsies, are incubated for a short time and after the determination of uninhibited O$_2$ consumption, a saturating concentration of ouabain is then added and immediately (5 min) the subsequent rate of decline in media O$_2$ content is indicative of other non Na$^+$,K$^+$-ATPase energy demands. By difference, then, the rate of O$_2$ use associated with Na$^+$,K$^+$-ATPase cycling can be determined.

Another useful tool in Na$^+$,K$^+$-pump activity determination involves the quantitative cellular uptake of [86]Ru (26,33). Ru is useful in that it is preferred over K$^+$ for the binding site on the Na$^+$,K$^+$-ATPase enzyme, and is not easily dislodged from the enzyme, making it a good indicator in the study of K$^+$ uptake (73). [86]Ru uptake is determined by means of an incubation of both uninhibited and ouabain-inhibited cells, with the difference being an indication of Na$^+$,K$^+$-ATPase activity. A potential liability of this method is that K^+ is not exclusively transported by Na^+,K^+-ATPase but may involve other routes (i.e., K^+,H^+-exchange).

Major Sites of Na$^+$,K$^+$-ATPase Activity

The contribution of Na^+,K^+-ATPase activity to whole tissue energy expenditures in various tissues was reviewed by Kelly and McBride (56) and Kelly et al. (57).

The major tissues accounting for whole body O_2 consumption are the skeletal muscle (largely because it is the largest tissue pool within the body; 96); liver (due to its myriad of functions including endocrine, detoxification, and regulatory processes and consequent high metabolic rate; 50,67), and the gastrointestinal tract (67). Na^+,K^+-ATPase action accounts for 9–45%, 16–51%, and 16.9–61.3% of the O_2 utilization of these organs under a variety of physiological and nutritional circumstances (67). Only one study has reported direct measurement of whole body contribution of Na^+,K^+-pump activity. Swaminathan et al. (120) intraperitoneally infused ouabain into guinea pigs and depressed whole-body O_2 used by 40%. This is higher than the value (18–23%) calculated in the model of sheep metabolism devised by Gill et al. (34). In a similar model, M. Summers, et al. (*unpublished data*) determined that 21–30% of O_2 use in the growing chicks fed diets of differing crude protein and sucrose content was due to Na^+,K^+-ATPase activity.

Endocrine Regulation of Na$^+$,K$^+$-ATPase

Endocrine regulation of cellular metabolism has dramatic effects on metabolic transductions within the cell. Insulin, thyroid hormones, and growth hormone alter O_2 consumption due to changed activity of the Na^+,K^+-pump, either by induction of Na^+,K^+-ATPase gene expression or post-translational alteration of existing pumps within the plasma membrane via receptor modification or secondary messengers (67,100).

In diabetic rats, the activity of Na^+,K^+-ATPase is decreased in skeletal muscles (59) and in the presence of elevated levels of glucose, neuroblastoma cells show a 25% decrease in transport activity of the Na^+,K^+-pump (127). It has been well established that insulin stimulates the Na^+,K^+-pump (129), however, it is not a direct effect and may be mediated through the actions of cyclic AMP (111). A potential mode of action of insulin includes the hyperpolarization of the cell membranes accompanied by stimulation of Na^+ efflux from the cell (129).

It appears that cells acquired from different species may also have differing sensitivities to the actions of insulin. For example, Early et al. (21,22,25) indicated that ruminant skeletal muscle is much less sensitive to insulin potentiation of Na^+,K^+-pump action than skeletal muscle acquired from nonruminants (78,129). This is important in that transport of nutrients such as amino acids and glucose may not be as affected in ruminants during periods of elevated plasma insulin concentrations.

Thyroid hormones have been implicated as major regulators of whole body heat production (53) partially through the control of Na^+,K^+-pump synthesis and activity in many different cell types including skeletal muscle cells and hepatocytes (52,55) and jejunal epithelial cells (63). Smith and Edelman (112) indicated that, in the adult rat, tissue Na,K^+-ATPase responses to T_3 in a variety of tissues (liver, kidney, jejunal epithelium, and skeletal muscle) were of similar magnitude to changes in QO_2. Gregg and Milligan (35) stated that hepatocyte O_2 consumption attributable to Na^+,K^+-pump action increased from 18% in thyroidectomized sheep in 24% in T_3-supplemented thyroidectomized sheep. Also, McBride and Early (65) found that ouabain-sensitive respiration accounted for 18.1% and 28.6% of in vitro O_2 consumption in skeletal muscle cells and hepatocytes from euthyroid sheep, however, corresponding values from hyperthyroid sheep were 26.5% and 35.7%, respectively, indicating substantial increases in the activity of Na^+,K^+-ATPase. There were also concomitant increases in the energy cost of protein synthesis (as measured by cycloheximide-inhibited respiration) in hepatocytes from the hyperthyroid sheep. Results from our laboratory have also shown that exposure to a cold environment, a condition associated with elevated thyroid status, is accompanied by an elevation in the energy expended in maintaining Na^+,K^+-pump activity (75). Differences among tissues exist, with the increases Na^+,K^+-ATPase activity paralleling those in skeletal muscle aerobic energy expenditure, while there was a disproportionate increase in this cost associated with the hepatocytes and gastrointestinal tissue (76).

Growth hormone, which in dairy cows elevates whole body heat production (124), has been investigated as an influence on ion transport in numerous tissues including skeletal muscle, liver, kidney, jejunum, and the brain (24,66). Skeletal muscle (external intercostal) is associated with no change in energetics in steers or dairy cows (probably due to the increased emphasis of nutrient partitioning to the mammary gland in dairy cows; 56). However hepatic tissue from steers treated with recombinantly derived growth hormone had a disproportionately greater amount of the increase in organ O_2 consumption associated with Na^+,K^+-ATPase activity (24). There was also an elevation in hepatic mass in the growth hormone treated steers (23) and, with the probable increase in the absolute numbers of Na^+,K^+-pumps, a greater proportion to increased maintenance energy costs.

Na^+,H^+-Exchange

The Na^+,H^+-antiport, which translocates Na^+ from the extracellular fluid to the cytosol at the same time exuding H^+ from the cytosol to the exterior with a stoichiometry of $1:1$ (38), exists in most cell membranes and plays a central role in regulating cell volume and intracellular pH (pH_i; 45). Sodium ions enter the cell down their electrochemical gradient established by Na^+,K^+-ATPase, perhaps causing a conformational change in the antiport, increasing its affinity for H^+. Grinstein et al. (37) demonstrated that the Na^+,H^+-antiport was activated when rat thymic lymphocytes were incubated in a hypertonic medium and also that the mode of activation of the antiport was similar to the response of phorbol esters [stimulators of protein kinase C (PKC)]. Those observations strongly suggested the relationship between PKC and the antiport; results which have been supported in many cell types. However, Chang and his colleagues reported the reverse effect of PKC on Na^+,H^+-antiport action in enterocytes isolated from mature chickens (15,82). Also Ahn et al. (1) observed that the activation of PKC caused a reduction of the antiport in the proximal colon of rabbits. Although the regulatory mechanism of the antiport is not yet fully understood, mitogens have stimulated the plasma Na^+,H^+-exchanger resulting in the influx of Na^+ and alkalinization of the cytosol (113). Stimulation of Swiss 3T3 cells with bombesin results in rapid elevation in Na^+,H^+-antiport and Na^+,K^+-ATPase activity and increased concentration of molecules related to signal transduction [diacylglycerol (DAG), Ca^{2+}, cAMP] with subsequent stimulation of DNA synthesis (102). Na^+ entry via the antiport could be a regulator of Na^+,K^+-ATPase activity, since Na^+ binding to this enzyme on the cytosolic side of the plasma membrane initiates its conformational change (90,121). In addition to the ability of the antiport in pHi regulation (122), the antiport is likely to be a key mediating factor in the rapid response to mitogenic stimulation. This could be due to altered Na^+ entry rates and pHi, which are possible cues of mRNA and protein synthesis (72). However, quantification of the energy costs supporting the Na^+,H^+-antiporter activity is difficult because of the questionable specificity of amiloride and its analogues in the inhibition of this process. Soltoff and Mandel (115) demonstrated that amiloride inhibited the ouabain-sensitive component of O_2 consumption in rabbit proximal tubules by about 50%, which is similar to what we have observed in various tissues (jejunoileum, kidney, liver, and skeletal muscle) from the young chick (H.S. Park et al., *unpublished observations*). Soltoff and Mandel (115) and Soltoff et al. (114) have concluded that amiloride not only inhibits the Na^+,H^+-antiport, but directly inhibits Na^+,K^+-ATPase. Therefore, inhibition of respiration by amiloride cannot be taken as a reliable measure of energetic costs resulting from operation of the Na^+,H^+-antiport.

Using $^{22}Na^+$ influx into intestinal epithelial cells, more than half of the total Na^+ entry occurred through the Na^+,H^+-antiporter (108) indicating that Na^+,H^+-dependent entry of Na^+ into the cell is probably a major component of the Na^+,K^+-ATPase-dependent energy expenditure. Even though quantification of Na^+,H^+-activity is not yet elucidated, the Na^+,H^+-antiporter could be a major candidate to explain unidentified Na^+,K^+-dependent QO_2 from tissues (gut and skeletal muscle) of the growing chick as modeled by Summers (117; Fig. 4).

Ca^{2+} Transport

Calcium ion transport partly occurs via an ATP-dependent process across the plasma, endoplasmic reticulum, and mitochondrial membranes against its electrochemical grádient. Calcium ion concentration in the cytosol is maintained by the sophisticated combination of active and passive transport systems. The role of Ca^{2+} in cell regulation is prominent, involving neuromuscular excitability, blood coagu-

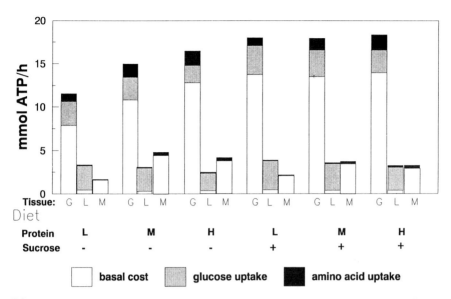

FIG. 4. Components of gut (G), liver (L) and muscle (M) Na,K transport-linked energy expenditures in chicks fed different levels of crude protein (CP: L, low; M, medium; H, high) and sucrose added (+) or not added (−) to the drinking water.

lation, secretion, and various enzyme reactions. Murphy et al. (81) demonstrated that changes in cytosolic Ca^{2+} have a profound effect on the rate of mitochondrial ATP production in hepatoma, as well as normal tissue, by measuring activation of the rate of ATP-generating respiration by mitochondria isolated from both cells in the presence of increasing cytosolic Ca^{2+}. Ca^{2+} did not appear to be significant in the control of rat thymocyte mitochondrial respiration (61). Further information on the role of Ca^{2+} in cellular regulation is available in recent reviews (14,93,104).

In normal eukaryotic cells, there may be at least seven Ca^{2+}-transporting systems; plasma membrane (Ca^{2+}-ATPase, Na^+/Ca^{2+} exchange, and Ca^{2+} channel), inner mitochondrial membrane (an electrophoretic uniporter and Na^+/Ca^{2+} exchanger) and endo(sarco)- plasmic reticulum (Ca^{2+}-ATPase and a Ca^{2+} channel) (13). The Ca^{2+}-ATPase system has a tenacious affinity for Ca^{2+} and consequently is mainly involved in the fine regulation of the ion. In the plasma membrane, Ca^{2+} is translocated from cytosol to extracellular fluid where the Ca^{2+} concentration is approximately 10,000 times greater than in the cytosol. In organelle membranes, the direction of the movement is from cytosol into the organelle lumen, where a high Ca^{2+} concentration is also maintained. Both of the above transport systems are mediated via ATP hydrolysis. In the plasma membrane, numerous studies suggested that Ca^{2+}-ATPase has two different ATP-binding sites—a high affinity binding site (K_m 1μM) and a low affinity binding site (K_m 0.1–0.3mM; 93).

Estimates for the stoichiometry of Ca^{2+} across various membranes exist in the literature. In reconstituted liposomal vesicles from human erythrocytes, a stoichi-

TABLE 2. Energy cost of Ca^{2+} transport

Tissue	Percentage of energy consumed	Reference
Rabbit reticulocytes	2.6	Siems et al. (130)
Skeletal muscle sarcoplasmic reticulum	7.0	Hasselbach and Oetliker (40)
Chick EDC muscle	13.0	Summers et al. (119)
Pancreatic islets	40.0	Owen et al. (131)
Ehrlich ascites cells	11.3	Muller et al. (80)
Hepatocytes	−1.8 to 2.9	Nobes et al. (87)

ometry between Ca^{2+} transported and ATP hydrolyzed approached 1 (85). However, across the sarcoplasmic reticulum membrane Kirtley et al. (58) indicated with certainty that hydrolysis of 1 mole ATP is required to pump two Ca^{2+}. For the plasma membrane, Garrahan and Rega (32) reported that several studies posted values ranging from 0.86 to 2.1 mol Ca^{2+} per ATP consumed but that these stoichiometrical estimates are as yet unconfirmed (32).

The magnitude of energy cost for supporting Ca^{2+}-ATPase has been questioned. To approach this problem, two techniques have been used; stoichiometric calculations and use of a specific inhibitor (Table 2). Hasselbach and Oetliker (40) calculated that 7% of the resting energy requirement in muscle supports Ca^{2+}-ATPase activity. Later, empirical measurements yielded slightly higher values supporting Ca^{2+} translocation by investigation O_2 consumption with or without ruthenium red or lanthanum, which both competitively block Ca^{2+}-ATPase-dependent Ca^{2+} translocation. Values of 11.3% in Ehrlich ascites tumor cells (80) and 13.0% in skeletal muscle (extensor digitorum communis) from week-old broiler chicks (119) have been reported. However, Nobes et al. (87) did not observe any La^+ inhibition of O_2 consumption for hepatocytes isolated from 24 hour fasted rats. Once these hepatocytes were supplemented with extra fatty acids (3 mM octanoate), the total respiration rate increased by 92% and La^+ inhibited 2.9% of O_2 consumption. Table 2 shows the energetic cost of Ca^{2+} cycling in several tissues. Although the extent of Ca^{2+}-dependent energy expenditure varies with tissue type, Summers et al. (119) speculated that the translocation of Ca^{2+} probably accounts for up to 10% of resting energy use by the whole body. Conversely, in the strenuously exercised muscle, O_2 consumption increased approximately 80 times over the corresponding resting muscle (83). This leads us to speculate that the associated energetic cost of Ca^{2+} translocation would also be enhanced and be a significant metabolic component of this increased O_2 consumption.

TRANSPORT OF ORGANIC COMPOUNDS

Amino Acids

Transport of macromolecules occurs by a number of specific, often energy requiring processes. Many specific amino acid transporters have been studied since the early 1960s and are largely classified into two groups (Na^+-dependent and -independent). In terms of cellular energetics, Na^+-dependent amino acid transport is significant because cotransport of amino acids entails movement of one Na^+ down its transmembrane concentration gradient; the gradient is actively regenerated by the action of Na^+,K^+-ATPase which catalyzes movement of three Na^+ for each ATP hydrolyzed.

Is the energy stored in the gradient of Na^+ electrochemical potential across the plasma membrane sufficient for amino acid transport? With cultured human fibroblasts, Dall'Asta et al. (18) provided a clear answer by showing the apparent efficiency of the energy transfer from the Na^+-electrochemical potential to the chemical gradient of 2-methylaminoisobutyric acid, a non-metabolizable amino acid analogue, is close to thermodynamic equilibrium, suggesting the electrochemical gradient of Na^+ is sufficient to energize intracellular amino acid accumulation. Further, Newsholme and Parry-Billings (84) calculated in muscle that the free energy change for the process of Na^+-dependent glutamine uptake by skeletal muscle was 12.3 kJ per mol glutamine (36.9 kJ per mol ATP) which may reflect, in another way, that the Na^+ electrochemical potential is the driving force to transport glutamine, assuming the free energy change of ATP hydrolysis is 52 kJ per mol.

Even though available information on the proportions of amino acids being transported into the cytosol via the Na^+-dependent systems is not available, the assumption of one ATP for transport of each amino acid, which is often adopted in the literature, may be an overestimate (76). From stoichiometric calculation, Waterlow and Millward (126) recently suggested that the total utilization of ATP for amino acid transport would be 10 mmol/kg/day (0.8 kJ/kg/day) by assuming the entry rate of amino acids is 30 mmol/kg/day in humans.

Recent work of Adeola et al. (2) led us to suspect that increased Na^+,K^+-ATPase may be closely related to increased Na^+-dependent amino acid transport by showing a linear relationship between Na^+,K^+-ATPase activity and protein synthesis in the muscle when pigs were offered different protein content diets. Similarly, Scandinavian researchers reported that higher Na^+,K^+-ATPase activity in the proximal tubules appeared in the high protein fed group suggesting increased Na^+ and amino acid symport (54). In tumor cells, however, increased energy consumption for protein synthesis in an amino acid fortified medium was not accompanied by increased energy consumption supporting the Na^+,K^+-pump, probably reflecting utilization of a greater proportion of Na^+-independent transport systems in this high extracellular amino acid environment (80).

Glucose

Glucose transport also occurs via cotransport of Na^+ in the brush border of gastrointestinal and proximal tubular epithelium. The free energy required for this process originates from the hydrolysis of ATP linked to Na^+,K^+-ATPase activity. Like the amino acid transporter, the proportion of glucose transport by the active mechanism may depend on the extracellular substrate concentration (48). From mathematical modeling, Summers (117) calculated the proportions of energy expenditure for amino acid and glucose transport linked to Na^+,K^+-ATPase energy cost in the growing chick (Fig. 4). As mentioned earlier, because the electrochemical potential established by Na^+,K^+-ATPase is the driving force of the transport of amino acids, glucose, and other ions, this work was aimed at segregating basal and transport-dependent energy costs across different tissues. Since the gastrointestinal tract absorbs amino acids and glucose, relatively high proportions of energy expenditure would be expected to be due to their respective transport. In skeletal muscle, although energy costs of amino acid transport and even Na^+,K^+-ATPase activity appear somewhat low, it must be noted that this is the single largest amino acid pool within the body accounting for a substantial ATP consuming process by amino acid uptake (56).

Transport Across Nuclear and Mitochondrial Membranes

Transport across the nuclear envelope, consisting of an inner and outer nuclear membrane, partially occurs by nucleoside triphosphate (NTP) consuming processes. After Agutter et al. (3) suggested that the nucleocytoplasmic transport of mRNA is an ATP-dependent process which is mediated by an NTPase on the nuclear envelope, the mode of mRNA transport has been intensively investigated. It has been suspected that the process may be one important step in gene expression in eukaryotic cells. Recently, Schroeder et al. (106) demonstrated that the efflux of two specific poly(A)-rich mRNAs (actin and β-tubulin) from isolated nuclei of mouse lymphoma cells is very much ATP-dependent. Further, their calculation for the activation energy of ATP-promoted efflux of poly(A)-rich RNA (51.5 kJ/mol) is quite close to the corresponding value for the activation energy of NTPase on the nuclear envelope (48.1 kJ/mol) strongly suggesting an involvement of NTPase in mediating nucleocytoplasmic mRNA efflux.

The ATP dependence of proteins transferred into the nucleus has recently been demonstrated with the following two step model; (i) binding to a receptor either on the nuclear envelope or in the cytoplasm and (ii) a following ATP-driven translocation through the nuclear pore (125). Garcia-Bustos et al. (31) showed direct evidence of ATP involvement for cytonuclear protein import using apyrase (which catalyzes the hydrolysis of ATP to AMP and two molecules of orthophosphate) or by substituting a nonhydrolyzable ATP analogue for ATP.

Most mitochondrial peptides are imported from the cytosol, requiring an electrochemical potential and the hydrolysis of NTP. Pfanner et al. (92) demonstrated that specific binding of the truncated precursor of the ADP/ATP carrier to the mitochondrial surface, and insertion into the outer membrane required NTPs but transport of the precursor from the outer membrane to the inner membrane required a membrane potential. Even though the translocation of RNA or protein into or across the membrane is biologically important, the energy consumed for this process would be minor in comparison to whole cellular expenses because only a small number of high energy phosphate bond equivalents are required for each macromolecule transported (119).

Protein

Synthesized protein in the cytosol destined for the cell surface, i.e., membrane bound or secretory proteins, is processed through the complex consecutive route; rough endoplasmic reticulum → Golgi apparatus → secretory vesicles → plasma membrane. A detailed discussion of this topic is clearly outside of the scope for this chapter. In summary though, secretory vesicles released from the Golgi apparatus attach to the cell surface, fuse with the cytoplasmic face of the plasma membrane, and expel macromolecules into the extracellular fluid by exocytosis. Exocytotic protein secretion can be divided into two classes: constitutive and regulated pathways (19). The former involves the export of newly synthesized proteins by a continuous flow of secretory vesicles without stimulation of secretagogues. The latter is described as exocytosis of secretory granules which is stimulated by the appropriate signal. Sanchez (103) indicated that the regulated pathway is ATP-dependent by demonstrating a reduction in secretion from human platelets due to agonists (DAG, phorbol-esters, and collagen) and ATP depletion. Upon repletion of ATP, the secretory activity was restored. The requirement for ATP for secretion has also been demonstrated by Holz et al. (46) using digitonin-permeabilized adrenal chromaffin cells. These authors showed that after a preincubation in a MgATP medium and subsequent membrane permeabilization, there are both MgATP-dependent, as well as MgATP-independent, secretory mechanisms. Although the extent of oxidative metabolism supporting exocytosis and secretion is still not available, Akkerman et al. (4) reported the rate of energy consumption for secretion in platelets. Unstimulated platelets utilized about 3.5 and 0.5 μmol ATP equivalents min^{-1} 10^{11} cells^{-1} at 37°C and 15°C, respectively. However, when the cells were incubated with thrombin, a secretagogue of platelets, 16 and 2 μmol ATP equivalents min^{-1} 10^{11} cells^{-1} at those temperatures were consumed indicating that the incremental ATP utilization is largely dependent upon secretion.

Receptor mediated endocytosis, an ATP-dependent process, usually occurs with the binding of ligands to their corresponding receptors on the plasma membrane. The accumulation of ligand-bound receptors at the clathrin-coated pit leads to the formation of coated vesicles and consequent budding off into the cytosol. In the cytosol, the ligand-bound receptors are either dissociated in sequential reactions with subsequent receptor recycling to the cell surface or subject to lysosomal degradation. Podbilewicz and Mellman (95) demonstrated that post-dissociation within the cytosol, the recycling of the receptor to the cell membrane requires ATP; ATP depletion resulted in the blockage of transferrin receptor transfer back to the basolateral membrane in MDCK cells.

Proton pumps appear to be very important in sustaining endocytosis and are responsible for maintaining a variety of intracellular acidic compartments. These include clathrin-coated vesicles, endosomes, lysosomes, Golgi-derived vesicles, and chromaffin granules (29). Acidification established by the proton pump (an ATP-dependent process) across the cell membrane plays a major role in the dissociation of the ligand-receptor complex, and the activation of proteases and solubilization of receptors and ligands within the lysosome. For a further discussion of the mechanisms and metabolic significance of receptor mediated endocytosis, the reader is referred to the recent review of Forgac (29).

Summers et al. (119) summarized the energy requiring steps in the receptor cycle: (i) cytoskeleton assembly and disassembly; (ii) H^+-ATPase activity; (iii) maintenance of cell surface and total cellular receptor activity; and (iv) protein phosphorylation. The proportional energetic costs of each step may vary with cell type.

Even though the amount of energy devoted to endo- or exocytosis and secretion remains to be answered, Summers et al. (119) speculated that it could be quantitatively significant because of the involvement of several energy-linked processes and very fast turnover time of plasma membrane.

TURNOVER OF PROTEIN AND PHOSPHOLIPIDS IN MEMBRANES

Protein

Membrane proteins (plasma, mitochondrial, and endoplasmic reticulum) continuously turnover somewhat in relation to their particular rates and functions as enzymes, channels, transporters, and receptors. Except for the nerve myelin, most membrane preparations contain more dry weight of protein than lipid (27). Mostly, the membrane of structures whose metabolic activity is high has a large protein content (for example, the sarcoplasmic reticulum and mitochondrial membranes). After Tweto and Doyle's (123) pioneering study investigating plasma membrane protein turnover in cultured hepatoma cells, investigators using either radioactive labeling or immunocytochemical labeling have observed that membrane proteins undergo degradation heterogeneously (39). Synthesized membrane protein at the ribosome is sorted via endoplasmic reticulum and Golgi apparatus processes and targeted to the membrane where the protein is inserted, possibly following the hydrophobicity of the signal segment. For instance, using the polarized epithelial cell line Caco-2, Le Bivic et al. (62) observed that the basolateral proteins were delivered directly and efficiently to the destined membrane (>97%), but the apical proteins reached the apical side by different routes with relatively low efficiency.

Unlike soluble proteins, membrane proteins are likely to be degraded by one or sometimes more than one system which Hare (39) described as: (i) lysosomal, (ii) cytosolic, (iii) extracellular, and (iv) mitochondrial proteinases. Generally, proteolysis of intracellular soluble proteins is mainly performed by two distinct processes: the ATP-dependent ubiquitin pathway and lysosomal proteolytic route (43). In the first system, the conjugation of ubiquitin, a 76-residue polypeptide, to the protein programmed for degradation requires ATP (28). As mentioned above, ATP is required to maintain an acid environment inside the lysosome for provision of a favorable milieu for proteinases.

Unfortunately, the quantitative importance of the turnover of membrane proteins to whole body energy is not yet clear nor is the regulation of the mechanism controls. Presumably, the process of membrane protein turnover could be substantively important energetically due to their relatively short half lives (39).

Phospholipids

Membrane structure has been described by the fluid mosaic model of Singer and Nicholson (109) where, within a bilayer of phospholipids, there are functional proteins which are capable of diffusing laterally (83). Phospholipids may also play a non-structural role in the regulation of protein turnover via Ca^{2+}/phospholipid-activated protein kinase C (116). The bilayer is subject to continual modification of structure and composition throughout the life of the membrane. Precursors for phospholipid bilayer synthesis can markedly affect membrane structure, potentially alter the energy required for synthesis, and modify the control function for both cellular and interorgan metabolism. For example, Clandinin et al. (16) showed that intake of diets of high versus low ratios of polyunsaturated to saturated lipid composition resulted in significant alteration in the fatty acid composition of plasma membranes from brain, liver, and intestinal mucosal tissues. Phospholipid turnover is characterized by rapid ATP-requiring synthesis and degradation (7). Phospholipid turnover has been considered important in accounting for erythrocytic O_2 consumption (97), but it appears to be a lesser component than protein turnover and ion transport in reticulocytes (130). Because of the rapid turnover rate of intestinal mucosa and liver (67), the energetic cost of phospholipid turnover in these tissues could be important. Summers et al. (119) also suggested that the recycling of lipid could be of quantitative significance within the hepatocyte, erythrocyte, and nervous tissue, but there are few studies examining its energy consuming metabolic significance.

THE ROLE OF THE PLASMA MEMBRANE IN CELLULAR ENERGETICS

Extracellular stimulation of the plasma membrane and subsequent effects on cellular metabolism have been the focus of considerable research during the past two decades. In this section, the mechanism of how cells transfer signals from the exterior to the cytosol and nucleus will be briefly discussed with insulin and catecholamine stimulation, which are probably the most important agonists in cellular energetics, used as examples.

On catecholamine binding to the adrenergic receptor on the plasma membrane, the α-subunit of GTP-binding protein (G protein) binds GTP possibly by conformationally changing the receptor. GTP bound G protein activates adenylate cyclase (a membrane bound protein and catalyst of cAMP biosynthesis) and then cAMP (the original second messenger) phosphorylated a wide range of enzymes to regulate metabolism. The most crucial step in this pathway is the amplification of the primary signals by G protein. Because the hydrolysis of GTP bound to the α-subunit by GTPase occurs relatively slowly (msec), G protein can still identify the original signal during this time (10). Although intracellular signaling via cAMP is a classic pathway, animal cells have several alternative second messengers (i.e., inositol triphosphate (IP$_3$) and Ca^{2+}). For example, when phospholipase C (PLC) activating factors (i.e., vasopressin, bombesin) bind their corresponding receptors on the plasma membrane, Gplc protein is primed and consequently PLC is activated (9). Phospholipase C hydrolyzes phosphatidylinositol 4,5-bisphosphate to IP$_3$ and 1,2-DAG. Diactylglycerol plays a role in activating PKC and IP$_3$ is capable of increasing cytosolic Ca^{2+} concentration by releasing intracellular Ca^{2+} stores (8). The roles of PKC and Ca^{2+} in cellular metabolism are referred to by Nishizuka (86) and Berridge (8), respectively.

Additionally, when some growth factors (epidermal growth factor and platelet-derived growth factor) and insulin bind the extracellular domain of their receptor on the plasma membrane, the cytosolic region undergoes autophosphorylation by tyrosine kinases at a tyrosine residue (99,105). Tyrosine kinase activity of skeletal muscle-derived insulin receptors was highly correlated with the serum insulin concentration and with in vivo glucose utilization rate (12). How then, does the insulin receptor remember and amplify the signals? Recently, Hayes et al. (41) tested a hypothesis to describe the amplification of the insulin-binding signal through the intermolecular phosphorylation of unoccupied receptors mediated by the ligand-bound receptors within the clustered cell-surface insulin receptors. Using insulin-occupied receptors isolated from rat livers as a source of activated kinase, they demonstrated that addition of activated receptors resulted in increased phosphorylation of the substrate receptors in the presence of a high concentration of non-phosphorylated human placenta insulin receptors (substrate receptors). This indicated the capability of the insulin receptor for intermolecular phosphorylation. However, there is little detailed information about the next step of signal transduction mediated by insulin (i.e., phosphorylation and dephosphorylation of regulatory enzymes). Dent et al. (20) discussed this matter by analogy with the mechanism for the stimulation of glycogen synthesis in mammalian skeletal muscle by insulin.

Furthermore, insulin activates PKC in various tissues (42,51). Using cultured fetal chick neurons, Heidenreich et al. (42) observed that insulin increased the activity of PKC in both cytosolic and membrane fractions and the mechanism of activation of PKC by insulin was not mediated by protein synthesis. Cycloheximide did not affect insulin-induced PKC activation. The activating mode of PKC was not accompanied by the translocation of the enzyme from the cytosol to the membrane. However, insulin induced the apparent translocation of PKC from the cytosol to the membrane in rat soleus muscles and adipocytes (51). Also Ishizuka et al. (51) found that insulin provoked rapid increases in DAG content and stimulated glucose transport in rat diaphragm and soleus muscle. After comparative studies with PKC activators (phorbol esters) and inhibitors (staurosporine and polymixin B), they suggested that the enhancement of glucose transport in the above tissues by insulin is partially mediated by PKC action.

Further, insulin is involved in the initiation of differentiation. Pulse dosing with insulin accelerates the differentiation of chick embryo myoblasts to myotubes and myofibers incubated in a serum-free medium (98). Those authors speculated that brief insulin contact with the component cells may trigger cells to memorize the information generated by insulin and mobilize signal transduction across the plasma membrane.

A number of peptides (i.e., growth factors and hormones) act as triggers to mitogenesis in quiescent cells by binding to their corresponding receptors on the plasma membrane and subsequently activate separate signal transduction pathways (101). As Bourne (10) stated, "no two cell types are stimulated by the same battery of mitogenic signals or show the same array of early responses," animal cells probably do have a certain capability to choose a particular signaling pathway in response to different mitogenic stimuli.

In consequence, the plasma membrane plays a pivotal role in the transmission of information generated by extracellular stimuli via various systems existing on/in the membrane and subsequently in the regulation of cellular metabolism (i.e., activation of triglyceride lipase by catecholamines). Although the energy expended on the actual phosphorylation and dephosphorylation of G proteins is quite small, there are certainly more far reaching effects on cellular metabolic regulation and consequently on cellular energetics.

CONCLUSIONS

In conclusion, reflection on the mechanism of oxidative phosphorylation serves to instantly underscore the principle of central involvement of ion movements across biological membranes in the energy transduction processes of mammals. Having done that, however, one rapidly encounters substantial issues of quantitative understanding. The very center-point of energy conservation, the quantitative linkage and constancy of this linkage between proton movement across the inner mitochondrial membrane and regeneration of the terminal pyrophosphate bond of ATP is not thoroughly understood in intact tissues of intact subjects. In mitochondria "slippage" in the effectiveness of proton pumping during electron transfer, leakage of protons down their electrochemical gradient after pumping and, in brown adipose tissue, direct facilitated and uncoupled passage of protons down the electrochemical gradient would contribute to heat and entropy yield from absorbed nutrients before metabolic regeneration of energy currency (ATP). Quite obviously, not all of these mechanisms are manifest in all tissues at all times. After phosphorylation of ATP, metabolic handling of ions, membrane events, and interactions of ions and membranes play a further and highly significant role in energy expenditure (Table 3). A considerable number of reports indicate that the energy cost of maintaining Na^+, K^+ distribution across cellular membranes in some species may be as great as that of protein turnover (56,57,119). However, there is certainly not unanimous agreement on a major energetic role for Na^+, K^+-transport (11). It is tempting to speculate that

TABLE 3. *Energy consuming processes within the cellular membrane*

Component		Percentage of total energy consumption	Reference
Ion transport			
Na$^+$,K$^+$-ATPase	Whole body	21–30%	Summers, France, Gill, and Milligan (*unpublished observations*)
Na$^+$,K$^+$-ATPase	Whole body	Up to 40%	Swaminathan et al. (120)
Na$^+$,K$^+$-ATPase	Whole body	18–23%	Gill et al. (34)
Ca^{2+}-ATPase	Whole body	Up to 10%	Summers et al. (119)
K$^+$-H$^+$-ATPase	Whole body	Negligible	
Na$^+$,H$^+$-antiport	Whole body	?	
H$^+$ leakage mitochondria	Hepatocyte	30%	Brand (11)
Organic compound transport			
Amino Acids	Whole body	Negligible (<1%)	Waterlow and Millward (126)
Glucose	Whole body	Substantial	Summers (117)
Nucleic Acids	Whole body	Negligible	Summers et al. (119)
Protein	Whole body	Negligible	Gill et al. (34)
Macromolecular turnover			
Membrane protein	Whole body	Substantial	
Phospholipids	Whole body	Substantial	

the energy expenditure via Na$^+$,K$^+$-transport that may occur in some species is not similarly expressed when other mechanisms (i.e., brown adipose tissue in smaller animals) are emphasized. However, the emphasis on and variation in Na$^+$,K$^+$-transport in gut tissue appears to play a role in nutritional energetics. Clearly the regulation of Ca^{2+} concentration by movement across membranes is essential to metabolic regulation of life and muscular contraction and is a meaningful (~10%) component of overall energy expenditure.

The manifold membrane processes including exo- and endocytosis, turnover and macromolecular transfer all entail energy costs which at best have only been tentatively estimated. The metabolic control system entailing inositol phospholipids in membranes and that involving G-protein also necessitate energy use, which, although totally essential in the regulatory process, are not expected to be numerically major components of whole-animal use.

Imaginative experimental approaches linked with effective integration of our understanding by means of modeling will take place. There is evidence in the literature of increasing emphasis upon approaches in metabolic studies that will yield greater quantitative understanding of in vivo energy metabolism (49,50). Non-destructive techniques such as in vivo nuclear magnetic resonance spectroscopy (30) for the study of metabolism are being employed to a greater extent in experimental biology.

We can look forward to the likelihood of imminent answers to many of the quantitative gaps that now exist in our knowledge of energy use in the whole organism. Presently, armed with the concept and belief that there are in fact metabolic mechanisms that accomplish excretion or dissipation of nutrient energy consumed in excess of standard requirements, one senses an underlying feeling that this could lead to more comfortable means of dealing with human obesity, and perhaps indulgence. The latter provides cause for anxiety. On the other hand, one can also look towards improved overall nutrient use resulting from greater knowledge of energy transformations in vivo.

REFERENCES

1. Ahn J, Change EB, Field M. Phorbol ester inhibition of Na-H exchange in rabbit proximal colon. *Am J Physiol* 1985;249:C527–C530.
2. Adeola O, Young LG, McBride BW, Ball RO. In vitro Na$^+$,K$^+$-ATPase dependent respiration and protein synthesis in skeletal muscle of pigs fed at three dietary protein levels. *Br J Nutr* 1989;61:453–465.
3. Agutter PS, McArdle HJ, McCaldin B. Evidence for involvement of nuclear envelope nucleoside triphosphatase in nucleocytoplasmic translocation of ribonucleoprotein. *Nature* 1976;263:165–167.
4. Akkerman JWN, Gorter G, Schrama L, Holmsen H. A novel technique for rapid determination of energy consumption in platelets. *Biochem J* 1983;210:145–155.
5. Atkinson DE. *Cellular energy metabolism and its regulation.* New York: Academic Press, 1977;239–263.
6. Balaban RS, Soltoff SP, Storey JM, Mandel L. Improved renal cortical tubule suspension: spectrophotometric study of O_2 delivery. *Am J Physiol* 1980;238:F50–F59.
7. Berridge MJ. Inositol triphosphate and as second messengers. *Biochem J* 1984;220:345–360.
8. Berridge MJ. Inositol lipids and intracellular communication. In: Fiskum G, ed. *Cell calcium metabolism* New York: Plenum, 1989;115–124.
9. Birnbaumer L, Abramowitz J, Brown AM. Receptor-effector coupling by G proteins. *Biochim Biophys Acta* 1990;1031:163–224.
10. Bourne HR. Summary: signals past, present, and future. *Cold Spring Harb Symp Quant Biol* 1988;8:1019–1031.
11. Brand MD. The contribution of the leak of protons across the mitochondrial inner membrane to standard metabolic rate. *J Theor Biol* 1990;145:267–286.
12. Bryer-Ash M. Rat insulin-receptor kinase activity correlates with in vivo insulin action. *Diabetes* 1988;38:108–116.
13. Carafoli E. Membrane transport of calcium: an overview. In: Fleischer S, Fleischer B, eds. *Methods in enzymology, vol. 157.* San Diego: Academic Press, 1988;3–11.
14. Carafoli E. Calcium pump of the plasma membrane. *Physiol Rev* 1991;71:129–153.
15. Chang EB, Drabik DL, Rao MC. Protein kinase C (PKC) inhibition of Na/H exchange in brush borders of small intestine. *Gastroenterology* 1987;92:A1341.
16. Clandinin MT, Foot M, Robson L. Plasma membrane: can its structure and function be modified by dietary fat? *Comp Biochem Physiol* 1983;76B:335–339.
17. Crabtree B, Taylor DJ. Thermodynamics and metabolism. In: Jones MN, ed. *Biochemical thermodynamics.* Amsterdam: Elsevier, 1979;333–378.
18. Dall'Asta V, Bussolati O, Guidotti GG, Gazzola GC. Energization of amino acid uptake by System A in cultured human fibroblasts. *J Biol Chem* 1991;266:1591–1596.
19. De Camilli P, Jahn R. Pathways to regulated exocytosis in neurons. *Annu Rev Physiol* 1990;52:625–645.
20. Dent P, Lavoinne A, Nakielny S, Caudwell FB, Watt P, Cohen P. The molecular mechanism by which insulin stimulates glycogen synthesis in mammalian skeletal muscle. *Nature* 1990;348:302–308.
21. Early RJ, McBride BW, Ball RO. Effects of plus insulin infusions on phenylalanine metabolism in

sheep. I. Effects on plasma concentration, entry rate and utilization by the hindlimb. *Can J Anim Sci* 1988;68:711–719.

22. Early RJ, McBride BW, Ball RO. Effects of plus insulin infusions on phenylalanine metabolism in sheep. II. Effects on *in vivo* and *in vitro* protein synthesis and related energy expenditures. *Can J Anim Sci* 1988;68:721–730.

23. Early RJ, McBride BW, Ball RO. Growth and metabolism in somatotropin-treated steers: II. Carcass and noncarcass tissue components and chemical composition. *J Anim Sci* 1990;68:4144–4152.

24. Early RJ, McBride BW, Ball RO. Growth and metabolism in somatotropin-treated steers: III. Protein synthesis and tissue energy expenditures. *J Anim Sci* 1990;68:4153–4166.

25. Early RJ, Thompson JR, Christopherson RJ. Net blood exchange of branched-chain amino and α-keto acids across the portal-drained viscera and hindlimb of cattle during infusions of leucine and insulin. *Can J Anim Sci* 1989;69:131–140.

26. Felber SM, Brand MD. Factors determining the plasma-membrane potential of lymphocytes. *Biochem J* 1982;204:577–585.

27. Finean JB, Coleman R, Michell RH. *Membranes and their cellular functions*. Oxford: Blackwell Scientific Publications, 1984.

28. Finley D, Varshavsky A. The ubiquitin system. Functions and mechanisms. *Trends Biochem Sci* 1985;10:343.

29. Forgac M. Structure and function of vacuolar class of ATP-driven proton pumps. *Physiol Rev* 1989;69:765–796.

30. Foster MA, Fowler PA. Non-invasive methods for assessment of body composition. *Proc Nutr Soc* 1988;47:375–385.

31. Garcia-Bustos JF, Wagner P, Hall MN. Yeast cell-free nuclear protein import requires ATP hydrolysis. *Exp Cell Res* 1991;192:213–219.

32. Garrahan PJ, Rega AF. Plasma membrane calcium pump. In: Bronner F, ed. *Intracellular calcium regulation*. New York: Alan R. Liss, 1990;271–303.

33. Gelehrter TD, Shreve PD, Dilworth VM. Insulin regulation of Na/K pump activity in rat hepatoma cells. *Diabetes* 1984;33:428–434.

34. Gill M, France JM, McBride BW, Milligan LP. Simulation of the energy costs associated with protein turnover and Na^+,K^+-transport in growing lambs. *J Nutr* 1989;119:1287–1299.

35. Gregg VA, Milligan LP. Thyroid induction of thermogenesis in cultured hepatocytes and sheep liver. In: Moe PW, Tyrrell HF, Reynolds PJ, eds. *Energy metabolism in farm animals*. Totowa, NJ: Rowman and Littlefield, European Association of Animal Products, publication no 32, 1987;10–13.

36. Grimaldi S, Pascale E, Pozzi D, D'Onofrio M, Giganti MG, Verna R. Effect of ouabain binding on the fluorescent properties of the Na^+/K^+-ATPase. *Biochim Biophys Acta* 1988;944:13–18.

37. Grinstein S, Cohen S, Goetz JD, Rothstein A. Osmotic and phorbol ester-induced activation of Na^+,H^+ exchange: possible role of protein phosphorylation in lymphocyte volume regulation. *J Cell Biol* 1985;101:269–276.

38. Grinstein S, Rotin D, Mason MJ. Na^+/H^+ exchange and growth factor-induced cytosolic pH changes. Role in cellular proliferation. *Biochim Biophys Acta* 1989;988:73–97.

39. Hare JF. Mechanisms of membrane protein turnover. *Biochim Biophys Acta* 1990;1031:71–90.

40. Hasselbach W, Oetliker H. Energetics and electrogenecity of the sarcoplasmic calcium pump. *Annu Rev Physiol* 1983;45:325–339.

41. Hayes GR, Lydon LD, Lockwood DH. Intermolecular phosphorylation of insulin receptor as possible mechanism for amplification of binding signal. *Diabetes* 1991;40:300–303.

42. Heidenreich KA, Toledo SP, Brunton LL, Watson MJ, Daniel-Issakani S, Strulovici B. Insulin stimulates the activity of a novel protein kinase C, PKC-ε, in cultured fetal chick neurons. *J Biol Chem* 1990;265:15076–15082.

43. Hershko A, Ciechanover A. Mechanisms of intracellular protein breakdown. *Annu Rev Biochem* 1982;51:335–364.

44. Himms-Hagen J. Brown adipose tissue thermogenesis: Interdisciplinary studies. *FASEB J* 1990;4:2890–2898.

45. Hoffmann EK, Simonsen LO. Membrane mechanisms in volume and pH regulation in vertebrate cells. *Physiol Rev* 1989;69:315–382.

46. Holz RW, Bittner MA, Peppers SC, Senter RA, Eberhand DA. MgATP-independent and MgATP-dependent exocytosis. *J Biol Chem* 1989;264:5412–5419.

47. Hootman SR, Ernst SA. Estimation of Na,K-pump numbers and turnover in intact cells with [^{3}H] ouabain. In: Fleischer S, Fleischer B, eds. *Methods of enzymology, vol. 156*. San Diego: Academic Press, 1988;213–228.

48. Hopfer U. Membrane transport mechanisms for hexoses and amino acids in the small intestine. In: Johnson LR, ed. *Physiology of the gastrointestinal tract.* New York: Raven Press, 1987;1499–1526.
49. Huntington GB. Energy metabolism in the digestive tract and liver of cattle: influence of physiological state and nutrition. *Reprod Nutr Dev* 1990;30:55–68.
50. Huntington GB, Eisemann JH. Regulation of nutrient supply by gut and liver tissues. *J Anim Sci* 1988;66(Suppl 3):35–48.
51. Ishizuka T, Cooper DR, Hernandez H, Buckley D, Standaert M, Farese RV. Effects of insulin on diacylglycerol-protein kinase C signalling in rat diaphragm and soleus muscles and relationship to glucose transport. *Diabetes* 1990;39:181–191.
52. Ismail-Beigi F, Bissell DM, Edelman IS. Thyroid thermogenesis in adult rat hepatocytes in primary monolayer culture: direct action of thyroid hormone in vitro. *J Gen Physiol* 1979;73:369–383.
53. Ismail-Beigi F, Edelman IS. Mechanisms of thyroid calorigenesis. Role of active sodium transport. *Proc Natl Acad Sci U.S.A.* 1970;67:1071–1078.
54. Jakobsson B, Larsson SH, Wieslanderm A, Aperia A. Amino acid stimulation of Na,K-ATPase activity in rat proximal tubule after high-protein diet. *Acta Physiol Scand* 1990;139:9–13.
55. Karin NJ, Cook JS. Regulation of Na$^+$,K$^+$-ATPase by its biosynthesis and turnover. *Curr Top Membr Trans* 1983;19:713.
56. Kelly JM, McBride BW. Symposium on Thermogenesis: mechanisms in large mammals. The sodium pump and other mechanisms of thermogenesis in selected tissues. *Proc Nutr Soc* 1990;49:185–202.
57. Kelly JM, Park HS, Milligan LP, McBride BW. Nonmammary metabolism in support of lactation and growth. Cellular energy metabolism and regulation. *J Dairy Sci* 1991;74:651–668.
58. Kirtley ME, Sumbilla C, Inesi G. Mechanisms of calcium uptake and release by sarcoplasmic reticulum. In: Bronner F, ed. *Intracellular calcium regulation* New York: Alan R. Liss, 1990;249–270.
59. Kjeldsen K, Braendgaard H, Sidenius P, Larsen JS, Norgaard A. Diabetes decreases Na$^+$-K$^+$ pump concentration in skeletal muscles, heart ventricular muscle, and peripheral nerves of rat. *Diabetes* 1987;36:842–848.
60. Klingenberg M. Mechanism and evolution of the uncoupling protein in brown adipose tissue. *Trends Biochem Sci* 1990;27:781–791.
61. Lakin-Thomas PL, Brand MD. Stimulation of respiration by mitogens in rat thymocytes is independent of mitochondrial calcium. *Biochem J* 1988;256:167–173.
62. Le Bivic A, Quaroni A, Nichols B, Rogriguez-Boulan E. Biogenetic pathways of plasma membrane proteins in Caco-2, a human intestinal epithelial cell line. *J Cell Biol* 1990;111:1351–1361.
63. Liberman UA, Asano Y, Lo CS, Edelman IS. Relationship between Na$^+$-dependent respiration and Na$^+$ + K$^+$ adenosine triphosphatase activity in the action of thyroid hormone on rat jejunal mucosa. *Biophys J* 1979;27:127–144.
64. Mandel LJ, Balaban RS. Stoichiometry and coupling of active transport to oxidative metabolism in epithelial tissues. *Am J Physiol* 1981;240:F357–F371.
65. McBride BW, Early RJ. Energy expenditure on sodium, potassium-transport and protein synthesis in skeletal muscle and isolated hepatocytes from hyperthyroid sheep. *Br J Nutr* 1989;62:673–682.
66. McBride BW, Burton JH, MacLeod GK. Skeletal muscle energy expenditures associated with Na$^+$,K$^+$-transport and protein synthesis in somatotropin-treated lactating cows. *J Dairy Sci* 1989;70(Suppl 1):175.
67. McBride BW, Kelly JM. Energy cost of absorption and metabolism in the ruminant gastrotestinal tract and liver: a review. *J Anim Sci* 1990;68:2997–3010.
68. McBride BW, Milligan LP. The effect of lactation on ouabain-sensitive respiration of the duodenal mucosa of cows. *Can J Anim Sci* 1984;64:817–824.
69. McBride BW, Milligan LP. Influence of feed intake and starvation on the magnitude of Na$^+$,K$^+$-ATPase (EC 3.6.1.3)-dependent respiration in duodenal mucosa of sheep. *Br. J Nutr* 1985;53:605–614.
70. McBride, Milligan LP. Magnitude of ouabain-sensitive respiration in the liver of growing, lactating and starved sheep. *Br J Nutr* 1985;54:293–303.
71. McBride BW, Milligan LP. Magnitude of ouabain-sensitive respiration of lamb hepatocytes (Ovis aries). *Int J Biochem* 1985;17:43–49.
72. Mehmet H, Moore JP, Sinnett-Smith JW, Evan GI, Rozengurt E. Dissociation of c-*fos* induction from protein kinase C-independent mitogenesis in Swiss 3T3 cells. *Oncogene Res* 1989;1:215–222.
73. Mendoza SA, Rozengurt E. Measurement of ion flux and concentration in fibroblastic cells. In: Fleischer S, Fleischer B, eds. *Methods in enzymology, vol. 146* New York: Academic Press, 1987;384–399.

74. Milligan LP. Energetic efficiency and metabolic transformations. *Fed Proc* 1971;30:1454–1458.
75. Milligan LP, McBride BW. Shifts in animal energy requirements across physiological and alimentational states: energy costs of ion pumping in animal tissues. *J Nutr* 1985;115:1374–1382.
76. Milligan LP, Summers M. The biological basis of maintenance and its relevance to assessing responses to nutrients. *Proc Nutr Soc* 1986;45:185–193.
77. Mitchell P. Keilin's respiratory chain concept and its chemiosmotic consequences. *Science* 1979;206:1148–1159.
78. Moore RD. Effects of insulin upon transport. *Biochim Biophys Acta* 1983;737:1–49.
79. Morowitz HJ. *Foundations of bioenergetics* New York: Academic Press, 1978.
80. Muller M, Siems W, Buttgereit F, Dumdey R, Rapoport SM. Quantification of ATP-producing and consuming processes of Ehrlich ascites tumour cells. *Eur J Biol Chem* 1986;161:701–705.
81. Murphy AN, Kelleher JK, Fiskum G. Submicromolar Ca^{2+} regulates phosphorylating respiration by normal rat liver and AS-30D hepatoma mitochondria by different mechanisms. *J Biol Chem* 1990;265:10527–10534.
82. Musch MW, Nahkla AF, Chang EB. Phorbol ester-stimulated secretion in chicken ileum: role of arachidonic acid metabolism. *Gastroenterology* 1990;99:393–400.
83. Newsholme EA, Leech AR. *Biochemistry for the medical sciences.* Chichester: John Wiley, 1983.
84. Newsholme EA, Parry-Billings M. Properties of glutamine release from muscle and its importance for the immune system. *J Parenter Enterol Nutr* 1990;14:63S–67S.
85. Niggli V, Adunyah ES, Penniston JT, Carafoli E. Purified $(Ca^{2+}-Mg^{2+})$-ATPase of the erythrocyte membrane. *J Biol Chem* 1981;256:395–401.
86. Nishizuka Y. Studies and perspectives of protein kinase C. *Science* 1986;233:305–312.
87. Nobes CD, Hay WW Jr, Brand MD. The mechanism of stimulation of respiration by fatty acids in isolated hepatocytes. *J Biol Chem* 1990;265:12910–12915.
88. Nobes CD, Lakin-Thomas PL, Brand MD. The contribution of ATP turnover by the Na^+/K^+-ATPase to the rate of respiration of hepatocytes. Effects of thyroid status and fatty acids. *Biochim Biophys Acta* 1989;976:241–245.
89. Norby JG, Jensen J. Determination of the ATP-binding capacity and the dissociation constant of the enzyme-ATP complex as a function of K^+ concentration *Biochim Biophys Acta* 1971;233:104–116.
90. Pedemonte CH, Kaplan JH. Chemical modification as an approach to elucidation of sodium pump structure-function relations. *Am J Physiol* 1990;258:C1–C23.
91. Pederson PL, Carafoli E. Ion motive ATPases. I. Ubiquity, properties, and significance to cell function. *Trends Biol Sci* 1987;12:146–150.
92. Pfanner N, Hoeben P, Tropschug M, Neupert W. The carboxyl-terminal two-thirds of the ADP/ATP carrier polypeptide contains sufficient information to direct translocation into mitochondria. *J Biol Chem* 1987;262:14851–14854.
93. Pietrobon D, Virgilio FD, Pozzan T. Structural and functional aspects of calcium homeostasis in eukaryotic cells. *Eur J Biochem* 1990;193:599–622.
94. Pietrobon D, Zoratti M, Azzone GF. Molecular slipping in redox and ATPase H^+ pumps. *Biochim Biophys Acta* 1983;723:317–321.
95. Podbilewicz B, Mellman I. ATP and cytosol requirements for transferrin recycling in intact and disrupted MDCK cells. *EMBO J* 1990;9:3477–3487.
96. Reeds PJ, Fuller MF, Nicholson BA. Metabolic basis of energy expenditure with particular reference to protein. In: Garrow JS, Halliday W, eds. *Substrate and energy metabolism in man.* London: CRC Press, 1985.
97. Reimann B, Klatt D, Tsamaloukas AG, Maretzki D. Membrane phosphorylation in intact human erythrocytes. *Acta Biol Med Germ* 1981;40:487–493.
98. Reiss K, Kajstura J, Korohoda W. The insulin signal initiating cellular differentiation is preserved by chick embryo myoblasts incubates at 2°C. *Eur J Cell Biol* 1990;53:42–47.
99. Rosen OM. Structure and function of insulin receptors. *Diabetes* 1989;38:1508–1511.
100. Rossier BC, Geering K, Kraehenbuhl JP. Regulation of the sodium pump: how and why? *Trends Biol Sci* 1987;12:483–487.
101. Rozengurt E. Signal transduction pathways in mitogenesis. *Br. Med Bull* 1989;45:515–528.
102. Rozengurt E, Fabregat I, Coffer A, Gil J, Sinnett-Smith J. Mitogenic signaling through the bombesin receptor: role of a guanine nucleotide regulatory protein. *J Cell Sci Suppl* 1990;13:43–56.
103. Sanchez A, Ca^{2+}-independent secretion is dependent on cytoplasmic ATP in human platelets. *FEBS Lett* 1985;191:283–286.

104. Schatzmann HJ. The calcium pump of the surface membrane and of the sarcoplasmic reticulum. *Annu Rev Physiol* 1989;51:473–485.
105. Schlessinger J, Ullrich A, Honegger AM, Moolenaar WH. Signal transduction by epidermal growth factor receptor. *Cold Spring Harb Symp Quant Biol* 1988;53:515–519.
106. Schroeder HC, Friese U, Bachmann M, Zaubitzer T, Muller WEG. Energy requirement and kinetics of transport of poly(A)-free histone mRNA compared to poly(A)-rich mRNA from isolated L-cell nuclei. *Eur J Biochem* 1989;181:149–158.
107. Schrodinger E. *What is life? The physical aspect of the living cell and mind and matter.* London: Cambridge University Press, 1967.
108. Semrad CE, Chang EB. Calcium-mediated cyclic AMP inhibition of Na-H exchange in small intestine. *Am J Physiol* 1987;252:C315–C322.
109. Singer SJ, Nicholson GL. The fluid mosaic model of the structure of cell membranes. *Science* 1972;175:720–731.
110. Skou JC. The ($Na^+ + K^+$) activated enzyme system and its relationship to transport of sodium and potassium. *Q Rev Biophys* 1975;7:401–434.
111. Skou JC. The energy coupled exchange of Na^+ for K^+ across the cell membrane. The Na^+,K^+-pump. *FEBS Lett* 1990:268:314–324.
112. Smith TJ, Edelman IS. The role of sodium transport in thyroid thermogenesis. *Fed Proc* 1979;38:2150–2153.
113. Soltoff SP, Cantley LC. Mitogens and ion fluxes. *Annu Rev Physiol* 1988;50:207–223.
114. Soltoff SP, Cragoe EJ Jr, Mandel JL. Amiloride analogues inhibit proximal tubule metabolism. *Am J Physiol* 1986;250:C744–C747.
115. Soltoff SP, Mandel LJ. Amiloride directly inhibits the Na,K-ATPase activity in rabbit kidney proximal tubules. *Science* 983;220:957–959.
116. Sugden PH, Fuller SJ. Regulation of protein turnover in skeletal and cardiac muscle. *Biochem J* 1991;273:21–37.
117. Summers M. *Energy metabolism in the broiler chick* [Thesis]. Guelph, Ontario, Canada: University of Guelph, 1991.
118. Summers M, Carter RR, Early RJ, Grovum WL, Milligan LP. The ovine parotid gland—a model to compare *in vitro* and *in vivo* energy expenditures on ion transport and protein synthesis. In: Van Der Honing Y, Close WH, eds. *Energy metabolism of farm animals* Wageningen, 1989;163–166.
119. Summers M, McBride BW, Milligan LP. Components of basal energy expenditure. In: Dobson A, Dobson M, eds. *Digestive physiology and metabolism in ruminants* (eds.) Ithaca, NY: Cornell University Press, 1988;257–285.
120. Swaminathan R, Chan ELP, Sin LY, Ng SKF, Chan AYS. The effect of ouabain on metabolic rate in guinea-pigs: estimation of energy cost of sodium pump activity. *Br J Nutr* 1989;61:467–473.
121. Sweadner KJ, Goldin SM. Active transport of sodium and potassium ions. *N Engl J Med* 1980;302:777–783.
122. Thomas RC. Cell growth factors. Bicarbonate and pHi response. *Nature* 1989;337:601.
123. Tweto J, Doyle D. Turnover of the plasma membrane proteins of hepatoma tissue culture cells. *J Biol Chem* 1976;251:872–882.
124. Tyrrell HF, Brown ACG, Reynolds PJ, et al. Effect of growth hormone on utilization of energy by lactating Holstein cows. In: Akern A, Sundstol F, eds. *Energy metabolism in farm animals*. Norway: The Agricultural University of Norway, 1982;46–49.
125. Wagner P, Kunz J, Koller A, Hall MN. Active transport of proteins into the nucleus. *FEBS Lett* 1990;275:1–5.
126. Waterlow JC, Millward, DJ. Energy cost of turnover of protein and other cellular constituents. In: Wieser W, Gnaiger E, eds. Stuttgart: Springer-Verlag, 1989;277–282.
127. Yorek MA, Dunlap JA, Ginsberg BH. Effect of increased levels on Na^+/K^+-pump activity in cultured neuroblastoma cells. *J Neurochem* 1988;51:605–610.
128. Zoratti M, Favaion M, Peitrobon D, Azzone GF. Intrinsic uncoupling of mitochondrial pumps. I. Non-ohmic conductance cannot account for the nonlinear dependence of static head respiration on H. *Biochem* 1986;25:760–767.
129. Muranaka Y. Relationship between ionic surroundings and insulin actions on glucose transport and Na,K-pump in muscles. *Comp Biochem Physiol* 1988;89A:103–112.
130. Siems W, Dubiel W, Dumdey R, Muller M, Rapoport SM. Accounting for the ATP-consuming processes in rabbit reticulocytes. *Eur J Biochem* 1984;134:101–107.
131. Owen A, Sener A, Malaisse WJ. Stimulus-secretion coupling of glucose-induced insulin release: LI divalent cations and ATPase activity in pancreatic islets. *Enzyme* 1983;29:2–14.

DISCUSSION

Dr. Hirsch: . . . timed to the total animal and energy metabolism. We have 10 minutes or perhaps even 15 for discussion of this. Dr. Newsholme is the official discussant. Eric, could we begin with your discussion and then open it up to everyone else.

Dr. Newsholme: I feel that you are considerably more courageous than I would be in trying to give numbers for energy expenditure of some of these processes. The second law of thermodynamics always puts my students off. I'm going to discuss the second law of thermodynamics, so back to Maxwell's demon. You remember, Maxwell posed the problem that if you have two cylinders of gas which are at equal temperature, the second law of thermodynamics effectively says that there will not be a spontaneous change in temperature. Suppose then that we put a little demon, Maxwell's demon, here with a little gating mechanism, a little trap door. And every time the demon sees a fast molecule coming this way, he opens the gate in that direction, and every time a slow molecule comes in this direction, he opens the trap door in the other direction. The result would be an increased temperature on one side and a decreased temperature on the other, disobeying the second law of thermodynamics. Now, the reason that can't happen is because somebody has to pay the demon. He's not going to stand there and do the trap door manipulation for nothing. And it depends, therefore, on how much you pay him as to how much it costs you or the animal to regulate. And I've been a little concerned that we do have to pay for the regulation that we see every time we measure a plasma glucose level after a carbohydrate meal. How much is it costing us, how much are we paying the demon, and of course it may well be that some societies are of the socialist trend and pay very little to the demon, and yet we may well have market force economies that pay the demon enormously and get very effective regulation. It may well be that this is part and parcel of the individual variation that we see. I have been trying to persuade some of my colleagues to take up that challenge, the sort of A.V. Hill challenge if you like. If you're paying the demon a lot so he's doing a very good job for you (this is the North American society)—he's doing a very good job for you in regulating the system, then the control of the blood glucose level, etc., etc., should be very efficient. Whereas if you have a rather poor socialist economy, then you pay the demon very little and you can see what happens in Eastern Europe, and the controls may then be out of line. So we wonder whether there is special importance to the second law of thermodynamics. Assume that we have a process in which our substrate is converted to an intermediate and then to a product Y, and those are what we call non-equilibrium processes. If you increase the activity of X to Y, it will not affect the overall flux of that system. All it will do is lower the concentration of X because it's the first step that limits the flux. Very straightforward, yet how many times do we read in the literature, as far as I can understand it, that we have a sodium leak mechanism, and this is an active process. It seems to me that the sodium leak process is the limiting process in all this, and the ATPase simply responds. So if you change the activity of the ATPase, you will not, if my assumptions are right, change the energetics of the system because the limiting process won't change. In a steady state, the rate of ATP hydrolysis will not change simply by activating the ATPase. You must of course also at the same time activate the leak. If you inhibit this process and stop the ATP utilization, then you can make assessments of what the capacity of the system is. But if you say, there is an increase of tenfold in activity when I measure it in my test tube; therefore, we have an increase of tenfold in the cycling rate, it may not be the case. It may be that what we're doing is to lower the sodium concentration and nothing else. Is this mechanism which we would like to call a translocation cycle, playing a role in regulating, the intracellular concentration of sodium ions? Think how difficult it would be to regulate the concentration of sodium ions if you only had the exit process, you only had the ATPase, if the concentration had to be 2.30 millimolar inside the cell, at 2.31 millimolar you would still have to have an E-flux. But at 2.30 the E-flux would have to stop, a total inhibition. And even though Eric Hultman this morning suggested that glycogenolysis was totally zero, I would like to argue, that may not be the case. I think it's enormously difficult if not impossible to inhibit one process totally. I believe the sodium leak mechanism allows you to have a system which in part will help to regulate the sodium concentration inside the cells, just as the idea of the leak mechanism for the protons in the electron transfer system would do exactly the same thing; that is, help to regulate the concentration, or help to regulate the capacity and the magnitude of the protonmotive force which must be important in terms of the function of that cell.

We wonder about the role of the intestine. I think in the rumen that there is this apparently large capacity for increasing energy utilization. We have noted that if we take the rat and we measure the capacity to use glucose by the absorptive cells of the small intestine, the capacity of the glycolytic pathway from glucose is perhaps greater than the amount of glucose that's normally taken into the body on the average diet of the rat. Presumably there has to be some inhibition of the glycolytic process. Glucose-6-phosphatase is allegedly present in the mucosal cells. Does this mean that there is a significant substrate cycle between glucose and glucose-6-phosphatase in those cells whose role is primarily to regulate the use of glucose by the intestinal cells? This may apply to some amino acids and to other agents, and may in part explain some of the reason for that rather high uptake of, and high stimulation of energy by that particular organ. I was also interested in the idea that we have the sodium proton exchange here and although it did not appear to be important energetically, it might be important in controlling the proton concentration within the cell. I've never actually seen that process given a capacity in terms of changing the proton concentration in the cell. If it's something that happens, it might change under different conditions while never being given a capacity. The capacity to generate protons by the process Eric Hultman was talking about, glucose to lactate, is enormous, as much perhaps as the type 2-B fibers that we heard about this morning. I would worry that if we place a lot of emphasis on that sodium proton transporter in terms of control of pH, we are ignoring a very basic metabolic process. It was music to my ears to hear Doctor Milligan emphasize the importance of attempting for nutritionists (and we call ourselves cellular nutritionists) to take on board the education of our colleagues in other disciplines in exactly this way.

ACKNOWLEDGMENT

The financial assistance of the Natural Sciences and Engineering Research Council of Canada for the preparation of this chapter is greatly appreciated.

TABLE 1. *Comparison of whole body protein synthesis rates with dietary protein allowances at different ages*[a]

Age group	Protein synthesis[b] (A)	Protein allowance[b] (B)	Ratio A/B
Infant (premature)	11.3, 14	~3	4.3
Newborn	6.7	1.85	3.6
Child (15 months)	6.3	1.3	4.8
Child (2–8 years)	3.9	1.1	3.5
Adolescent (~13 years)	~5	1.0	~5
Young adult (~20 years)	~4.0	~0.75	~5.3
Elderly (~70 years)	~3.5	0.75	4.7

[a] Extended slightly from Young et al., ref. 1, where original references are given. The protein synthesis rate for the newborn is based on Denne and Kalhan, ref. 2.
[b] g protein/kg^{-1}/day^{-1}

and that of Millward and his colleagues, may not, in the final analysis, be fundamentally different, we believe that a consideration of amino acid utilization and needs in relation to oxidative metabolism, serves a useful focus, for a number of reasons:

First, amino acid oxidation is accomplished easier than that of carbohydrate and fat, as emphasized by Krebs (5) a number of years ago. His studies provide us with an understanding of how fuels are selected in mammals. Briefly, he pointed out that, owing to the high K_m values of enzymes initiating the degradation of amino acids, a rise in their concentration automatically increases their rates of degradation. In support of this, our ^{13}C-tracer studies in young men receiving graded intakes of test amino acids including leucine and lysine, have shown that there is a highly significant correlation between their rates of amino acid oxidation and the plasma (and presumably tissue) concentration of the amino acid (5). Because tissue amino acid concentrations would change, or at least tend to rise, with ingestion of protein-containing meals, assuming an adequate supply of both energy and indispensable amino acids, it appears to us that a higher than minimal, or obligatory, oxidative loss of amino acids is an inevitable fate when consumed at adequate but not excessive levels. Parenthetically, the selection of and proportionate contribution made by the major respiratory fuels to energy flux and expenditure will depend on the diet and host nutritional and hormonal balance (6) but for the immediate argument we are just interested in the fate of amino acids in the healthy subject in relation to overall energy and nitrogen balance.

Second, the importance of amino acid oxidation has been discussed by us previously, with particular reference to the partitioning of the amino acid requirement into that immediately associated with new protein deposition and that related to oxidative catabolism. For example, we (1) estimated that only approximately 20%, or less, of the daily leucine and lysine requirement in the 6-month-old infant is deposited in new tissue protein. Hence, the major fraction of the requirement can be explained by a loss due to oxidative catabolism. Amino acid oxidation is of primary and overriding metabolic importance in setting the quantitative dietary need. This being true, then if amino acid oxidation were to be diminished, and with other metabolic processes remaining essentially the same, it would follow that the daily amino acid requirement would be lowered.

Evidence in strong support for the above view emerges from the recent amino acid kinetic studies by Thompson et al. (7,8) in patients with maple syrup urine disease (MSUD). These investigators showed that, despite significant elevations of plasma leucine in MSUD subjects, mean rates of whole body protein synthesis and catabolism were similar to control values as was also their growth rates. However, leucine oxidation rates in the MSUD subjects were about 5 to 10 times lower than the rates expected in healthy subjects who receive adequate, but not excessive, intakes of leucine (Table 2). This is a convincing demonstration that the status of oxidative catabolism is a primary determinant of the requirement value for the indispensable amino acid. In further support of this interpretation are the results of the growth studies of infants with inborn errors of amino acid metabolism. These individuals are not able to tolerate the intake amounts of specific amino acids that are usual for infants with a normal complement of enzymatic capacity to oxidize specific amino acids. Hence, dietary therapy is aimed at restricting intake of the specific amino acid so as to "normalize" the plasma concentration but without impairing growth and other functions. Thus, Ruch and Kerr (9) estimated that, for normal growth, the requirements for phenylalanine in patients with phenylketonuria (PKU) and for leucine in infants with MSUD were about 58% and 38%, respectively, of those in healthy infants. Similar findings were reported by Kindt and Halvorsen (10) for leucine, but not for phenylalanine, perhaps because in this latter case the PKU patient still might be able to achieve a significant conversion of phenylalanine to tyrosine, despite the very low, *in vitro*, activity level of hepatic phenylalanine hydroxylase (11). Nevertheless, these observations emphasize that if the oxidative capacity of body tissues and organs is reduced, at least for the case where it is due to defective gene expression, this leads to a lower rate of amino acid catabolism in relation to the rate of uptake into pathways leading to protein anabolism. We take

TABLE 2. *Significance of oxidative activity as determinant of requirement: studies in children with maple syrup urine disease (MSUD)*[a]

	MSUD	Control	Healthy adults[b]
Plasma Leucine (μmol/l^{-1})	351	91	~120
Leucine Oxidation (μmol/kg^{-1}/h^{-1})	1.1	10–20[c]	~12
Protein Turnover[d] (g/kg^{-1}/24h^{-1})			
Catabolism	4.1	4.1	~3.5
Synthesis	3.8	3.7	~3.3

[a] From Thompson et al., ref. 7.
[b] Approximate values at an adequate but not excessive leucine intake of 40 mg/kg^{-1}/day^{-1}. Based on MIT studies.
[c] Estimated, assuming a protein intake of ~1g/kg^{-1}/day^{-1}.
[d] For postabsorptive state in children.

these various findings with infants suffering from a limited capacity to oxidize specific, indispensable amino acids, to mean it is the catabolic side of amino acid metabolism that plays a major and primary role in establishing the quantitative value for the dietary requirement. Hence, it follows that factors capable of altering the activity of specific enzymes of cells and organs, with one of these being the energy status of the organism (12,13), will likely have a profound affect on amino acid utilization and, thus, the minimum dietary intakes needed to maintain a given protein nutritional status.

While we are concerned with the oxidative catabolism of amino acids, it might also be worth giving some initial mention to the formation and fate of urea, the major nitrogen end-product of amino acid metabolism. It is now evident that urea is not just a terminal metabolite of amino acid catabolism but it is also subject to regulation and to further metabolism, depending upon host nutritional conditions. Thus, in the context of nitrogen-energy interactions it is pertinent to ask "what regulates urea synthesis" and "how does energy intake or status influence urea formation and its fate?" Although, a detailed consideration of urea metabolism and its regulation goes beyond the scope of this presentation (see ref. 14 for a recent review), in brief, there are a number of recent stable-isotope tracer studies that are relevant to point out here. First, Jahoor and Wolfe (15) find that both the nitrogen supply (e.g., alanine, glutamine) and availability of energy substrate (e.g., glucose) affect urea production. They propose that an effect on the integrity of urea cycle enzyme activity might account for the influence of glucose *per se* in diminishing urea production.

Second, Jackson and colleagues (16) have made important contributions to our understanding of urea kinetics in relation to nutritional issues. They have shown, for example, that there is an effective salvaging of some urea-N via its metabolism within the bowel. According to these investigators (16) the dominant dietary factor that influences the hydrolysis of urea within the gastrointestinal tract and the subsequent recycling of urea-derived N, for purposes of N retention, is the supply of dietary protein and that the form of dietary energy seems to have little effect, except perhaps when protein intakes are low. Of importance here, however, is that a precise description of N-balance relationships between protein and energy intake is, or might be, complicated by the further metabolism of urea. There is considerable room for further studies of urea nitrogen kinetics, to gain a more complete understanding of the impact of energy intake and status on the metabolic flow of nitrogen and its eventual loss from the body.

NITROGEN AND ENERGY INTERACTIONS: RELEVANCE TO AMINO ACID REQUIREMENTS

The interactions between protein/amino acid and energy metabolism have a profound effect on estimations of nutrient requirements, especially because nitrogen balance is so sensitive to the level of energy intake and status of body energy metabolism.

TABLE 3. *1985 FAO/WHO/UNU (17) estimates of amino acid requirements at different ages (mg/kg per day)*

Amino acid	Infants (3–4 months)	Children (2 years)	School boys (10–12 years)	Adults
Histidine	28	?	?	8–12
Isoleucine	70	31	28	10
Leucine	161	73	44	14
Lysine	103	64	44	12
Methionine and cystine	58	27	22	13
Phenylalanine and tyrosine	125	69	22	14
Threonine	87	37	28	7
Tryptophan	17	12.5	3.3	3.5
Valine	93	38	25	10
Total	714	352	216	84
Total per g protein[a]	434	320	222	111

[a] Total mg per g crude protein. From Table 38 in ref. 17, and based on all amino acids minus histidine.

As summarized in Table 3, the most recent FAO/WHO/UNU (17) estimates of indispensable amino acid requirements at various stages of life in human subjects show that the needs decline, when expressed per unit body weight, and if expressed in reference to the dietary protein allowance, the fall is even more precipitous since the ratio of the total indispensable amino acid need to the protein allowance also declines. The latter value changes from about 43% of the total protein requirement being in the form of a balanced mixture of indispensable amino acids for infants to only about 11% in the adult (Table 3). While this decline, in the proportion of in-dispensable amino acids-to-total-nitrogen (IAA/TN ratio), could reflect a funda-mental, biologically significant change in amino acid metabolism during develop-ment, we believe this picture of change in the IAA/TN ratio is more likely the consequence of inadequate experimental design and inappropriate interpretation of previous N balance data. The earlier studies, especially those carried out four or five decades ago by Rose and collaborators (18), and whose investigations supply much of the basis for present, internationally accepted requirement values, were confounded by lack of sufficient attention to protein-energy interactions. For ex-ample, as summarized in Table 4 (19), based on body weight changes of his exper-imental subjects the level of energy supplied by the experimental diet in some, if not all, of Rose's studies (18) was clearly excessive. This would have had a major affect on N balance as indicated earlier and, in consequence, it would lead to an underestimate of dietary N or amino acid needs, when based on N balance criteria. We have considered this topic earlier (20) and there is little reason to repeat details. Perhaps, suffice it to say, for our present purpose, that we have carried out a series of studies, using stable isotope probes, to reassess the requirements for indispensable amino acids in adults given adequate but not excessive energy intakes (20). Fur-thermore, we have concluded that the requirement values we present in Table 5 are

TABLE 4. *Body weight change in two of Rose's experimental subjects: an illustration of the effects of an excess energy intake*

Period (days)	Subject RLW body wt (kg)	Period (days)	Subject GAP body wt (kg)
6	82.1	6	67.6
4	83.1	4	68.0
6	83.4	6	68.1
8	84.0	4	68.5
6	84.2	6	68.2
4	84.7	4	68.9
6	85.3	6	68.6
4	86.0	4	68.9
6	86.1	6	69.2
4	86.5	4	69.0
6	87.5	6	69.4

From Rose and Wixon, ref. 19.

a more appropriate approximation of actual physiological needs for this age group than those values (Table 3) that were accepted by the 1985 FAO/WHO/UNU (17) international expert group. When expressed per unit of protein need the amino acid requirements for the adult are similar to those for the young child (Tables 3 and 5). We should state, in the interests of a balanced review, that the adult requirement values shown in Table 5 have been criticized by some investigators and are not yet universally accepted (21–23). The fundamental point at issue, however, is that because inadequate consideration has been paid to the metabolic consequences of nitrogen (protein)-energy interactions in the past this may well have confused and

TABLE 5. *Tentative, amino acid requirement estimates for the adult and corresponding requirement pattern for the preschool child*

| Amino acid pattern[c] | Adult | | 1985 FAO/WHO preschool (mg/g protein) |
	Tentative requirement[a] (mg/kg/day)	Amino acid pattern[b] (mg/g protein)	
Isoleucine	23	35	28
Leucine	40	65	66
Lysine	30	50	58
Total SAA[d]	13	25	25
Total AAA[e]	39	65	63
Threonine	15	25	34
Tryptophan	6	10	11
Valine	20	35	35

[a] From Young et al., ref. 20.
[b] Values rounded to nearest 5.
[c] From FAO/WHO/UNU, ref. 17.
[d] Sulfur amino acids.
[e] Aromatic amino acids.

misdirected, an important component of the field of human protein and amino acid nutrition. Furthermore, this also means that the nutritional requirement data base from which to judge, and understand, the consequences of pathologic states on the protein (nitrogen, amino acid) and energy relations with which we are concerned here, is both limited and may very well be misleading.

PROTEIN TURNOVER IN DISEASE AND ENERGY/NITROGEN RELATIONSHIPS

As summarized by various investigators (24–27) many studies in animal and man have now been carried out to determine the responses of protein turnover in the whole body and specific organs to injury, sepsis, or other states including organ failure. The findings reported in the literature are diverse but major injury and sepsis appear to be characterized by increases in both whole body protein synthesis and breakdown, with the changes generally being greater with more severe stress (28–29), although perhaps not always (30).

We (31) and now many others (see ref. 32 for review) have used the measurement of urinary N^τ-methylhistidine (3-methylhistidine) to determine whether, and to what extent, the skeletal muscles contribute to the increased rate of whole body protein breakdown. It is apparent that there is a quantitatively important, enhanced rate of muscle protein breakdown and, frequently, there is a significant loss of nitrogen from muscles under these unfavorable conditions (27,33,34). The mechanism(s) responsible for the alteration in the turnover of muscle proteins remains a matter of speculation and an important problem to resolve because it has therapeutic value in relation to design of optimum nutritional and pharmacological strategies. For example, it is possible that both lysosomal (35,36) and nonlysosomal (37) processes are involved and that products of activated macrophages may serve as a signal. However, it is not yet clear how interleukin-1 (38) or tumor necrosis factor (TNF) (39,40) affect muscle protein synthesis and breakdown, whether directly or through intermediate processes (41). Nevertheless, when TNF is given intravenously to patients there is an increased rate of body protein turnover and increased efflux of amino acids from the forearm (42). Furthermore, these cytokines appear to be responsible, at least partially, for the alterations in energy metabolism that occur in injury and sepsis (43).

Of relevance to our focus on energy-nitrogen relations, concerns the possible reasons for the enhanced net rate of muscle protein degradation and whether nutritional therapy should simply be aimed at lowering the turnover rate. Some of the reasons for a higher turnover rate have been summarized by Newsholme et al. (44) and they include; (i) it supplies amino acids for protein synthesis required by the repair processes and by cells of the immune system; (ii) it provides amino acids for hepatic gluconeogenesis, in order to supply glucose as an obligatory energy substrate required for cells involved in repair and the immune system; (iii) it provides branched-chain amino acids that will be oxidized in muscle, to serve as an additional energy source for this tissue. Furthermore, it has been reported that under conditions of trauma, sepsis, and burns both the muscle and plasma concentrations of glutamine decrease (44–46) whereas the activity of muscle glutamine synthetase is elevated (47,48) and its net release is elevated (48). Hence, Newsholme et al. (44) have proposed that an increased net rate of protein degradation in muscle provides branched-chain amino acids which provide part of the nitrogen for the synthesis of glutamine in the muscle; this glutamine, after release by the muscle, will then be used to support function of immunocompetent cells and those involved in tissue repair.

In summary, it appears that the enhanced rate of body protein turnover, especially in skeletal muscle in trauma and disease states, confers on the organism a mechanism for survival, carrying a significant cost, due to high rates of amino acid oxidation, or losses, of indispensable amino acids.

ENERGY SOURCE AND THE NITROGEN ECONOMY

Glucose Versus Lipid in Healthy Subjects

The impact of changes in total energy intake on N balance was evaluated in the chapter by Young et al., *Whole Body Energy and Nitrogen (Protein) Relationships* and now it is of both metabolic and practical, nutritional interest to determine whether the different energy-yielding substrates exert similar or specific effects.

There is not an obligatory requirement for dietary carbohydrate, since for those tissues that normally show a preference for glucose as a major fuel (brain, erythrocytes, renal medulla) (49) it can be obtained via hepatic gluconeogenesis from amino acids and the glycerol derived from hydrolysis of triglycerides (50,51). It would be expected that under conditions of a very low or absent carbohydrate intake gluconeogenesis would be high and there would be decline in the efficiency of dietary N retention. Indeed, the studies conducted earlier in this century by Cathcart (52) revealed that a relatively small carbohydrate load (about 400 kcal/day) markedly reduced the loss of N in fasted subjects. However, he also observed that an isocaloric level of fat did not have this same sparing effect (Fig. 1), although we now appreciate that conservation of body protein and reduced N excretion during prolonged starvation depends upon the continued availability of lipid fuels (53–55). It may also be of interest to note, Cathcart's early findings have been enlarged through recent studies of leucine oxidation in obese volunteers, both before and after they consumed low energy diets, based on either carbohydrate or fat, or a combination of the two. Thus, Vasquez et al. (56) found that during caloric restriction dietary carbohydrate reduced the catabolism of leucine. Lipid, on the other hand, increased leucine oxidation. Assuming that leucine oxidation, in this case, mirrors overall amino acid or nitrogen catabolism then the findings of Cathcart (52) and of Vasquez et al. (56) are entirely consistent and suggest that we might usefully continue with some emphasis on N balance data, at least for the moment.

As stated by Munro (57) in 1964, carbohydrate has specific actions on protein

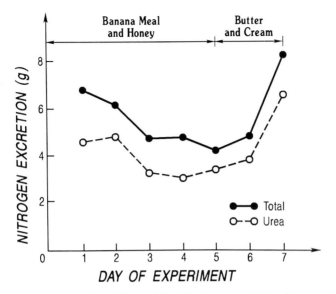

FIG. 1. Urinary nitrogen excretion while an adult subject consumed a low-nitrogen, carbohydrate diet (consisting of banana meal and honey) for 5 days followed by a fat diet (consisting of 65 g butter and 340 g 55% cream) for 2 days. Drawn from the data of Cathcart, ref. 52.

metabolism and N balance not equally shared with fat; administration of carbohydrate lowers body N output in the fasting subject, whereas fat does not (Fig. 1), as mentioned above, and isocaloric substitution of fat for carbohydrate results in a transient increased N output. Also, separation of meals containing dietary carbohydrate from those containing protein causes a transient rise in N output whereas this does not occur when fat is separated from protein intake. From these findings Munro (57) concluded that carbohydrate exerts a specific action on the utilization of amino acids during their absorption from protein-containing meals, in addition to an effect shared by fat and carbohydrate on the metabolism of amino acids during the postabsorptive period.

Because the practical, protein-nutritional significance of many of the earlier N balance studies was difficult to judge, especially for those carried out at supra-maintenance intakes of protein, we (58) also studied the quantitative effect, on protein utilization at barely adequate protein intakes, of an isoenergenetic exchange of dietary fat for carbohydrate in healthy young men. The results are depicted in Fig. 2, with the N-balance data obtained from 21-day dietary experimental periods involving one of two dietary ratios of carbohydrate to fat calories: for diet A (Fig. 2), the ratio was an equal proportion of energy from carbohydrate and from fat, and for diet B, the ratio was such that twice as much energy was from carbohydrate as from fat. This latter ratio was chosen in view of recommendations by various professional and authoritative groups (59) for the US population to reduce the total amount of fat in the diet. As shown in Fig. 2, nitrogen (N) balance and dietary protein utilization

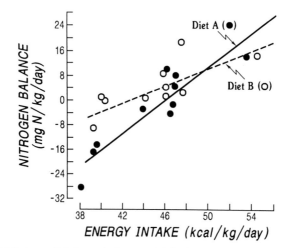

FIG. 2. Relation between N balance and energy intake in young men receiving a 0.6 g protein/kg/day diet for 21 days which supplied a carbohydrate:fat energy ratio of either 1:1 (diet A) or 2:1 (diet B). From Richardson et al., ref. 58.

were significantly better with the higher carbohydrate diet. Also of possible interest, the protein-sparing effect of the carbohydrate was greater in those subjects who were on marginal energy and protein intakes and who were losing weight.

Whether or not these "longer-term" effects of a change in dietary carbohydrate:fat ratio on N metabolism are mediated through the action of insulin, as Munro (57) postulated for acute experiments, remains to be determined. However, some observations would support the contention that the favorable effect of dietary carbohydrate on body N balance is mediated, in part by the effects of insulin. Thus, Fuller et al. (60) used a continuous infusion of physiological amounts of exogenous insulin together with glucose in well-nourished pigs. The glucose was infused with insulin at a rate sufficient to maintain plasma glucose concentrations within the normal physiological range, and to avoid the normal hypoglycemic and counter-regulatory response in body metabolism. The response to this treatment over a period of 3 to 7 days was a two- to seven-fold increase in plasma insulin, a 50% decrease in plasma glucose, a 40% decrease in plasma urea concentration, and a 30% fall in urinary excretion of urea N. After terminating the insulin infusion, plasma urea levels rapidly returned to those of the control period. These authors (60) concluded that a major component of the protein-sparing effect, achieved by a surfeit feeding of carbohydrate, is mediated by insulin. We will return to this later. So far, however, the data suggest to us that at high sub-maintenance or adequate energy intakes there is a small but greater sparing effect on overall N retention due to carbohydrate, compared with fat, when total N intakes are marginally adequate. However, at more generous N intakes and with initially adequate energy intakes, the protein-sparing effects of glucose and lipid would appear to be essentially comparable and of little or no significance, for protein nutrition, *per se*.

Glucose Versus Lipid in Disease States

The immediate foregoing discussion applies to the healthy subject and so it is important for us to survey the N-sparing effects of carbohydrate (glucose) and fat in hospitalized patients suffering from varying disease conditions. This is pertinent for us to examine because glucose turnover is increased and endogenous glucose production shows limited suppressibility in injury, sepsis, and other disease (61–64), and there is enhanced lipid oxidation (65) and altered ketone body metabolism (66,67), with some evidence indicating that there might be a resistance to the normal protein anabolic effect of insulin, but this needs further study (68). Finally, although it is unclear whether there may be a particular preference for glucose or lipid as a fuel under specific disease conditions (69), many of these observations suggest that the impact of glucose and fat on the nitrogen and energy economies of the host could differ according to the pathologic condition. For example, it is of possible interest that obese trauma patients show a greater mobilization of protein compared with non-obese multiple trauma patients (70).

The literature presents an array of findings and conclusions and so we find it difficult to construct a solid, quantitative picture concerning the comparative effects of glucose-derived versus lipid-derived calories on body nitrogen metabolism and the overall balance of body protein. Thus, some studies suggest that lipid-based parenteral systems are not as effective in promoting N balance and retention as those where glucose is a sole or major energy-yielding source (71). On the other hand, there are now a number of studies showing that these principal energy sources are equivalent, or of little nutritional or clinical difference, in their effects on N balance (e.g., 72–79), when total energy intakes are relatively adequate. Complicating the picture, however, is the condition of the patient and levels of energy intake used for comparative purposes. It appears (71) that when the daily level of glucose of intake exceeds about 2 g/kg or higher fat is used with the same efficacy as measured by N balance in the catabolic or depleted patient. Furthermore, since the level of nitrogen intake can influence both the protein and energy balance (80) this adds another level of difficulty in drawing comparisons between sources of energy on N utilization.

Some Possible Physiologic Mechanisms for N-Sparing and a Comparison of Carbohydrate Versus Fat

Even if it can be accepted that glucose and fat have an equivalent impact on whole body N retention when intakes of glucose are non-limiting (or above that necessary to suppress endogenous glucose production maximally), it remains desirable to learn how these energy sources bring about their N-sparing effects.

Although glucose and lipid might well be equally effective in promoting body nitrogen retention, the study by Shaw and Holdaway (74) illustrates that these exogenous fuel sources have different effects on metabolism. Using short-term tracer studies they showed that lipid did not affect glucose oxidation and production whereas glucose did. This might be a somewhat different situation to that for normal, healthy subjects (81). Furthermore, Baker et al. (72) found differences in blood plasma amino acid and hormonal profiles between lipid and glucose-based systems, despite equivalent effects on overall body N balance or, in the Shaw and Holdaway (74) case, on net protein catabolism as judged by the isotopically measured rate of urea production. Also, Ferranini et al. (82) found that lipid infusion, in healthy volunteers, had a hypoaminoacidemic effect of its own and distinct from that due to glucose. Again, this indicates differences between glucose and lipids in terms of their specific metabolic effects, despite a possible similar impact on total body N balance. The fate of amino acids and their detailed metabolic consequences in terms of providing energy in the form of lipid or carbohydrates can only be partly understood by observing changes, or differences, in plasma amino acid levels. Thus, we turn to some tracer studies of whole body and regional amino acid kinetics, to gain a better appreciation for the comparative metabolic effects of carbohydrate and lipid fuels on the nitrogen economy of the host. First, mainly using leucine kinetics, that we will assume to be a reasonable index of the dynamic status of whole body amino acid metabolism, it may be possible to construct a preliminary picture of the impact of insulin, carbohydrate, and fat on whole body and regional aspects of protein and amino acid metabolism, as presented in the following section.

Emphasis on Glucose, Insulin, and Other Hormones

Because changes in energy and nitrogen metabolism are undoubtedly dependent upon a complex of interrelated mechanisms involving, in part, the hormonal regulation of substrate mobilization, utilization, and interconversion, it is necessary to examine energy-nitrogen relations in reference to a number of key hormones. Among these, insulin is taken to be of superior importance.

In general, the net effects of insulin on whole body protein regulation appear to be a distinct decrease in proteolysis and a stimulation (perhaps small) of protein synthesis, although there have been differences, both qualitative and quantitative, in the reported findings.

Hence, in Table 6 we present a selected survey of the studies concerned with whole body amino acid (mainly leucine) kinetics in adults and the effects of insulin or glucose and/or amino acid administration, by vein. It is reasonable to conclude from the listing of results given in this table, that whole body leucine (and tyrosine) kinetics are sensitive to insulin and glucose administration and that insulin generally exerts an inhibitory effect on protein breakdown, often associated with a reduced rate of amino acid oxidation (89,90,94). This fall in whole body protein breakdown occurs in an insulin dose-dependent manner (84,86). Because skeletal muscle is a tissue that is sensitive to insulin action this reduction in whole body protein breakdown might be attributed, at least, to a decrease in the output of amino acids from the skeletal muscles.

TABLE 6. *A selected survey of effects of insulin, glucose, and amino acids on* in vivo *amino acid kinetic in human adults: whole body*

Authors	Tracer approach	Conditions	Outcome
Robert et al. (83)	Continuous ^{13}C-leu	Glucose alone; insulin; euglycemic	PS ↓; PB ↓; leu ox—
Fukagawa et al. (84)	Continuous ^{13}C-leu	Euglycemic insulin clamp	PS ↓; PB ↓; leu ox—
Wolfe et al. (85)	Continuous ^{13}C-ala and ^{15}N-urea	Glucose infusion with constant insulin and glucagon	Ala flux ↑; urea production ↓
Tessari et al. (86)	Continuous ^{3}H-leu; ^{14}C-kic	Postabsorptive: variable insulin with euglycemia	PS ↓; PB ↓; leu ox ↓
Fukagawa et al. (87)	Continuous ^{13}C-leu and ^{15}N-ala	Postabsorptive; euglycemic insulin clamp	PB ↓, leu ox—
Tessari et al. (88)	Continuous ^{3}H-leu; ^{14}C-kic	Type 1 diabetics; insulin without glucose	↓ PB
Shangraw et al. (89)	Continuous ^{13}C-leu	Postabsorptive; euglycemic insulin clamp	↓ PB; leu ox ↓
Castellino et al. (90)	Continuous ^{14}C-leu	Insulin with low, basal and elevated plasma amino acids	↓ PB; ↓ leu ox
Arfvidsson et al. (91)	Continuous U-^{14}C-tyr	Postabsorptive: insulin with euglycemic	Tyr flux ↓
Tessari et al. (92)	Continuous ^{3}H-leu; ^{14}C-kic	1. Hyperinsulinemia with euglycemia	↓ PB
		2. Hyperaminoacidemia	↑ PS
		3. Hyperaminoacidemia with euglycemic hyperinsulinemia	↑ PS; ↓ PB
Fukagawa et al. (93)	Continuous ^{13}C-leu	Amino acids alone	↑ PS
		AA with euglycemic hyperinsulinemia	↑ PS; ↓ PB
Flakoll et al. (94)	Continuous ^{14}C-leu	Insulin with hypoaminoacidemia ⎫⎬⎭	↓ PS; ↓ PB ↓ leu ox
		Amino acids plus insulin with euglycemia and euaminoacidemia ⎫⎬⎭	↓ PB; PS—
Frexes-Steed et al. (95)	Continuous ^{14}C-leu	Postabsorptive and 4-day fast. Variable leucine with euglycemia and euleucinemia	↓ PB

PS, protein synthesis; PB, protein breakdown; Leu ox, leucine oxidation; ↓, decrease; ↑, increase; —, no change.

A summary of findings from a number of investigations concerned with the effects of insulin on *in vivo* aspects of protein and amino acid metabolism in the skeletal musculature of adult humans is presented in Table 7. It is evident that the consistency of the observations regarding insulin's suppression of whole body proteolysis (Table 6) do not carry over to the *in vivo* studies on skeletal muscle (Table 7); some have found a decrease in muscle protein breakdown whereas others have not, despite an improved overall amino nitrogen balance across the organ when insulin and glucose are given (96,97). Whether these variable findings are due to the fact that different tracer models have been used, whether the insulin is given locally or systemically, or whether the forearm responds differently to the hind-limb, for example, is not at

TABLE 7. *A selected survey of effects of insulin, glucose, and amino acids on* in vivo *amino acid kinetics in humans: muscle*

Authors	Model	Conditions	Outcome
Pozefsky et al. (96)	Foream: A-V balance	Local hyperinsulinemia	↑ AAN balance
Elia et al. (97)	Foream: A-V balance	Glucose infusion	↓ Ala output; ↑ AAN balance
Gelfand and Barrett (98)	Forearm: ^{3}H-phe; 1-^{14}C-leu exchange	Local hyperinsulinemia	↓ MPB
Bennet et al. (99)	Anterior tibialis; ^{13}C-leu; biopsy	Fasting and amino acids	↑ MPS with amino acids
Bennet et al. (100)	Leg: A-V difference ^{15}N-Phe; 1-^{13}C-leu	AA alone AA + insulin with euglycemia	Insulin augmented leu uptake; MPB?
Fryburg et al. (101)	Forearm: ^{3}H-phe; ^{14}C-leu	12 + 60h fast + local insulin	Insulin ↓ MPB
Tessari et al. (88)	Forearm: ^{3}H-leu; ^{14}C-kic	Type 1 diabetic; peripheral insulin and amino acids	No effect on muscle
Arfvidsson et al. (91)	^{14}C-tyr: leg exchange	Physiologic hyperinsulinemia	MPS— MPB—

AAN, amino acid nitrogen; MPB, muscle protein breakdown; MPS, muscle protein synthesis; —, no change.

all clear. Also, there is still little *in vivo* evidence that insulin stimulates muscle protein synthesis, the recent study by Bennet et al. (100) indicates that insulin promotes synthesis when the availability of amino acids is not limiting. Additionally, a muscle-related decrease in whole body protein breakdown may not apply to the insulin-deficient, type 1 diabetic patient, since Tessari et al. (88) propose that, in this condition, skeletal muscle is not a major site of an insulin-induced acute suppression of proteolysis.

Thus, these various investigations provide an incomplete and uncertain picture; it should be recognized also that the effect of insulin on the overall body protein economy depends upon whether an exogenous amino acid supply accompanies insulin administration. When amino acids are supplied, whole body (92,93) and muscle protein (100) (see Table 6) synthesis, which require available amino acids, may be stimulated. Nevertheless, the effect of insulin in stimulating synthesis appears to be small. Also, insulin's suppression of proteolysis appears to be augmented by amino acids (94).

In general, although somewhat tentative in terms of specific mechanisms, the various actions of insulin and glucose on leucine (amino acid, protein) kinetics are consistent with the fact that maximum nitrogen retention is achieved when both protein and carbohydrate intakes are consumed together at generous intakes. We appreciate, however, that the relations between insulin, carbohydrate, and amino acids are probably more complex than our discussion implies; for example, insulin-induced hypoglycemia can result in an *increased* whole body leucine flux, perhaps due to increased protein breakdown in the intestinal tissues (102). Additionally, the level of plasma amino acids can affect glucose uptake by human forearm tissue (103). In consequence, amino acids might potentially compete with glucose as a fuel, depending in this case on plasma concentrations. Indeed, this complexity in the interrelations between insulin, glucose, amino acids, and amino acid kinetics, depending upon their concentrations in body fluids and their availability to sustain an anabolic response, is reminiscent of the relationships between energy intake and nitrogen balance. As reviewed in the chapter by Young et al., *Whole Body Energy and Nitrogen (Protein) Relationships*, the N balance data can be schematically depicted in relatively simple form (Fig. 3) but this undoubtedly camouflages, as the foregoing suggests, the more complex set of metabolic processes that operate to achieve a given N balance within the intake ranges of energy and nitrogen considered. Basically, the quantitative, and even qualitative, role played by insulin in relation to the underlying components of the N balance responses discussed above cannot yet be stated with any degree of confidence. Much further *in vivo* study remains to be undertaken on this aspect of the regulation of body protein and amino acid metabolism.

In relation to the overall anabolic action of insulin on body protein balance it is also pertinent to question the possible involvement of the counter regulatory ("anti-insulin") hormones, glucagon, catecholamines, and the glucocorticoids, in energy-

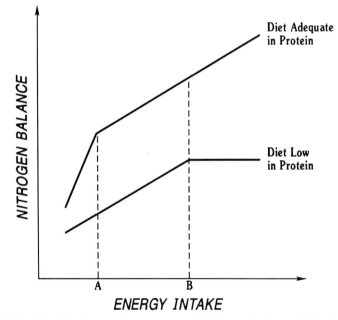

FIG. 3. Relationship of N balance and energy intake with diets of differing protein levels. Between energy intake A (low) and B (higher) the two lines are parallel. From Munro, ref. 57, with permission.

TABLE 8. *Effects of various hormones on* in vivo *amino acid kinetics in adult humans*

Authors	Model and approach	Outcome
Glucagon		
Nair et al. (106)	^{13}C-leu infusion: glucagon with insulin deficiency	↑ PB; ↑ leu ox
Couet et al. (107)	^{13}C-leu infusion: glucagon excess with maintenance of insulin	PB—
Epinephrine		
Miles et al. (120)	^{15}N-leu; ^{2}H-ala; ^{2}H-leu and epinephrine infusion	↓ leu ox; ↓ PAA
Lamont et al. (121)	β-adrenergic blockade (propanolol 80 mg b.i.d.) 1-^{13}C-leu infusion	↑ leu ox; PB— urea N/ creatinine ↑
Kraenzlin et al. (122)	^{13}C-leu infusion epinephrine infusion with constant insulin and glucagon	↓ PB; ↓ leu ox; *But* net forearm leu release ↑
Matthews et al. (123)	Infusions of ^{13}C-leu; ^{2}H$_5$-phe; ^{15}N-glu(NH$_2$); epinephrine infusion for 8.5 h	PB—; little change in ↑ glu(NH$_2$) flux; leu ox—; ↓ PAA
Glucocorticoids		
Gelfand et al. (133)	^{13}C-leu; 72 h infusion cortisol (6 mg/m^2 per h)	leu flux— leu ox—
Simmons et al. (134)	^{2}H$_3$-leu; 8 h hydrocortisone infusion	↑ PB
Darmaun et al. (135)	^{13}C-leu; ^{2}H$_5$-phe; ^{15}N-glu (NH$_2$); ^{13}C-ala; hydrocortisone infusion for 64 h	PB ↑, Ala flux ↑ Glu (NH$_2$) flux ↑
Beaufrere et al. (136)	^{13}C-leu; ^{15}N-glu (NH$_2$); ^{13}C-ala; 20 mg 3× daily prednisone	↑ leu ox; ↑ PB ↑ glu (NH$_2$) flux and synthesis ↑ ala flux and synthesis

PB, whole body protein breakdown; PAA, plasma amino acid concentration; leu ox, leucine oxidation; ↑, increase; ↓, decrease; —, no change.

nitrogen relations. For example, ingestion of carbohydrate suppresses and protein intake stimulates glucagon secretion. It is also clear that the circulating glucagon concentration depends on the ratio of protein to carbohydrate in meals (104,105).

As summarized in Table 8, when glucagon is infused, during a state of insulin deficiency, there is an increased rate of whole body leucine oxidation and proteolysis (106). Thus, glucagon's effect is opposite that of insulin in this condition (Table 6). However, hyperglucagonemia does not appear to have an effect on whole body leucine flux (proteolysis) when this co-exists with maintained or "normal" insulin levels (107). Hence, the more favorable impact on body N retention by a dietary mixture of carbohydrate and protein as compared with dietary protein alone might be due, in part, to these interactions between glucagon and insulin on amino acid utilization.

The activity of the sympathetic nervous system increases when carbohydrate (glucose) is consumed but not when protein or fat are ingested (108–110). Epinephrine stimulates hepatic glucose production (111,112), impairs glucose disposal (113), and it is a potent lipolytic agent (114). For these reasons, the effect of catecholamines on *in vivo* aspects of protein and amino acid metabolism is of potential importance. This point of view is supported by the suggestion made a number of years ago that epinephrine could reduce proteolysis (115), whereas an acceleration of proteolysis by catecholamines was earlier assumed, possibly because physical trauma and infection is characterized by a protein catabolic state (116) as well as hyperepinephrinemia (117). To date, there are a limited number of studies that have reported findings about the relationships between epinephrine and dynamic aspects of *in vivo* amino acid metabolism. Epinephrine causes plasma amino acids to decline (118,119) and from this response it is to be expected that amino acid oxidation rates would also be reduced (1). From the summary in Table 8, it is reasonable to draw the tentative conclusion that β-agonists reduce whole body leucine oxidation, and possibly protein breakdown, whereas β-blockade increases leucine oxidation. If these alterations in plasma leucine kinetics reflect the global response of body amino acid metabolism, then a reasonable interpolation of the data leads to the conclusion that the overall effects of SNS activation are similar, but may not be identical, to that of insulin. It is intriguing to speculate that the potentially greater nitrogen sparing effect of carbohydrate relative to lipid is related to a cooperative or synergistic action of insulin and the sympathetic nervous system on amino acid metabolism.

Whether the glucocorticoids modulate the physiologic effects of energy and exogenous amino acids on nitrogen retention and sparing, as discussed above, is not clear. It has been appreciated for some time that administration of pharmacological amounts of corticoids in man causes muscle wasting (1). Animal studies have revealed that both the stimulation of muscle proteolysis (124–126) and inhibition of protein synthesis (125,127–129) are consequences of glucocorticoid administration and these changes have been implicated in the loss of body protein and increased output of urinary nitrogen (130,131) due to hormone administration. It is also relevant that plasma cortisol concentrations show a diurnal variation during a brief fast, with peak concentrations occurring at 0800 h and the lowest at around midnight (132), varying over about a three- to five-fold range. As summarized in Table 8, Gelfand et al. (133) did not find a change in leucine flux (protein breakdown) when four obese subjects received a cortisol infusion for 72 h but three other studies involving glucocorticoid administration in normal subjects have reported increases in postabsorptive whole body proteolysis (134–136) and, where measured, in leucine oxidation (136). However, there seems to be some disagreement concerning the extent to which glucocorticoids might continue with these same effects during the fed period (compare ref. 136 and ref. 137).

Alanine (134,135) and glutamine (135) fluxes are also increased by glucocorticoids. However, the enhanced whole body proteolysis may not be due to increased muscle (myofibrillar) protein breakdown, since urinary 3-N$^\tau$-methylhistidine is apparently, not affected (136). It is likely that the length, as well as dose, of corticoid administration is important. At least this is the case in the rat where a temporal response of an increased muscle proteolysis occurs which reaches a peak at about 4 days followed by a return to normal rates of turnover as hormone administration is prolonged (124–126).

Although the glucocorticoid effects noted above (134–136) are exerted within a physiologic range of hormone levels it is not yet possible to state whether this counter-regulatory hormone can be implicated in the normal regulation of whole body protein and amino acid metabolism or account, in mechanistic terms, for the nitrogen-sparing actions of energy and protein that we have so far covered.

Emphasis on Alanine and Glutamine

It is pertinent here to recall that alanine and glutamine account for 60–80% of the amino acids released from the skeletal musculature (138–141), with muscle serving as the major source of plasma alanine in postabsorptive human subjects (142). In view of the important roles played by these amino acids in interorgan nitrogen transport and because alanine is qualitatively the most important gluconeogenic amino acid (143) and an important determinant of urea production (144), the N-sparing effects of energy sources on nitrogen balance might be exerted by a significant influence on the release of these amino acids from muscle and their subsequent fate in splanchnic nitrogen metabolism and hepatic gluconeogenesis.

Short-term infusion of glucose does suppress alanine release from forearm muscle, as noted earlier (97). Alanine infusion increases urea production (144). Large doses of oral glucose and intravenous glucose restrain alanine uptake by the splanchnic bed (145–147). These responses of alanine metabolism are generally consistent with the decrease in loss of nitrogen from the whole body during long-term glucose infusion (148,149). However, glucose infusion has been shown to increase whole body alanine flux (83) which suggests that tissues other than muscle, possibly the gut, account for an increased rate of alanine formation and entry into plasma. Nevertheless, the important point is that this effect does not correlate with the diminished rate of urea production (89). This is also the case where a carbohydrate-rich, low-protein diet is consumed (150). Hence, the role that the glucose-induced, diminished output of muscle alanine plays in relation to the body nitrogen-sparing property of glucose remains unclear to us and more extensive and elegant studies on the fate of alanine nitrogen need to be performed.

In light of these findings for alanine, it might be that the regulation of glutamine release from skeletal muscle offers a further clue concerning the metabolic basis for the favorable effect of glucose administration on nitrogen retention. This latter amino acid accounts for more than 60% of the free amino acid pool in skeletal muscle (151,152), it serves as a precursor in biosynthetic processes and as an important vehicle for nitrogen and carbon transport between body tissues. Furthermore, it may have regulatory functions in relation to the synthesis (153,154) and breakdown (155,156) of proteins, and it serves as a gluconeogenic precursor (157). However, although glutamine efflux from muscle increases with early starvation (158) glucose infusion does not alter glutamine release from skeletal muscle (97), nor does the output change after a protein meal (139). Thus, it does not appear that altered glutamine flux and interorgan flow is responsible for the N-sparing effect of glucose, at least in reference to its net output from the periphery and the consequences of short-term glucose administration. Perhaps the impact of glucose or energy substrates on glutamine is more subtle, possibly via an effect on the glutamine translocation cycle (159). This cycle regulates the intracellular glutamine environment and, under favorable conditions, perhaps promotes improved protein balance via mechanisms responsible for protein synthesis and breakdown. Thus, the role of glutamine, despite its known and major function in N-homeostasis, remains to be clarified in relation to its energy-nitrogen relations.

Lipids and Amino Acid Kinetics

Briefly with regard to the effect of lipid sources, it was observed some years ago by Sherwin et al. (160) that an infusion of β-hydroxybutyrate in non-obese and obese subjects reduced urinary N excretion, and this has been confirmed (161). This effect of the ketone bodies is apparently attributable to a stimulation of amino acid incorporation into proteins, accompanied by, or causally related to, a diminished amino acid oxidation (162,163), which may be exerted at the level of the skeletal muscle (164–167). Of possible interest is the finding that whole body proteolysis does not seem to be affected by ketone bodies (162,168), whereas triglyceride (LCT) and medium chain fatty acids appear to reduce both amino acid (leucine) oxidation as well as protein turnover (169,170). Thus, fatty acids and ketone bodies may exert their N-sparing effects via different mechanisms. This tentative conclusion is drawn, however, from a limited *in vivo* data base and it would be useful to have additional evidence from further comparative investigations (171) to better define the mechanisms underlying the effects of different lipid-energy sources on whole body, organ, and interorgan N metabolism.

Practical Correlates

These various metabolic observations considered here both raise and may well provide guidance and answers to questions of practical and therapeutic importance. One of these is the desirable relationship between the protein (nitrogen, amino acid) intake and the sources and level of the energy supply, for purposes of achieving optimal body energy and protein balance and for supporting tissue and organ function over the long-term. In arriving at sound recommendations and for establishing effective therapeutic stages recognition must now be given to the significant metabolic and physiologic costs due either to excessive or "imbalanced" nutritional support in the stressed patient. These potentially include further increases in insulin when levels might already be high (172), excessive hepatic lipogenesis and fatty liver (173), and relatively high rates of CO_2 production when energy (carbohydrate) intake is excessive with a precipitation of respiratory stress (174,175). These problems might be minimized with a partial replacement of the carbohydrate with fat. It is hoped that our metabolic exposé provides a partial basis for ultimately making a rational decision regarding how much fat should be used with what effect on metabolic function. Overfeeding (176) induced by non-volitional refeeding or precipitation of the refeeding syndrome might also be an undesirable outcome of inappropriate nutritional therapy.

Also, the extent to which the contribution of protein made by catabolism and amino acid oxidation to total energy expenditure and balance will, of course, dictate the desirable ratio of the protein to non-protein energy intake and, as discussed above, it appears to us that in catabolic states the additional losses of nitrogen generally exceed the degree of change occurring in energy expenditure. However, it also seems that the contribution made by protein rarely exceeds about 20% of the total energy substrate oxidized. This might serve as a pointer for the formulation of a nutritional supplement intended to cover the deficit that might exist with free-choice food intakes (177).

With reference to lipid we have given little attention to its metabolism *per se*, but we did mention the protein sparing effects of fatty acids and of ketone bodies and how they might bring about their effects. The studies that we have reviewed were in non-stressed and fasting subjects. As Rich (178) has pointed out recently, the effect of infusions of ketones in stress and sepsis is still unclear. Hence, it remains for future studies to establish whether it would be desirable to include them as part of optimal nutritional therapy. Nevertheless, their water solubility characteristics and independence on insulin action must mean that, together in an appropriate balance with glucose and fatty acids, they could be used to achieve effective protein balance and nitrogen sparing in stressed patients.

Additionally, in the context of lipid-derived calories it is now appreciated that the fatty acid pattern of triacylglycerols can have important metabolic and cellular consequences. Thus, whether the lipid used to supply a significant proportion of the energy should be in the form of mixture of both medium- and long-chain triacylglycerols is an important and still unresolved question, but this issue is now receiving attention (179). Also, the dietary environment (180) and specific fatty acid composition of the lipid are of importance since they can influence the fatty acid composition of membranes and, in consequence, modify the actions of cytokines (181) and the metabolic response to thermal injury (182), for example.

Thus, not only are the sources and amounts of energy yielding substrate determinants of the characteristics of *in vivo* energy-nitrogen relations but the qualitative nature of the lipids, especially their constituent fatty acids, is likely to be a modifying influence under differing pathophysiological states. This possibility and its nutritional and clinical implications deserve further metabolic and clinical investigation.

SUMMARY AND CONCLUSION

In conjunction with the material covered in our earlier chapter [*Whole Body Energy and Nitrogen (Protein) Relationships*], the relations between energy and nitrogen (protein) have been reviewed and it is now well documented that both the amount and source of the dietary energy as well as the nitrogen supply have profound effects on body protein balance. It is also evident that these various interrelations are dependent upon a complex of interrelated mechanisms and we have discovered that our understanding of these mechanisms is still quite rudimentary, despite the potential practical and clinical importance of these aspects of metabolism and nutrition. For example, how an infusion of glucose brings about its nitrogen-sparing effect in the intact host is not yet clear, at least in terms of the principal organs involved, the actions and quantitative importance of various hormonal signals, possibly with insulin being of major significance, and the major pathways of carbon and nitrogen trafficking that are affected. Much exciting research on *in vivo* aspects of amino acid and fuel substrate metabolism and their interactions remains to be performed, despite the useful beginnings outlined above.

It is clear to us that a comprehensive treatment and understanding of energy-nitrogen relations, particularly with regard to an eventual concern for practical nutritional issues, demands that we now both broaden and deepen our inquiry. This presents a real challenge but at the same time it is one that can be decorated with intriguing metabolic and physiologic issues and which must be integrated eventually within the context of the nutritional needs and characteristics of the patient or individual.

ACKNOWLEDGMENTS

The senior author's unpublished studies were supported by NIH grants DK15856 and DK42101. Studies were conducted at the general Clinical Research Center at the Massachusetts Institute of Technology funded by a grant (M01-44-00088) from the National Center of Research Resources—NIH.

REFERENCES

1. Young VR, Meredith C, Hoerr R, Bier DM, Matthews DE. Amino acid kinetics in relation to protein and amino acid requirements: the primary importance of amino acid oxidation. In: Garrow JS, Halliday D, eds. *Substrate and energy metabolism in man*. London: John Libbey, 1985;119–133.
2. Denne SC, Kalhan SC. Leucine metabolism in human newborns. *Am J Physiol* 1987;253:E608–E615.
3. Millward DJ, Rivers JPW. The need for indispensible amino acids: The concept of the anabolic drive. *Diabetes Metab Rev* 1989;5:191–211.
4. Millward DJ, Jackson AA, Price G, Rivers JPW. Human amino acid and protein requirements: current dilemmas and uncertainties. *Nutr Res Rev* 1989;2:109–132.
5. Krebs HA. Some aspects of the regulation of fuel supply in omnivorous animals. *Adv Enzyme Regul* 1972;10:397–420.
6. Randle PJ. Fuel selection in animals. *Trans Biochem Soc* 1986;14:799–806.
7. Thompson GN, Bresson JL, Pacy PJ, et al. Protein and leucine metabolism in maple syrup urine disease. *Am J Physiol* 1990;258:E654–E660.
8. Thompson GN, Walter JH, Leonard JV, Halliday D. In vivo enzyme activity in inborn errors of metabolism. *Metabolism* 1990;39:799–807.
9. Ruch T, Kerr D. Decreased essential amino acid requirements without catabolism in phenylketonuria and maple syrup urine disease. *Am J Clin Nutr* 1982;35:217–228.

10. Kindt E, Halvorsen S. The need of essential amino acids in children: an evaluation based on the intake of phenylalanine, tyrosine, leucine, isoleucine and valine in children with phenylketonuria, tyrosine aminotransferase defect, and maple syrup urine disease. *Am J Clin Nutr* 1980;33:279–286.

11. Thompson GN, Halliday D. Significant phenylalanine hydroxylation in vivo in patients with classical phenylketonuria. *J Clin Invest* 1990;86:317–322.

12. Kaplan JH, Pitot HC. The regulation of intermediary amino acid metabolism in animal tissues. In: Munro HN, ed. *Mammalian protein metabolism* New York: Academic Press, 1970, 387–443.

13. Harper AE. Enzymatic basis for adaptive changes in amino acid metabolism. In: Taylor TG, Jenkins NK, eds. *Proceedings of the XIII International Congress of Nutrition.* London: John Libbey, 1986;409–414.

14. Meijer AJ, Lamers WH, Chamuleau RAFM. Nitrogen metabolism and ornithine cycle function. *Physiol Rev* 1990;70:701–748.

15. Jahoor F, Wolfe RR. Regulation of urea production by glucose infusion *in vivo. Am J Physiol* 1987;253:E543–E550.

16. Jackson AA, Doherty J, DeBenoist M-H, Hibbert J, Persaud C. The effect of level of dietary protein, carbohydrate and fat on urea kinetics in young children during rapid catch-up weight gain. *Br J Nutr* 1990;64:371–385.

17. FAO/WHO/UNU. Energy and protein requirements. Report of a joint FAO/WHO/UNU consultation. *Technical report series No 724,* Geneva: World Health Organization, 1985.

18. Rose WC. The amino acid requirements of adult man. *Nutr Abstr Rev* 1957;27:631–647.

19. Rose WC, Wixom RL. The amino acid requirements of man. XVI. The role of the nitrogen intake. *J Biol Chem* 1955;217:997–1004.

20. Young VR, Bier DM, Pellett PL. A theoretical basis for increasing current estimates of the amino acid requirements in adult man, with experimental support. *Am J Clin Nutr* 1989;50:80–92.

21. Millward DJ, Rivers JPN. The role of indispensable amino acids and the metabolic basis for their requirements. *Eur J Clin Nutr* 1988;42:367–393.

22. Millward DJ. Amino acid requirements in adult man. *Am J Clin Nutr* 1990;51:492–494.

23. Young VR, Bier DM, Pellett P. Amino acid requirements in adult man. Reply to J. Millward. *Am J Clin Nutr* 1990;51:494–496.

24. Waterlow JC. Protein turnover with special reference to man. *Q J Exp Physiol* 1984;69:409–438.

25. Kinney JM, Elwyn DH. Protein metabolism and injury. *Annu Rev Nutr* 1983;3:433–466.

26. Winters RW, Greene HL; eds. *Nutritional support of the seriously ill patient.* New York: Academic Press, 1983, 303p.

27. Rennie MJ. Muscle protein turnover and wasting due to injury and disease. *Br Med Bull* 1985;41:257–264.

28. Jahoor F, Desai M, Herndon DN, Wolfe RR. Dynamics of the protein metabolic response to burn injury. *Metabolism* 1988;37:330–337.

29. Shaw JHF, Wolfe RR. Energy and protein metabolism in sepsis and trauma. *Aust N Z J Surg* 1987;57:41–47.

30. Winthrop AL, Wesson DE, Pencharz PB, Jacobs DG, Heim T, Filer RM. Injury severity, whole body protein turnover, and energy expenditure in pediatric trauma. *Metabolism* 1987;22:534–537.

31. Bilmazes C, Kien CL, Rohrbaugh DK, et al. Quantitative contribution by skeletal muscle to elevated rates of whole-body protein breakdown in burned children as measured by N$^\tau$methyl/histidine output. *Metabolism* 1978;27:671–676.

32. Sjölin J. Skeletal muscle protein metabolism in human infection—evaluation of 3-methylhistidine as a marker of myofibrillar protein degradation. *Acta Universitatis Upsaliensis* (Uppsala, Sweden) 1988;159.

33. Young VR. The role of skeletal and cardiac muscle in the regulation of protein metabolism. In: Munro HN, ed. *Mammalian protein metabolism,* vol IV. New York: Academic Press, 1970; 585–674.

34. Sjölin J, Stjernstrom H, Friman G, Larsson J, Wahren J. Total and net muscle protein breakdown in infection determined by amino acid effluxes. *Am J Physiol* 1990;258:E856–E863.

35. Hummel RP, James H, Warner BW, Hasselgren P-O, Fischer JE. Evidence that cathepsin B contributes to skeletal muscle protein breakdown during sepsis. *Arch Surg* 1988;123:221–224.

36. Odessey R. Regulation of lysosomal proteolysis in burn injury. *Metabolism* 1987;36:670–676.

37. Furuno K, Goldberg AL. The activation of protein degradation in muscle by Ca^{2+} or muscle injury does not involve a lysosomal mechanism. *Biochem J* 1986;237:859–864.

38. Goldberg AL, Kettlehut JC, Furuno K, Fagan JM, Baracos V. Activation of protein breakdown

and prostaglandin E_2 production in rat skeletal muscle in fever is signaled by a macrophage product distinct from interleukin-1 or other known monokines. *J Clin Invest* 1988;81:1378–1383.

39. Kettlehut IC, Goldberg AL. Tumor necrosis factor can induce fever in rats without activating protein breakdown in muscle or lipolysis in adipose tissue. *J Clin Invest* 1988;81:1384–1389.
40. Moldawer LL, Lowry SF, Cerami A. Cachectin: its impact on metabolism and nutritional status. *Annu Rev Nutr* 1988;8:585–609.
41. Kettlehut IC, Wing SS, Goldberg AL. Endocrine regulation of protein breakdown in skeletal muscle. *Diabetes Metab Rev* 1988;4:751–772.
42. Starnes HF Jr, Warren RS, Jeevanandam M, et al. Tumor necrosis factor and the acute metabolic response to tissue injury in man. *J Clin Invest* 1988;82:1321–1325.
43. Tredget EE, Yu M-Y, Zhong S, Burini R, et al. Role of interleukin 1 and tumor necrosis factor on energy metabolism in rabbits. *Am J Physiol* 1988;255:E760–E768.
44. Newsholme EA, Newsholme P, Curie R, Challoner E, Ardawi MSM. A role for muscle in the immune system and its importance in surgery, trauma, sepsis and burns. *Nutrition* 1988;4:261–268.
45. Askanazi J, Carpentier YA, Michelsen CB, et al. Muscle and plasma amino acids following injury. *Ann Surg* 1980;192:78–85.
46. Aulick LH, Wilmore DS. Increased peripheral amino acid release following burn injury. *Surgery* 1979;85:560–565.
47. Ardawi MSM. Skeletal muscle glutamine production in thermally injured rats. *Clin Sci* 1988;74:165.
48. Ardawi MSM, Majzoub MF. Glutamine metabolism in skeletal muscle of septic rats. *Metabolism* 1991;40:155–164.
49. Young VR. Energy metabolism and requirements in the cancer patient. *Cancer Res* 1977;37:2336–2347.
50. Kaloyianni M, Freedland RA. Contribution of several amino acids and lactate to gluconeogenesis in hepatocytes isolated from rats fed various diets. *J Nutr* 1990;120:116–122.
51. Brennan MF, Fitzpatrick GM, Cohen KH, Moore FD. Glyerol: major contributor to the short-term protein sparing effect of fat emulsions in normal man. *Ann Surg* 1975;182:386–393.
52. Cathcart EP. The influence of carbohydrates and fats on protein metabolism. *J Physiol* 1909;39:311–330.
53. Cahill GF Jr. Starvation in man. *Clin Endocrinol Metab* 1976;5:397–415.
54. Saudek CD, Felig P. The metabolic events of starvation. *Am J Med* 1976;60:117–126.
55. Goodman MN, Larsen PR, Kaplan MM, Aoki TT, Young VR, Ruderman NB. Starvation in the rat. II. Effect of age and obesity on protein sparing and fuel metabolism. *Am J Physiol* 1980;239:E277–E286.
56. Vazquez JA, Morse EL, Adibi SA. Effect of dietary fat, carbohydrate and protein on branched chain amino acid catabolism during caloric restriction. *J Clin Invest* 1986;76:737–743.
57. Munro HN. General aspects of the regulation of protein metabolism by diet and by hormones. In: Munro HN, Allison JB, eds. *Mammalian protein metabolism*. New York: Academic Press, 1964;381–481.
58. Richardson DP, Wayler AH, Scrimshaw NS, Young VR. Quantitative effect of an isoenergetic exchange of fat for carbohydrate on dietary protein utilization in healthy young men. *Am J Clin Nutr* 1979;32:2217–2226.
59. National Research Council. *Diet and health: implications for reducing chronic disease risk: Food and Nutrition Board*. Washington, DC: National Academy Press, 1989;749p.
60. Fuller MF, Weekes TEC, Cadenhead A, Bruce JB. The protein-sparing action of carbohydrate. 2. The role of insulin. *Br J Nutr* 1977;38:489.
61. Long CL. Energy balance and carbohydrate metbolism in sepsis. *Am J Clin Nutr* 1977;30:1301–1310.
62. Shaw JHF, Wolfe RR. Determination of glucose turnover and oxidation in normal volunteers and in patients with severe pancreatitis using stable and radioisotopes: the response to substrate infusion and total parenteral nutrition. *Ann Surg* 1986;204:665–672.
63. Shaw JHF, Holdaway CM. Protein-sparing effect of substrate infusion in surgical patients is governed by the clinical state and not by the individual substrate infused. *J Parent Enteral Nutr* 1988;12:433–440.
64. Shaw JHF, Humberstone DM, Wolfe RR. Energy and protein metabolism in sarcoma patients. *Ann Surg* 1988;207:283–289.
65. Golster AD, Bier DM, Cryer PE, Monafo WW. Plasma palmitate turnover in subjects with thermal injury. *J Trauma* 1984;24:938–944.

66. Lanza-Jacoby S, Rosato E, Broccia G, Tabarea A. Altered ketone body metabolism during gram-negative sepsis in the rat. *Metabolism* 1990;39:1151–1157.
67. Hartl WH, Jauch K-W, Kimmig R, Wicklmayr M, Gunther B, Heberer G. Minor role of ketone bodies in energy metabolism by skeletal muscle tissue during the postoperative course. *Ann Surg* 1988;207:95–101.
68. Jahoor F, Shangraw RE, Miyoshi H, Wallfish H, Herndon DN, Wolfe RR. Role of insulin and glucose oxidation in mediating protein catabolism of burns and sepsis. *Am J Physiol* 1989;275:E323–E331.
69. Long CL, Nelson RM, Akin JM, Griger JW, Merrick HW, Blakemore WS. A physiologic basis for the provision of fuel mixtures in normal and stressed patients. *J Trauma* 1990;30:1077–1085.
70. Jeevanandam M, Young DH, Schiller WR. Obesity and the metabolic response to severe multiple trauma in man. *J Clin Invest* 1991;87:262–269.
71. Long JM, Wilmore DW, Mason AD, Pruitt BA. Effect of carbohydrate and fat intake on nitrogen excretion during total intravenous feeding. *Ann Surg* 1977;185:417–422.
72. Baker JP, Detsky AS, Stewart S, Whitwell J, Marliss EB, Jeejeebhoy KN. Randomized trial of total parenteral nutrition in critically ill patients; metabolic effects of varying glucose-lipid ratios as the energy source. *Gastroenterology* 1984;87:53–59.
73. Gazzanigan AB, Day AT, Sankary H. The efficiency of a 20 percent fat emulsion as a peripherally administered substrate. *Surg Gynecol Obstet* 1985;160:387–392.
74. Shaw JHF, Holdaway CM. Protein-sparing effect of substrate infusion in surgical patients is governed by the clinical state, and not by the individual substrate infused. *J Parenter Enteral Nutr* 1988;12:433–440.
75. Woolfson AMJ, Heatley RV, Allison SP. Insulin to inhibit protein catabolism after injury. *N Engl J Med* 1979;300:14–17.
76. Bark S, Holm K, Hakamsson I, Wretlind A. Nitrogen-sparing effect of fat emulsion compared with glucose in the postoperative period. *Acta Chir Scand* 1976;142:423–427.
77. Paluzzi M, Meguid MM. A prospective randomized study of the optimal source of non-protein calories in total parenteral nutrition. *Surgery* 1987;102:711–716.
78. Nordenstrom J, Askannazi J, Elwyn DH, et al. Nitrogen balance during total parenteral nutrition. Glucose vs. fat. *Ann Surg* 1983;197:27–33.
79. Jeejeebhoy KN, Anderson GH, Nakhoodu AF, Greenberg GR, Sanderson I, Marliss EB. Metabolic studies in total parenteral nutrition with lipid in man. Comparison with glucose. *J Clin Invest* 1976;57:125–136.
80. Shaw SN, Elwyn DH, Askanazi J, Iles M, Schwarz Y, Kinney JM. Effects of increasing nitrogen intake on nitrogen balance and energy expenditure in nutritionally depleted adult patients receiving parenteral nutrition. *Am J Clin Nutr* 1983;37:930–940.
81. Felley CP, Felley EM, vanMelle GD, Frascarolo P, Jéquier E, Felber J-P. Impairment of glucose disposal by infusion of triglycerides in humans: role of glycemia. *Am J Physiol* 1989;256:E747–E752.
82. Ferrannini E, Barrett EJ, Bevilaequa S, et al. Effect of free fatty acids on blood amino acid levels in humans. *Am J Physiol* 1986;250:E686–E694.
83. Robert J-J, Bier DM, Zhao XH, Matthews DE, Young VR. Glucose and insulin effects on de novo amino acid synthesis in young men: studies with stable isotope labeled alanine, glycine, leucine and lysine. *Metabolism* 1982;31:1210–1218.
84. Fukagawa NK, Minaker KL, Rowe JW, et al. Insulin-mediated reduction of whole body protein breakdown: dose-response effects on leucine metabolism in postabsorptive men. *J Clin Invest* 1985;76:2306–2311.
85. Wolfe RR, Shaw JHF, Jahoor F, Herndon DN, Wolfe RR. Response of glucose infusion in humans: role of changes in insulin concentration. *Am J Physiol* 1986;250:E306–E311.
86. Tessari P, Trevison R, Inchiostro S, et al. Dose-response curves of effects of insulin on leucine kinetics in humans. *Am J Physiol* 1986;251:E334–E342.
87. Fukagawa NK, Minaker KL, Rowe JW, Matthews DE, Bier DM, Young VR. Glucose and amino acid metabolism in aging man: differential effects of insulin. *Metabolism* 1988;37:371–377.
88. Tessari P, Biolo G, Inchiostro S, et al. Effects of insulin on whole body and forearm leucine and KIC metabolism in type I diabetes. *Am J Physiol* 1990;259:E96–E103.
89. Shangraw RE, Stuart CA, Prince MJ, Peters EJ, Wolfe RR. Insulin responsiveness of protein metabolism *in vivo* following bedrest in humans. *Am J Physiol* 1988;255:E548–E558.
90. Castellino P, Luzi L, Simonson DC, Haymond M, DeFronzo RA. Effect of insulin and plasma amino acid concentrations on leucine metabolism in man: the role of substrate availability on estimates of whole body protein synthesis. *J Clin Invest* 1987;80:1784–1793.

91. Arfvidsson B, Zachrisson H, Moller-Loswick A-C, Hyltander A, Sandstrom R, Lundholm K. Effect of systemic hyperinsulinemia on amino acid flux across human legs in postabsorptive state. *Am J Physiol* 1991;260:E46–E52.

92. Tessari P, Inchiostro S, Biolo G, et al. Differential effects of hyperinsulinemia and hyperaminoacidemia on leucine-carbon metabolism in vivo. Evidence for distinct mechanisms in regulation of net amino acid deposition. *J Clin Invest* 1987;79:1062–1069.

93. Fukagawa NK, Minaker KL, Young VR, Matthews DE, Bier DM, Rowe JW. Leucine metabolism in aging humans: effect of insulin and substrate availability. *Am J Physiol* 1989;256:E288–E294.

94. Flakoll PJ, Kulaylat M, Frexes-Steed M, et al. Amino acids augment insulin's suppression of whole body proteolysis. *Am J Physiol* 1989;257:E839–E847.

95. Frexes-Steed M, Warner ML, Bulus N, Flakoll P, Abumrad MN. Role of insulin and branched-chain amino acids in regulatory protein metabolism during fasting. *Am J Physiol* 1990;258:E907–E917.

96. Pozefsky T, Felig P, Tobin JD, Soeldner JS, Cahill GF. Amino acid balance across tissues of the forearm in postabsorptive man. Effects of insulin at two dose levels. *J Clin Invest* 1969;48:2273–2282.

97. Elia M, Neale G, Livesey G. Alanine and glutamine release from the human forearm: effects of glucose administration. *Clin Sci* 1985;69:123–133.

98. Gelfand RA, Barrett EJ. Effect of physiologic hyperinsulinemia on skeletal muscle protein synthesis and breakdown in man. *J Clin Invest* 1987;80:1–6.

99. Bennet WM, Connacher AA, Scrimgeour CM, Smith K, Rennie MJ. Increase in anterior tibialis muscle protein synthesis in healthy man during mixed amino acid infusions: studies of incorporation of $[1\text{-}^{13}\text{C}]$leucine. *Clin Sci* 1989;76:447–454.

100. Bennet WM, Connacher AA, Scrimgeour CM, Jung RT, Rennie MJ. Euglycemic hyperinsulineamia augments amino acid uptake by human leg tissues during hyperaminoacidemia. *Am J Physiol* 1990;259:E185–E194.

101. Fryburg DA, Barrett GJ, Louard RJ, Gelfand RA. Effect of starvation on human muscle protein metabolism and its response to insulin. *Am J Physiol* 1990;259:E477–E482.

102. Hourani H, Williams P, Morris JA, May ME, Abumrad NN. Effect of insulin-induced hypoglycemia on protein metabolism in vivo. *Am J Physiol* 1990;259:E342–E350.

103. Schwenk WF, Haymond MW. Decreased uptake of glucose by human forearm during infusion of leucine, isoleucine, or threonine. *Diabetes* 1987;36:199–204.

104. Krezowski PA, Nuttal FZ, Gannon MC, Bartosh NH. The effect of protein ingestion on the metabolic response to oral glucose in normal individuals. *Am J Clin Nutr* 1986;44:847–856.

105. Westphal SA, Gannon MC, Nuttall FQ. Metabolic response to glucose ingested with various amounts of protein. *Am J Clin Nutr* 1990;52:267–272.

106. Nair KS, Halliday D, Matthews DE, Welle SL. Hyperglucagonemia during insulin deficiency accelerates protein catabolism. *Am J Physiol* 1987;253:E208–E213.

107. Couet C, Fukagawa NK, Matthews DE, Bier DM, Young VR. Plasma amino acid kinetics during acute states of glucagon deficiency and excess in healthy adults. *Am J Physiol* 1990;258:E78–E85.

108. Welle SL, Lilavivathana V, Campbell RG. Increased plasma norepinephrine concentrations and metabolic rates following glucose ingestion in man. *Metabolism* 1980;29:806–809.

109. Young JB, Rowe JW, Pallotta, et al. Enhanced plasma norephinephrine response to upright posture and oral glucose administration in elderly human subjects. *Metabolism* 1980;29:532–539.

110. Welle S, Lilavivathana V, Campbell RG. Thermic effect of feeding in man: increased plasma nor-epinephrine levels following glucose but not protein or fat consumption. *Metabolism* 1981;30:953–958.

111. Rizza RA, Cryer PE, Haymond MN, Gerich J. Adrenergic mechanisms for the effects of epinephrine on glucose production and clearance in man. *J Clin Invest* 1980;65:682–689.

112. Soman V, Shamoon H, Sherwin RS. Effect of physiologic infusion of epinephrine in normal humans: relationship between the metabolic response and β-adrenergic binding. *J Clin Endocrinal Metab* 1980;50:294–297.

113. Rizza R, Haymond M, Cryer P, Gerich J. Differential effects of epinephrine on glucose production and disposal in man. *Am J Physiol* 1979;237:E356–E362.

114. Steinberg D, Vaughan M. Release of free fatty acids from adipose tissue *in vitro* in relation to rates of triglyceride synthesis and degradation. In: *Handbook of physiology, adipose tissue*. Washington, DC: American Physiological Society; 335–347.

115. Garber AJ, Karl JE, Kipnis DM. Alanine and glutamine synthesis and release from skeletal muscle. III. β-Adrenergic inhibition of amino acid release. *J Biol Chem* 1976;251:851–857.

116. Wolfe RR, Jahoor F, Hartl WH. Protein and amino acid metabolism after injury. *Diabetes Metab Rev* 1989;5:149–164.
117. Wilmore DW, Long JM, Mason MC, Skreen RW, Pruitt BA. Catecholamines: mediators of the hypermetabolic response to thermal injury. *Ann Surg* 1974;180:653–669.
118. Shamoon E, Jacob R, Sherwin RS. Epinephrine-induced hypoaminoacidemia in normal and diabetic subjects. Effect of beta blockade. *Diabetes* 1980;29:875–881.
119. Del Prato S, DeFronzo RA, Castellino P, Wahren J, Alvestrand A. Regulation of amino acid metabolism by epinephrine. *Am J Physol* 1990;258:E878–E887.
120. Miles JM, Nissen SL, Gerich JE, Haymond MW. Effects of epinephrine infusions on leucine and alanine kinetics in humans. *Am J Physiol* 1984;247:E166–E172.
121. Lamont LS, Patel DG, Kalhan SS. β-Adrenergic blockade alters whole-body leucine metabolism in humans. *J Appl Physiol* 1989;67:221–225.
122. Kraenzlin ME, Keller V, Keller A, Thelin A, Arnaud MJ, Stauffacher W. Elevation of plasma epinephrine concentrations inhibits proteolysis and leucine oxidation in man via β-adrenergic mechanisms. *J Clin Invest* 1989;84:388–393.
123. Matthews DE, Pesola G, Campbell RG. Effect of epinephrine on amino acid and energy metabolism on humans. *Am J Physiol* 1990;258:E948–E956.
124. Tomas FM, Munro HN, Young VR. Effect of glucorticoid administration on the rate of muscle protein breakdown in rats as measured by the urinary excretion of N^τ-methylhistidine. *Biochem J* 1979;178:139–146.
125. Kayali AG, Young VR, Goodman MN. Sensitivity of myofibrillar proteins to glucocorticoid-induced muscle proteolysis. *Am J Physiol* 1986;252:E621–E626.
126. Kayali AG, Goodman MN, Lin J, Young VR. Insulin- and thyroid hormone-independent adaptation of myofibrillar proteolysis to glucocorticoids. *Am J Physiol* 1990;E699–E705.
127. Odedra BR, Bates PC, Millward DJ. Time course of effect of catabolic doses of corticosterone on protein turnover in skeletal muscle and liver. *Biochem J* 1983;214:617–627.
128. Rannels SR, Jefferson LS. Effects of glucocorticoids on muscle protein turnover in perfused rat hemocorpus. *Am J Physiol* 1980;238:E564–E572.
129. Shoji S, Pennington RJR. The effect of cortisone on protein breakdown and synthesis in rat skeletal muscle. *Mol Cell Endocrinal* 1977;6:159–169.
130. Wise JK, Hendler R, Felig P. Influence of glucorticoids on glucagon secretion and plasma amino acid concentrations in man. *J Clin Invest* 1973;52:2774–2782.
131. Sapir DG, Pozefsky T, Knochel JP, Walser M. The role of alanine and glutamine in steroid-induced nitrogen wasting in man. *Clin Sci Mol Med* 1977;53:215–220.
132. Haymond MW, Karl IE, Clarke WL, Pagliara AS, Santiago JV. Differences in circulating gluconeogenic substrates during short-term fasting in men, women and children. *Metabolism* 1982;31:33–42.
133. Gelfand RA, Matthews DE, Bier DM, Sherwin RS. Role of counterregulatory hormones in the catabolic response to stress. *J Clin Invest* 1984;74:2238–2248.
134. Simmons PS, Miles JM, Gerich JE, Haymond MW. Increased proteolysis. An effect of increases in plasma cortisol within the physiologic range. *J Clin Invest* 1984;73:412–420.
135. Darmaun D, Matthews DE, Bier DM. Physiological hypercortisolemia increases proteolysis, glutamine and alanine production. *Am J Physiol* 1988;255:E366–E373.
136. Beaufrere B, Horber FF, Schwenk WF, et al. Glucocorticoids increase leucine oxidation and impair leucine balance in humans. *Am J Physiol* 1989;257:E712–E721.
137. Horber FF, Haymond MW. Human growth hormone prevents the protein catabolic side effects of prednisone in humans. *J Clin Invest* 1990;86:265–272.
138. Felig P. Amino acid metabolism in man. *Annu Rev Biochem* 1975;44:933–955.
139. Elia M, Livesey G. Effects of ingested steak and infused leucine on forelimb metabolism in man and the fate of the carbon skeletons and amino groups of branched chain amino acids. *Clin Sci* 1983;64:517–526.
140. Aoki TT, Brennan MF, Meuller WA, et al. Amino acid levels across normal forearm muscle and splanchnic bed after a protein meal. *Am J Clin Nutr* 1976;29:340–350.
141. Marliss EB, Aoki TT, Pozefsky T, Most AS, Cahill GF. Muscle and splanchnic glutamine and glutamate metabolism in postabsorptive and starved man. *J Clin Invest* 1971;50:814–817.
142. Consoli A, Nurjhan N, Reilly JJ, Jr., Bier DM, Gerich JE. Contribution of liver and skeletal muscle to alanine and lactate metabolism in humans. *Am J Physiol* 1990;259:E677–E684.
143. Felig P, Marliss M, Pozefsky T, Cahill GF Jr. Amino acid metabolism in the regulation of gluconeogenesis in man. *Am J Clin Nutr* 1970;23:986–992.

144. Wolfe RR, Jahoor F, Shaw JHF. Effect of alanine infusion on glucose and urea production in man. *J Parenter Enteral Nutr* 1987;11:109–111.
145. Felig P, Wahren J, Hendler R. Influence of oral glucose ingestion on splanchnic glucose and gluconeogenic substrate metabolism in man. *Diabetes* 1975;24:468–475.
146. Ferrannini E, Wahren J, Felig P, DeFranzo RA. The role of fractional glucose extraction in splanchnic glucose metabolism in normal and diabetic man. *Metabolism* 1980;29:28–35.
147. Felig P, Wahren J. Influence of endogenous insulin secretions on splanchnic glucose and amino acid metabolism in man. *J Clin Invest* 1971;50:1702–1711.
148. O'Connell RC, Morgan AP, Aoki TT. Nitrogen conservation in starvation in graded responses to intravenous glucose. *J Clin Endocrinol Metab* 1974;39:555–563.
149. Wolfe BM, Culebras JM, Sim AW, Ball MR, Moore FD. Substrate interactions in intravenous feeding. *Ann Surg* 1977;186:518–540.
150. Yang RD, Matthews DE, Bier DM. Wen Z-M, Young VR. Response of alanine metabolism in humans to manipulation of dietary protein and energy intakes. *Am J Physiol* 1986;250:E39–E46.
151. Askanazi J, Carpentier JA, Michelsen CB, et al. Muscle and plasma amino acids following injury. *Ann Surg* 1980;192:75–85.
152. Bergstrom J, Furst P, Noreel O, Vinnars M. Intra-cellular free amino acid concentrations on human muscle tissue. *J Appl Physiol* 1974;36:693–697.
153. MacLennan PA, Braun RA, Rennie MJ. A positive relationship between protein synthetic rate and intracellular glutamine concentration in perfused rat skeletal muscle. *FEBS Lett* 1987;215:187–191.
154. Jepson MM, Bates PC, Broadbert P, Pell JM, Millward DJ. Relationship between glutamine concentration and protein synthesis in rat skeletal muscle. *Am J Physiol* 1988;255:E166–E172.
155. Wu G, Thompson JR. The effect of glutamine on protein turnover in chick skeletal muscle *in vitro*. *Biochem J* 1990;265:593–598.
156. Millward DJ, Jepson MM, Omer A. Muscle glutamine concentration and protein turnover *in vivo* in malnutrition and in endotoxemia. *Metabolism* 1989;38:(Suppl 1):6–13.
157. Smith RJ. Glutamine metabolism and its physiological importance. *J Parenter Enteral Nutr* 1990;14:40S–44S.
158. Goldstein LA. Interorgan glutamine relationships. *Fed Proc* 1986;45:2176–2179.
159. Newsholme EA, Parry-Billings M. Properties of glutamine release from muscle and its importance for the immune system. *J Parenter Enteral Nutr* 1990;14:63S–67S.
160. Sherwin RS, Hendler RG, Felig P. Effect of ketone infusions on amino acid and nitrogen metabolism in man. *J Clin Invest* 1975;55:1382–1390.
161. Pawan GLS, Semple SJG. Effect of 3-hydroxybutyrate in obese subjects on very-low-energy diets and during therapeutic starvation. *Lancet* 1983;1:15–17.
162. Miles JM, Nissen SL, Rizza RA, Gerich JE, Hayward WW. Failure of infused β-hydroxybutyrate to decrease proteolysis in man. *Diabetes* 1983;32:197–205.
163. Nair KS, Welle SL, Halliday D, Campbell RG. Effect of β-hydroxybutyrate on whole-body leucine kinetics and fractional mixed skeletal muscle protein synthesis in humans. *J Clin Invest* 1988;82:198–205.
164. Buse MG, Biggers JF, Friderics KH, Buse JF. Oxidation of branched-chain amino acids by isolated hearts and diaphragms of the rat: the effect of fatty acids, glucose, and pyruvate respiration. *J Biol Chem* 1972;248:697–706.
165. Wagenmakers AJM, Veerkamp JH. Interactions of various metabolites and agents with branched-chain 2-oxo acid oxidation in rat and human muscle *in vitro*. *Int J Biochem* 1984;16:971–976.
166. Palmer TN, Caldecourt MA, Warner JP, Sugden MC. Modulation of branched-chain amino acid oxidation in rat hemidiaphragms *in vitro* by glucose and ketone bodies. *Biochem Int* 1985;11:407–413.
167. Wu G, Thompson JR. Ketone bodies inhibit leucine degradation in chick skeletal muscle. *Int J Biochem* 1987;19:937–942.
168. Umpleby AM, Chubb D, Boroujerdi MA, Sonksen PH. The effect of ketone bodies on leucine and alanine metabolism in dogs. *Clin Sci* 1988;74:41–48.
169. Beaufrere B, Tessari P, Cattalini M, Miles J, Haymond MW. Apparent decreased oxidation and turnover of leucine during infusion of medium-chain triglycerides. *Am J Physiol* 1985;249:E175–E182.
170. Tessari P, Nissen SL, Miles JM, Haymond MW. Inverse relationship of leucine flux and oxidation to free fatty acid availability in vivo. *J Clin Invest* 1986;77:575–581.
171. Pencharz P, Beesley J, Sauer P, et al. Total body protein turnover in parenterally fed neonates:

effects of energy source studied by using [^{15}N]glycine and [1-^{13}C]leucine. *Am J Clin Nutr* 1989;50:1395–1400.
172. Frayn KN, Little RA, Stoner HB, Galasko CB. Metabolic control in non-septic patients with musculo-skeletal injuries. *Injury* 1984;16:73–79.
173. Sheldon GF, Petersen SR, Sanders R. Hepatic dysfunction during hyperalimentation. *Arch Surg* 1978;113:504–508.
174. Greig PD, Elwyn DH, Askanazi J, Kinney JM. Parenteral nutrition in septic patients: effect of increasing nitrogen intakes. *Am J Clin Nutr* 1987;46:1040–1047.
175. Askanazi J, Rosenbaum SH, Hyman AI, Silverberg JM-E, Kinney JM. Respiratory changes induced by the large glucose loads of total parenteral nutrition. *JAMA* 1990;243:1444–1447.
176. Casper K, Matthews DE, Heymsfield SB. Overfeeding: cardiovascular and metabolic response during continuous formula in adult humans. *Am J Clin Nutr* 1990;52:602–609.
177. Jallut D, Tappy L, Kohut M, et al. Energy balance in elderly patients after surgery for a femoral neck fracture. *J Parenter Enterol Nutr* 1990;14:563–568.
178. Rich AJ. Ketone bodies as substrates. *Proc Nutr Soc* 1990;49:361–373.
179. Carpentier YA, Richelle M, Haument D, Deckelbaum RJ. New developments in fat emulsions. *Proc Nutr Soc* 1990;49:375–380.
180. Feingold KR, Adi S, Staprans I, et al. Diet affects the mechanisms by which TNF stimulates hepatic triglyceride production. *Am J Physiol* 1990;259:E177–E184.
181. Bibby DC, Grimble LF. Dietary fat modifies some metabolic actions of human recombinant tumor necrosis factor α in rats. *Br J Nutr* 1990;63:653–668.
182. Hirschberg Y, Pomposelli JJ, Blackburn GL, Istfan NW, Babayan V, Bistrian BR. The effects of chronic fish oil feeding in rats on protein catabolism induced by recombinant mediators. *Metabolism* 1990;39:397–402.

Energy Metabolism: Tissue Determinants and
Cellular Corollaries, edited by J. M. Kinney
and H. N. Tucker. Raven Press, Ltd.,
New York © 1992.

The Energetic Cost of Regulation: An Analysis Based on the Principles of Metabolic-Control-Logic

*E. A. Newsholme, †B. Crabtree, and *M. Parry-Billings

*Cellular Nutrition Research Group Department of Biochemistry, University of Oxford,
Oxford, OX13QU, United Kingdom; and †Rowett Research Institute, Aberdeen,
AB2 9SB, Scotland

Energy expenditure is increased under a variety of conditions when the body carries out either physical or chemical work; but not all the energy is converted into useful work, and the implicit assumption is that all of the energy not transformed into work can be classified as wasted. However, this represents a myopic view of energy consumption since it does not take into account the energy that is expended to provide for control and regulation of *all* the processes involved in the expenditure of energy. Indeed, such energy usage in control is essential for the precision that characterizes the control of processes from, for example, energy provision in physical activity to doubling of the cell content of DNA in the cell cycle.

The importance of precision in regulation is illustrated by referring to one relatively simple metabolic process, the everyday occurrence of synthesizing glycogen from blood glucose. The pathway of conversion of glucose to glycogen involves four to five enzymes, but the control of the pathway may require ten or more separate enzymes. This illustrates the importance of precise regulation of the rate of this pathway. And why is this precision so important? The capacity to synthesize glycogen is sufficiently high that if fully activated under the wrong conditions it could lead to severe hypoglycemia: but if the pathway were not activated sufficiently, it could lead to hyperglycemia. Indeed this may be part of the reason for hyperglycemia in type II diabetes.

This chapter will describe, in particular, the principles underlying the processes involved in precision of control from which, eventually, we may be able to provide a better quantitative assessment of the energy expended in control. The principles will be illustrated by examples that range from recovery from exercise through burns or sepsis to the cell cycle. First, however, it is necessary to have an understanding of how knowledge of control is achieved and to appreciate what is meant by *metabolic-control-logic*.

METABOLIC-CONTROL-LOGIC

An approach for provision of a qualitative model of control involves the following stages (1).

1. Identification of the equilibrium nature of all the reactions in the pathway;
2. Identification of the flux-generating step;
3. A study of the properties of the enzymes or systems in the pathway; identify internal communication system: comparing substrate concentrations with K_m and inhibitor concentrations with K_i, predict possible control sites;
4. Identification of reactions regulated by external regulators;
5. Formulation of a theory of control;
6. Testing of the theory;
7. Acceptance, modification or rejection of the theory.

The authors consider that this 7-point approach provides the *best* means for identifying effectors of enzymes or transport processes; knowledge of these effectors permits the formulation of a hypothesis of control of changes in flux through a pathway or of the concentration of an important intracellular signal. It should be brought to the attention of readers that enzymes in the test tube can interact with many compounds that change the activity but which have no known physiological significance. Such promiscuous behavior of enzymes can only be identified by a careful testing of the qualitative hypothesis based on the properties discovered in stage 4 of the above approach. It is unfortunate and misleading when hypotheses of control are based solely on the behavior of enzymes in the test tube. Since this behavior may be promiscuous or capricious, such hypotheses must always be rigorously tested before they are accepted. It should be emphasized that the above 7-point plan applies to both qualitative and quantitative approaches to metabolic control.

Once the qualitative theory has been tested and accepted it is then possible and indeed important to provide a quantitative model to test the hypothesis *in detail*. However, to provide a quantitative model, mechanisms for improving sensitivity in control have to be identified and, if they are present, incorporated into the model. In order to understand the mechanisms by which sensitivity can be increased, the subject of sensitivity must be understood.

Sensitivity in Metabolic Regulation

Sensitivity in metabolic regulation can be defined as the quantitative relationship between the relative change in enzyme activity and the relative change is concentration of the regulator. (If the concentration of a regulator (X) changes by $\triangle X$, the relative change is $\triangle X/X$; similarly if the flux (J) changes by $\triangle J$, the relative change is $\triangle J/J$. The sensitivity of J to the change in concentration of (X) is given by the ratio $(\triangle J/J):(\triangle X/X)$ and this sensitivity is indicated by the symbol s (see Fig. 1; ref.

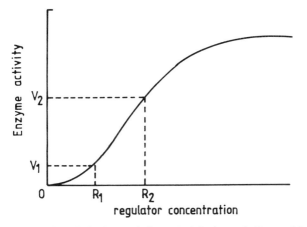

FIG. 1. A definition of sensitivity in metabolic control. A change in the regulator concentration, R, produces a change in the enzyme activity, V. An increase in concentration of R from R_1 to R_2 increases the activity from V_1 to V_2. Sensitivity can be defined as the relationship between these changes such that $(R_2 - R_1)/R_1$ produces a change $(V_2 + V_1)/V_1$. Sensitivity is the quantitative relationship between these two values.

2). For example, if the concentration of a regulator increases twofold, the question arises as to how large an increase in enzyme activity will this produce? The greater the response of enzyme activity to a given increase in regulator concentration, the greater is the sensitivity. To understand more clearly what may be involved in providing sensitivity it is necessary to begin with the simplest way in which a protein can interact with a small regulator–that is, equilibrium-binding.

Equilibrium-Binding of a Regulator to an Enzyme

It is likely that all regulators modify the activity of an enzyme by binding in a reversible manner to a protein. [This protein may not be the immediate target enzyme but may be an enzyme involved in an interconversion-cycle that controls the target enzyme by covalent modification (1).] Such binding, which is described as equilibrium-binding, will control the activity of the enzyme as follows:

$$E + R \leftrightharpoons E^*R$$

where E is the inactive form of the enzyme and E* is the active form. The asterisk indicates that the binding of the effector molecule R has changed the conformation of the catalytic site of the enzyme to produce the active form of the enzyme. The normal response of enzyme activity to the binding of the regulator is hyperbolic. Unfortunately, this response is relatively "inefficient" for metabolic regulation; for example, a twofold change in regulator concentration will change the enzyme activity by no more than twofold (i.e., the maximum sensitivity is unity). This may be difficult to accept when simply observing the steepness of the initial part of a hyperbolic

TABLE 1. *The relative change in concentration of regulator that is necessary to increase the activity of an enzyme from 10% to 90% of maximum activity when change in activity is due to equilibrium binding of a regulator*

Degree of sigmoidity of response of enzyme activity to regulator concentration	Concentration of regulator providing		Relative change in regulator concentration necessary to increase activity from 10% to 90%
	10% Activity	90% Activity	
Hyperbolic (no sigmoidity)	0.11	9.0	81.0
+	0.18	8.0	44.4
+ + +	1.20	9.8	9.2
+ + + + +	2.60	12.6	4.8
+ + + + + +	5.00	19.6	3.9
+ + + + + + + +	9.60	32.6	3.4

The reaction that is described by a hyperbolic response is $E + R \rightleftarrows E*R$ and to obtain an increase in enzyme activity from 10% to 90% of maximum requires a change in regulator concentration of 81-fold. The reaction that would produce a nonhyperbolic response is $E + nR \rightleftarrows E(R)n$—that is more than one molecule of regulator bound to the enzyme. If the Monod, Wyman, Changeux model for a sigmoid curve is used for calculation of the relationship between regulator concentration and activity, the calculation shows that for a change from 10% to 90% the relative change in the concentration of regulator is less than 81-fold and for an exaggerated sigmoid curve much less than 81-fold ($\sim$ fourfold) (28). Note by reference to Fig. 1 that this improvement in sensitivity is achieved largely by a decrease in the activity at the lower concentrations of regulator—that is only 10% of the activity is achieved at $\sim$ 100-fold greater concentration of regulator for an exaggerated sigmoid response in comparison to a hyperbolic response.

curve. However, it must be appreciated that sensitivity is defined on the basis of relative changes and not absolute changes in concentration. It will be seen that many means of improving sensitivity tend to decrease the activity of the system at low concentrations of substrate (see below) (see Fig. 1).

The hyperbolic response is the simplest relationship between a protein and its regulator, or between a hormone and its receptor or a neurotransmitter and its receptor. It can therefore be considered as the basic response with which any mechanism for improving sensitivity can be compared. The basic limitation of this mechanism is given in Table 1. Not surprisingly, nature has provided mechanisms for improving sensitivity in control over that provided by the hyperbolic curve. These are described below.

Mechanisms for Improving Sensitivity at Non-Equilibrium Reactions

Multiplicity of Regulators

It has been assumed, in the previous section, that there is only one regulator for the enzyme. However, it is possible for an enzyme to be regulated by several different regulators which bind at different sites on the enzyme. In this case, provided the concentrations of all the regulators change in the same direction (or in directions to change the activity of the enzyme in the same way) the effect of all the regulators will be additive. A good example is 6-phosphofructokinase in muscle which may be influenced by at least 8 effectors (see ref. 1).

Co-Operativity

For many enzymes that play a key role in metabolic regulation, the response of their activity to the substrate or regulator concentration is sigmoid. This phenomenon is known as positive cooperativity. For part of the concentration range of the regulator, the sensitivity will be greater than that provided by the hyperbolic response, i.e., greater than unity, and the quantitative significance of this can be calculated by using a simple molecular model of cooperativity (Table 1) (1).

The classic example of a sigmoid relationship is the binding of oxygen to hemoglobin. Despite the fact that most biology students know the molecular basis for its sigmoid nature, the physiological advantage over that of the hyperbolic curve of myoglobin is not often appreciated. It is not due to a difference in the lungs: the extent of binding of oxygen at the partial pressure of oxygen in the lungs is similar for the two proteins. However, myoglobin releases most of its oxygen at the very low partial pressure of oxygen close to the mitochondrion within the muscle fiber whereas, in contrast, hemoglobin releases it at the much higher partial pressure in the capillaries. Note that this is not an explanation—only a description of the two curves. The high oxygen partial pressure ensures a high rate of oxygen diffusion from the capillary to the muscle (or other cell): this then ensures that aerobic metabolism can occur at a sufficiently high rate to provide for the *normal* functioning of the tissues of the body. Mammalian life as we know it would not be possible if myoglobin was the transport protein for oxygen.

It should be noted that proteins that exhibit cooperativity are, in general, more complex than those which exhibit a hyperbolic response and this requires an increase in genetic information. The energetic cost of this is, of course, very difficult to assess.

Interconversion Cycles

A number of enzymes (e.g., glycogen phosphorylase, pyruvate dehydrogenase) are known to exist in two forms, conventionally designated a and b, one being a covalent modification of the other. The conversion of one form to the other can be brought about, for example, by reaction with ATP so that one form is a phosphorylated modification of the other. In general, only one of the two forms (a) has significant catalytic activity so that the activity of the enzyme and hence the flux through the reaction can be regulated by altering the proportion of the enzyme in any one form. The interconversions between the forms are carried out by enzymes, one for each direction; and each enzyme catalyzes a non-equilibrium reaction (Fig.

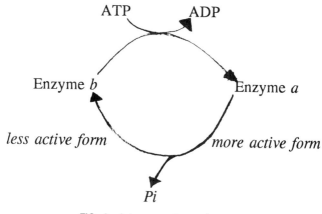

FIG. 2.   Interconversion cycles.

2). The activity of one or both of these interconverting enzymes can be altered by regulators. Although the improvement in sensitivity provided by such cycles is likely to be large, it is dependent upon the kinetic properties of *both* interconverting enzymes and very few of these enzymes have received a sufficiently detailed kinetic analysis that would be necessary to allow an estimation of the improvement in sensitivity. Highest sensitivity is achieved when the K_m values of both interconverting enzymes for their substrates are much lower than the concentration of the substrates, which are the enzymes that are to be covalently modified. This has been termed zero-order ultrasensitivity (3). In other words, both interconverting enzymes catalyze processes that approach saturation with substrate (4).

The covalent modification of an enzyme overcomes one of the limitations of the equilibrium binding—that is, the dependence upon mass action, i.e., the change in concentration of effector which can only change the target enzyme activity by equilibrium binding (Table 1). The response of the target enzyme, which is now controlled by the proportion of the enzyme in the active (or inactive form), is dependent upon a covalent reaction—that is, one in which the overall reaction is thermodynamically favored and is much less dependent upon concentration changes.

This mechanism requires a complex interplay of kinetics of the two interconverting enzymes and hence a considerable increase in genetic information will be required to generate such a process. Again, the energetic cost of this is unknown.

Substrate Cycle

A totally different mechanism for improving sensitivity is known as the substrate cycle. This is discussed at some length, since it is considered to be important in the dissipation of chemical energy (see below).

It is possible for a reaction that is non-equilibrium in the forward direction of a pathway (i.e., A → B) to be opposed by a reaction that is non-equilibrium in the

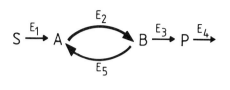

FIG. 3. A hypothetical substrate cycle. In this hypothetical pathway, enzyme E_2 catalyzes a key regulatory reaction and to improve the sensitivity of control at this reaction, a reverse reaction catalyzed by enzyme E_5 is present in the tissue and both enzymes are simultaneously catalytically active. And it is proposed that the activities of both enzymes can be increased to increase the rate of substrate cycling and hence provide an improvement in sensitivity for metabolic control.

reverse direction of the pathway (i.e., B → A). Both reactions must be chemically distinct (different reactions) so that they will be catalyzed by separate enzymes (Fig. 3). A substrate cycle between A and B occurs if the two enzymes are simultaneously catalytically active. For every molecule of A converted to B and back again to A, chemical energy must be converted to heat, which is lost to the environment. The role of substrate cycles in improving sensitivity should be appreciated by reference to Table 2.

An example of a substrate cycle is the fructose 6-phosphate/fructose 1,6-bisphosphate cycle (Fig. 4). This cycle is considered to be important in the control of the rate of degradation of glycogen to lactate, which provides energy for muscle under anaerobic or hypoxic conditions (e.g., at the beginning of exercise, climbing stairs, sprinting). The operation of this cycle results in the hydrolysis of adenosine triphosphate (ATP) to adenosine diphosphate (ADP) and phosphate (Pi), as fructose 6-phosphate is converted to fructose 1,6-bisphosphate and back again, so that the chemical energy available in the ATP molecule is converted into heat. Consequently,

TABLE 2. *Effect of a small increase in regulator concentration on net flux through a reaction controlled by a substrate cycle*

	Enzyme activities[a]		Net flux	Relative fold
Concentration of regulator	E2	E5	A to B	increase in flux
Situation 1[b]				
Basal	10	9.8	0.2	
Fourfold above basal	90	9.8	81.2	406
Situation 2[c]				
Basal	10	9.8	0.2	
Fourfold above basal	90	1.0	89.0	445

Note the dramatic improvement in sensitivity over that provided by equilibrium binding (Table 1).

[a] The activities are hypothetical and are based on the situation described in Fig. 3.

[b] In situation 1, the regulator has no effect on the reverse reaction catalyzed by E_5. The ratio, cycling rate/flux in the basal state is 49.

[c] In situation 2, the regulator not only increases the activity of E_2 but decreases that of E_5. The improvement in the relative change of the net flux is, however, not much greater than that in situation 1 (445-fold compared with 406).

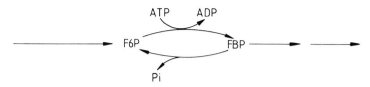

FIG. 4. The fructose 6-phosphate/fructose bisphosphate cycle in muscle. The forward reaction is catalyzed by phosphofructokinase and the reverse reaction by fructose bisphosphatase. Both enzymes are present in skeletal muscle (2) and there is now evidence that they are simultaneously active and that the rate of cycling can be increased by catecholamine hormones (5).

the greater the rate of cycling, the greater the rate of conversion of chemical energy into heat, which is then lost to the environment.

The role of substrate cycling in the provision of sensitivity and flexibility in metabolic regulation has been discussed in detail in several reviews (1,2,5). The role of a cycle can best be understood when it is appreciated that, in some conditions, an enzyme activity may have to be reduced to values closely approaching zero. Even with a sigmoid response this would require that the concentration of an activator be reduced to almost zero or that of an inhibitor increased to an almost infinite level (due to the relatively ineffectual nature of equilibrium binding). Such enormous changes in concentration are not common in living organisms, since they would cause catastrophic osmotic and ionic problems and unwanted side-reactions. However, the net flux through a reaction can be reduced to very low values (approaching zero) via a substrate cycle. Thus, as the concentration of the product of the forward enzyme (E_2) (i.e., B in Fig. 3) increases, it is converted back to substrate A by the reverse enzyme (E_5), which maintains a low concentration of the product (B). This ensures that the *net* flux (i.e., A to B) is very low despite a finite activity of the forward enzyme and a moderate concentration of the activator of the enzyme. Now if the concentration of this activator is increased, by only a small amount above that at which the activities of the two enzymes are almost identical (and the flux is almost zero), the activity of E_2 will increase so that the net flux through the reaction will increase from almost zero to a moderate rate. Such a cycle, therefore, provides a large improvement in sensitivity; indeed, it can be seen as a means of producing a threshold (or almost threshold) response.

And, of importance, the cycle provides an improvement in sensitivity without changing the properties or characteristics of the enzyme catalyzing the forward reaction in the pathway and for this reason can be seen to be different from the other mechanisms for improving sensitivity: this has also been shown to be the case when the precise quantitative role of substrate cycles in metabolic control is considered (4).

One advantage of the substrate-cycling mechanism for increasing sensitivity is that the sensitivity can be varied very quickly and very effectively. This is achieved by varying the rate of cycling; sensitivity is proportional to the ratio, cycling rate/flux (2). In contrast, the increase in sensitivity provided by, for example, cooperativity (see above in Table 1) is not variable, since it is dependent on the fixed properties of the enzyme. It is considered that the variability of sensitivity in regulation provided

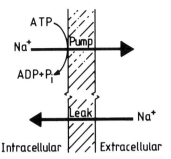

FIG. 5. The Na^+-translocation cycle. The presence of an Na^+ leak and an $(Na^+ + K^+)$-activated ATPase in many tissues suggests that the "Na^+-translocation substrate cycle" is a general phenomenon. We consider that the role of this cycle in tissues is to provide a sensitive mechanism for the precise regulation of the intracellular concentration of Na^+. It is known that the concentration difference between intracellular and extracellular cations is biologically very important.

by cycling is a *major* advantage. Such variations can be controlled by hormones or nerves. In addition, when the sensitivity is increased by increased cycling rates, this does not interfere in the basic cellular control mechanism. Further, the increase in genetic information necessary to provide this mechanism may be small, but the investment in energy when the cycle is operating to provide sensitivity in control may be large.

The above discussion has focused attention on the role of substrate cycles in regulation of metabolic flux. However, control of metabolic flux is only one aspect of the phenomenon of homeostasis: control of the concentration of certain ions (e.g., intracellular Na^+ or Ca^{2+}), control of the concentration of key proteins (e.g., many regulatory enzymes) and control of the concentration of key metabolites (e.g., plasma glucose, plasma glutamine, intracellular cholesterol) must also occur. These concentrations may be maintained by what is in essence a substrate cycle: the Na^+ concentration in many, if not all, cells is probably precisely regulated by the balance between the Na^+-leak process and the Na^+-pump process which has been described as a "translocation cycle" (Fig. 5) (2). Indeed it is difficult to conceive of a process as effective as this translocation cycle for the regulation of the *precise* intracellular Na^+ concentration; furthermore, it provides a specific physiological function for the Na^+-leak process.

Similarly, the Ca^{2+} ion concentration in the cytosol and especially in the mitochondrial matrix may be regulated by a similar translocation cycle; and the cycle may provide a threshold response to the uptake of Ca^{2+} by the mitochondrion in response to an increase in cytosolic Ca^{2+} concentration (6). In some cells, the intracellular cholesterol concentration may be regulated by the balance between esterification of cholesterol and hydrolysis of cholesterol ester (1). And a translocation cycle in the release of glutamine from muscle may play an important role in the control of the plasma concentration of glutamine, which is an important fuel for the immune system (see below).

Branched Point Sensitivity and Precision in Control

Much of metabolism is branched and although this may be necessary as an essential part of the diversity of reactions in the body, it is considered that branched-points may also have been adapted for precision in regulation, as described next.

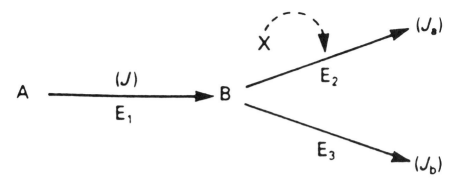

FIG. 6. The theory of enhanced sensitivity in control afforded by branch-points in pathways. In this system there are three fluxes, J, J_a, and J_b, such that $J = (J_a + J_b)$; X is a regulator of E_2 and, since there is no *direct* feedback from E_2 to E_1, X changes J_a at the expense of J_b, leaving J unchanged. Let us assume that J_a represents a biosynthetic pathway for which B is a precursor (e.g., J_a could represent the generation of purine and pyrimidine nucleotides for DNA and/or RNA synthesis and B the precursor glutamine). As J_a is increased (by regulator X), the concentration of B will tend to decrease and "deflect" flux from J_b to J_a. However, assuming that E_2 is not saturated with B, this decreased concentration of B will also reduce the flux through E_2 and hence reduce J_a. Consequently, the increased J_a brought about by regulator X will be "opposed" by the decreased concentration of B, resulting in a less effective response of J_a to X. This will decrease the precision of control of the flux through J_a by X. If, during the cell cycle, a *precise* increase in the rate of *de novo* pathways for purine and pyrimidine nucleotide synthesis was required, this may not be provided by this system due to the opposition effect. There are two solutions to this problem. One is to provide a sensitive feedback regulatory mechanism to increase the flux through the pathway when required. The other is to increase massively the flux through J and J_b. In other words, the highest sensitivity for the flux J_a is achieved when the fluxes J and J_b are much greater than J_a. Under these conditions the biosynthetic pathway (J_a) does not become seriously limited by changes in precursor concentration during the "deflection" of the flux from J_b to J_a and is therefore most sensitive to the action of regulator X.

The increased sensitivity in control provided by the branched point mechanism is similar in principle to that achieved in the substrate cycle; a continuous high flux in one branch of a pathway provides optimal conditions for the precise regulation of the (much smaller) flux in the other branch. Thus, the sensitivity in the arm which has the smaller flux depends upon the ratio of fluxes in the two branches. This is equivalent to the sensitivity improvement in cycling which is produced by the cycling rate/flux (see above). The process is discussed below.

It can be shown that if a metabolic influx, J, divides into two fluxes J_a and J_b, and J_a is regulated by factor X, the highest sensitivity of flux J_a to changes in the regulator X is achieved when $J_b \gg J_a$ (see Fig. 6). In non-mathematical terms, high sensitivity is achieved because the rate of the low-flux pathway (that is, J_a) can be increased markedly without decreasing significantly the concentration of the metabolic intermediate(s) of the main pathway (B). A large decrease in the concentration of B would "oppose" the stimulation of the rate of the low-flux pathway. Thus the system also serves to stabilize the concentration of B. The significance of this is illustrated by reference to nutrition of the immune system.

TABLE 3. *Rates of utilization of glucose or glutamine by lymphocytes and macrophages and other tissues in mouse, rat, and man*

Animal	Tissue	Rates of utilization (nmol/hr per mg protein)	
		Glucose	Glutamine
Mouse	Macrophages	355	186
Rat	Mesenteric lymphocytes	42	223
	Maximally-working heart	1,000	—
Man	Peripheral lymphocytes	65	190
	Brain	200	—

It should be noted that the rate of utilization of glutamine by lymphocytes in man may be equivalent to the rate of glucose utilization by the brain—and since the amount of tissue is approximately the same (~1,400g) the demand for glutamine by cells of the immune system may be similar to that of the brain for glucose. It is therefore not inconsequential!
Data are taken from Newsholme and Leech, ref. 1, and Newsholme et al., ref. 11.

Cellular Nutrition and the Immune System

There is now considerable evidence that rapidly dividing cells [e.g., fibroblasts, tumor cells (7)], those with the potential for rapid cell division [e.g., lymphocyte (8,9)] and those with a high protein-synthesizing capacity [e.g., macrophages (10)] utilize both glutamine *and* glucose (and probably fatty acids) at very high rates (for reviews, see refs. 10–12; Table 3). However, little of the carbon of the glutamine, glucose, or fatty acid is completely oxidized by the Krebs cycle (9,11). The role of partial oxidation of glutamine (glutaminolysis) in rapidly-dividing cells has been considered previously to be the provision of energy *and/or* the provision of both nitrogen and carbon for precursors for synthesis of macromolecules (e.g., purine and pyrimidine nucleotides for DNA and RNA). However, there are problems with both explanations. Quantitative studies show that the rate of glutaminolysis is markedly in excess (>2500-fold) of that of the precursor requirements (Table 4) (13). But it has been shown that enzymes of the Krebs cycle, necessary for complete oxidation, *are*

TABLE 4. *Maximal activity of carbamoylphosphate synthetase II (CPS-II), rates of synthesis of uridine nucleotides, and rate of glutamine utilization by lymphocytes*

Rates (nmol/h per mg protein)		
CPS-II activity	[^{14}C]-incorporation from HCO_3 into uridine nucleotides	Glutamine utilization
6.3	0.08	223

CPS-II activity represents the maximum capacity for pyrimidine nucleotide synthesis in these cells, which is considerably less than the actual measured rate of uridine nucleotide synthesis under the conditions of the experiment.
Data are taken from Szondy and Newsholme, ref. 13.

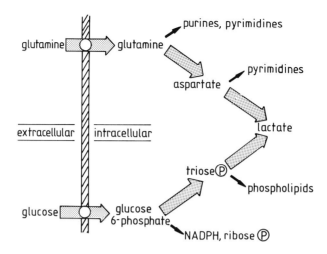

FIG. 7. The oxidative and biosynthetic branches of the glutaminolytic and glycolytic pathways in lymphocytes and other rapidly dividing cells. For glutaminolysis, glutamine provides nitrogen for both the purine and pyrimidine rings and aspartate provides both nitrogen and carbon for the pyrimidine ring. For glycolysis, glucose 6-phosphate is the substrate for the pentose phosphate pathway, which provides both ribose and NADPH, and triose phosphate provides glycerol 3-phosphate, which is a component of phospholipids in membranes. It has been shown that the fluxes through glutaminolysis and glycolysis are massively in excess of the rates and even the maximum capacities of the biosynthetic pathways. This is indicated by the breadth of the arrows in the diagram.

indeed present in these cells (9,11) so that if energy generation *per se* was the major reason for high rates of glutamine utilization, it would be expected that more of the carbon skeleton of glutamine would be converted to acetyl-CoA for complete oxidation via the Krebs cycle (i.e., that glutamine oxidation rather than glutaminolysis would occur).

So why is glutamine used at such a high rate? On the basis of control theory (4) it has been suggested that the high rates of glutaminolysis (and glycolysis) provide optimal conditions for the *precise* and sensitive control of the rate of use of the intermediates of these pathways for biosynthesis *precisely* at the time required by the synthetic processes during the cell cycle (e.g., glutamine for pure and pyrimidine nucleotide synthesis (14,15) (Fig. 7). This, therefore, is an example of branched point sensitivity. Consequently, any decrease in the flux through this glutamine pathway—even if small—could impair the functioning of the immune system (11): indeed, a decrease in the level of glutamine in the culture medium has been shown to decrease markedly the rate of proliferation of rat lymphocytes (13) (Table 5) and human lymphocytes (16); and a decrease in the concentration of glutamine has been shown to decrease the rate of phagocytosis in macrophages (16). It is important to appreciate that the high rate of glutamine utilization (and also those of glucose and fatty acids) and its partial oxidation plus the effects of decreases in the concentration of glutamine are predicted by the theoretical work (4).

In non-mathematical terms, high sensitivity is achieved because the rate of the

TABLE 5. *The half time required to cause a maximal rate of incorporation of ^{3}H-thymidine into DNA in rat mesenteric lymphocytes and circulating lymphocytes of man stimulated by concanavalin-A at different concentrations of glutamine*

Concentration of glutamine (mM)	~ Half times for maximum rate of incorporation (hour)	
	Rat	Man
0.01	>60	>60
0.05	50	>48
0.3	39	30
0.6	—	27
1.0	27	—

The normal concentration of glutamine in rat plasma is 0.9 mM and that in man is 0.6 mM: therefore a decrease below this physiological value would be expected to increase the time it takes to reach the maximum rate of proliferation of T-lymphocytes. Invading organisms would gain an advantage if they invaded when the plasma glutamine level was decreased. Is this an explanation for opportunistic infections?

Data are from Szondy and Newsholme, ref. 13, and Newsholme and Crabtree, ref. 14.

biosynthetic pathway (e.g., purine or pyrimidine nucleotide synthesis) can be increased markedly without decreasing significantly the concentration of the metabolic precursors (e.g., glutamine, aspartate) which are constituents of the main pathway: a decrease in concentration of glutamine, for example, could "oppose" the stimulation of the biosynthetic pathway for synthesis of purine and pyrimidine nucleotides. In lymphocytes, this high sensitivity will be particularly important when macromolecular synthesis is required during proliferation in response to an immune challenge; but, in the terminally differentiated macrophage, it is likely to be for synthesis of mRNA for producing secretory and receptor proteins and enzymes when demanded by an immune challenge (10).

Furthermore, this explanation provides an answer to the question of why these cells do not appear to allow pyruvate, generated from either glucose or glutamine, or acetyl-CoA generated from β-oxidation of fatty acids to be oxidized. If fully oxidized, a large amount of energy would be produced (via the Krebs cycle and electron-transport process) and, since a high ATP concentration inhibits key reactions in both glycolysis (e.g., 6-phosphofructokinase) and glutaminolysis (e.g., oxoglutarate dehydrogenase), high rates of these latter processes would not be possible: and thus the advantage of precision in control of the rates of biosynthesis would be lost. (It is, however, possible that, at some stage of the cell cycle, when the demand for ATP becomes very large, the rate of the complete Krebs cycle will increase dramatically.)

The principle of branched point sensitivity may be of considerable importance in understanding some of the unusual characteristics of rapidly dividing cells and further theoretical and practical work is required in this area. Thus, there is evidence in lymphocytes that high but partial rates of fatty acid oxidation may be important in provision of a dynamic buffering system for acetyl-CoA, which has an extremely important biosynthetic function in such cells (Fig. 8) (17). This may be the *raison*

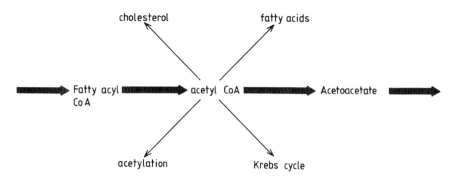

FIG. 8. Branched-point sensitivity for the ketogenic pathway in lymphocytes. It has been shown that rat mesenteric lymphocytes have a high rate of formation of acetoacetate from endogenous substrate that is presumed to be fatty acids (35). The role of this ketogenic pathway in lymphocytes is considered to be the maintenance of a constant level of acetyl-CoA despite marked variations in its rate of utilization by these cells for synthesis of specific fatty acid (e.g., myristic acid for myristylation of proteins) for chain extension of fatty acids to produce specific long chain fatty acids that may be required for membrane structure, for cholesterol synthesis for new membranes, for acetylation of proteins (e.g., histones) that may play a role in control of cell cycle activity and of course for extra ATP generation by the Krebs cycle if required at some specific time during the cell cycle.

d'être for the apparent conversion of fatty acids to ketone bodies in these cells but the significance of this phenomenon in the whole animal is unknown.

It is, however, unclear as to how much energy may be required to maintain such branched-point sensitivity in these cells. The maintenance of the plasma glutamine concentration will require energy (see below) but whether branched-point sensitivity imposes a rate of metabolism that is expensive, in energetic terms, is unclear. The high rate of glycolysis in tumor cells and in immune cells has been proposed by the authors to provide branched-point sensitivity. The process involves the conversion of glucose to lactate and unless lactate can be completely oxidized by other tissues it will be converted to glucose in liver. The conversion of glucose to lactate in one tissue (immune cells) and re-conversion to glucose in the liver is known as the Cori cycle and is equivalent to a large inter-tissue substrate cycle. It therefore leads to expenditure of energy. Its quantitative importance in energy expenditure is, however, still uncertain but it may be quite large. Further work is needed on the fate of the endproducts of glutaminolysis and of β-oxidation of fatty acids in these cells. It is possible that if glutamate and ketone bodies, which are released by immune cells, are reconverted to glutamine and fatty acids, respectively, the extra energy expenditure required for these biosynthetic processes would be high.

SOURCE OF GLUTAMINE FOR THE IMMUNE SYSTEM

If glutamine is required at such a high rate by the immune system, from where does it arise? Glutamine will be made available in the lumen of the intestine from the digestion of protein. However, studies demonstrate that little of this glutamine enters the bloodstream; the absorptive cells of the small intestine utilize glutamine at a high rate and probably utilize almost all that is absorbed from the lumen of the gut. Hence, to satisfy the high demand for glutamine by the immune system (and other tissues, such as kidney, colon, and the small intestine), it must be provided within the body. There is now considerable evidence that the major tissue involved in glutamine production is skeletal muscle: it contains a high concentration of glutamine, it has the enzymic capacity to synthesize glutamine, it is known to release glutamine into the bloodstream at a high rate, and *in vitro* studies indicate that this rate can be controlled (18,19).

Control of Glutamine Release by Skeletal Muscle

Using the 7-point approach to understanding control of processes, it appears that both glutamine synthetase and the outward transport of glutamine are non-equilibrium processes. However, it appears that glutamine transport, rather than glutamine synthesis, is the flux-generating step—that is, the outward transport of glutamine approaches saturation with substrate (intracellular glutamine). The evidence that transport is the flux-generating process for the release of glutamine into the extracellular space and, therefore, into the bloodstream is as follows:

1. A comparison of the rates of release of glutamine from isolated incubated soleus muscle of the rat in relation to the variations in the concentration of intracellular glutamine provides a very approximate K_m value for outward transport of glutamine of less than 0.3 mM glutamine; yet, in rat soleus muscle, the concentration of glutamine is normally >4 mM (20).

2. There is no relationship between the change in muscle glutamine concentration and the change in the rate of glutamine release by isolated incubated muscle: that is, the rate of release is independent of the glutamine concentration.

The simplest interpretation of these findings is that a decrease in the intracellular concentration of glutamine will not cause a significant decrease in the rate of release, that is, the process approaches saturation with its substrate, intracellular glutamine.

What is the physiologic importance of this piece of biochemistry? First, it suggests that the rate of *synthesis* of glutamine in muscle will normally have no effect on the rate of glutamine *release* from muscle: that is, the rate of glutamine release is "protected" from variations in the intracellular glutamine concentration. Thus, although the activity of glutamine synthetase may be increased in conditions associated with an increase in the rate of muscle glutamine release (e.g., burns, cancer cachexia, high levels of glucocorticoids), this enhancement functions not to *control* the rate of release but to maintain a steady-state concentration of glutamine in the muscle. It is, of course, possible that the rate of glutamine synthesis could, under some conditions, be so much lower than that of release that the intracellular glutamine level would fall to such low levels that the rate of release would be decreased; in this case, the release process would no longer be flux-generating and glutamine synthesis might *then* control the rate of release: this, however, may be a *pathological* rather than a *physiological* condition.

Second, factors that control the rate of glutamine release from muscle must affect the flux-generating step, that is, the outward transport of glutamine. To identify physiologic factors that control rates of glutamine release by skeletal muscle, this transport rather than glutamine synthetase process must be studied in depth (stage 4 of the 7-point approach described above).

Third, since the process of glutamine utilization by lymphocytes and macrophages does not approach saturation with glutamine, at the normal plasma levels of this amino acid, the transport of glutamine out of muscle will act as the flux-generating step for the process of glutamine utilization in cells of the immune system. Consequently, control of this transport process in muscle will influence the rate of glutamine utilization and, hence, the function of cells of the immune system, particularly during an immune challenge.

The extremely important conclusion that stems from this application of metabolic-control-logic is that *muscle* must play a vital role in maintenance of the rate of the key process of glutamine utilization in the *immune cells* and, consequently, skeletal muscle can be considered to be part of the immune system (Fig. 9). This may therefore be important in understanding why skeletal muscle is broken down under conditions of burns, sepsis, trauma, or surgery: it is suggested that this is to provide amino acids for synthesis of glutamine (11).

The above discussion has focused attention on the process of transport of glutamine out of muscle and has emphasized that it plays a vitally important role in the immune system. For this reason, perhaps, it is not surprising that the control of glutamine release from muscle may be subject to mechanisms for improving its sensitivity to metabolic control by physiological factors, such as hormones and/or lymphokines. One means of increasing the sensitivity is described below.

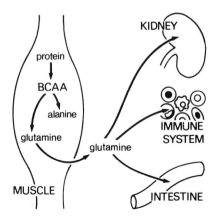

FIG. 9. The relationship between glutamine production in muscle and glutamine utilization in various tissues. The flux-generating step for glutamine utilization in kidney, lymphocytes, and intestine may be in muscle, so that glutamine metabolism can be considered as a branched metabolic pathway which is initiated in muscle and is completed in several other tissues. The clinical implications of this relationship may be considerable, especially in that control of glutamine release by muscle may be a major site of hormonal regulation.

TABLE 6. *Properties of the processes of release and uptake of glutamine by muscle*

	K_m (mM)	V_{max} (nmol/min per mg protein)
Glutamine release	<0.3	100
Glutamine uptake	7.0	1020

Data for release are approximate (Parry-Billings, ref. 20) and data for uptake taken from Hundal et al., ref. 29.

A Translocation Cycle in the Release of Glutamine by Muscle

Glutamine can be both released (19) and taken up by skeletal muscle (18). The properties of these two processes are given in Table 6.

Some workers have tacitly assumed that the *inward* transport of glutamine is the same process as glutamine release from muscle (18). It does not appear to have been considered that uptake and release could be two *separate* processes and this, perhaps, has led to some confusion. Thus, it has been suggested that glutamine transport across the membrane is "symmetrical"; this implies that both processes are near-equilibrium, that is, the same process that transports glutamine out also transports it into the muscle. However, calculations of the free energy change for glutamine uptake and the release process indicate that they are both non-equilibrium. If both processes are non-equilibrium, transport cannot be "symmetrical." Consequently, it is concluded that the processes of glutamine uptake and release by muscle are distinct, that is, that two different transporters are involved and that they provide a *translocation cycle* between the extracellular and intracellular glutamine pools.

It is predicted that this cycle will enhance the sensitivity of the mechanism(s) that controls the rate of glutamine release from muscle. Indeed, given the proposed importance of glutamine release from skeletal muscle (see above and below), it would be expected that the sensitivity of control of this process would be enhanced by such a mechanism. It would also allow feedback control by the plasma glutamine level which would serve to maintain the plasma concentration constant.

This cycle is, therefore, predicted to play, in principle, a role in the regulation of the plasma glutamine similar to that of the cycle between glucose and glucose 6-phosphate in the liver in the regulation of the plasma glucose level or the cycle between triglyceride and fatty acid in adipose tissue in the regulation of the plasma fatty acid level (Fig. 10).

SUBSTRATE CYCLES: THEIR RANGE AND QUANTITATIVE IMPORTANCE IN THERMOGENESIS

A substrate cycle requires the presence of enzymes in a cell that catalyzes the forward and back reactions (different reactions and different enzymes): hence the enzymatic potential exists for a large number of cycles. However, the potential for

control of plasma glucose level by the liver

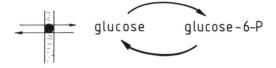

control of plasma FFA level by adipose tissue

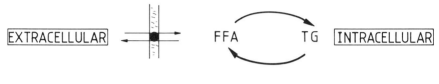

control of plasma glutamine level by muscle

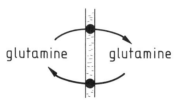

FIG. 10. The substrate cycles proposed to regulate the rate of mobilization of liver glycogen, adipose tissue, triglyceride, and muscle glutamine. In liver, the glucose/glucose 6-phosphate cycle catalyzed by glucokinase and glucose 6-phosphatase appears to play a role in the regulation of glucose uptake and release by the liver (1). In adipose tissue, the triglyceride/fatty acid cycle is considered to play an important role in the regulation of the rate of the mobilization of fatty acids from adipose tissue. And in muscle, it is considered that the glutamine translocation cycle plays a role in the control of the precise rate of glutamine release by this tissue for other use by other tissues as shown in Fig. 9.

substrate cycling does not prove that they exist: this must be demonstrated experimentally. This was first done for the triacylglycerol/fatty acid substrate cycle *in vivo* in 1959 (21) and *in vitro* in 1963 (22). In 1973, the use of dual-isotopic labeling was developed for the measurement of the glucose/glucose 6-phosphate and the fructose 6-phosphate/fructose 1,6-bisphosphate cycle (for review see ref. 5). Since that time, the rates of several other cycles have been measured.

A very important question is the rate of substrate cycling in man. A survey of some cycles in man and their rates in some conditions is presented in Table 7. These results demonstrate the existence of some such cycles in man; and the results have only been obtained in the last few years. Eventually, when a larger number of cycles have been investigated quantitatively, including for example the glutamine translocation cycle in skeletal muscle, it should be possible to indicate more precisely the quantitative importance of substrate cycles in thermogenesis: the presently available results not only indicate that they can account for considerable rates of thermogenesis but that the rates of such cycles change under conditions in which ther-

TABLE 7. *The rates of some substrate cycles in man*

Substrate cycle	Condition	Rate
Glucose/glucose 6-phosphate plus fructose 6-phosphate/fructose bisphosphate	Euthyroid	6.8 μmol/kg/min
	Hyperthyroid	7.7 μmol/kg/min
	Hypothyroid	1.1 μmol/kg/min
Glucose/glucose 6-phosphate	Basal	1.8 μmol/kg/min
Fructose 6-phosphate/fructose bisphosphate	Basal	0.7 μmol/kg/min
Glucose recycling (Cori cycle)	Euthyroid	1.3 μmol/kg/min
	Hyperthyroid	4.7 μmol/kg/min
Triacylglycerol/fatty acid	Injured	3.3 μmol/kg/min
	Basal	1.1 μmol/kg/min
	Glucose infusion	2.5 μmol/kg/min
	Normal	0.6 μmol/kg/min
	Burn injury	10.1 μmol/kg/min

For details see Newsholme and Challiss, ref. 5.

mogenesis is known to change in man. Three conditions in which cycles may play an important role are described below.

Postexercise Oxygen Consumption

Termination of exercise can occur almost instantaneously but this is also accompanied by a time-lag in the change in oxygen consumption. During this "recovery period," oxygen is consumed in excess of that required to support the metabolism of the resting muscle. This extra oxygen consumption in recovery was noted in the early 1920s and for many years has been ascribed to the payment of an oxygen debt. More recently it has been termed "postexercise recovery oxygen" or "extra postexercise oxygen consumption" (EPOC). The old name "debt" implied that it involved some form of reversal of the anaerobic processes that "saved' oxygen at the beginning of activity. However, this plays a minor role in explaining the magnitude of recovery oxygen after exercise.

A calculation has been carried out on the amount of oxygen that would be consumed by all of the processes considered to occur after exercise. It indicates a large difference between that calculated and that observed (Table 8). Despite the obvious inaccuracies inherent in such calculations, the oxygen not accounted for by "classical" processes is large: the authors consider that some of this oxygen may be accounted for by stimulation of the rates of substrate cycles which would require energy and therefore oxygen. The significance of increased rates of cycling would be to increase the sensitivity of metabolic control so that the increased rates of metabolism that occur during exercise can return gradually and smoothly to the normal resting level during the recovery period, and that fuel reserves, for example, glycogen can be restored to normal as quickly and effectively as possible but without

TABLE 8. Calculations on oxygen consumption required to restore metabolism to normal during a recovery period of 60 min following hard intermittent exercise

Recovery process requiring O_2 consumption	Calculated O_2 required	
	mmol/man	Percentage of EPOC
ATP and phosphocreatine resynthesis[a]	56.0	4.1
Lactate conversion to glycogen[b]	392	29
Repletion of oxymyoglobin plus oxyhemoglobin[c]	7.5	0.6
Increased work of heart[d]	43.0	3.2
Increased work of respiratory muscles[e]	17.5	1.3
Total	516	38.2

The total measured extra postexercise oxygen consumption (EPOC) during a 60 min period after exhaustive exercise was 1350 mmol O_2 (30).

The changes are taken from study by Karlsson and Saltin, ref. 30: the calculations provide similar results if data are taken from studies by Hermansen and Vaage ref. 31 and by Hultman et al. ref. 32.

In all the calculations a P/O ratio of 3.0 is assumed: hence 1 mmole of O_2 consumed is assumed to be equivalent to 6 mmole of ATP synthesized.

[a] 12 mmol of $\sim$ P per kg wet wt of muscle is required to restore ATP and phosphocreatine levels to pre-exercise values: therefore assuming all muscles are affected by the exercise equally, which is very unlikely, this is equal to $12 \times 40/100 \times 70/6 = 56$ mmol O_2, assuming 40% of body wt is muscle.

[b] 21 mmol of lactate was removed from 1 kg of muscle during 60 min: formation of glycogen from 2 mmoles of lactate requires 8 mmoles ATP. Therefore, 21 mmole lactate requires $8/6 \times 0.5 \times 21 = 14$ mmol O_2/kg muscle = 392 mmol O_2/man (that is, 28 kg muscle).

[c] Calculations were based on studies in dog (33): 1.5 ml/kg body wt estimated to have been released from venous blood; 0.9 ml/kg estimated to be released from stores of oxymyoglobin. Assuming this would be the same for 70 kg man oxygen required would be 168 ml or 7.5 mmol/man.

[d] Assuming that the increased work of heart is due to carrying increased O_2 needed as recovery O_2: this is 30.2 liter and assuming a utilization coefficient of O_2 in blood as 60% and an oxygen capacity of blood of 18.5 vol. %, the amount of blood required to transport the extra O_2 is about 300 liter. The heart has to work against a mean pressure of 100 mg Hg which is 0.132 atmos. Work done by heart = $100 \times 0.112 = 39.6$ liter atmos. = 965 kcal. Assuming an efficiency of heart of 25% – the amount of energy required is 3860 kcal or 772 ml of O_2. If further 25% is required for pulmonary circulation this is 0.96 liter or 43 mmoles O_2.

[e] It is assumed that for the utilization of 1 liter of O_2, 35 liters of air are inspired (34). Assuming the mean pressure in the pleural cavity is 15 mmHg the work done by the respiratory muscles in inspiring 35 liters is $35 \times 15/760 = 0.69$ liter atmos. = 16 kcal. Therefore, for 30.2 liter of O_2 = $16 \times 30.2 = 483$ kcal. Assuming 25% efficiency of respiratory muscle = 1852 kcal = 370 ml O_2 or 17.5 mmoles.

causing hypoglycemia. A speculative suggestion of the role of the fructose 6-phosphate/fructose bisphosphate cycle before, during, and after exercise is given in Fig. 11.

In the 1980s, a very carefully controlled and systematic study was carried out by a research group in Oslo. They showed that, after 60–90 minutes of exercise (at about 70% of VO_2max) in human volunteers, oxygen consumption was elevated for at least 12 hours after cessation of exercise (23). Similar findings were observed for this same level of exercise but lasting for shorter periods of time (20 and 40 minutes).

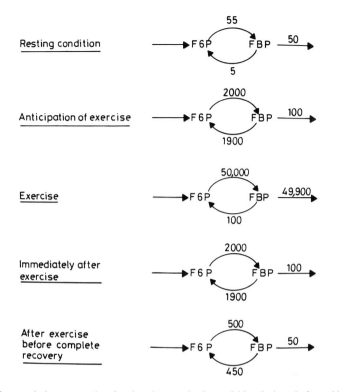

FIG. 11. A speculative suggestion for the changes in the activities 6-phosphofructokinase and fructose bisphosphatase during the 3 periods of exercise anticipation, activity, and recovery. In the resting condition, prior even to anticipation of exercise, the muscle is resting and the activity of phosphofructokinase is low and that of fructose bisphosphatase is even lower, that is the cycling rate is very low. Anticipation of exercise, especially of the sprint-type activity ("fight or flight" phenomenon) will, via stress hormones and nervous control, it is suggested, increase the activities of both enzymes and that of bisphosphatase will be close to its maximum. This means that the cycling rate is high and much greater than the glycolytic flux (since the muscle is still at rest, in the example the cycling rate/flux ratio is 19. Once exercise begins, changes in the concentration of regulators, which are related to an increased rate of ATP utilization, increase the activity of phosphofructokinase and decrease those of bisphosphatase so that the flux increases from 100 to 49,900 or almost 500-fold although the activity of phosphofructokinase is increased by only 25-fold. Immediately after exercise, both enzyme activities decrease but not to resting values. This allows more precise control of the rate of glycolysis as it approaches the resting value but also causes increased rates of ATP hydrolysis and therefore a greater energy demand than expected. This increased rate of cycling may take several hours to return to the original resting values. There is some evidence that the rate of this cycle is increased after exercise in muscle (36).

Indeed there is a linear relationship between the extent of recovery oxygen and the time of exercise (24). Of considerable importance is the fact that the respiratory exchange ratio was found to be lowered for the whole of the recovery period indicating a greater rate of fat oxidation after exercise (23). Since these subjects were allowed to eat only simple carbohydrate meals after exercise, and since the plasma glycerol and fatty acid levels were elevated, these findings suggest that triacylglycerol is being mobilized from the adipose tissue depots and the fatty acids are being utilized by muscle and perhaps other tissues: this would allow the carbohydrate in the diet to be converted to glycogen in muscle and liver rather than being oxidized. It also suggests that the rate of the triacylglycerol/fatty acid cycle is enhanced. This is now known to be the case: Bahr et al. (25) have now measured the rate of the triacyl-glycerol/fatty acid cycle and they have shown that, for the extra oxygen consumed at 3 hours after cessation of exercise, at least 50% can be explained from the increased rate of this cycle. This is in general agreement with the discrepancy shown in Table 8. The advantage of maintaining the activity of the cycle for several hours after exercise may be to ensure satisfactory rates of fatty acid mobilization and also buffering of the fatty acid level. After prolonged exercise glycogen levels will be low so that some fatty acid release from adipose tissue will be necessary. However, since the subject is resting—too high a rate of release would lead to dangerously high levels of fatty acids in the bloodstream.

Thermic Response to Food

The increase in heat production that occurs after a meal (the thermic response to food) has been divided into two parts: obligatory and facultative. The obligatory thermogenesis is that released in the processes of transport, metabolism and assimilation of the metabolites absorbed after digestion; for example, conversion of one molecule glucose to glycogen requires the hydrolysis of three molecules of ATP to ADP. The remainder of the thermogenesis is described as facultative. However, much of this may be due to control and therefore cannot be described, in meaningful terms, as facultative. Such control may include the operation of substrate cycles, which have many properties that are consistent with their playing a role in the thermic response to food (2).

The authors suggest that one role of the increased sympathetic activity after a meal is to provide higher rates of substrate cycling for improved sensitivity of processes that control the rates of synthetic and degradative processes. This would result in thermogenesis, but such thermogenesis cannot be considered as the primary role of the thermic response to food. The primary role, we argue, is to provide for sensitivity in control. That is, a significant proportion of the energy ingested in the meal must be lost as heat to provide for sensitivity in metabolic control to permit the proper assimilation of the molecules absorbed from the food. It should be noted that these rates of cycling will vary from condition to condition, from time to time, and from individual to individual. And indeed it is known that facultative thermogenesis shows such variability.

Substrate Cycling and Aging

While the process of aging is not yet understood at a molecular level, its effects can be seen in structural changes affecting some proteins such as collagen and elastin.

These structural changes may be caused by errors in the translation process, but it is also possible that they may arise during transcription and so become incorporated into the messenger-RNA. Such changes are likely to be detrimental to the well-being of the animal. So far, however, only one or two examples are known of changes in protein structure which can explain some of the very obvious macroscopic changes that characterize aging (e.g., the changes in protein structure of the lens which underlies deterioration in sight). The following speculative hypothesis seeks to provide a molecular explanation for some of the characteristic macroscopic changes of aging.

We have already seen that sensitivity in control can only be improved by a limited number of mechanisms. Two of these could be described as dynamic, in that they depend upon the kinetics of an enzyme or enzymes involved in regulation; they are the substrate cycle and the interconversion cycle (see above). If the efficiency of these two types of cycles deteriorated with aging, they would progressively fail to provide the high level of sensitivity required for normal metabolic control. This might come about in the following way.

The normal role of the substrate and interconversion cycles is to improve the sensitivity of the regulatory process, so that, when a regulator concentration alters, the change in enzyme activity will be sufficiently large to meet the demands of the new physiological situation. The regulator(s) could be operative within the cell (e.g., changed adenine nucleotide levels during exercise) or from outside (e.g., changed concentration of a hormone which mediates its effect through an intracellular second messenger). The kinetics of the interconversion cycle or the rate of substrate cycling may provide the necessary degree of amplification. However, if the maximum rates of these cycles are reduced, caused by aging, sensitivity to the regulator could be markedly reduced—with at least three consequences.

1. If the change in regulator concentration cannot produce a sufficient response from the metabolic system, then the physiological response will not be adequate. For example: the energy for the contractile process in sprinting comes mainly from glycolysis; if the sensitivity of the control mechanisms of phosphorylase and 6-phosphofructokinase are decreased, then the increase in the rate of glycolysis will not be sufficient to meet the energy demands of the contractile process. The rate of energy utilization by the contractile process must then be curtailed—by the sprinter reducing speed or at least curbing acceleration. This is, of course, a well-known phenomenon of aging.

2. In an attempt to increase the rate of the metabolic process to meet physiological demand, the concentration of regulator may rise much higher than normal—to try and overcome the lack of sensitivity in the regulatory process. A very large increase in regulator concentration could be detrimental to the physiology of a particular tissue. An increase in the concentration of a reactive intermediate could lead to the accumulation of side products which might be detrimental and even dangerous to the well-being of the cell. For example, a large increase in concentration of intracellular glucose can lead to the accumulation of the less readily metabolized sugars, fructose and sorbitol via the polyol pathway. These may be responsible for damage to nerves and to the lens in diabetes mellitus.

3. Substrate cycles not only regulate the flux through metabolic pathways but also the precise concentration of intracellular ions (e.g., sodium and calcium ions). A reduction in the rate of such cycles could decrease the precision of regulation, to produce large fluctuations in the intracellular concentrations of such ions. The resultant ionic and osmotic imbalances could eventually lead to cell damage and even death.

Since a large number of processes in all tissues of the body may be controlled by interconversion or substrate cycles, gradual impairment in the rate of such cycles with age could lead to a generalized decline in the responsiveness of tissues and of physiological processes within those tissues. This would produce a general deterioration in what might be termed the "efficiency" of the many and varied physiological processes in the tissues and organs of the body.

The author has discussed elsewhere how a reduction in the rate of substrate cycles could, in particular, account for obesity; since this is common in middle and old age, it would be consistent with the hypothesis outlined above (5). Further, the syndrome of accidental hypothermia, which is very prevalent in debilitated elderly people in no more hostile an environment than their own home, could also be explained by inability to increase the rate of substrate cycles in response to hypothermia. A marked decrease in the capacity of such cycles, due to old age, would preclude adequate heat generation when they are stimulated. Thus, even healthy elderly subjects seem to be less able than young adults to maintain their core temperature (and therefore muscle temperature) when exposed to a low ambient temperature (26). Among elderly subjects, those who are thinnest are most at risk, showing a fall in core temperature (and therefore in muscle temperature) after only a mild degree of cooling. This is not merely because of their poorer insulation but because they are less able to mount a protective increase in their metabolic rate (27). This may be due to a decreased ability to stimulate substrate cycles in tissues such as liver, adipose tissue, and muscle. Perhaps the catecholamine sensitivity of thermogenic cycles is even lower in cachectic elderly people than in well-nourished elderly people. This is an interesting question and of considerable importance for the future, especially since the average age of the population in the Western world is increasing markedly and the health of the elderly population will become of major economic importance in the relatively near future.

REFERENCES

1. Newsholme EA, Leech AR. *Biochemistry for the medical sciences.* Chichester: John Wiley, 1983; 233–234.
2. Newsholme EA, Crabtree B. Substrate cycles in metabolic regulation and in heat generation. *Biochem Soc Symp* 1976;41:61–110.
3. Koshland DE, Goldbeter A, Stock JB. Amplification and adaptation in regulatory and sensory systems. *Science* 1982;217:220–225.
4. Crabtree B, Newsholme EA. A quantitative approach to metabolic control. *Curr Top Cell Regul* 1985;25:21–76.
5. Newsholme EA, Challiss RAJ. A common mechanism to explain decreased rates of thermogenesis and insulin resistance in obesity. In: Bjorntorp P, ed. *Obesity.* (*in press*).

6. Nicholls DG, Crompton M. Mitochondrial calcium transport. *FEBS Lett* 1980;111:261–268.
7. Board M, Humm S, Newsholme EA. Maximum activities of key enzymes of glycolysis, glutaminolysis, pentose phosphate pathway and tricarboxylic acid cycle in normal, neoplastic and suppressed cells. *Biochem J* 1990;265:503–509.
8. Ardawi MSM, Newsholme EA. Glutamine metabolism in lymphocytes of the rat. *Biochem J* 1983; 212:835–842.
9. Ardawi MSM, Newsholme EA. Metabolism in lymphoyctes and its importance to the immune response. *Essays Biochem* 1985;21:1–44.
10. Newsholme P, Gordon S, Newsholme EA. Rates of utilization and fates of glucose, glutamine, pyruvate, fatty acids and ketone bodies by mouse macrophages. *Biochem J* 1987;242:631–636.
11. Newsholme EA, Newsholme P, Curi R, Challoner E, Ardawi MSM. A role for muscle in the immune system and its importance in surgery, trauma, sepsis and burns. *Nutrition* 1988;4:261–268.
12. Newsholme EA, Newsholme P, Curi R, Crabtree B, Ardawi MSM. Glutamine metabolism in different tissues. In: Kinney JM, Borum PR, eds. *Perspectives in clinical nutrition.* Baltimore-Munich:Urban & Schwarzenberg, 1989;71–98.
13. Szondy Z, Newsholme EA. The effect of glutamine concentration on the activity of carbarmoyl-phosphate synthase II and on the incorporation of [^{3}H]thymidine into DNA in rat mesenteric lymphocytes stimulated by phytohaemagglutinin. *Biochem J* 1989;261:979–983.
14. Newsholme EA, Crabtree B, Ardawi MSM. The role of high rates of glycolysis and glutamine utilisation in rapidly-dividing cells. *Biosci Rep* 1985;4:393–400.
15. Newsholme EA, Crabtree B, Ardawi MSM. Glutamine metabolism in lymphocytes, its biochemical, physiological and clinical importance. *Q J Exp Physiol* 1985;70:473–489.
16. Parry-Billings M, Evans J, Calder PC, Newsholme EA. Does glutamine contribute to immunosuppression after burns? *Lancet* 1990;336:523–525.
17. Curi R, Williams JF, Newsholme EA. Formation of ketone bodies by resting lymphocytes. *Int J Biochem* 1989;21:1133–1136.
18. Rennie MJ, Hundal HS, Babij P, et al. Characteristics of a glutamine carrier in skeletal muscle have important consequences for nitrogen loss in injury, infection and chronic disease. *Lancet* 1986;1:1008–1011.
19. Parry-Billings M, Leighton B, Dimitriadis GA, Vasconcelos PRL, Newsholme EA. Skeletal muscle glutamine metabolism during sepsis in the rat. *Int J Biochem* 1989;21:419–423.
20. Parry-Billings M. *Studies in glutamine metabolism in muscle* [Thesis]. Oxford: Oxford University, 1989.
21. Leboef B, Flint RB, Cahill GF. Effect of epinephrine on glucose uptake and glycerol release by adipose tissue *in vivo. Proc Soc Exp Biol Med* 1959;102:527–537.
22. Steinberg D. Fatty acid mobilization—mechanisms of regulation and metabolic consequences. *Biochem Soc Symp* 1963;24:111–144.
23. Maehlum S, Grandmontagne M, Newsholme EA, Sejersted OM. Magnitude and duration of excess post-exercise oxygen consumption in healthy young subjects. *Metabolism* 1986;35:425–429.
24. Bahr R, Ignes I, Vaage O, Newsholme EA, Sejersted OM. Effect of duration of exercise on excess postexercise oxygen consumption. *J Appl Physiol* 1987;62:485–490.
25. Bahr R, Hansson P, Sejersted OM. Triglyceride/fatty acid cycling is increased after exercise. *Metabolism* 1990;39:993–999.
26. Collins KJ, Easton JC, Belfield-Smith H, Exton-Smith AN, Pluck RA. Effects of age on body temperature and blood pressure in cold environments. *Clin Sci* 1985;69:465–470.
27. Fellows IW, Macdonald IA, Bennett T, Allison SP. The effect of undernutrition on thermoregulation in the elderly. *Clin Sci* 1985;69:525–532.
28. Newsholme EA, Start C. *Regulation of metabolism.* Chichester: John Wiley, 1973.
29. Hundal HS, Watt PW, Rennie MJ. Amino acid transport in perfused rat skeletal muscle. *Biochem Soc Symp* 1986;14:1070–1071.
30. Karlsson J, Saltin B. Oxygen deficit and muscle metabolites in intermittent exercise. *Acta Physiol Scand* 1971;82:115–122.
31. Hermansen L, Vaage O. Lactate disappearance and glycogen synthesis in human muscle after maximal exercise. *Am J Physiol* 1977;233:E432–E429.
32. Hultman E, Bergstrom J, McLennan-Anderson N. Breakdown and resynthesis of phosphorylcreatine and adenosine triphosphate in connection with muscular work in man. *Scand J Clin Lab Invest* 1967; 19:56–66.
33. Piiper J, di Prampero PE, Cerretelli P. Oxygen debt and high-energy phosphates in gastrocnemius muscle of the dog. *Am J Physiol* 1968;215:523–531.

34. Hill AV, Long CNH, Lupton H. Muscular exercise, lactic acid and the supply and utilisation of oxygen. *Proc R Soc Lond [Biol]* 1925;97:96–138.
35. Curi R, Williams JF, Newsholme EA. Formation of ketone bodies by resting lymphocytes. *Int J Biochem* 1989;21:1133–1136.
36. Challiss RAJ, Arch JRS, Newsholme EA. The rate of substrate cycling between fructose 6-phosphate and fructose 1.6-bisphosphate in skeletal muscle from cold exposed, hyperthyroid or acutely exercised animals. *Biochem J* 1985;31:217–220.

DISCUSSION

Dr. Wolfe: Doctor Newsholme and his colleagues have summarized specific examples in which they have assessed metabolic control using a 7-stage process. The two general areas of application of this approach have been the assessment of substrate cycling and the development of the branched-point mechanism theory. The theory behind the increased sensitivity resulting from the latter process is similar to that for substrate cycling—a high continuous flux in one branch of a pathway provides optimal conditions for the precise regulation of the (much smaller) flux in the other branch. The example of the branched-point mechanism involves the role of the high rate of catabolism of glutamine in the cells of the immune system in enabling precise control of intermediates in the catabolism pathway for important biosynthetic processes, such as purine and pyrimidine nucleotide synthesis. Experimental assessment of the physiological importance of this theory is facilitated by the ease with which the immune system can be studied *in vitro* in a manner that may be quantitatively relevant to the *in vivo* situation. In this example, it has been possible to experimentally validate the branched-point mechanism of control.

The assessment of the physiological control of substrate cycling has been much harder to ascertain from *in vitro* experiments. For example, the authors point out that the first experimental data demonstrating substrate cycling was from isolated adipocytes. Indeed, much of the quantitative work on substrate cycling to this date has been on the TG/FA cycle in isolated fat cells. However, there is a good chance that these studies have been hindered by the difficulty in maintaining FFA efflux via binding to albumin, since there is no flow to take away newly-bound albumin-FFA complexes. This would result in the exaggeration of intracellular cycling. Thus, although TG/FA cycling within the fat cell is well-established *in vitro*, in a wide variety of studies in human studies, it has been difficult to demonstrate any TG/FA cycling within the adipocyte. In a variety of circumstances (overnight fast ± various hormone infusions, 3-day fast, exercise, recovery from exercise) the rate of release of fatty acids (Ra FFA) is almost exactly three times the rate of lipolysis, as reflected by Ra glycerol. Only during the infusion of glucose, which stimulates reesterification more than it inhibits lipolysis, and in severe injury or sepsis, can a high rate of intracellular TG/FA cycling be demonstrated.

Even when substrate cycles have been identified to exist in normal man, amplification of the control of net substrate flux has not always been found to correspond to that predicted from the theoretical $1 + C/J$. A number of authors, including several experiments by our group, have shown that the hepatic glucose cycle (glucose $\rightarrow$ glucose-6-P $\rightarrow$ glucose) functions in normal man (about 40% of flux recycles). However, in virtually all circumstances tested to date, the percent recycled remains roughly constant. Thus, although in theory a high rate of cycling can amplify control, this necessitates that when one pathway is stimulated there is not corresponding increase in the reciprocal pathway. Yet, this is precisely what occurs with the glucose cycle in man. Thus, the amount of glucose cycling back into the liver is roughly a constant percentage of the glucose put out into the blood.

The difficulty in demonstrating some cycles in man, and the failure in other cases for a functioning substrate cycle to amplify control in man, does not mean that the theory underlying substrate cycling is invalid. Rather, there is a limited domain of validity that can only be ascertained by testing *in vivo*. In that regard, we have shown the cycling of FA from adipocytes into plasma, clearance from plasma and reesterification, secretion into plasma as (VLDL) triglyceride, clearance and peripheral reesterification ("extracellular" TG/FA cycling) not only accounts for approximately 70% of total lipolysis under normal conditions (yielding a value for $1 + C/J$ of greater than two), but provides an amplification of the availability of fatty acids in response to exercise of about two-fold—almost exactly that predicted. Furthermore, in recovery, a high rate of reesterification (as much as 90% of lipolysis) can account for 13% of the extra energy expenditure of the recovery from exercise.

Thus, perhaps I can underscore point 6 of the approach to the development of a model of metabolic control: testing of theory. The general notion of substrate cycling has been a great advance in the understanding of metabolic control. However, it does not appear to consistently function in humans in the predicted manner, and therefore empirical testing (in humans) is ultimately essential for step 6 to be employed sufficiently to enable acceptance of a model.

Energy Metabolism: Tissue Determinants and Cellular Corollaries, edited by J. M. Kinney and H. N. Tucker. Raven Press, Ltd., New York © 1992.

Assessment of Substrate Cycling in Humans Using Tracer Methodology

Robert R. Wolfe

Metabolism Unit, Shriners Burns Institute, and Departments of Anesthesiology and Surgery, University of Texas Medical Branch, Galveston, Texas 77550

Substrate cycles exist when opposing, non-equilibrium reactions, catalyzed by different enzymes, are active simultaneously. On the basis of both *in vitro* and *in vivo* studies of cycling in animals (1,2), it has been proposed that substrate cycling plays a role in the regulation of body weight, thermogenesis, and altered sensitivity of flux to hormonal regulation (1–4). However, prior to our application of stable isotope tracer methodology to the problem, there was no evidence that substrate cycling occurred in humans. Furthermore, the extent of hormonal control of cycling (even in animals) was uncertain, and no pathophysiological situation had been identified in humans in which alterations in substrate cycling could be demonstrated to be of potential physiological importance. This chapter presents a review of our past studies in this area.

GLUCOSE CYCLING

Based on activity measurements of enzymes of opposing reactions in potential substrate cycles, it appears that cycling between fructose-6P and fructose-bi-P in muscle is likely to be the most important cycle in the metabolism of glucose (4,5). However, to date it has not been feasible to quantify this process dynamically *in vivo*. On the other hand, there are three potential substrate cycles in the liver that are involved in the metabolism/production of glucose that can be assessed *in vivo*. The glucose cycle involves the simultaneous conversion of glucose to glucose-6P and glucose-6P to glucose; the fructose cycle is the same as in muscle; and the PEP cycle involves the simultaneous conversions of pyruvate to oxaloacetate, oxaloacetate to phosphoenolpyruvate (PEP), and PEP to pyruvate. It has been possible, using tracer methodology, to assess the rates of all of these cycles. However, the methodology for the assessment of the glucose cycle is the least controversial, and the cycle that has received the most attention. Consequently, the primary focus of this section will be the glucose cycle.

METHODS

Assumptions for Tracer Studies

The results described in this chapter have all been obtained using the primed-constant infusion technique. This is the traditional non-compartmental approach to kinetic analysis. There are several assumptions implicit in the use of the non-compartmental analysis using tracers. With regard to the kinetic analysis, the total rate of appearance (Ra) of substrate can only be quantified if the substrate appears directly into the sampled compartment, or if all irreversible loss occurs from the sampled compartment (6). Also, the infused tracer must be treated identically to the endogenously-occurring tracee; the infused tracer must not substantially affect the endogenous kinetics of the tracee; isotopic exchange between tracer and other compounds most reflect true reaction rates; recycling of tracer does not occur; and the isotope infusion and sampling site must be appropriate to reflect isotopic enrichment subsequent to complete mixing of tracee and tracer. Each of these assumptions is discussed briefly below as they apply to the quantitation of glucose kinetics.

The first assumption we will consider is that new glucose is released directly into plasma. The liver is the predominant site of glucose production, and the two major compartments of glucose distribution are the plasma and the interstitial fluid (7). The initial site of appearance of newly produced glucose (i.e., plasma versus interstitial fluid) can be ascertained by observation of the temporal relationship between the hepatic vein, arterial, and interstitial fluid glucose concentration following acute stimulation of glucose production. We accomplished this in a conscious sheep model prepared with chronic catheters that enabled the sampling of the arterial blood, hepatic venous blood, and the thoracic duct lymph. The latter value is representative of a mixed sample of the lymph (8). Glucose production was then stimulated acutely by a bolus injection of glucagon. Glucose concentration rose rapidly in the hepatic vein, followed by a more moderate increase in the arterial concentration, and a slower and even smaller increase in the thoracic duct (interstitial fluid) concentration (Fig. 1). These results can most easily be interpreted as showing that glucose essentially enters the blood directly from the liver, this validating the calculation of the rate of production using non-compartmental analysis.

The assumption that isotopically-labeled tracers are treated the same as their more abundant, naturally-occurring counterparts has been generally accepted for a wide variety of compounds for at least 40 years. It was therefore surprising when the possibility of isotopic discrimination of certain species of labeled glucose during the hyperinsulinemic, euglycemic clamp technique was claimed (9). However, it appears that much of the basis for that notion derived from the use of a contaminated infusate (10). Thus, although it is still not possible to entirely rule out the possibility of isotopic discrimination having a significant impact on calculated results in such extreme, unphysiological conditions as the infusion of pharmacological amounts of insulin (11), in most situations it is not likely to be a problem. This is not to say that isotope discrimination does not occur, as this phenomenon is well established in the bio-

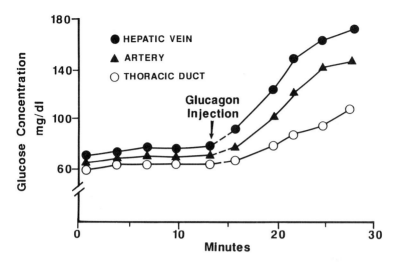

FIG. 1. Experiment in conscious sheep in which samples were obtained from the hepatic vein, artery, and thoracic duct (as representative of interstitial fluid) prior to and following the injection of glucagon.

logical world (12). However, the magnitude of discrimination is likely to be trivial in relation to the other sources of error in the determination of glucose kinetics *in vivo*.

It can reasonably be assumed that the small moler amounts of radioactive glucose infused for tracer studies have no effect on the endogenous kinetics. This is because the sensitivity of detection by scintillation counting enables the administration of a sufficient amount of label with the administration of only a trivial amount of total compound, relative to the rate of endogenous production of the tracer. In the case of stable tracers, however, the lower sensitivity of detection of enrichment by mass spectrometry generally requires the administration of a sufficiently large amount of labeled compound so that the tracer cannot be considered to be "massless." Furthermore, the natural occurrence of stable isotopes in glucose prior to tracer infusion must also be considered in the calculations of substrate kinetics (13). This is particularly a potential problem with the bolus injection technique (14). The possible influence of infused "tracer" on endogenous kinetics might especially be expected to be a problem in the case of glucose, owing to the extreme sensitivity of the regulation of glucose Ra by the liver. For example, the intravenous infusion of (unlabeled) glucose at the rate of 1 mg/kg/min, which is only half the normal production rate, results in a sustained suppression of endogenous production almost exactly equal to the infusion rate, even though the peripheral glucose and insulin concentrations are unaffected (15). However, under most circumstances it should not be necessary to infuse a stable isotope tracer of glucose at a rate greater than 0.07 mg/ kg/min under even the most extreme circumstances, and such an infusion would have minimal effects on endogenous kinetics.

The assumption that isotopic exchange between the tracer and other compounds reflects true reaction rates is the most difficult to assess experimentally, since the tracer is used because of the difficulty in directly quantifying reaction rates by other means. Whereas there is little reason to doubt this assumption with regard to glucose, it must be realized that this assumption has not been critically assessed.

The general assumption that label does not recycle is common to all tracer studies. However, this assumption in fact is not only known to be untrue for various glucose tracers, it is in fact the occurrence of recycling that enables calculation of the rate of glucose cycling. This point will be discussed in more detail below.

The effect of tracer infusion site/sampling site on the calculated kinetics has received considerable attention, since differences in calculated production rates as great as 50% can result with some substrates (16). However, due to the large plasma pool of glucose, relative to its rate of production, the exact infusion and sampling site has little effect on the calculated kinetics (17). Even under the extreme conditions of the hyperinsulinemic clamp, when the importance of the infusion and sampling sites is increased, it is not a major problem for the accurate calculation of glucose Ra.

Site of Loss of ^2H from the 2, 3, and 6 Positions of Glucose

Figure 2 shows the major sites at which ^2H in the 2, 3, and 6 positions are lost in the process of glycolysis and gluconeogenesis. ^2H in the 2 position is lost in the hexose-isomerase reaction (glucose-6P $\leftrightarrow$ fructose-6) (Fig. 2). Any 2-^2H-glucose-6P that enters the hexose monophosphate shunt will also lose its label. In the aldolase cleavage of fructose-6P, the 3-^2H appears on the C-1 of di-hydroxyacetone phosphate (DHAP). In the isomerization to glyceraldehyde 3P (G3P), the 3-^2H is exchanged with protons of water (Fig. 2). Also, any 3-^2H-glucose-6P entering the hexose monophosphate shunt will lose its label in the oxidation of 6-phosphogluconic acid to ribulose 5-phosphate, thereby ultimately producing unlabeled fructose-6P. ^2H in the 6 position of glucose is not lost in the process of glycolysis, but can be lost at two possible sites in the process of gluconeogenesis. One ^2H in the 6 position is lost in the pyruvate carboxylase reaction, and there is also the likelihood of loss of ^2H from the 6 position in equilibration with the hydrogen pool of the mitochondria during the equilibration between oxaloacetate, malate, and fumarate (Fig. 2). It is evident from Fig. 2 that the extent to which infused ^2H-labeled glucose is involved in tracer recycling depends on the specific site of labeling of the molecule. These different rates of recycling of ^2H-labels can be capitalized upon to determine the rate of hepatic glucose cycling.

Figure 3 shows the sites of loss of ^2H from glucose initially labeled in the 2, 3, and 6 positions, in relation to potential substrate cycles of glucose in the liver. If the different potential substrate cycles shown in Fig. 3 are functional, then it is clear that the site of labeling of glucose will affect the subsequent calculation of Ra glucose. For example, a multi-labeled molecule that enters the liver and is metabolized as far as fructose-6P, and is then recycled back out into the blood as glucose, will lose its

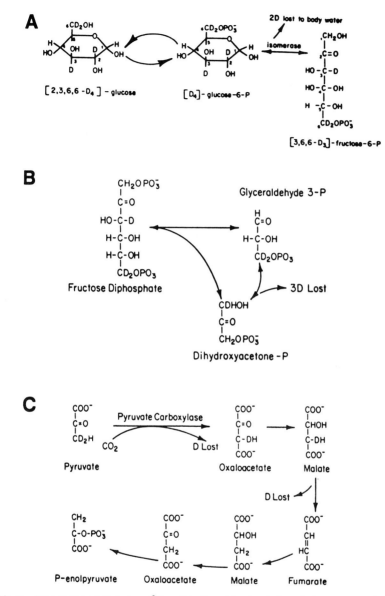

FIG. 2. Sites of loss of deuterium (^{2}H, or D in figure) in glycolysis and gluconeogenesis from the 2 position **(A)**, 3 position **(B)**, and 6 position **(C)**.

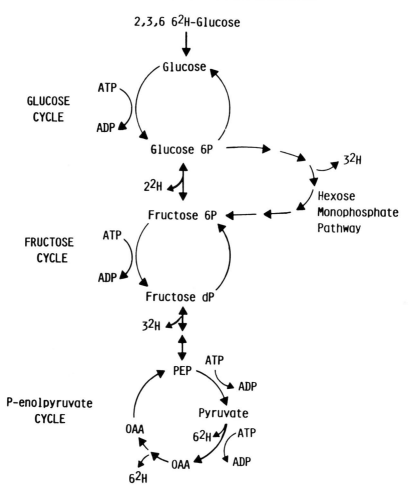

FIG. 3.   Loss of deuterium from the 2, 3, and 6 positions of glucose in relation to potential sites of substrate cycles in the liver.

2-^{2}H, but retain the ^{2}H in the 6 position. In this example, a higher value for Ra glucose would be obtained with the 2-^{2}H than the 6-^{2}H tracer.

Extension of the general considerations outlined above to quantitation of hepatic glucose substrate cycling requires the assumptions that the rate of the glucose-6P isomerase reaction is high relative to the net flux of glycolysis. If so, the rate of the glucose cycle can be calculated by determining the Ra glucose using a 2-^{2}H-glucose, as a tracer, and subtracting from that value the value for Ra glucose determined simultaneously with 6, 6-^{2}H-glucose. The value for Ra glucose determined with 6, 6-^{2}H-glucose represents the total new hepatic production of glucose from glycogen and gluconeogenesis. It will not include any glucose output resulting from glucose cycle activity, since the 6 label is not lost in that cycle. The Ra glucose determined with 2-^{2}H-glucose, on the other hand, includes not only the true value for total new glucose production, but also reflects the rate of glucose cycle activity, since the 2-^{2}H-label would be lost in the glucose cycle (presuming, as stated above, that the isomerase activity is high relative to the net rate of metabolism of glucose-6P). The rate of the fructose cycle would not affect the rate of the glucose cycle calculated from Ra glucose (2-^{2}H) – Ra glucose (6, 6-^{2}H), since neither the 2-^{2}H or the 6-^{2}H of glucose is lost in the fructose cycle.

The extent of loss of ^{3}H label from the 2-position of glucose-6P in the isomerase reaction with fructose-6P was assessed in humans by Wajngot et al. (18), by infusing 2-^{3}H, ^{14}C-galactose and measuring the ^{3}H/^{14}C ratio in plasma glucose. The rationale of this approach is shown in Fig. 4. In the production of glucose from galactose, both the 2-^{3}H and 2-^{14}C will be retained to the step in which glucose-6P is produced. Then, the 2-^{14}C will be retained in glucose that is produced and released into the

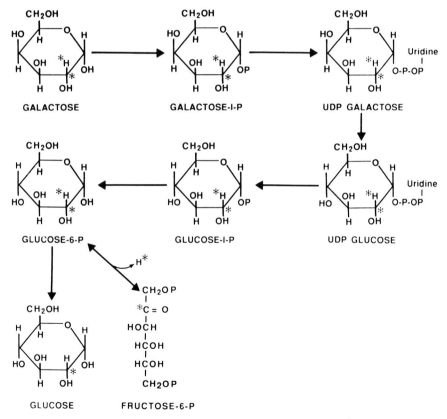

FIG. 4. Using the ratio of ^{3}H/^{14}C(*) in glucose to assess the extent to which ^{3}H label in the second position is lost in the isomerase reaction between glucose-6P and fructose-6P.

blood, but 2-^{3}H will be lost via the isomerase reaction. If, as is assumed in the calculation of the glucose cycle using the approach described above, the loss of the ^{3}H in the isomerase reaction is extremely rapid relative to the glucose-6-phosphatase reaction in which glucose is produced, then the ^{3}H/^{14}C ratio in glucose would be 0, since all ^{3}H would be lost before glucose is produced (Fig. 4). However, after 3 h of tracer infusion the ratio ranged from 0.12 to 0.20, indicating extensive, but not complete, loss of the 2-^{3}H.

These results were confirmed by these authors in a second experiment in which [2-^{3}H, 2-^{14}C]-glucose was infused, and the ^{3}H/^{14}C ratio determined in excreted acet-aminophen-glucuronide. The rationale for this experiment is shown in Fig. 5. Acet-aminophen (e.g., Tylenol) is conjugated in the liver with UDP-glucuronate. Glu-curonate is produced from glucose, with loss of ^{3}H occurring again at the isomerase reaction between glucose-6P and fructose-6P (Fig. 5). Consequently, the ratio of ^{3}H/^{14}C in the excreted acetaminophen-glucuronate should reflect the extent of loss of the ^{3}H label in the isomerase reaction. As with the galactose experiment, the ratios ranged from 0.10 to 0.23, again indicating that about 90% of the 2-^{3}H is lost in the isomerase reaction. Since in the calculation of Ra (2-^{3}H) it is assumed that any glucose that goes through the glucose cycle will lose all the label, but in fact only 80% is lost, then the calculated rate will be approximately 20% below the true value.

Accurate calculation of Ra (6H) depends on the assumptions that not only is [6-^{3}H] not lost in the glucose cycle, but also that all label is lost in the *de novo* production of glucose. To test this hypothesis, Wajngot et al. (18) infused 3-^{3}H, ^{14}C-lactate, and determined the ^{3}H/^{14}C ratio in glucose relative to the ^{3}H/^{14}C in the blood lactate. Complete loss of the ^{3}H-label in gluconeogenesis (Fig. 2C) would result in a ratio of 0. The observed ratio was about 0.10, meaning that 10% of the label is not lost. This may or may not result in an underestimation of the true value for Ra (6H), depending on the analytical technique used. Whereas the original labeled glucose has two enriched hydrogens attached in the 6-position, any recycled label will be singly-labeled in that position, because one H has to be lost in the pyruvate car-boxylase reaction (Fig. 2). With ^{3}H and scintillation counting, a single-versus double-labeled 6-^{3}H-glucose molecule cannot be distinguished, and thus incomplete detri-tiation will result in a 10% underestimation of the true value for Ra (6H). On the other hand, GCMS analysis of isotopic enrichment when 6, 6-^{2}H$_2$-glucose is used as a tracer will distinguish that tracer from 6-^{2}H$_1$-glucose, since the latter (recycled) molecule will be one mass unit lighter than the original tracer. In our experience, we find that the excess singly enriched glucose is about 20% of the amount of the original doubly labeled tracer, which corresponds to 10% total recycling of tracer reported by Wajngot et al. (18). However, that recycled glucose is excluded from the analysis, and therefore there is good reason to believe that production measured with 6, 6-^{2}H-glucose will be closer to the true value than when 6-^{3}H-glucose is used.

If 6-^{3}H, is used, some label is lost in the fructose-6P cycle, thereby contributing to the overestimation of the true value of Ra (6H). The reason for this is shown in Fig. 6. 6-^{3}H-fructose-6P forms [3, 3-^{3}H$_2$]-GAP, which isomerizes to [3, 3-^{3}H$_2$]-DHAP. In the formation of glucose, GAP and DHAP condense, forming some [1, 1-^{3}H$_2$]-

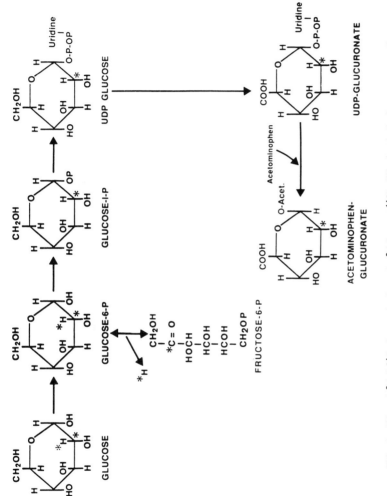

FIG. 5. When 2-^{3}H, 2-^{14}C-glucose is given, the ^{3}H (but not ^{14}C) will be lost in the isomerase reaction, between glucose-6P and fructose-6P. If this reaction is fast, relative to other fates of glucose-6P, then ^{14}C-labeled UDP-glucuronate will be produced. This latter value can be determined as urinary acetaminophen-glucuronate.

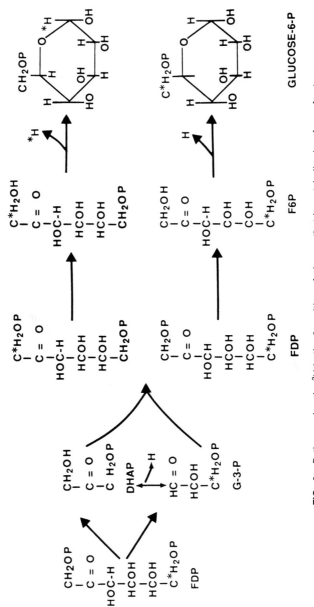

FIG. 6. Pathway whereby ^3H in the 6 position of glucose that is metabolized as far as fructose-bi-P can be lost if that molecule recycles back to glucose.

FDP and about the same amount of [6, 6-^{3}H$_2$]-F-6P. One ^{3}H on the one-position of F-6P is then lost during isomerization to F-6P, meaning that about one fourth of the [6, 6-^{3}H$_2$]-glucose that cycles through the fructose-6P cycle will lose its label. The actual extent of the loss of the 6-^{3}H will then depend on the rate of the fructose-6P cycle relative to the rate of hydrolysis of glucose-6P to glucose. If, for example, each molecule cycles through the fructose an average of 3 times before the 6, 6P leaves as glucose, then about half of the ^{3}H-label in the 6 position would be lost ($\frac{3}{4} \times \frac{3}{4} \times \frac{3}{4} = \frac{27}{64}$ remains). Consequently, when 6-^{3}H- or 6, 6-d$_2$-glucose is used, the rate of Ra (6H) will be overestimated by an amount dependent on the rate of the hepatic fructose-6P cycle to the rate of the conversion of 6, 6P to glucose.

The above consideration obviously creates a problem in the quantitation of the fructose cycle with 6-^{3}H-glucose. Although the difference between Ra (3H) and Ra (6H) has been used as an estimate of the rate of fructose cycling (e.g., 18,19), it is obvious that the assumption is not valid that no label from the [6-^{3}H$_2$]-glucose is lost in the cycle. Furthermore, loss of the *H in the 3-position in the fructose-6P cycle does not appear to be complete. When 3-^{3}H, 1-^{14}C-fructose was infused into volunteers, if detritiation was complete, the ratio of ^{3}H to ^{14}C in blood glucose would have been zero. This is because the [3-^{3}H, 1-^{14}C]-fructose is converted in the liver to [1-^{3}H, 3-^{14}C]-DHAP, just as [1-^{3}H, 3-^{14}C]-DHAP would be produced from the metabolism of [1-^{3}H, 3-^{14}C]-glucose (Fig. 2). However, the observed ratio of ^{3}H/^{14}C in glucose was 14–27% of that in the infused fructose, indicating that detritiation is only about 75–85% complete. Thus, Ra$_{(3H)}$ will include all newly produced glucose, but only about 75–85% of glucose that goes through the fructose-6P cycle. The difference of Ra$_{(3H)}$ − Ra$_{(6H)}$ will thus underestimate the extent of the cycle. This is consistent with the fact that it is difficult to demonstrate significant fructose-6P cycling in man with this approach (e.g., 18,19,20).

Thus, the difference between Ra$_{(2H)}$ and Ra$_{(6H)}$ will provide a reasonable estimate of the rate of the glucose cycle, since about 80% of the 2-*H, but none of the 6*H, is lost in the cycle. The calculated value will be about a 20% underestimate of the true value, depending on whether [6-^{3}H] or [6, 6-d$_2$]-glucose is used, with the latter tracer theoretically resulting in the larger underestimate of the glucose cycle (because the [6-^{3}H]-tracer underestimates the true value for Ra$_{(6H)}$). On the other hand, the quantitation of the fructose-6P cycle by the difference between Ra$_{(3H)}$ and Ra$_{(6H)}$ underestimated.

There is little possibility that this method of estimating the rate of glucose cycling will overestimate the true values by virtue of glucose going to glycerol-6P, being incorporated into triglyceride, then released as glycerol and reincorporated into glucose. Although, this pathway would theoretically add to the calculation of Ra2-Ra6 (since the 2-d would be lost but the 6-d would be retained), the quantitative aspect of this cycle is virtually nil. Using a high rate of infusion of [1-^{13}C]-glucose, we found that <1% of the glycerol flux is derived from labeled plasma glucose (21). Since the percentage contribution of glycerol to glucose output in postabsorptive man is <5% (22), the amount of apparent glucose substrate cycling is insignificant that might actually be an artifact due to the occurrence of this alternative route.

Analysis of Isotopic Enrichment

The rate of the glucose cycle can be ascertained by simultaneously infusing [2-*H]- and [6-*H]-glucose, where the labeled tracers can be either the radioactive tritium or the stable isotope deuterium. When radioactivity is used, anion and cation exchange chromatography is used to isolate the plasma glucose from other, potentially labeled, compounds in the plasma. Then, chemical degradation is necessary to distinguish radioactivity in different positions (i.e., C-2 vs C-6) of the plasma glucose. Different approaches have been used (9,20). In all approaches, the counts in the 6 position are determined separately from the 2 position. However, in the method used by Karlander et al. (20), the radioactivity in the 1 position is not distinguished from that in the 2 position, thus the possibility of recycled ^3H from the 6 position contributing to the apparent enrichment at the 2 position is not excluded. This would cause an underestimation of $Ra2^3H$. In contrast, the detritiation procedure used by Bell et al. (9) to determine the specific activity in position 2 should exclude any enrichment in position 1.

Beyond the potential overestimation of activity of [2-^3H]-glucose if the 1 position is not excluded, there are other problems with the analysis of specific radioactivity of the specific positions of glucose. Regardless of the method of separation of the 2 and 6 positions, the untestable assumption must be made that with each sample ion exchange chromatography successfully eliminates 100% of other labeled compounds, such as lactate and alanine. If this is not accomplished, the difference between Ra2 and Ra6 will be underestimated. Another potential problem in the radioactive techniques is the uncertain extent to which complete separation of the activity of the 2 and 6 positions is accomplished. This was reported to vary between 86% and 97% by Karlander et al. (20), but it is not clear how the recovery of each individual sample processed was determined. Also, due to limitations in the amount of radioactivity that can be administered to human subjects, low counts are obtained, leading to less precision in determining specific activity.

The stable isotope methodology we have used first involves the isolation of plasma glucose by ion exchange chromatography. Then, the pentaacetate derivative is formed for the analysis of the enrichment of [6,6-d_2]-glucose, and the tri-methylsilyl derivative is formed for the analysis of 2-d_1-glucose enrichment. Measurement of isotopic enrichment of the two derivatives is performed by means of selected ion monitoring using a gas-chromatograph mass-spectrometer (GCMS). The ions at mass/charge ratio (m/e) 171:170:169 are selectively monitored using the chemical ionization mode with methane as the reactant gas to determine the [6,6-d_2]-glucose enrichment. The ion at m/e 170 is monitored to account for the existence of any singly labeled glucose in the calculation of the enrichment due to the doubly labeled tracer (23). Ions at m/e 205:204 are selectively monitored using electron impact ionization to determine [2-d]-glucose enrichment in the tri-methylsilyl derivative. By using these ions, the molecular fragments included the carbon position of interest (e.g., the 6 position), while excluding the other labeled position in the molecule (e.g., the 2 position).

In contrast to the approach necessary when radioactive tracers are used, this stable isotope approach eliminates any possibility of cross contamination of isotopic enrichment at the two positions. The fragment used to analyze the enrichment of 2-d-glucose has a structure of $[(CH_3)_3SiO^2CH^3CHOSi(CH_3)_3]^+$, whereas the structure of the fragment used to analyze 6, 6-d_2-glucose enrichment is $(C_2H_3O_2C^6H_2C^5C^4C^3HC_2O_2H_3)$.[+] Thus, enrichment at the 2 position could not affect the apparent enrichment at the 6 position, or vice versa. Since both fragments exclude the 1 position, any deuterium that was not lost from the 6 position and was subsequently recycled into glucose would not be considered in the measurement of the enrichment of 2-d-glucose. Furthermore, the 6-d enrichment would not be significantly affected by such recycling either, since the mass increase due to recycling is reflected by an increase in the ratio of m/e 170:169, and this is accounted for in the calculation of the ratio of m/e 171:169, which was used to monitor the enrichment of 6, 6-d_2-glucose. The technique we used to measure isotopic enrichment can reliably determine the known levels of natural abundance of stable isotopes of a glucose standard, and the co-efficient of variation on five repeat analyses of the same sample (in the range of isotopic enrichment used in this study) is consistently below 2%. Finally, because of mass spectrum identification, there is little possibility of contamination of the glucose peak with another compound that would cause spurious analysis of glucose enrichment.

Role of Substrate Cycling in Thermogenesis and Amplification of Substrate Flux

Since heat production owing to ATP dissipation occurs during operation of substrate cycling, it has been hypothesized that substrate cycling may count for a significant fraction of the basal metabolic rate (BMR). The rate of heat production from substrate cycling can be estimated from the equation:

$$dh_t/dt = h_tnc,$$

where ht is the heat released by the hydrolysis of 1 mol of ATP and rephosphorylation of 1 mol of ADP, n is the number of ATP molecules hydrolyzed to ADP per revolution of the cycle, and c is the rate of cycling in mols/unit time (4). It has been shown that for each mol of ATP synthesized and hydrolyzed, 17.4 kcal of heat are released when the substrate is carbohydrate (4).

A substrate cycle can potentially amplify the control of net flux by an amount equal to $1 + C/J$, when C = the rate of cycling, and J = the rate of net flux (4). In the case of the glucose cycle, $Ra_{(2H)} - Ra_{(6H)}$ equals the rate of cycling, and $Ra_{(6H)}$ equals the rate of net flux.

EXPERIMENTAL RESULTS

Basal Rate of Glucose Cycling

We have studied a total of 24 normal volunteers under similar resting conditions (19,24–26). The overall average rate of cycling is 4.7 ± .03 μmol/kg/min, in comparison to a rate of net flux of 11.2 ± 0.48 μmol/kg/min. Thus, at rest the daily energy expenditure attributable to the hepatic glucose cycle (for a 70 kg man) is (17.4 kcal/mol ATP) × (1 mol ATP/1 mol glucose cycled) × (0.473 mol glucose cycled/day) = 9.23 kcal/day. Thus, as compared to a total daily energy expenditure of about 1,600 kcal/day, only a minimal amount (less than 1%) can be attributed to the hepatic glucose cycle.

Response in Burn Injury

Severe burn injury is characterized metabolically by an elevation in resting energy metabolism, as well as an accelerated rate of basal glucose production (28). Therefore, we determined the rate of glucose cycling in a group of nine severely burned patients ($\overline{X}$ burn size of 74% of body surface) by the methods described above. We found the rate of glucose cycling to be increased to 9.3 ± 2.8 μmol/kg/min, as compared to the control value for that experiment of 4.0 ± 0.4 μmol/kg/min.

Despite this large increase in cycling, however, the energy cost of the cycle was still less than 1% of total energy expenditure, and $1 + C/J \sim 1.3$.

Hormonal Control of the Glucose Cycle

We have investigated the role of a number of hormones in controlling the glucose cycle (19,24). Some of the results are summarized in Table 1. The cycling data are presented as the peak response to the hormone infusion, because the response to many hormones, such as glucagon, was transient. Glucose cycling was markedly stimulated by 1 h of glucagon infusion. The increase in glucagon necessary to induce this response was in the physiological range (approximately 400 pg/ml), but a maximal (pharmacological) dose of glucagon further stimulated cycling. A total of 5 days of prednisone treatment had no significant effect on glucose cycling, nor did 1 h of epinephrine infusion at 0.03 μg/kg per min (enough to raise the plasma concentration to about 400 pg/ml). The lack of a response to epinephrine was consistent with the fact that adrenergic blockade in severely burned patients, while diminishing sympathetic stimulation, had no effect on the rate of glucose cycling (26). In normal volunteers, the elevation of glucose concentration, with maintenance of basal levels of insulin and glucagon by somatostatin and hormone infusions, also had no effect on glucose cycling. Hypothyroid patients had a decreased rate of cycling associated with the hypometabolic state. However, whereas 1 week of T_3 infusion restores the normal metabolic rate, the rate of cycling was still depressed. On the other hand, 6 months of T_4 treatment restored the normal rate of cycling. Hyperthyroid patients with increased metabolic rates did not have significantly altered rates of glucose cycling.

In all cases, the amount of energy necessary to re-synthesize the ATP used in the glucose cycle was a small fraction of total resting energy expenditure (REE) (Table 1). When glucagon was infused at a high dose (yielding plasma concentrations greater

TABLE 1. *Hormonal control of glucose cycle*

	Control value		
	Cycling (μmol/kg/min)	% REE	1 + C/J
Glucagon (low dose)	5.3 ± 0.9	0.4	1.4
Glucagon (high dose)	4.4 ± 0.8	0.4	1.4
Prednisone	5.3 ± 0.9	0.5	1.4
Epinephrine	3.4 ± 0.8	0.3	1.3
Hyperthyroid	6.8 ± 1.9	0.4	1.4
Hypothyroid	6.8 ± 1.9	0.4	1.4
Glucose + somatostatin	6.4 ± 1.3	0.3	1.4
	Peak response		
	Cycling (μmol/kg/min)	% REE	1 + C/J
Glucagon (low dose)	18.0 ± 1.9[a]	1.8	1.9
Glucagon (high dose)	25.8 ± 6.0[a]	2.5	1.7
Prednisone	4.9 ± 0.7	0.5	1.5
Epinephrine	6.9 ± 2.3	0.7	1.5
Hyperthyroid	7.7 ± 1.3	0.7	1.5
Hypothyroid	1.1 ± 3.0[a]	0.2	1.1
Glucose + somatostatin	6.9 ± 2.8	0.9	6.3

[a] Significantly different from control data, $p < 0.05$.
REE, resting energy expenditure.

than 1,000 pg/ml), the energy requirement of the glucose cycle rose to 2.5% of total REE, but that response was transient. On the other hand, if this one hepatic cycle is considered representative of other cycles in glucose metabolism occurring throughout the body, it could mean that this type of cycling is important physiologically.

The values for $1 + C/J$ are also presented in Table 1. The normal value was 1.4, and this value was not markedly affected by any perturbation. In other words, cycling generally changed in proportion to net flux. The only exception was during glucose infusion. In this case, the value C/J approached infinity because of the suppression of net glucose flux as measured with 6, 6-d_2-glucose ($J = 0$). Nonetheless, the actual amplification expected in this circumstance would not be expected to be large in an absolute sense, due to the low rate of total flux rate. The fact that the rate of cycling changes in relation to net flux enables the development of the hypothesis that there is no specific control of the reserve direction of the glucose cycle (i.e., glucose → glucose-6P), but rather it is simply a function of the amount of glucose produced (or infused). The extrapolation from this observation is that despite the potential for amplification indicated by the normal resting value of $1 + C/J$ of 1.4, in reality no amplification of control of the net rate of glucose release would occur because of changes in the extent of cycling. We tested this latter hypothesis by observing the response to exercise, in which there is a rapid and large change in requirement for energy substrates.

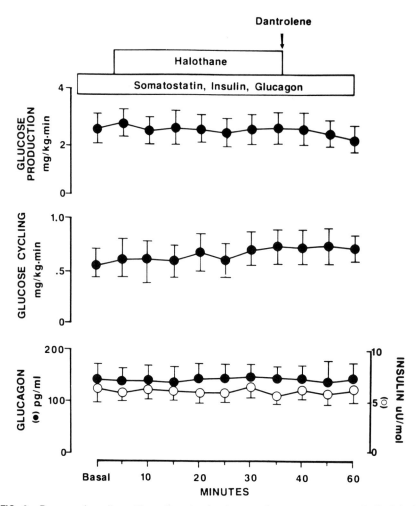

FIG. 9. Response in malignant hyperthermia when hormonal response was controlled by infusion of somatostatin, insulin, and glucagon.

tion increased to a level slightly (but not significantly) above the basal level. The pattern of glucose cycling followed the rate of glucose production, falling to an undetectable rate during MH, and after dantrolene increasing abruptly back to the normal percent of total production (Fig. 8). When hormones were not controlled, both plasma glucagon and plasma insulin concentration decreased during MH, and both rose immediately after dantrolene (Fig. 8). In a separate set of experiments, changes in insulin and glucagon in MH were prevented by the infusion of somatostatin, insulin, and glucagon at constant rates throughout (Fig. 9). In this circumstance, plasma glucose concentration, glucose production, and glucose cycling were not significantly affected by either halothane or dantrolene despite the usual MH syndrome responses in terms of body temperature and other physiological factors.

The results of this study confirmed again the primacy of glucagon as a physiological regulator of glucose production, and also that glucose cycling is a direct function of the rate of production. It also indicated that increased body temperature (via a non-specific Q_{10} effect) is of minimal importance, relative to hormone concentration, in the regulation of the glucose cycle. This implies that in other circumstances, such as severe burn injury (26), in which increases in glucose cycling and body temperature occur concomitantly, the glucose cycling is stimulated by hormones (i.e., elevated glucagon), rather than simply occurring in response to an increase in body temperature caused by another mechanism.

Triglyceride/Fatty Acid Cycling

Triglyceride/fatty acid (TG/FA) cycling involves the reesterification into TG of fatty acids that have been initially released as a consequence of the lipolysis (i.e., the hydrolysis of TG). There are two routes of recycling *in vivo* (Fig. 10):

1. Intracellular, wherein fatty acids are reesterified within the adipocyte in which the lipolysis occurred; and
2. Extracellular, where the fatty acid is released into the plasma and transported to another tissue (predominantly liver) for clearance and reesterification.

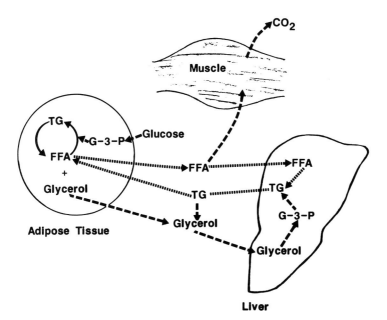

FIG. 10. Intracellular (dashed line) and extracellular (bold dashed line) routes of triglyceride/fatty acid substrate cycling.

In the latter route, the newly produced TG may be subsequently released into plasma (mainly as VLDL) and transported back to the adipose tissue for storage. The quantitation of TG/FA cycling can be accomplished with a combination of stable isotope tracer methodology and indirect calorimetry. The total rate of lipolysis is determined by means of d5-glycerol. The hydrolysis of triglyceride is accurately reflected by the rate of release of glycerol since:

1. Glycerol cannot be re-utilized within the adipocyte (30);
2. It is not produced metabolically by any other pathway (21); and
3. The gut output is small (31).

The release of one glycerol molecule must coincide with the simultaneous release of three fatty acids. Thus, the total rate of release of fatty acids is equal to three times the rate of appearance of glycerol (Ra glycerol).

The difference between the total release of fatty acids and the rate of appearance of fatty acids into the plasma (RaFFA) is equal to the rate of reesterification of fatty acids within the adipocyte. The RaFFA can be determined by means of a labeled tracer of any individual FFA (e.g., [1-^{13}C]-palmitate), and then converted to total FFA turnover by dividing Ra palmitate by the fraction of the total FFA concentration represented by palmitate (determined by gas-chromatography). This calculation presumes that all fatty acids released by lipolysis either enter the plasma or are reesterified. It is also possible that fatty acids might be "directly" oxidized without entering the plasma. This would cause an overestimation of the intracellular recycling of FFA. However, it seems unlikely that this pathway of oxidation occurs to a great extent. Over a large number of experiments, the ratio of RaFFA/Ra glycerol is about $\frac{3}{1}$ (21,24,32–34). Biopsy data indicate that virtually all fat is in the form of triglyceride (35), meaning that no partial hydrolysis of TG occurs. Since "direct" oxidation of FFA would therefore also involve the release of glycerol into the plasma, the ratio of RaFFA/Ra glycerol would be significantly less than three if there was much of this type of oxidation. On the other hand, it is well known that the rate of plasma FFA oxidation, as determined by the collection of $^{13}CO_2$ during the infusion of [1-^{13}C]-palmitate, underestimates the total rate of fat oxidation (as determined by indirect calorimetry) by about 50% (36). One possible explanation for this is that about half of the fatty acid pool comes from "direct" oxidation of fatty acids that do not enter the plasma pool. However, as discussed above, this would result in a ratio of RaFFA/Ra glycerol equal to 1.5 in the absence of any intracellular recycling, which is approximately half the actual value. A more likely explanation is that the tracer experiment underestimates the true rate of oxidation. A major reason why this could occur is loss of label to routes other than CO_2 once labeled acetyl-CoA enters the TCA cycle. When the two carbons of acetyl-CoA enter the TCA cycle, two carbons are lost to CO_2. Thus, for a label to accurately reflect the oxidation rate of a substrate whose terminal oxidation involves entry into the tricarboxylic acid (TCA) cycle, a $^{13}CO_2$ molecule must be recovered for every labeled acetyl-CoA molecule that enters the cycle. However, this does not occur. When [1-^{13}C]-acetate is infused as tracer, [1-^{13}C]-acetyl-CoA is produced, virtually all of which enters the TCA cycle in the fasting state. However, only about 50% of the label is recovered as $^{13}CO_2$, even after accounting for labeled CO_2 retained in the bicarbonate pool (37). Label can be lost from the cycle via a number of pathways other than CO_2, most notably involving label moving from alpha-ketoglutarate to glutamate and glutamine, and from oxaloacetate ultimately to glucose. Therefore, it is likely that the traditional means of measuring plasma FFA oxidation using the collection of labeled CO_2 underestimates the true value by as much as 50%. Thus, it is possible that the entire discrepancy between the rates of total fat oxidation and isotopically determined plasma FFA oxidation is an artifact. Consistent with this possibility, RaFFA virtually always exceeds the total rate of fat oxidation.

Once FFAs have entered the plasma, there are two possible fates; oxidation by a tissue distant from the site of release (e.g., muscle), or reesterification. The extent of reesterification, or recycling of fatty acids, via this extracellular route is equal to RaFFA minus total fat oxidation. Total fat oxidation is determined by indirect calorimetry.

Assessment of the Physiological Significance of TG/FA Cycling

As discussed above in relation to glucose cycling, there are two aspects of TG/FA cycling of potential physiological significance; (i) thermogenesis; and (ii) amplification of control of net substrate flux. The role of TG/FA cycling in thermogenesis is quantifiable, in that eight high-energy phosphate bonds are required per mol of triglyceride recycled (38). Because approximately 18 kcal of heat are released per mol of ATP hydrolyzed and synthesized (4), the total energy cost is approximately 144 kcal mol^{-3} triglyceride recycled.

The equation to calculate the amplification of control of net flux resulting from substrate cycling $(1 + C/J)$ can be applied to the TG/FA cycle. When calculating this value for the intracellular route of recycling, J = RaFFA, and C = [(3 × Ra glycerol) − RaFFA]. In the case of the extracellular route of the TG/FA cycle, the rate of cycling (C) equals the total rate of reesterification, and net flux (J) is equal to the difference between total flux and reesterification. In this special case, net flux is equal to substrate (fatty acid) oxidation. Total flux via the extracellular route is the rate of appearance of FFA in plasma, which in turn is determined by the rate of lipolysis minus the amount of fatty acids recycled intracellularly. The impact of changes in percentage reesterification on the rate of fat oxidation can best be evaluated by comparing the actual rate of fat oxidation with the rate that would have occurred had there been no change in the percentage reesterification. In an analogous manner, the effect of a change in percentage reesterification on plasma concentration can be evaluated by comparing the actual FFA concentration with the value that would have occurred if the percentage of reesterification had not changed. In the latter case, it must be assumed that all fatty acids not oxidized or reesterified remain in a plasma volume of 3 liters.

Physiological Significance of TG/FA Cycling

Fasting is the most extreme circumstance in which normal, resting man must rely on fatty acids as an energy substrate. This has prompted us to perform a series of studies to investigate the mechanisms responsible for the increased availability of FFA that occurs in this circumstance (32–34). Common to all of these studies is the observation that, in the basal state, short-term (3-day) fasting causes a doubling in the rate of TG/FA cycling (Table 2). Associated with this increased cycling is a modest increase potential amplification of the control of net flux in response to an acute stimulation $(1 + C/J)$. This potential amplification of control is gained at little cost in terms of energy metabolism, since even with the elevated rate of cycling in fasting, only 2% of the REE is due to TG/FA cycling. As would be anticipated from these data, the infusion of epinephrine caused a significantly greater increase in plasma FFA after a 3-day fast than before (32).

We have investigated the effect of a variety of clinical states on TG/FA cycling (26,39–44). The most consistent, dramatic effect is seen in severe burn injury, in which the total rate of cycling is increased almost fivefold (Table 2) (26). This is associated with a significant increase in $1 + C/J$ (Table 2) (as predicted from the increased $1 + C/J$), an increase in the response of plasma FFA to epinephrine infusion (42). Although the energy cost of this increased cycling is markedly greater than in normal volunteers, it still consists of less than 2% of the total REE (Table 2).

The primary mechanism responsible for increased TG/FA cycling in most circumstances is increased adrenergic activity. We have investigated the response to numerous perturbations in normal man, including increases in the concentration of epinephrine, glucagon, and cortisol; blocking adenosine activity; and changes in glucose and insulin concentration (21,24). Epinephrine consistently caused an increase in TG/FA cycling, while also causing an increase in total flux. Hyperglycemia also increased intracellular TG/FA cycling, but lipolysis decreased (21).

TABLE 2. *Physiological changes in total triglyceride/fatty acid cycling*

	Rate of Cycling (μmol/FA kg^{-1}/min^{-1})	Energy cost kcal kg^{-1}/h^{-1}	% REE	Amplification $(1 + C/J)$
Fasting[a]				
12 h fast	3.9 ± 0.3	11.1 ± 0.2	1.3 ± 0.06	2.09
84 h fast	6.8 ± 0.2[c]	18.4 ± 0.4[c]	2.0 ± 0.02	2.30
Burn injury (12 h fast)[b]				
Normal volunteers	3.5 ± 0.4	9.4 ± 0.4	1.4 ± 0.5	2.10
Burn patients	15.8 ± 1.34	42.6 ± 5.4	1.7 ± 0.09	2.74

[a] From Wolfe et al., ref. 32; Klein et al., ref. 33; and Klein et al., ref. 34 ($n = 12$).
[b] From Wolfe et al., ref. 26.
[c] Significantly different from 12 h fast ($p < 0.05$).
REE, resting energy expenditure.

Response of TG/FA Cycling to Exercise

The transition from rest to exercise, and then from exercise to recovery, represents the most dramatic change in energy expenditure that can be encountered under normal conditions. If the TG/FA cycle plays any role in matching FA availability and energy requirements, one would anticipate that the response to exercise would be one such circumstance. We have therefore investigated the response of normal volunteers to 4 h of moderate exercise (40% $\dot{V}O_2$max) (45). This exercise intensity and duration was chosen to maximize the reliance on fat as an energy substrate. If TG/FA cycling amplifies responsiveness, one would expect the percentage reesterification to fall during exercise in conjunction with the stimulation of lipolysis (to amplify the availability of fatty acids for oxidation). In recovery, the percentage reesterification should rise as the rate of lipolysis falls (to reduce the elevated plasma FFA level more rapidly than could be accomplished by only a reduction in lipolysis).

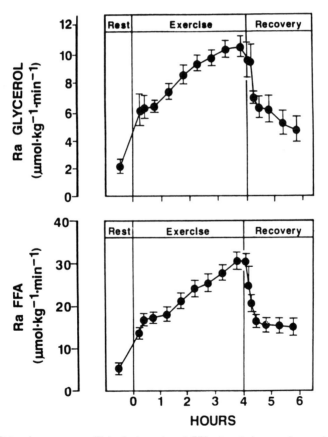

FIG. 11. Rate of appearance (Ra) of glycerol and FFA at rest, in exercise, and in recovery ($n = 5$).

Lipolysis was stimulated significantly at the start of exercise, but did not reach its maximal level until 4 h of exercise, despite the constant energy requirement throughout. In recovery, lipolysis gradually declined, but 2 h after exercise had stopped the value was still significantly greater than the resting value (Fig. 11). Changes in RaFFA corresponded to the stimulation of lipolysis (Fig. 11). Accompanying these responses of lipolysis, there were reciprocal changes in the percentage reesterification. The value dropped from the resting value of 70% to 25–35% throughout exercise. In recovery, almost 90% of the fatty acids released by lipolysis were reesterified (Fig. 12). In exercise, approximately 55% of total fatty acid oxidation was attributable to the decrease in the percentage reesterification (Fig. 13). This figure agrees quite closely with the theoretical amplification due to cycling in normal man ($1 + C/J = 2$, Table 2). In other words, fatty acid oxidation increased by twice as much as it would have, had the same stimulation of lipolysis occurred in a system in which total flux = net flux in the resting state. In recovery, the increased reesterification was important in enabling the fatty acids to return towards the basal level, despite the sudden decrease in demand for energy substrates and the sluggish responsiveness of the rate of lipolysis. The amplification of control was achieved almost entirely via changes in the percentage reesterification via the extracellular route. The rate of intracellular recycling was low in all phases of the experiment.

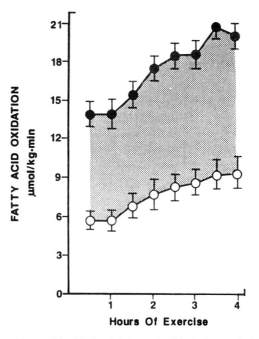

FIG. 12. Rate of total fatty acid oxidation (●) determined by indirect calorimetry and calculated rate of fatty acid oxidation (○) had there been no change in percent reesterification from resting value (70%). Shaded area represents increased oxidation in exercise accounted for by changes in percent reesterification, and it is >50% of total fat oxidation.

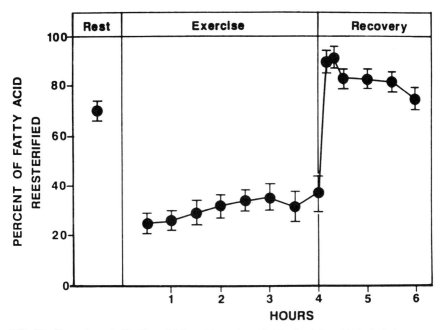

FIG. 13. Percent reesterification of fatty acids made available via triglyceride hydrolysis.

Factors Controlling Intracellular and Extracellular Recycling

The total flux of the intracellular route of recycling is determined by the rate of lipolysis. The primary factors determining the extent of reesterification within the adipocyte are the ability of the plasma to carry away released FFA (i.e., adequate albumin-binding sites), and the availability of glucose to produce glycerol-3-phosphate for reesterification. The normally low rates of intracellular recycling indicate that adipose tissue blood flow is usually adequate to clear away fatty acids released by lipolysis. The only situation in which we have not found this to be the case is in patients who are critically-ill with sepsis (39). Hypoalbuminemia and adrenergic-mediated reduction of adipose tissue blood flow may combine to limit FFA transport in this circumstance. Excess glycerol-3-phosphate production, leading to increased intracellular recycling, only occurs in situations of stimulated glucose uptake, such as hyperglycemia or hyperinsulinemia (21).

The regulation of the extracellular pathway of recycling is somewhat different from the general case considered by Newsholme and Crabtree (4) in their discussion of the contribution of substrate cycling to the control of net flux. The rate of total flux is equal to the rate of release of fatty acids into plasma (RaFFA), which is equal to the rate of lipolysis minus the intracellular recycling of FFA. Extracellular recycling is equal to the rate of reesterification of FFA cleared from the plasma, and the net flux is the difference between total flux and recycling, which is the same as the rate of fat oxidation. Thus, the possible sites of control of the extracellular TG/FA route of recycling include:

1. Lipolysis;
2. Reesterification within the adipocyte;
3. Reesterification of FFAs that have entered the plasma; and
4. Fatty acid oxidation.

The roles of factors 1 and 2, above, are no different in extracellular cycling than intracellular cycling. In contrast to the situation with intracellular reesterification, changes in the extent of reesterification of FFA that enter the plasma can be extremely important in determining the overall response to a stimulus, such as exercise. However, it is unlikely that changes in the percentage reesterification are generally accomplished by direct regulation of reesterification. For example, although in exercise the fraction of flux recycled decreased, the absolute amount of reesterification via the extracellular route doubled, and this amount corresponded with the expected change in FFA delivery to the liver due to altered hepatic blood flow (46). Changes in the oxidation of fatty acids in tissues such as muscle, coupled with changes in the delivery of FFA to the liver, are at least in part responsible for changes in the fraction of flux that is reesterified via the extracellular route. However, in contrast to the notion of the liver reesterifying a constant fraction of delivered FFAs, in recovery both the absolute and relative rate of reesterification increased dramatically, despite a decrease in the delivery of FFA to the liver as the plasma concentration fell. The most plausible explanation is that there was accelerated clearance and reesterification of FFA in peripheral adipose tissue, but the signal for this type of peripheral clearance and reesterification is unclear. Also, an increased efficiency of reesterification within the liver cannot be excluded.

The unique aspect of the extracellular TG/FA cycle, as compared to other substrate cycles, is that the rate of net flux is not simply passively determined by the difference between the total rate of flux and the amount that is recycled. Rather, the rate of net flux, which is actually the rate of fat oxidation, can be directly regulated. For example, in response to exercise, the large increase in the energy requirement of the exercising muscles was undoubtedly responsible for the accelerated rate of fat oxidation, and thus decreased availability of fatty acids for reesterification. This was reflected by an increased percentage of FFA flux that was oxidized, and decreased percentage that was reesterified. The reverse situation occurred in recovery. Thus, a significant component of TG/FA cycling could be considered to be "passively" regulated. Nevertheless, this does not diminish the importance of this cycle in enabling the matching of FFA availability and tissue requirements for energy substrates.

ACKNOWLEDGMENTS

Supported by NIH grant DK34817 and a grant from the Shriner's Hospital and NIH Clinical Research Center grant 00073.

REFERENCES

1. Hue H. The role of futile cycles in the regulation of carbohydrate metabolism in the liver. *Adv Enzymol Relat Areas Mol Biol* 1980;52:247–331.
2. Katz J, Rognstad R. Futile cycles in the metabolism of glucose. *Curr Top Cell Regul* 1976;10:237–289.
3. Newsholme EA, Gevers W. Control of glycolysis and gluconeogenesis in liver and kidney cortex. *Vitam Horm* 1967;25:1–87.
4. Newsholme EA, Crabtree B. Substrate cycles in metabolic regulation and in heat generation. *Biochem Soc Symp* 1976;41:61–109.
5. Clark MG, Williams CH, Pfeiffer WF, et al. Accelerated substrate cycling of fructose-6-phosphate in the muscle of malignant hyperthermic pigs. *Nature* 1973;245:99–101.
6. Cobelli C, Toffolo G. Compartmental versus non-compartmental modeling for two accessible pools. *Am J Physiol* 1984;247:R488–R496.
7. Schwarz J-M, Caveggion E, Honeycutt D, et al. Interstitial fluid is a mathematically-identifiable compartment of glucose kinetics. *FASEB J* 1991 (*submitted*).
8. Guyton AC. *Textbook of medical physiology*, 4th ed. Philadelphia: WB Saunders, 1971.
9. Bell PM, Firth RG, Rizza RA. Assessment of insulin action in insulin-dependent diabetes mellitus using 6-^{14}C-glucose, 3-^{3}H-glucose and 2-^{3}H-glucose: differences in the apparent pattern of insulin resistance depending on the isotope used. *J Clin Invest* 1986;78:1479–1486.
10. McMahon MM, Schwenk WF, Haymond MW, Rizza RA. Accumulation in plasma of a radioactive contaminant present in 6-^{3}H but not 6-^{14}C-glucose leads to a systematic underestimation of glucose turnover. *Diabetes* 1989;38:97–107.
11. Finegood DT, Bergman RN, Vranic M. Modeling error and apparent isotope discrimination confound estimation of endogenous glucose production during euglycemic glucose clamps. *Diabetes* 1988;37:1025–1034.
12. Jacobson BS, Smith BN, Epstein S, Laties GG. The prevalence of carbon-13 in respiratory carbon dioxide as an indicator of the type of endogenous substrate. *J Gen Physiol* 1970;55:1–17.
13. Rosenblatt JI, Wolfe RR. Calculation of substrate flux using stable isotopes. *Am J Physiol* 1988;254;E526–E531.
14. Cobelli C, Toffolo G, Bier DM, Nosadini R. Models to interpret kinetic data in stable isotope tracer studies. *Am J Physiol* 1987;253:E551–E564.
15. Wolfe RR, Allsop JR, Burke JF. Glucose metabolism in man: responses to intravenous glucose infusion. *Metabolism* 1979;28:210–220.
16. Layman DL, Wolfe RR. Sample site selection for tracer studies applying a unidirectional circulatory approach. *Am J Physiol* 1987;253:E173–E178.
17. Jahoor F, Klein S, Miyoshi H, Wolfe RR. Effect of isotope infusion and sampling sites on glucose kinetics during a euglycemic clamp. *Am J Physiol* 1988;255:E871–E874.
18. Wajngot A, Chendramouli V, Schumann WC, Kumaran K, Efendic S, Landau BR. Testing of assumptions made in estimating the extent of futile cycling. *Am J Physiol* 1989;19:E668–E675.
19. Shulman GI, Ladenson PW, Wolfe MH, Ridgway EC, Wolfe RR. Substrate cycling between gluconeogenesis and glycolysis in euthyroid, hypothyroid and hyperthyroid man. *J Clin Invest* 1985;76:757–764.
20. Karlander S, Roovete A, Vranic M, Efendic S. Glucose and fructose-6-phosphate cycle in humans. *Am J Physiol* 1986;251:E530–E536.
21. Wolfe RR, Peters EJ. Lipolytic response to glucose infusion in human subjects. *Am J Physiol* 1987;252:E218–E223.
22. Bortz WM, Paul P, Hoff AG, Holmes WL. Glycerol turnover and oxidation in man. *J Clin Invest* 1972;51:1537–1546.
23. Rosenblatt JI, Wolfe MH, Wolfe RR. Stable isotope tracer analysis by gas chromatography mass spectrometry, including quantitation of istopomer effects. *Am J Physiol* 1990 (*in press*).
24. Miyoshi H, Shulman GI, Peters EJ, Wolfe MH, Elahi D, Wolfe RR. Hormonal control of substrate cycling in humans. *J Clin Invest* 1988;81:1545–1555.
25. Weber JM, Klein S, Wolfe RR. Role of the glucose cycle in control of net glucose flux in exercising humans. *J Appl Physiol* 1990;68:1815–1819.
26. Wolfe RR, Herndon DN, Jahoor F, Miyoshi H, Wolfe MH. Effect of severe burn injury on substrate cycling by glucose and fatty acids. *N Engl J Med* 1987;317:403–408.

27. Wolfe RR. Nutrition and metabolism in burns. In: *Critical Care*, Fullerton, CA: Society in Critical Care Medicine, 1986;7:19–63.
28. Nelson TE, Flewellen EH. The malignant hyperthermia syndrome. *N Engl J Med* 1983;309:416–418.
29. Wolfe RR, Nelson TE. Hepatic glucose and fructose cycling in malignant hyperthermia. *Am J Physiol* 1990 (*in press*).
30. Dixon M, Webb EL. *Enzymes*. New York: Academic Press, 1979;842–843.
31. Wasserman DH, Lacy DB, Goldstein RE, Williams PE, Cherrington AP. Exercise-induced fall in insulin and increase in fat metabolism during prolonged muscular work. *Diabetes* 1989;38:484–491.
32. Wolfe RR, Peters EJ, Klein S, Holland OB, Rosenblatt JI, Gary H Jr. Effect of short-term fasting on the lipolytic responsiveness in normal and obese human subjects. *Am J Physiol* 1987;252:E189–E196.
33. Klein S, Peters EJ, Rosenblatt JI, Holland OB, Wolfe RR. Effect of short- and long-term beta-adrenergic blockade on lipolysis during fasting in humans. *Am J Physiol* 1989;257:E65–E73.
34. Klein S, Holland OB, Wolfe RR. Importance of blood glucose concentration in regulating lipolysis during fasting in humans. *Am J Physiol* 1990;258:E32–E39.
35. Arner P, Ostman J, Mono and di-acyl glycerols in human adipose tissue. *Biochim Biophys Acta* 1974; 369:209–221.
36. Wolfe RR. *Tracers in metabolic research: radioisotope and stable isotope/mass spectrometry techniques*. New York: Alan R. Liss, 1983;81–98.
37. Wolfe RR, Jahoor F. Recovery of labeled CO_2 during the infusion of C-1 versus C-2-labeled acetate: implications for tracer studies of substrate oxidation. *Am J Clin Nutr* 1990;51:248–252.
38. Wolfe RR and Peters EJ. Lipolytic response to glucose infusion in human subjects. *Am J Physiol* 1987;252:E218–E223.
39. Ella M, Zed C, Neale G, Livesey G. The energy cost of triglyceride-fatty acid recycling in non-obese subjects after an overnight fast and four days of starvation. *Metabolism* 1987;36:252–255.
40. Shaw JHF, Wolfe RR. Fatty acid and glycerol kinetics in septic patients and in patients with gastrointestinal cancer: the response to glucose infusion and parenteral feeding. *Ann Surg* 1987;205:368–376.
41. Shaw JHF, Wolfe RR. An integrated analysis of glucose, fat and protein metabolism in severely traumatized patients. Studies in the basal state and the response to total parenteral nutrition. *Ann Surg* 1989;209:63–72.
42. Shaw JHF, Croxon M, Holdaway L, Collin JP, Wolfe RR. Glucose, fat and protein kinetics in patients with primary and secondary hyperparathyroidism. *Surgery* 1988;103:526–532.
43. Wolfe RR, Herndon DN, Peters EJ, Jahoor F, Desai M, Holland OB. Regulation of lipolysis in severely burned children. *Ann Surg* 1987;206:214–221.
44. Wolfe RR, Herndon DN, Jahoor F, Miyoshi H, Wolfe MH. Effect of severe burn injury on substrate cycling by glucose and fatty acids. *N Engl J Med* 1987;317:403–408.
45. Klein S, Peters EJ, Shangraw RE, Wolfe RR. Lipolytic response to metabolic stress in critically-ill patients. *Crit Care Med* 1990 (*in press*).
46. Klein S, Wolfe RR. Whole-body lipolysis and triglyceride-fatty acid cycling in cachetic patients with esophageal cancer. *N Engl J Med* 1990 (*in press*).
47. Wolfe RR, Weber JM, Klein S, Carraro F. Role of triglyceride-fatty acid cycle in controlling fat metabolism in humans during and after exercise. *Am J Physiol* 1990;258:E382–E389.
48. Rowell LB, Blackmon JR, Martin RH, Mazzarella JA, Bruce RA. Hepatic clearance of endocyanine green in man under thermal and exercise stress. *J Appl Physiol* 1965;20:384–394.
49. Shaw JHF, Wolfe RR. Glucose, fatty acid, and urea kinetics in patients with severe pancreatitis: the response to substrate infusion and total parenteral nutrition. *Ann Surg* 1986;204:665–672.

DISCUSSION

Dr. Bier: I think the main issue that I'd like to address is just the one of tracer kinetics and the models that one has to use to deal with the issue of cycling from the point of tracer. Bob has done a lot of work with the glucose cycle, and there we have a relatively simple circumstance in the sense that all of the traces leaves the liver and enters the plasma compartment. The principal problem that one has to deal with in any of the other cycles is whether or not all of the tracer and all of the tracee are mixing and appearing in the sampled compartment. That assumption is being applied to that problem is a non-compartmental approach, which is only valid for describing the kinetics in the system if the sampled compartment sees all of the tracer and all of the tracee. I think that in each of these other cases one has the possibility that this doesn't happen. Now, Bob has some very good evidence with the fatty acid cycle, particularly finding in his resting subjects that the ratio of FFA/glycerol flux was 3, close to 3. Other individuals have not been that lucky, but I don't think anyone has measured it as consistently as Bob. I think that's fairly good evidence that one actually has an indication of all the appearance of FFA. The other thing I think that supports the calculation is the fact that most of the very low density triglyceride fatty acids that the liver puts out, are the source of the plasma FFA. So again this would support the use of plasma sampling. But I do think that we have to be cautious because in most of the other kinds of cycles that we deal with there is the potential (which does exist in the fatty acid cycle) that if tracee doesn't appear in plasma or if fatty acids are reesterified inside the cell that do appear in the plasma compartment, we will seriously underestimate the nature of the cycling.

Energy Metabolism: Tissue Determinants and Cellular Corollaries, edited by J. M. Kinney and H. N. Tucker. Raven Press, Ltd., New York © 1992.

Overview: Cellular Corollaries of Energy Expenditure

Jules Hirsch, Rudolph L. Leibel, and Neile K. Edens

The Rockefeller University, New York, New York 10021

This summary is a review and comment on the presentations of Park et al., Newsholme et al., Young et al., and Wolfe. All presentations deal with the thermodynamics of heat production and energy utilization in man. There is great danger in supposing that biologic systems operate differently from that predicted by the laws of thermodynamics. Indeed, much of the early history of the science of nutrition was the step-by-step validation of the laws of thermodynamics in experimental animals and in man. A fundamental experiment for nutritional science was the demonstration that oxidation inside or outside of living systems is equivalent and thus, the concept of "vital" heat as a unique heat produced by the organism, is forever discredited. The casual observer of human energy metabolism will nevertheless occasionally entertain a small, residual flight into the old, enemy territory of vitalism. Thus, a liquid diet isocaloric with a diet of solid foods may be considered to have special powers superior to a diet of solid foods for use in reducing the stored calories of adipose tissue. A more serious and often debated issue is whether the fundamental cellular machinery responsible for thermogenesis operates differently from person-to-person and thus whether the caloric need for the maintenance of cellular processes varies widely from one individual to another. To examine such issues, the resting thermogenesis (RMR), often the largest component of energy expenditure by the organism, must be carefully examined.

The resting metabolic rate is reminiscent of the entropy term of thermodynamic equations. It is the minimum amount of work that must be performed to maintain tissue integrity and a body temperature of 37°C. Like entropy, which is the heat equivalent of all the spins, oscillations, and orbits of the atoms and molecules in a substance at a given temperature, resting metabolism is not available for work, but it is a necessary condition for life. Of course, the many reactions which summate to create resting metabolism, each must donate free energy to the living system, thus, RMR is inevitably associated with rising entropy. Hence, life has been described as a massive drain on negentropy, i.e., foods laden with molecules which undergo rapid increases in entropy as they donate energy to the organism.

The presentations on cellular corollaries of energy expenditure have focused on

525

three varieties of chemical reactions which are major producers of resting thermogenesis. They are: (i) the maintenance of ionic and hence electrochemical integrity across cell membranes, (ii) protein turnover, and (iii) the so-called futile metabolic cycles. Of each of these, one might ask: What is the exact chemical nature of the activity? How costly is it in an energetic sense; and thus, how much does it contribute to resting heat production? And finally, what adaptive value does it have? Answers to each of these questions are of direct clinical relevance.

ENERGETICS AND CELL MEMBRANES

For proper cellular function, ionic concentrations and pH within cells must be maintained within narrow ranges and at levels different from extracellular fluids. Furthermore, different intracellular organelles have pHs and ionic concentrations different from each other and specially suited to their particular functions in degrading, oxidizing, or synthesizing molecules. Extraordinarily minute spaces must therefore have carefully guarded ionic territories separated by lipid membranes. The continuous leakage of fluid and ions across these membranes is opposed by a myriad of ionic pumps. Pumping is costly: The expenditure for non-ionic pumping is proportional to the logarithm of the concentration gradient and for ionic substances there is the additional cost of moving electrically charged substances across an electrical field. The energy for these processes is derived from that made available when an electron pair released from the oxidation of a carbon atom moves along a mitochondrial transport chain to a less energetic level in the oxygen of water. This motion along the electron transport chain generates a proton gradient, the energy of which is transferred to ATP, available throughout the body to fuel ionic pumps. The necessary heat and entropy changes which occur in the mitochondrion indicate that this is a less than perfectly efficient process. This very inefficiency is capitalized on in a special tissue, brown adipose tissue, to generate heat by virtue of a protein present in the mitochondrion of the brown adipocyte which enables the proton conductance pathway to become uncoupled from ATP production. The heat which is generated makes brown adipose tissue a specifically thermogenic organ. Brown adipose tissue is in fact the major locus of non-shivering thermogenesis in the hibernator and in the very young, but its functional capacity in adult man remains uncertain.

In most cells, remarkable feats of ionic pumping occur. It is notable, for example, that the intracellular concentration of free calcium is roughly 10,000 times less than the extracellular concentration. The maintenance of such very low and carefully controlled calcium levels are essential for the mechanisms of intracellular signaling. Of course, no pumping system is 100% efficient and the conversion of free energy from ATP into ionic gradients involves heat production as well as entropic change.

What is the energy cost of these processes? At the source of ATP production, the proton gradient across the inner mitochondrial membrane, there is a continuous slow leak. This particular inefficiency generates heat and entropy change which can account for as much as 30% of the resting heat production of isolated rat hepatocytes.

Efforts have been made to evaluate the overall energy cost in the entire organism for the maintenance of ionic integrity. The typical experimental approach utilizes a special pump inhibitor, for example, the inhibition of the sodium-potassium ATPase by ouabain. The sudden decline in oxygen consumption when ouabain is placed in contact with a tissue preparation is a rough indicator of the energy required for this particular pump function.

Estimates of the percent of resting metabolic rate attributable to sodium-potassium pumping vary widely from 9% to 61% depending on the organ under consideration and the physiological and nutritional state. The maintenance of calcium gradients are estimated to account for an additional 7–20% of resting energy needs. Transporting energy substrates such as glucose, amino acids, and fatty acids in and out of cells, and also, the transfer of RNA across nuclear membrane make for additional energy cost. The cell membrane contains an elaborate array of pumps and receptors and therefore the cost of maintenance of the integrity of the pumping system and the structure of the membrane itself must be considered. The receptors are modulated in their activity by the action of phosphorylases or kinases in which ATP and GTP are important donors of energy. Were the cost of all of the processes outlined above to be summed, a major fraction of resting metabolic rate would surely result.

ENERGETICS AND TURNOVER

The plan for protein structure is locked in the nucleus of cells and the steps whereby the plan is executed and the protein transported to its appropriate structural or functional site, are chemically elegant and numerous. One might expect that so important an end product as a protein would remain unchanged for very long periods of time. Instead, a continuous cycling of protein occurs within the organism and one must ask how costly this cycling is and what adaptive ends it serves.

The amount of protein cycling can be estimated in different ways. The fact that about 50 mg of nitrogen per kg body weight per day are excreted in an average individual on a eucaloric diet, indicates that in a 70 kg individual 22 g of protein is destroyed and replaced each day. Studies of amino acid turnover by labeled isotopic techniques show that protein cycling occurs in most proteins in the body, but at different rates depending on the protein under consideration. Thus, an estimate of skeletal muscle protein turnover which can be made either by isotopic techniques or by measuring the excretion rate of 3-methylhistidine will not provide the same estimate of protein turnover per unit of lean body mass as that provided by measures of total body protein turnover in nitrogen balance studies. The nitrogen balance technique has the obvious advantage of giving an estimate of turnover without compartmental or kinetic assumptions that must be made when other techniques are used.

Data using any method of calculating protein turnover show that diet has a profound effect on turnover. Thus, balance is achieved at very different levels of protein feeding depending on the level of dietary carbohydrate and fat as well as total caloric intake. It seems, furthermore, as though the commonest disequilibrium is that of increased protein turnover. Disease states varying from sepsis, trauma, and burns to cancer can result in manyfold increases in protein turnover. Increased turnover must be the end result of a large number of coordinated chemical events which begin with the making of a DNA transcript through attachment of amino acids to tRNA, translation, and then the many post-translational, trafficking events to which proteins are subjected: glycosylation, changes in size, motions through the cell, and ultimate positioning. In the case of some regulatory proteins, there is the additional cost of altering protein configuration by GTP binding or other chemical shaping so that functional activity of the protein can be controlled. The exact cost of cycling is nearly impossible to estimate, but, the basal or lowest estimates of the cost of protein degradation and synthesis needed to achieve the levels of turnover as estimated by nitrogen excretion, suggest that at least 15% of resting metabolic rate is needed for this purpose.

What adaptive ends could be served by what seems to be so wasteful a process? There are, to be sure, obligate losses of protein in urine, the shedding of the skin, etc., but these are small and relatively little protein synthesis would be required to replace these losses. Another possible utility of cycling is the correction of errors in protein production. Rarely, a processing error might be made not only in transcription and translation, but in the ultimate shape and positioning of protein, but the evidence for such errors is meager. More importantly, there may be age-associated effect which lead to a deterioration in protein function making replacement advantageous. A frequently described example is the non-enzymatic glycosylation of hemoglobin which occurs at highest rates when blood glucose levels are elevated, as in diabetes. But other proteins may undergo age-associated, oxidative attack or other chemical changes. The replacement of these "worn" proteins could be advantageous.

A totally different, potential adaptive value of cycling has recently kindled the interest of investigators and clinicians. The frequent enormous increase in cycling with disease suggests that proteins may be reservoirs for special mixtures of amino acids which are of particular utility in some disease states. Much has been made of the particular utility of branch chain amino acids for oxidation in muscle and also the need for these amino acids as donors of nitrogen for the synthesis of glutamine in muscle. A special role of glutamine in the metabolism of cells with immune function may make the availability of this amino acid particularly important in disease.

The control of protein turnover rate during various disease states, whether mediated via cytokines or hormones remains an active research pursuit. From the standpoint of the clinical nutritionist, it is important to develop correct information on what mixture of amino acids is of particular utility for alimentation in a given disease state. If any random mixture of amino acids would be sufficient to handle the special needs of fever or sepsis one might have expected that such states would be accompanied by a ravenous appetite for the ingestion of protein. Evidently there are special needs and these are better met by some selective reshaping process in which specific amino acid mixtures are provided. Clinical nutritionists and the industries which supply nutrient mixtures for treatment will be increasingly concerned with research endeavors which define the special nutritional needs in various disease states. Blunt edged tools such as hyperalimentation of all nutrients or even all amino acids have been helpful but not fully satisfactory. Similarly, the administration of sympathetic antagonists or other pharmacologic or hormonal agents in an effort to reduce the cycling of proteins have not been satisfactory in optimizing the level of catabolism in disease.

METABOLIC CYCLES IN CELLULAR CONTROL

In every chemical reaction, the reactants and products continuously exchange, but as equilibrium is approached, the concentrations of each reactant and the products approach fixed levels, determined by the dictates of the second law of thermodynamics. However, in body systems there are some reactions, often involving a series of steps, in which the reactants and products cycle back and forth in an energy-dependent fashion. This constitutes a so-called futile metabolic cycle. Notable examples are the glucose-glucose 6 phosphate cycle, the fructose phosphate-fructose diphosphate cycle, and the circulation of fatty acids from triglyceride released by lipolysis to the extracellular space and their return to the adipocyte for reesterification.

There are various ways to analyze the possible utility of such cycles. At the simplest level one might suppose that if there were a sudden metabolic demand for the product or reactant of a cycle, continuous cycling would assure immediate availability. Furthermore, when a given amount, e.g., one unit, of a material is required, there is an advantage to producing this not by a change from 1 to 2 units, but rather from 99 to 100 units of continuously produced materials. Less percentage deviation in concentration is apt to be less disruptive of the chemical milieu within the cell. These simple considerations of the utility of futile cycles can be supplemented with mathematically described and more subtle considerations, but one needs no further information to be assured that cycling could have adaptive value.

There are extraordinary situations in which inefficiency in a cycle is particularly advantageous as has been described in the case of non-shivering thermogenesis in brown adipose tissue, but usually, cycling is not very costly. It is possible by an examination of isotopically labeled substrates to measure the level at which cycling is occurring and to deduce from that the cost of cycling. Cycling related to glucose and fructose consume no more than several percent of the resting metabolic rate; however, the cycling of free fatty acid may be more costly. The total cost for metabolic cycling, although variously estimated, is not likely to exceed 10% of the resting metabolic rate.

This examination of the elements that give rise to resting metabolic rate and their assessment as to energy cost does not indicate the importance of each element. It is as though the value of a man were judged exclusively by the amount of money he can expend. The reason for attempting such an analysis and summation is simply to indicate that there are fixed and essential costs which summate to make resting metabolic rate and these are costs which are not likely to be very flexible. Thus, one cannot enhance the efficiency of caloric utilization by closing down ionic pumping systems and permitting potassium to leach from cells. There are abundant additional examples of processes whose costs are part of the resting metabolic rate and without which there would be a rapid demise of the organism. By examining these various processes, we have accounted for at least two-thirds of resting metabolic rate. If the cost of maintaining blood flow by the cardiovascular system, respiration, peristalsis, and similar organ functions were added to our energy account, then the total RMR should be reached. This, then, represents the energy cost of keeping the organism alive and functional at a temperature of 37°C before any useful work against the environment can be performed. In this limited sense, it is similar to the entropy term of thermodynamics which accounts for the heat trapped within all matter, but unavailable for useful work against the environment.

If one accepts the essentiality for life of the resting metabolic rate, which accounts for from 50% to 70% of total caloric need of the organism, then it becomes relevant to consider the sources of fuel for this necessary expenditure. It may be that the necessary maintenance of resting thermogenesis is the reason that life has been described as a massive consumer of negentropy and, why one must carry a bag of negentropy in the form of adipose tissue triglyceride, sufficient to maintain resting metabolic rate for 30 or more days. Our laboratory has been concerned with the reasons why a third of all individuals in the United States carry with them an enlarged triglyceride store creating the disease state of obesity. As a part of this interest, we have examined the effects on energy metabolism of carrying more or less fuel in adipose tissue. When the amount of fuel carried is increased there is clearly a small and calculable additional cost to energy metabolism, simply the additional work required to carry increased mass in adipose tissue. This is not sufficiently great, however, to account for some of the aberrations we have found when caloric storage is changed.

There is of course the well known lawful relationship in man and other organisms between 24 hour caloric need and some exponent of body mass. Body mass to the three-fourths power or some appropriate indicator of active cytoplasmic mass such as surface area or measured lean body mass all relate linearly to 24 hour energy need (1). With obese individuals this same lawful relationship is maintained except for the small additional cost of carrying an excess of fatty tissue. However, when obese individuals lose adipose tissue by dieting and reestablish a new level of body weight, many will develop a persistent decline in caloric need greater than that anticipated with a change in body weight alone. In this circumstance, the anticipated relationship between caloric need and some exponent of body weight, is no longer found. The difference between observed caloric need and anticipated caloric need on the basis of body mass is of the order of 15% of total caloric expenditure (2).

We have examined this situation in individuals who are of normal body weight or who are obese, and who under experimental conditions are caused to gain 10% above usual body weight or to have a similar decline in body weight. When body weight is increased, there is a reciprocal finding to that described above, i.e., an unanticipated increase in 24 hour caloric need above that predicted by the usual relationship of lean body mass to caloric need. This is found in many but not all individuals and likewise, the lean and the obese when either caused to gain or lose weight show similar increases and decreases in caloric requirement. It appears therefore, that usual body weight for either obese or non-obese individuals, is that body weight at which the predicted relationship between caloric need and lean body mass pertains. When body weight is experimentally changed, unanticipated perturbations in caloric requirements are observed. These act in a direction to restore the individual to former, usual weight, i.e., the individual who is caused to gain weight develops an increase in caloric expenditure and the individual who has lost weight shows apparently increased efficiency or diminished caloric need.

Our preliminary observations of this phenomenon indicate that these changes in caloric requirement are not primarily in resting metabolic rate nor in that category of energy expenditure referred to as the thermic effect of food. Rather the change is found mainly in the caloric expenditure during physical activity. This is perhaps not surprising since the thermogenesis that is occurring in the resting state is the result of essential life reactions as described above. It would be surprising if regulatory mechanisms tending to maintain a fixed level of caloric storage would operate by changing such essential activities as pumping for ionic equilibrium, protein cycling, futile cycling, etc.

At this time it still remains unclear how the mass of adipose tissue is controlled. It may well be that the amount of stored energy in adipose tissue is secondary to some controlled variable outside of adipose tissue, e.g., in the central nervous system or autonomic nervous system. However, the possibility of some element in adipose tissue being involved in the control remains an attractive hypothesis.

In the course of examining possibilities of how adipose tissue mass might be regulated, the efflux of substrates, namely free fatty acids and glycerol, under various basal and stimulated conditions, have been examined. We have shown that the cycling of free fatty acid through the lipolysis of triglyceride and its reesterification in the cell occurs briskly in man as it does in all animal species examined, and that lipolysis and recycling can be measured accurately *in vitro* (3). We have also been able to show that very little if any of the cycling occurs intracellularly. There is now evidence that the free fatty acid which is lipolyzed leaves the adipocyte completely and then reenters for reesterification (4). Thus very little of the futile cycle can be laid at the door of intracellular lipolysis and reesterification; there is a necessary passage outside of the cell. It is not clear what meaning if any, this has for potential signaling of adipose storage level. But it suggests that local circulatory factors which can rapidly wash free fatty acids from the exterior of the adipocyte may be involved in the control of adipose tissue metabolism. It could be, therefore, that the particular adverse consequences of having fat in one or another site in the body may be as much related to local circulatory phenomena as to differences in the intrinsic functioning of the adipocytes.

SUMMARY

The careful evaluation of cellular contributions to resting thermogenesis uncovers an unusually fertile area of clinical investigation. Questions ranging from the nature of the catabolism of trauma and sepsis to the biologic roots of obesity emerge from such consideration. The advances in our understanding of biochemistry now coupled with molecular genetics and immunology can be applied to new clinical investigations which address important clinical problems. It is likely that the physiologic basis for many adverse clinical states will be found in this detailed study of the thermodynamics of man and that improved methods of alimentation specific for each disorder will become part of the science of clinical nutrition.

ACKNOWLEDGMENTS

This work was supported in part by NIH grant 2RO 1 DK30583 and NIH GCRC RR 00102.

REFERENCES

1. Kleiber M. *The fire of life*. New York: Robert E. Krieger Publishing, 1975;179–222.
2. Leibel RL, Hirsch J. Diminished energy requirements in reduced-obese patients. *Metabolism* 1984; 33:164–170.
3. Leibel RL, Hirsch J. A radioisotopic technique for the analysis of free fatty acid reesterification in small fragments of human adipose tissue. *Am J Physiol* 1985;248:E140–E147.
4. Edens NK, Leibel RL, Hirsch J. Mechanism of free fatty acid reesterification in human adipocytes in vitro. *J Lipid Res* 1990;31:1423–1432.

Subject Index